ACNE AGORAPH
ANOREXIA NERVOSA ANXIETY BACK
BREASTFEEDING BREAST LUMPS: BENIGN OF
CERVICAL CANCER CESAREAN BIRTH CHILDBI
CRAMPS AND OTHER PREMENSTRUAL MIS
DEPRESSION DIAPHRAGM DRESSING F
ENDOMETRIOSIS ESTROGEN REPLACE
FATIGUE FEMININE HYGIENE FIBRO
GYNECOLOGISTS AND THEIR A
HEALTH CLUBS HEART DISEASE HEMC
HOT FLASHES HOUSEHOLD HEALT
INTRAUTERINE DEVICE (IUD)
MARIJUANA MASTECT
MENSTRUATION MI
ORAL CONTRA
PREGNANCY

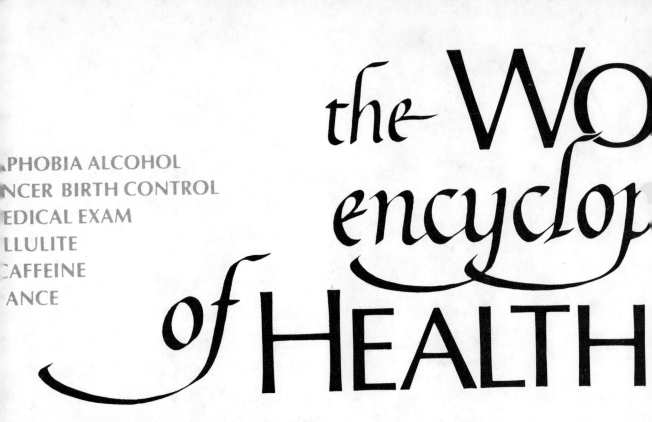

the WOMEN'S encyclopedia of HEALTH

...PHOBIA ALCOHOL
...NCER BIRTH CONTROL
...EDICAL EXAM
...LLULITE
...CAFFEINE
...ANCE

...GUE FEMININE HYGIENE
...ORS FITNESS GALLBLADDER DISEASE
...IVES HAIR CARE HAIR LOSS HEADACHES
...E HEMORRHOIDS HERBS FOR WOMEN HERPES
...RDS HYSTERECTOMY INFERTILITY

research associate *Takla Gardey*

MAN'S
dia
&NATURAL HEALING

ANOREXIA NE
BREASTFEEDING BREAS
CERVICAL CANCER CESAR
COOKING FOR HEALTH CRA
DEPRESSION DIAPHR
ENDOMETRI

Emrika Padus

senior editor, Prevention® magazine

RODALE PRESS   EMMAUS, PENNSYLVANIA

Library of Congress Cataloging in Publication Data

Padus, Emrika
    The woman's encyclopedia of
health and natural healing.

    Bibliography: p.
    Includes index.
    1. Women—Health and hygiene.
    2. Gynecology—Popular works.
    I. Gardey, Takla. II. Title
        RA778.P23   616'.008042   81-8610
        ISBN 0-87857-330-5 hardcover   AACR2

2   4   6   8   10
9   7   5   3   1   hardcover

This book is meant to supplement the advice and guidance of your physician. No two medical conditions are the same. Medical treatment varies from region to region and is changing constantly. Therefore, we urge you to seek out the best medical resources available to help you make informed decisions.

NOTICE

FOREWORD

ALICE ROTHCHILD, M.D.
Clinical instructor,
Harvard Medical School
Obstetrician/gynecologist,
Jamaica Plain, Massachusetts

WHY SHOULD YOU READ THIS BOOK? Why is it dangerous to leave your health solely in the hands of your doctor? Why is it important, particularly for us as women, to obtain more information about our bodies?

For centuries women have been the major source of health care in the community. As mothers they are often responsible for the diets and lifestyles of their families. They monitor the health of their children, and frequently older relatives. They decide when it is time to call the doctor and how to carry out his or her recommendations. They combine remedies from their grandmothers and the latest modern medicine has to offer. They are a major target for the advertising of an enormous variety of health-related merchandise. In addition, women see health care providers for contraception and pregnancy as well as when they are sick. And yet, who is in charge of this health care system? Who is the source of advice and information? Who has much of the power?

Despite the recent changes in medical school admissions, more than 90 percent of physicians in the United States are men. Traditionally, medicine is also surrounded by a powerful mystique in which patients, and women patients in particular, are often at a significant disadvantage. The doctor sometimes behaves as a benevolent father or a busy, important professional who doesn't have time for "your silly questions." Often clients are bewildered by big medical words: "myocardial infarction" rather than "heart attack"; or patronized by condescending tones: "Don't worry your head about that, honey. You wouldn't understand." One of the major concerns is that the medical problems of women are a special case of the social and political problems of women. Thus the dynamics between physician and client often reflect the issues between men and women in the society at large. Women's subservience in this setting is reinforced by their ignorance. The best patient is like a good child. "The doctor always knows best." Women's advice is frequently dismissed as old wives' tales.

Why is this a problem? Control over the structure, practice and norms in medicine gives the controller a major impact on people's lives. Take the field of obstetrics, for example. Childbirth was once solely the domain of women and their midwives. In the early 1900s in the United States, university-trained physicians were increasing in strength, developing licensing laws, and establishing medicine as a branch of higher learning accessible only through lengthy, expensive training. The field

was becoming increasingly closed to minorities, the lower class, and women. In keeping with this trend, the newly organized profession began attacking midwives, both in the name of science and reform. Interestingly enough, obstetricians at that time had little knowledge or skill that made them any safer than midwives. Sometimes they were even more dangerous because they would intervene more quickly. Male professionals thus took over women's health care long before the development of scientific technology.

With this change from women midwives to male physicians, pregnancy and labor began to be viewed as a dangerous, pathological event. Women were increasingly seen as suffering, helpless creatures needing to be rescued from the travails of childbirth. Heavy sedation and routine episiotomies and forceps deliveries became the norm. Breastfeeding was often discouraged by doctors. Women and their families became more and more disassociated from the experience of childbirth. Papers were published defending forceps deliveries as safer than spontaneous vaginal deliveries. Thus even the *definition* of a healthy, normal experience changed and remained so for several decades.

The natural childbirth movement

developed in reaction to these attitudes and practices. Women realized that they had relinquished control over a central event in their lives in the name of science and modernization. And yet, what had they gained? A long tradition of labor and birth support had been broken. Women had been redefined as not being strong enough to give birth without frequent intervention. While the technological advances that developed during the 20th century have been very important to the health and safety of many women and children, it is clear that an unquestioning acceptance of the doctor's advice is not without hazard. Women have found that understanding labor and being an active and educated participant have led to a marked reduction in medication and forceps deliveries. They have found that major improvements in the health of infants is more often related to improved nutrition, better spacing of children, and breastfeeding, than to x-rays or fetal monitors.

There is clearly a place for obstetric intervention and medical expertise. But these decisions cannot be left solely in the hands of the medical providers. The social and political attitudes of these providers have a serious impact on the practice of medicine. It is thus essential for each woman to learn as much as she can about her own health care and to be persistent in asking questions and obtaining information.

This awareness developed particularly during the 1970s within the women's movement. Women came together at first to discuss issues in their lives, or problems in their jobs or relationships. Contraception, sexuality, pregnancy and general health care quickly became important topics because every woman has had to confront these issues in her own life. Women realized that the more they knew about their bodies, the more control they had in their interactions with the health care system. Some women organized self-help groups in which they shared information and experiences regarding their bodies, learned to do exams, exchanged remedies for menstrual cramps, and provided a supportive group for further discussion. Other women read books like *Our Bodies, Ourselves*, magazines like *Prevention*, or became involved in women's clinics where education and explanation were major priorities. At the same time there was a rebirth of interest in nutrition, vitamins and exercise. In the lay press there has been a steady stream of information on the risks of cigarette smoking, the dangers of caffeine and sugar, the pros and cons of jogging, and the importance of preventing illness before it starts. Discussion continues on the appropriate use of vitamins, the impact of vitamins on a person's general health, susceptibility to colds, and so forth. Clearly all the answers are not in, but an important and lively debate is underway.

This book, *The Woman's Encyclopedia of Health and Natural Healing*, gives women a tremendous advantage. The book recognizes the important role women can and should play in their own health care and provides the guidance they'll need to confidently and effectively take on a more active role in maintaining their health, easing themselves through illness, and seeking out the best medical care when needed.

What makes this book different from most others on this subject is that it not only provides information about one's body and health, but it also offers practical, commonsense advice that is supported by scientific backing and a sensitivity to women's health issues. *The Woman's Encyclopedia of Health and Natural Healing* brings together the latest health and medical information available with the experience and opinions of women and women's health care professionals of all types: from

gynecologists, psychologists, pharmacologists, pathologists, dermatologists, surgeons, and scientific researchers to certified nurse-midwives, ob-gyn nurse practitioners, herbalists, nutritionists, therapists, and fitness experts. The result is an excellent balance of "modern medicine" and the natural commonsense approach to women's health reminiscent of the days when women were more in control of their health needs. For the reader, of course, this means having the benefit of weighing various viewpoints and considering medical options as well as natural alternatives in the treatment of both major and minor health problems.

Another important point is that this work is well organized and easy to use. Set up as a resource book, it clearly translates the medical jargon into understandable language. It focuses on prevention and diet as well as more traditional medical approaches. It can be used as a reference guide and as a resource to help in interactions with health care providers. It represents part of the ongoing struggle to redistribute the power between doctor and client, to demystify medicine by supporting an aware and informed consumer.

Editor: Mark Bricklin

Assistant Editor: Jim Nechas

Special Contributions by:
Eileen Mazer and
Marian Wolbers

Additional Contributions by:
Sharon Faelten
John Feltman
William Gottlieb
Jane Kinderlehrer
John Yates
Linda Shaw
Kerry Pechter
Laurie Lucas
Virginia Castleton
Porter Shimer
Carl Sherman
Dominick Bosco
Elaine Ruttle

Research Chief: Carol Baldwin

Research Associates:
Carol Matthews
Martha Capwell
Sue Ann Gursky
Christy Kohler
Carol Munson
Susan Rosenkrantz
Joann Williams

Copy Editor: Marian Wolbers

Office Personnel:
Carol Petrakovich
Barbara Hill
Brenda Peluso
Pat Hasik

Book Design: Joan Stoliar

Illustrations by: Jean Gardner

Photos by: Margaret Smyser

Calligraphy and Herbal Illustrations by:
Virginia Stone Dickinson

To the many physicians, researchers, and other health care professionals who so freely volunteered their energies and expertise, the scores of women who shared their personal experiences with us, and the entire *Prevention* staff who contributed to the preparation of this manuscript, I offer my sincere gratitude. Also, I'd like to recognize those professionals who took time away from their busy schedules to sit down with me and share their perspectives on women's health: that is, Stanley Birnbaum, M.D., Irma Denson, Philip Kingsley, Albert Kligman, M.D., Nan Koehler, Deborah Szekely Mazzanti, John Mikuta, M.D., Steven Paul, Ph.D., John Seybolt, M.D., Donald Solomon, M.D., and Dyveke Spino, Ph.D. Thanks too to Gideon Panter, M.D., and Albert Haverkamp, M.D., who made themselves available to answer our continual questioning.

My very special thanks go out to Mark for his confidence, inspiration, and motivation; to Joan for her brilliant design and tremendous insight; to Takla, Jim, Eileen, and Laura for their enthusiasm and moral support.

Here, too, I wish to remember Ella and Walter for a lifetime of encouragement; Lore and Walter for their interest and never-ending optimism; and especially Tom, my nearest and dearest supporter, without whose patience, pep talks, and TLC, this enormous and often overwhelming project would never have been possible.

ACKNOWLEDGMENTS

CONTENTS

IN THIS BOOK, TOPICS ARE ARRANGED
ALPHABETICALLY FOR EASY ACCESS.
WE'VE DESIGNED THE FOLLOWING AS
A GUIDE TO RELATED SUBJECTS.

THE
WOMAN'S
ENCYCLOPEDIA OF
HEALTH AND
NATURAL
HEALING

Nothing says women are more acne-prone than men. If anything, the opposite may be true. According to New York City dermatologist Irwin I. Lubowe, M.D., adolescent boys are more likely to get it—and get it more severely—than adolescent girls.

But, at least when I was in high school, it was the girls who worried most about it. We were the ones who hung around the bathroom mirror after lunch bemoaning our blemished chins. And, what's worse, we're the ones who continue to break out long after our 25th birthday—usually a week or so before a menstrual period.

What's a woman to do?

Unfortunately, entrusting your face to the hands of today's typical dermatologist may prove worse than doing nothing at all. Remember when x-ray treatment for acne was in vogue? Thyroid cancer turned out to be the unforgivable long-term aftereffect. Well, today we find the same M.D.'s recommending a whole slew of suspicious therapies—including antibiotics and synthetic hormones—with the same abandon that they dished out radiation a decade ago.

The funny thing is, those who go in for these heroic measures don't always look better than those who do nothing at all. And those who adopt sensible living habits (that is, exercise regularly, get plenty of sleep, practice some form of stress release, enjoy a moderate amount of sunshine, use a minimum amount of cosmetics, and eat a diet high in natural foods and low in sweet and fast foods) generally have clearer complexions naturally without all the hassle and hazards of weekly trips to the dermatologist.

Learn to Read Your Face

Your face is an amazing barometer of things going on inside your body. Learn to read it. Acne can be a signal of some kind of self-abuse. A face full of pimples following a tension-filled week is a clue that you've been bottling up stress. A rigorous exercise program or some form of daily meditation could provide a more becoming way to cope (see Anxiety).

Similarly, if your face repeatedly breaks out after a french fry-and-hamburger binge, there's a good chance that fried foods are your forbidden fruit. Despite word from the medical establishment that diet has nothing to do with acne, it's not uncommon for fried foods, as well as chocolate, nuts, iodized salt and all other sources of iodine including shellfish and kelp to aggravate acne. So who are you going to believe? Your face—or some medical research study funded in part by chocolate manufacturers? In our opinion, you can't do anything better for yourself, or your face, than to adopt a good natural foods diet.

Vitamin and mineral supplements, too, have saved many a face. And women's acne problems in particular respond especially well to the following nutrients.

Vitamin A. Through the years, medical research has repeatedly pointed to the importance of vitamin A in the treatment of acne. In fact, Albert Kligman, Ph.D., M.D., professor of dermatology at the University of Pennsylvania Medical School, recently reported his success with a vitamin A acid treatment. Vitamin A *acid* is a synthetic but directly absorbable form of vitamin A which is applied to the skin. While it can produce initial redness and burning (plus a couple of weeks' worth of peeling), Dr. Kligman says results have been promising.

Still, to our knowledge, no one has suggested that vitamin A taken orally might be useful in treating those predictable premenstrual acne eruptions. Perhaps it's of no special value here. But related information hints to us that there just may be a link.

It is generally believed that the female hormone estrogen helps to keep acne at bay. This, we are told, is the reason why men are somewhat more susceptible to severe acne and why women often break out just prior to menstruation when estrogen levels dip to their lowest point. This is also the reason why women who take birth control pills are often spared these monthly breakouts

and why women with severe cases are occasionally given prescriptions of synthetic estrogen.

Now, here comes the tie-in with vitamin A. Researchers have demonstrated that vitamin A levels in women fluctuate in a cyclic pattern during the menstrual cycle, which corresponds to the cyclic changes in female hormone production.

Interestingly enough, vitamin A has been successfully used to treat menorrhagia, heavy menstrual bleeding—another problem possibly related to an imbalance in female hormones.

Zinc. Evidence that the trace mineral zinc could clear acne first appeared at University Hospital in Uppsala, Sweden—quite by accident. It seems that one patient receiving zinc treatment there for acrodermatitis enteropathica, an inherited and sometimes fatal skin disease, also had acne. After the course of zinc therapy his acne almost completely cleared.

This fact, combined with the knowledge that in some animals zinc helps maintain vitamin A levels in the blood, led Gerd Michaëlsson, M.D., and two other hospital physicians to conduct a full-scale study on the effects of zinc and vitamin A supplements on acne.

Sixty-four patients between the ages of 13 and 25 took part in their study. They were divided into four groups. Group I was treated with 45 milligrams of zinc in tablet form three times daily. Group II was treated with similar-tasting tablets without zinc. Group III was given 150,000 to 200,000 international units (I.U.)—depending on body weight—of vitamin A twice daily. And Group IV took both the zinc and the vitamin A.

It is no surprise that the zinc groups came out on top in every category of evaluation. After only 4 weeks on zinc therapy, 65 percent of their pimples cleared, and after 12 weeks 87 *percent disappeared*! By contrast, those taking blank tablets improved by a chance 25 percent. The vitamin A group fared slightly better than that group but did not approach the improvement noted with zinc.

More patients in the zinc groups noticed a distinct improvement in their condition than did those in either of the other groups. Eight persons remarked that their facial skin was much less oily than before the zinc treatment. In addition, 9 out of 13 patients who hadn't had any luck with previous antibiotic treatment did very well on zinc. Many declared that their results were "definitely superior" to those obtained with tetracycline (antibiotic) treatment.

We, too, have heard nothing but grateful praise from women who have used zinc.

Vitamin B$_6$ (pyridoxine). This may be just what the dermatologist ordered for female acne complaints.

A skin specialist in Erie, Pennsylvania, B. Leonard Snider, M.D., gave daily B$_6$ supplements of 50 milligrams to 106 teenagers whose acne was under control, except for monthly flareups just prior to menstruation. In many cases the vitamin was taken for one week preceding and during the time of menstruation for an average of three menstrual periods. Seventy-six of the girls reported that B$_6$ reduced their acne flareup anywhere from 50 to 75 percent (*Ob. Gyn. News*, May 1, 1974).

Jonathan V. Wright, M.D., a nutrition-oriented physician in Kent, Washington, and author of *Dr. Wright's Book of Nutritional Therapy* (Rodale Press, 1979), also reports tremendous results with B$_6$. In a typical case, a 26-year-old woman came to him after having struggled through countless medical acne treatments since she was in sixth grade. "Mrs. Kraft's face was, honestly speaking, a mess," Dr. Wright recalls. "It was reddened over the cheeks and nose, and slightly puffy. The skin appeared coarse, a little like a pigskin football, and the redness was deepened in patches. There were pimples scattered all over, and many cysts and deep infected areas, called pustules. Her forehead was nearly as bad as her cheeks; the redness extended into her hairline, and seemed to terminate in a slightly greasy dandruff.

"Overall it appeared like an especially bad case of acne—but somehow, worse.

"Her trouble began about a year or so before her menstrual periods had begun. Initially, it seemed 'like a regular case of acne' with small pimples and cysts scattered about her face. But once her menses started, 'it really hit bad.' She noted that before her first few periods her face blossomed with pimples and cysts all over. For a while, the condition settled down for one to three weeks between cycles, but at age 15 or 16, it became constant: 'bad all the time, but awful before periods.' Since that time, it had remained as it now appeared.

"She'd used a variety of medications, mostly containing cortisone or one of its synthetic relatives. These 'did better than anything but still not much.' So she stopped them. For the infectious part of her skin condition, she'd been put on a variety of antibiotics, including tetracycline, erythromycin, and different types of penicillin. These had also only helped a little, and she'd stopped when she began to get frequent yeast infections. 'After that, I gave up on dermatologists,' she said. 'Nothing helped.'"

ANTI-ACNE SKIN CARE

Cleansers: Wash your face twice a day with a mild soap. Before bedtime, treat yourself to a gentle scrub with about a teaspoon of finely ground almonds, oatmeal (not the instant type), or cornmeal mixed into a paste with a few drops of warm water. Rinse with warm water.

Astringents: Commercially prepared astringents contain alcohol, which is extremely drying to the skin and also alters the natural pH (acid-alkali balance). Instead, dab a mixture of two teaspoons of apple cider vinegar per cup of water on blemishes after washing.

Poultices: The herb dock, which is a member of the sorrel family, has a unique drying quality which can be put to use as a gentle astringent tonic. If you're able to obtain a root from an herbalist's shop, botanical supply house or health food store, steam it to a mashable softness, gather it up between gauze squares (double thickness), and place on the troubled area of skin to draw out impurities. When the dock mash cools, replace with another filled gauze. Keep this up for half an hour or so.

Sun: Sunshine, in moderation, of course, can be a real bonus to a complexion problem. But remember, the dry heat that goes with it on an August afternoon can quickly undo all the benefits. Also, protect yourself from burning by using a good sunscreen containing para-aminobenzoic acid (PABA). **Note:** Be very cautious about sunning yourself if you're taking tetracycline. In some people, this antibiotic has a photosensitizing effect, meaning that sunlight can bring on a possibly severe rash.

Masks: If your acne is accompanied by oily skin (as is most often the case), try a clay mask. Fuller's earth or kaolin is available in most pharmacies and health food stores. Just mix a teaspoon of powdered clay with enough warm water to make a paste. Smooth on your face, avoiding the area around your eyes. Let dry for 10 minutes. Then rinse with warm water. A brewer's yeast mask also halts the formation of excess oil on the skin. Make a thin, loose mixture using a teaspoon of brewer's yeast with some plain yogurt. Pat thoroughly on the face, again avoiding the area around the eyes; let dry for 15 minutes, and then rinse. Follow each mask treatment with a splash of cool water to close the pores.

Facial Packs: Papaya mint tea is an excellent treatment for an acne explosion. Brew a pot. Then saturate a white washcloth in the extremely warm tea (it will stain) and hold to the affected area at least twice a day for 15 minutes.

Saunas: Dry heat such as Swedish sauna can be a disaster for acned skin, according to Irwin I. Lubowe, M.D. But many women find that moist steam helps to open clogged pores and benefits a badly blemished face. This steam is especially helpful when mingled with the gentle healing properties of herbs. Just drop a handful of burdock, camomile, fennel, nettle or linden (lime flowers) into two cups of cold water. Bring to a boil. Then shut off the heat and simmer. Place your face over the steamy liquid (not too close, now) and drape a towel over your head. Enjoy the warm refreshment for 5 to 10 minutes. Then rinse your face with cool water.

Dr. Wright decided to try vitamin B₆.

"So much research has in fact been done on the relationship of vitamin B₆ to cyclic women's health problems that it can and has filled volumes," he told us.

In addition, Dr. Wright's own clinical work has shown that vitamin B₆ eliminates many other symptoms that recur fairly regularly before menstrual cycles.

He asked Mrs. Kraft to take 100 milligrams of pyridoxine four times a day. Since research at the University of Cincinnati, Ohio, had shown that sometimes B₆ was effective only if applied externally, he asked her pharmacist to compound a cream with 100 milligrams of pyridoxine per gram of ointment. To "cover all the bases," he also asked the nurse to give Mrs. Kraft 300 milligrams of pyridoxine by injection.

Mrs. Kraft was skeptical, but when she had made certain that all of this was harmless, she agreed to give it a try.

Two months later when Mrs. Kraft checked back, she was much more talkative. "I never would have believed it," she confided, "but that vitamin B₆ has cleared up so many of my problems that I feel like a new person."

She looked like a new person, too, Dr. Wright told us. Once her infection was gone, she found that by taking 400 to 600 milligrams of pyridoxine daily, she could keep her face completely free of the rash. She even proved it to herself by not taking the vitamin for 48 hours, whereupon the rash started to reappear. She immediately began taking it again, and the rash cleared. "I won't stop again. I'm convinced," she said. She'd also found that, in her case, the vitamin B₆ cream wasn't necessary. The tablets "took care of everything."

Another woman told us of the good results she had with vitamin B₆.

"I've had acne since age 13 and have been on various antibiotics and creams. Nothing worked except a certain type of birth control pill, but its side effect was a 20-pound weight gain. So I stopped taking them and my complexion became hopeless.

"Then my mother gave me an article on vitamin B₆. I was skeptical and pessimistic but desperate. I took three a day and within six weeks my complexion glowed like a baby's. My dermatologist claims it was coincidence (a hormonal change) but I'm convinced it's the vitamins."

Of course, dosages should be determined for your individual condition. But to give you some idea of what to aim for, Dr. Lubowe generally recommends 50 milligrams of zinc gluconate twice a day, 25,000 I.U. of water-soluble vitamin A once a day, 400 I.U. of vitamin E twice a day, and, for premenstrual acne, 100 milligrams of vitamin B₆ twice a day.

AGORAPHOBIA

Panic. Terror. Fear. Fortunately, for most people, these feelings only rarely get a grip—and when they do, it's often in response to some voluntary confrontation like one of Hitchcock's greatest hits. But for a growing number of people—of which as many as 80 percent are women—a disabling panic attack complete with pounding heart, rapid pulse and cold sweat can strike anytime, anywhere. And, usually, it is in response to nothing at all—just a fleeting concern gone absolutely haywire.

It's called agoraphobia, which, literally translated, means fear of places of assembly but which actually encompasses a fear of many things. Fear of being hemmed in by crowds. Fear of disease and death. Eventually, even fear of leaving the house lest an attack should strike in unfamiliar surroundings.

In an article on agoraphobia in the *Harvard Medical School Health Letter* (August, 1979), David V. Sheehan, M.D., assistant professor of psychiatry at the Massachusetts General Hospital, Harvard Medical School, describes the variety of symptoms and diverse fears involved:

> Patients with this condition have usually visited many physicians over several years for relief. The cardiologist may be consulted to investigate a rapid pulse, pounding heart, and chest pain; the neurologist for lightheadedness and headaches; the ENT [ear, nose and throat] specialist for a lump in the throat and dizziness; the gynecologist for hot flashes; the endocrinologist for possible thyroid disease or low blood sugar; and the pulmonary specialist because of difficulty breathing or hyperventilation. Often the cancer specialist is consulted because of a preoccupation concerning malignant disease. When no underlying disease can be found, the person with agoraphobia attracts such diagnostic labels as "hysteria," "anxiety neurosis," "cardiac neurosis," "hypochondriasis," "depression," and even "autonomic epilepsy."

What brings on this curious array of symptoms is not entirely understood. But it appears to be triggered by stress. For example, a major operation, especially a gynecological one in which hormone balance is suddenly disturbed. An accident. A drastic life change—such as the birth of a child or the death of a loved one. Or even the more gradual stress of an upsetting life situation such as an unhappy marriage, or stressful work condition. Much hinges, of course, on how sensitive the person is and how well she can cope with stress.

"Your Emotional System Bulges at the Seams"

A person with an excitable personality and very strong feelings soon learns that our world doesn't tolerate intensity or people who dramatize, explains Arthur Hardy, M.D., director of the Territorial Apprehension Program, Inc. (TERRAP), a desensitization program for agoraphobics (see *Appendix*). "When you keep your feelings in, your body keeps score. Eventually your emotional system begins to bulge at the seams. When suppressed feelings finally come out in the open, they lead to a severe anxiety attack or panic."

Dr. Hardy says agoraphobia is a growing problem—1 out of every 100 persons may be affected to some degree. "We move faster. The world is more complicated. We have to know more people and go to school to know more things. Life requires a lot more coping skills than it used to."

Despite the increase in the number of cases, doctors often don't even know that any kind of treatment is available for the disorder. "It's like a secret disease," says Dr. Hardy. "Agoraphobia affects a lot more people than muscular dystrophy. It cripples more people than arthritis, and devastates more lives than other diseases, but it is not researched. You'd think an enlightened society like ours would know more about it, wouldn't you?"

With all of the mystery surrounding agoraphobia, some facts are known.

Only a small percentage of agoraphobics become totally housebound, for instance. "A lot of agoraphobics get around and do things but at a great expense," says Dr. Hardy. "They feel nervous, upset, tense and tightened up all the while they're doing things."

A woman also is more likely to become an agoraphobic than a man. "About 76 percent of the patients we see are women," says Dr. Hardy. He has several theories on why it strikes females so often. Among them, he suggests that our culture requires more perfection from women. "They are taught to be ladylike and told not to swear or do naughty things," he says. There may be other cultural reasons or it may stem from biological differences between the sexes, he adds.

Although some people associate the condition with older women, agoraphobia actually begins at an average of 23.9 years. The problem is that young people may ignore early warning signs thinking they will outgrow them. Shyness or an extreme sensitivity to ordinary things in the world, like noise, may foreshadow problems that could get worse, says Dr. Hardy. Yet people can have agoraphobia for years before they finally get help.

The interesting thing about all this is that agoraphobia with its easily misunderstood symptoms and difficulty in diagnosis is primarily a problem that affects women. And, at least according to one survey conducted by Dr. Sheehan, 98 percent of the agoraphobia victims are being treated with minor tranquilizers—most commonly Valium, the one prescribed more than twice as frequently for women as for men.

Do Tranquilizers Really Help?

Now you might say tranquilizers are intended to ease anxiety and there's probably no one filled with more anxiety than an agoraphobia victim. But the truth of the matter is, once again, that Valium isn't the answer. According to Dr. Sheehan's article, the hoopla over minor tranquilizers like Valium for the treatment of agoraphobia is greatly exaggerated. In his study, 57 patients together had consumed a total of nearly two-thirds of a million minor tranquilizer tablets and still continued to be stricken by the panic attacks. What's more, he adds, "No reliable evidence supports the use of antipsychotic drugs (so-called *major* tranquilizers), although they are prescribed for nearly half of all persons afflicted with agoraphobia."

What, then, does provide effective treatment?

Dr. Hardy, working with TERRAP for the past 18 years, has provided desensitization techniques for agoraphobics with notable success.

"We educate people about their agoraphobia and assure them that there is nothing wrong with their mind or their body," says Dr. Hardy. Patients are taught some basic psychology and relaxation techniques. Slowly their inhibited feelings come to the surface.

"They must be able to recognize and identify their feelings and to learn how to express them in socially acceptable ways to avoid criticism," says Dr. Hardy. "We tell them if they can openly express themselves, stay in contact with their feelings and speak up for themselves, they will have no problems. If they begin to inhibit themselves again, they'll revert back to their old habits."

It takes a lot for some agoraphobics to

go through a desensitization program. "It can be frightening to even attempt it," a recovered agoraphobic working at TERRAP told us. She had suffered from agoraphobia for nine years, spending the last year housebound. "It took me a long time to be able to walk into a TER-RAP meeting," she recalls. "I stood outside the door and listened for two months. I didn't want to walk into a room with so many people in it. It was too frightening for me." Now she travels, skis and throws parties without any difficulty.

"We have a success rate of 80 to 85 percent," says Dr. Hardy. People with agoraphobia don't go crazy, and panic attacks do not injure their bodies or minds in any way. Agoraphobia also is not fatal, he adds. He attributes his success rate to using psychological techniques to treat a "personality disorder." But what about the other 15 to 20 percent? Is it possible that some of those agoraphobics might respond favorably to a nutritional approach?

Laraine Abbey, R.N., a nurse practitioner who specializes in orthomolecular nutrition and clinical ecology in East Windsor, New Jersey, thinks so.

Nutritional Deficiencies and Fear

"I think all agoraphobics probably have nutritional deficiencies of one kind or another," Laraine Abbey told us. "I previously had worked with a number of people who had fears and anxieties and found they invariably cleared up on a nutritional program."

Sandra Leffler, of North Brunswick, New Jersey, was one of Laraine Abbey's patients. In November, 1978, Sandra started experiencing terrible pressure headaches. From then on, she began feeling constantly dizzy and out of whack.

"I was always afraid I was going to faint, so I stopped driving and didn't go out," she recalls. "I had my husband drive me to the store, but I wouldn't see my friends or even talk on the phone."

She went to three different doctors. The first one told her she wasn't getting any younger. (She was 33.) The second gave her a prescription for Valium. The third told her she was nervous and needed to lose weight. Feelings of depression had led her to a steady diet of junk food and had pushed her weight up to 182 pounds.

"I felt like I was going crazy. I felt like I was going to die," Sandra told us. "I started to lose my appetite and weight along with it, but I kept getting worse. I wouldn't set foot out of the house. I did all of my Christmas shopping through a catalog. I became obsessed with fear. I was afraid that the apartment was going to catch on fire, so I began sleeping on the couch. We had two cars, but no matter which one I was riding in, I thought it was going to explode."

People at a local health food store told Sandra about Laraine Abbey. And after several months, she was finally convinced to make an appointment with her.

"Sandra was my most outstanding case of agoraphobia," recalls the nurse practitioner, who counsels patients with a variety of disorders in her practice. "Blood and urine studies we did showed some abnormalities. For one thing, she was not getting enough vitamin B_1. Either her genetic requirement made her B_1 requirement higher than normal, or she was not absorbing it properly, or she was not getting enough from her diet. Whatever the case, she needed more B_1."

Sandra also was hypoglycemic, which means her blood sugar level was erratic. "The few agoraphobics I have seen have all had the standard hypoglycemic symptoms: depression, anxiety, tremors and a sense of impending doom," says Laraine Abbey. "When someone has severe hypoglycemia, I test for food allergy. In Sandra's case, she was very allergic to mushrooms. She also was allergic on a lesser scale to milk, eggs, mustard, onions, squash, pork, tomatoes, garlic, baker's yeast and tobacco."

Sandra began taking supplements, including a multivitamin and mineral tablet, vitamin C, B complex, lecithin, brewer's yeast and vitamin E. Since she was hypoglycemic, she started following a high-protein, low-carbohydrate diet and ate six times a day to keep her blood sugar level steady. She eliminated sugar and refined starchy foods like white rice from her diet. What happened? She lost 47 pounds and her fear.

"I'm driving and able to enjoy seeing people. I have made new friends around the neighborhood and I have found out that I *want* to go places," says Sandra. "My eyes are bright and clear, and my hair became sparkly shiny. People even compliment me on it now, and I say, 'That's from the wheat germ.'

"I guess I owe mostly everything to Laraine Abbey. She took the time and made me realize what was wrong. I realize how important nutrition is now. Your diet makes all of the difference in the world."

Sandra eventually will reduce her supplements to maintenance doses, and as her health stabilizes, she may gradually introduce foods to which she is mildly allergic back into her diet. "I guess I'll always have to stay away from sugar, though. Whenever I have a piece of 'regular' cake the headaches, tiredness and dizziness return," she says. "But I'm happy with my diet as it is. I feel so much better, I don't think I'd want to go back to the old way of eating."

Although Sandra's bout with agoraphobia caused her much unhappiness and even broke up her marriage, she did not seek psychological counseling for her disorder. Laraine Abbey believes some agoraphobics, however, may need both nutritional and psychological counseling in order to fully recover. A person's psychological health is very dependent on his or her biochemical health, and we should try to work with both areas simultaneously, she explains.

"I never believe you can separate the mind from the body," she says. "The same nutrients that feed the left kneecap feed the brain."

ALCOHOL: Social Drinking

Bloody Marys invade the Monday morning bridge club. Screwdrivers are a young mother's most valuable tool for coping with a rambunctious preschooler. And a carafe of chablis unabashedly replaces a pitcher of iced tea on the luncheon table of four female executives.

Chalk it up to women's liberation or just a sign of more permissive times, but women are now competing in the barroom as well as in the boardroom. True, men still command the lead in the liquor department. In a 1976 poll, 77 percent of all men questioned said they drank. Women weren't far behind, however, with 66 percent saying yes—up from 45 percent in 1958. Even worse, a recent study by the U.S. Department of Health and Human Services (HHS), formerly the Department of Health, Education and Welfare, reveals that nearly all women between the ages of 18 and 35 drink.

It's no wonder talk of "drying out" among women's circles today has turned from laundry on the line to women on the wagon!

Well, you can hardly put all the blame on women. Practically everybody drinks these days—even if it's only on those "special" occasions like weddings, anniversaries, birthdays, Christmas and New Year's Eve. Alcohol provides that temporary respite from the pressures of the real world. It may make you feel good for the moment. But that doesn't mean it's good for you.

To understand why alcohol has a lot in common with that proverbial wolf in sheep's clothing, let's first look at how our bodies must cope with it. When you have a cocktail, it sloshes to your stomach where a good portion of it is absorbed directly into your bloodstream. The remainder travels further along your digestive tract, but eventually it, too, winds up in the blood. From there about 80 percent of this liquid is sped to a detoxification center in the liver. The 20 percent that's left over is scattered throughout tissues of the intestines, stomach, kidney, lungs, spleen, retina, and, in men, the prostate and testes as well.

You can easily see which organs are likely to take the brunt of the damage over a long period of heavy drinking. But even sporadic drinking sprees can cause some congestion in the system. The liver is capable of metabolizing only so much alcohol at a time. For most

women, the rate is somewhat less than half a drink (or ¾ ounce of alcohol) per hour.

Preventing an overload can be achieved in part by slowing the absorption of alcohol into the bloodstream. The rate of absorption and the effect of a drink depends on several things.

1. *What you drink.* Generally speaking, the alcohol in diluted beverages like beer and wine and to a lesser degree, mixed drinks, is absorbed at a slower rate, which produces lower peak alcohol levels in the blood. Concentrated drinks such as martinis and straight-up shots send a surge of alcohol into the bloodstream. And that's what you don't want. But there are even some exceptions to that rule: when diluted to the same alcohol concentration, gin was found to be absorbed more rapidly than whiskey, and both more slowly than sweet red wines.

Many people suspect that the fizz in carbonated mixers speeds alcohol absorption. That's true to a certain extent. In studies, champagne was absorbed more rapidly than white wine, which generally takes a pretty poky route to the blood. But plain water had little advantage over carbonated water when mixed with gin or whiskey—probably because hard liquor is absorbed more rapidly anyway.

2. *How fast you drink it.* The faster you gulp, the faster your blood alcohol levels rise and the faster you get drunk. And while alcohol levels can reach the same peak in sippers as in guzzlers, studies have shown that those who guzzle stay drunker for longer periods of time.

3. *Whether or not there's food in your stomach.* It makes sense—the more food that mingles with the alcohol you drink, the less alcohol will be

directly absorbed into the bloodstream from the stomach. Studies have also shown that the type of food eaten can make the difference. Proteins and fats seem to slow the rate of alcohol absorption more than carbohydrates.

4. *The fact that you're female.* Perhaps you're already aware that it takes considerably less alcohol to get the same effect in you as it does in your husband or male companion. Of course, his tipping the scale at 170 pounds next to your 120 has something to do with it. But that's not the whole story. It seems that when a man and a woman are given equivalent doses of alcohol (calculated according to their body weights), the woman's blood alcohol levels will rise to a higher peak. The reason? Researchers cite body composition. A man's body is more muscle than fat, they say, and muscle tissue contains more water than fatty tissue. For women, it's just the opposite: we have more fat than muscle, and, consequently, less water. As a result, the same dose of alcohol will be watered down in a man, and relatively concentrated in a woman. Of course, you can't change your sex—but you can keep this fact in mind and limit your alcohol intake accordingly.

5. *Your emotional state.* Actually, this probably has more to do with the fact that you're female than you may realize. For a long time authorities on alcohol have known that a person who's emotionally upset, tense or tired is likely to receive a stronger impact from a given amount of alcohol. But no one could explain why. Now, new evidence suggests that at least in women, the female hormone estrogen may have something to do with it. In tests, a woman given a designated dose of alcohol under controlled circumstances experiences varying peak blood alcohol levels

depending on the stage of her menstrual cycle. Generally, alcohol levels peak and pack more of a wallop just before her period when estrogen levels are low. A low estrogen level is also responsible for premenstrual bouts with anxiety and depression.

Alcohol and Your Health

Actually, there's one school of thought that says moderate drinking is better than no drinking at all. An occasional swig or a slight daily indulgence helps you sleep better and makes your heart healthier, says Morris Chafetz, M.D., who was founding director of the National Institute on Alcohol Abuse and Alcoholism (NIAAA).

Indeed, a recent study confirms that one or two ounces of alcohol a day may slightly decrease your risk of coronary heart disease (*American Journal of Epidemiology*, March, 1978). But the whys and wherefores are kind of sketchy. Some say the preventive role of alcohol is related to its effect on high-density lipoproteins (HDL)—the fraction of cholesterol that seems to protect against coronary heart disease. Others favor alcohol's calming effects. Alcohol helps us cope with stress, they say, and stress is a major risk factor in coronary heart disease. And with regard to female complaints, many women say they drink during the premenstrual phase to relieve cramps and ease depression.

All of that is fine. But you can't convince us that drinking alcohol is a plus for our health and happiness. For example:

• Statistics show the most common cause of death for women under age 29 is the automobile accident. But according to J. Donald Miller, M. D., D.T.P.H., assistant director for Public Health Practice at the Centers for Disease Control, Atlanta, Georgia, at least half of those deaths are related to drinking. And it's not only the drinking driver who suffers; sometimes a person is killed as a consequence of somebody else's drinking and driving.

- Two recent studies on alcohol and sexual pleasure note that as blood levels of alcohol go up, women's ability to become aroused and reach orgasm goes down. And women don't even need to act tipsy for alcohol to reduce pleasure, researchers G. Terence Wilson, Ph.D., of Rutgers University, New Brunswick, New Jersey, and Victor J. Malatesta, Ph.D., of the University of Georgia have found.

- The latest study on alcohol and the mental performance of women social drinkers says moderate drinking may damage your memory. Researchers at the University of Oklahoma Health Sciences Center found that alcohol affects mental performance in such a way that moderate drinkers aren't as sharp even when they're sober. And age seems to boost the damage done by alcohol. The older the woman and the more alcohol she drinks, the worse she does on memory tests (*Journal of Studies on Alcohol*, January, 1980).

- Numerous reports indicate the combination of drinking and smoking poses a serious health risk. One such report released by Irwin J. D. Bross, Ph.D., and Jeanne Coombs, Ph.D., at Roswell Park Memorial Institute in New York reveals that women who smoke at least one pack of cigarettes and consume at least one alcoholic drink a day are 18 times more likely to get mouth and tongue cancer than women who avoid the combination. The researchers studied 2,000 women before coming to that conclusion, and they explain the results this way: when two carcinogens (cocarcinogens) act on the same target cells, malignant cells tend to develop more quickly.

Besides, any problem that alcohol seems to remedy, other more natural methods can heal better. For example, you can turn to the section Sleep and learn how to get a good night's rest without alcohol. To raise HDL in your blood, vitamin C, brewer's yeast and exercise are every bit as good as the big A. If it's relaxation you're searching for, you could find it bottled up in green glass but you'd be better off checking out our natural stress-relievers under Anxiety. And, for premenstrual complications, see Cramps and Other Premenstrual Miseries for more sensible solutions.

What we're trying to get across is that every excuse for drinking alcohol is just that—an excuse. You can't fight fire with fire. And you can't douse your physical or mental complaints with alcohol, which has its own set of built-in health hazards.

Obviously, the worst hazard of social drinking is alcoholism. Of course, not every woman who drinks socially develops that uncontrollable craving which we associate with alcoholism. But approximately 12 out of every 100 do. And we don't know why—or who might be more susceptible.

What we know is that every alcoholic begins the same way: with a drink. It's not as difficult as you may think to slip into heavy drinking patterns. The ultimate consequences are devastating. Liver damage. Disease of the pancreas. Anemia. Malnutrition. Ulcers. Brain damage. Memory loss. Sleep disturbances. Nervous system disorders. Psychosis. And even death. Alcoholics are 2½ times more likely to commit suicide or die prematurely than nonalcoholics, and are 7 times more likely to get into accidents (notably on the highways). According to HHS, alcoholism shortens life expectancy by 10 to 15 years.

The Effects of Light Drinking

Lighter drinkers will, of course, be affected to a lesser degree. But they are certainly not immune from the ill effects. They suffer from memory changes, sleep disturbances, headaches, digestive system disorders and even nutritional deficiencies. For example, every time you indulge in a before-dinner cocktail containing one jigger, or 1½ ounces, of liquor, you're reducing your intake of nutritious foods containing important vitamins, minerals and amino acids by 97 calories. That may not sound like much, but on a weekly basis (two drinks a day with a binge at week's end is typical of a moderate drinker), that amounts to about 1,500 to 2,000 calories.

Not only that, alcohol has a tendency to destroy certain vitamins—especially the B's such as thiamine (vitamin B₁) and folate. And for women—who, after all, are more prone to B vitamin deficiencies and anemia in the first place— even moderate drinking could be the straw that broke the camel's back.

If you do drink, at least make sure your diet is more than adequate and that you're safely supplemented with all nutrients but especially the B vitamins and vitamin C, which has been shown to protect against some of the toxic effects of alcohol (*Nutrition Reports International*, April, 1978).

It's also a good idea to stock up on zinc and bone meal or dolomite.

And be especially cautious about mixing alcohol with any type of drug. Even one or two drinks can have serious consequences for a person taking various prescription or over-the-counter drugs—including aspirin.

What happens very often is that alcohol inhibits enzymes that help the body metabolize other drugs. We have only to remember the well-publicized case of Karen Ann Quinlan to see the ultimate consequence.

See the accompanying chart of drug-alcohol interactions. Or consult your doctor before you mix *any* drug with any amount of alcohol.

Alcohol and Dieting

The most obvious reason to reduce your alcohol intake while you're trying to reduce your weight is that alcohol is fattening. One gin and tonic contains a jigger of 1½ ounces of 80-proof gin (that's 98 calories) and 6 ounces of tonic water (another 66 calories). That makes for a grand total of 164 calories. Empty calories no less. No protein. No vitamins. No minerals. Just plain old "just-what-you-don't-need"-type calories.

Of course you can juggle the ingredients. Perhaps dilute your shot with something more nutritious like fresh-squeezed orange juice or tomato juice. Or opt for a mixer with no calories like club soda or Perrier water. But you just can't get away from it. If you're talking alcohol, you're talking calories. And if it's calories that you're counting, remember, a stolen cocktail at noon robs you of a more nourishing baked potato or spinach omelet with lunch. Nutritious foods are never more important

14

HOW MANY CALORIES ARE YOU DRINKING?

Beverage	Measure (fluid ounces)	Calories
BEER		
Regular	12	155
Light	12	96
LIQUEUR		
Anisette	1½	123
Benedictine	1½	168
Creme de menthe	1½	165
Drambuie	1½	165
Kirsch	1½	125
Tia Maria	1½	138
LIQUOR		
Whiskey, gin, rum, vodka (80 proof), etc.	1½ (1 jigger)	98

MIXED DRINKS		
Bloody Mary	3	103
Daiquiri	3	190
Manhattan	3	161
Margarita	3	176
Martini	3	176
Screwdriver	3	111
Whiskey sour	3	190

MIXERS		
Bitter lemon	6	96
Club soda	6	0
Coke	6	72
Cream[a]	1 tablespoon	30
Fruit-flavored sodas	6	86
Ginger ale	6	64
Lemon juice	4	31
Orange juice	4	55
Tomato juice	4	22
Tonic water	6	66

WINE		
Red (Burgundy)	3½ (a wine-glass)	76
Rose (sparkling)	3½	84
White (chablis)	3½	58

SOURCES: Beverage values were adapted from *Calories and Carbohydrates*, by Barbara Kraus (New York: Grosset & Dunlap, 1971) except:
[a] Catherine F. Adams, *Nutritive Value of American Foods in Common Units*, Agriculture Handbook No. 456 (Washington, D.C.: Agricultural Research Service, U.S. Department of Agriculture, 1975).

than when you're dieting and calorie intake is cut to the bare essentials.

But let's face it, a widening waistline isn't the only pitfall in drinking and dieting. According to J. Murray McLaughlan, M.D., and his group at the Health Protection Branch of Canada's Department of National Health and Welfare in Ottawa, even normal people on a low-calorie diet for as little as 36 to 72 hours may develop significant hypoglycemia (low blood sugar) after a couple of alcoholic drinks.

Dr. McLaughlan put 12 volunteers on a 650-calorie-a-day diet for three days. On the third day, each volunteer drank a jigger of whiskey at 9 A.M., one at 10, and a third slug at 11. On a normal diet, three drinks like that would have shot their blood glucose or sugar levels up after lunch. But on the low-calorie diet, their blood glucose values fell to their lowest levels around 1 P.M. What's more, most subjects reported sudden tiredness, weakness or nervousness, nausea or headaches. Two complained of being ill, sweated profusely, and their pulse rates climbed to 140. One could not go on and had to eat a chocolate bar to coax his glucose level back up (*Nutrition Reports International*, November, 1973).

In a more recent study, the combination of alcohol with sweet mixers like tonic water or lemonade was found to be a more potent cause of hypoglycemia than either alcohol or a sweet drink alone (*Lancet*, June 18, 1977). No doubt this is the reason why one woman we spoke with said she suddenly passed out at a luncheon party after she drank just one gin and tonic on an empty stomach.

Alcohol and Pregnancy

Probably the most devastating implication of a woman drinking alcohol doesn't really have anything to do with her. Rather, it's the effect her drinking has on her unborn child.

According to statistics, miscarriages and stillbirths are much more common among heavy drinkers than among non-drinking mothers. And that's just the tip of the iceberg.

Maybe you've already heard the term Fetal Alcohol Syndrome, or FAS. It's a hot subject for women's and family magazines lately, and for good reason. With drinking becoming more socially acceptable for women and with more women of childbearing years drinking, it's about time we were enlightened about FAS.

In fact, FAS is now recognized as the third leading cause of birth defects—and the leading cause of mental deficiency—in the Western world. What's so disturbing, though, is that it is the only one that's entirely preventable. All it takes is nine months of abstinence, and yet at least one study indicates that 80 percent of middle-class women drink some alcohol during pregnancy. You'd think it was too much to ask!

And heaven knows FAS is worth preventing! FAS children come into this world with more than one serious handicap. For one thing, they have an unusual appearance. In fact, only six years ago, before this defect was linked to alcohol, FAS kids were simply diagnosed as FLKs—funny-looking kids. With small heads, short eye slits, narrow upper lips, feet deformities, crossed eyes, and deep creases in the palms of their hands, these little children defied typical diagnosis. In addition, they often had heart murmurs, cleft palates, and cleft chins. But what really set them apart from other children was their low intelligence quotient. A study conducted by the National Institutes of Health of such children until they were seven years old showed that 46 percent had IQs under 79. Average is about 100. Placing these children in an improved environment, giving them proper food and loving care had no major effect on their IQs or on their physical growth. Both remained deficient.

Of course, children of alcoholic mothers run the greatest risk of FAS. But—before you start to feel too smug— you don't have to be an alcoholic to leave your loved one with a legacy of grief.

Every time a pregnant woman has a cocktail, her unborn baby has one, too. One drink—whether a 12-ounce can of beer, a 3- to 5-ounce glass of wine, or a mixed drink containing 1½ ounces of alcohol—circulates through her baby's system.

No one knows whether that's enough to put an unborn child in any danger. But evidence does suggest that even if a woman usually drinks very little but drinks a lot in one day, she could cause irreparable damage.

What's especially frightening about this is that a developing fetus is particularly susceptible to the damaging effects of alcohol in the initial weeks of gestation—perhaps even before a woman realizes she is pregnant.

Take Sandy Weiss as an example. Sandy (not her real name) was not a heavy drinker—by any stretch of the imagination. She and her husband, Peter, rarely drank. If they were feeling particularly extravagant on an occasion, they might share a bottle of wine with a special Saturday night dinner.

Sandy's periods were always irregular. So, she never even gave it a second thought when her period was late the week of her best friend's wedding.

Saturday night there was a formal rehearsal dinner, with cocktails and wine. Sunday morning, before the wedding, Sandy had a drink to steady her nerves. Then there was the reception, with more cocktails, wine and champagne. After the excitement subsided and the bride and groom were whisked away in a shower of rice, Sandy joined the wedding party for an evening of drinks and dinner.

By the end of the 24-hour period, Sandy had consumed a total of 11½ drinks!

About a week later, Sandy got the word from her doctor that she was pregnant. Delighted, she didn't drink for the remainder of the pregnancy. Yet, despite her noble intentions, Sandy's daughter was born with a cleft lip and weighed only 5½ pounds. Later, when she was about to enter kindergarten, Sandy and Peter found out that their daughter's IQ was considerably below normal.

Actually, Sandy's alcohol binge was a pretty potent one. But recent research by Sterling Clarren, M.D., at the University of Washington, has shown that women who reported having as few as five drinks at one time have produced babies with malformations of the brain.

Can "Safe" Drinking Cause Birth Defects?

Kenneth L. Jones, M.D., a physician from the University of California Medical Center in San Diego, went even one step further in his 1978 speech to the American Medical Association. He insisted that an alcohol intake as low as one to two ounces per day (a level regarded as "safe" by the NIAAA) may cause malformation of the fetal brain tissue or decrease birth weight. No safe level of alcohol consumption can be determined, he said, because each woman's metabolism when pregnant varies, and blood alcohol levels vary also. What's safe for one woman may not be safe for another.

Not only that, drinking immediately before becoming pregnant may put the yet-to-be-conceived child at risk. According to research by Ruth E. Little, Sc.D., an average intake of one ounce of alcohol daily *before* pregnancy was associated with an average decrease in birth weight of almost a quarter pound (*American Journal of Public Health*, December, 1977). Low birth weight, by the way, has been linked to a whole host of physical and mental deficiencies.

After pregnancy, breastfeeding and drinking don't mix either, says Alison Young, R.N., of the Pregnancy and Health Program at the University of Washington. She advises no drinking while breastfeeding. "We're immovable on that issue," she says. "We feel that because the brain and liver are prime targets for alcohol in the adult, and because alcohol is reaching the infant in the milk, his immature organs must be under attack, too."

We do know for a fact that the amount of alcohol in breast milk is almost the same as the mother's blood alcohol level. Absorption is rapid and alcohol reaches the milk almost immediately. If the mother has a martini, then the baby has one, too. We also know from animal studies that alcohol from any kind of drink—hard liquor, beer or wine—inhibits oxytocin, the female hormone that helps the milk get to the nipple.

Our advice: if you are pregnant or breastfeeding, abstain from drinking alcohol. If you are planning to become pregnant, don't drink. And if you are a sexually active woman of childbearing age, be extremely cautious about drinking more than one or two drinks a day.

Social Drinking without Regrets

Still bent on a nip from the bottle every now and then? Well, we certainly can't stop you. But do yourself a favor and keep in mind the following hints to avoid the post-cocktail-party blues.

First of all, before you even leave your house, or reach for the corkscrew (if you're drinking at home), set a limit for yourself at, say, two mixed drinks or a maximum of three ounces of alcohol. If you know from experience that your tolerance is lower than that, pledge your limit accordingly. For some women, two small glasses of wine is tops. For others, one mug of beer is enough to take the edge off the day without pushing them off the brink. Also keep in mind that if your period is due next week, you'd probably do well to reduce your normal limit somewhat.

Once you've set your limit, though, stick with it—no matter what. For example, if you know from the start that it's going to be a long evening, make your first drink a nonalcoholic one. It doesn't have to be boring, you know. There are plenty of suitable beverages on the bar to choose from. Try a sparkling glass of water with a lime zest. Or a glass of orange juice with a sprig of mint. Who knows, you may even find that you prefer your Bloody Marys minus the vodka.

Then, pace yourself. Intersperse your gin and bitter lemons with a plain club soda on the rocks with a twist.

POTENTIAL DRUG PLUS ALCOHOL INTERACTIONS*

TYPE OF DRUG + ALCOHOL =	POSSIBLE SIDE EFFECT
ANTIBIOTICS Flagyl	Rapid heart rate, pounding headache, flushing of face, dizziness, nausea, vomiting, rapid breathing, faintness.
griseofulvin	Rapid heartbeat and flushing of face.
tetracycline	Impaired body detoxification process, resulting in enhanced effects of drug.
ANTIHISTAMINES *(used in allergic reaction such as hay fever)*	Enhanced side effects of drug, notably drowsiness.
BIRTH CONTROL PILLS (ESTROGEN)	Apparent decrease in breakdown of alcohol.
CIRCULATORY DRUGS	
nitroglycerin *(used to reduce blood pressure)*	Severe hypotension (low blood pressure) which could lead to cardiovascular collapse.
warfarin *(used to reduce blood clotting)*	Increased breakdown of drug resulting in its reduced effectiveness.
COLD MEDICINE	
Benylin	Same as for antihistamine.
CoTylenol Cold Formula Tablets	None reported with recommended doses.

SOURCES: Ainley, Wade, ed., *The Extra Pharmacopoeia*, 27th ed. (London: Pharmaceutical Press, 1977).
Eric W. Martin et al., *Hazards of Medication* (Philadelphia: J. B. Lippincott, 1978).
Physicians' Desk Reference, 34th ed. (Oradell, N.J.: Medical Economics Company, 1980).
Ben Morgan Jones and Marilyn K. Jones, "Interaction of Alcohol, Oral Contraceptives and the Menstrual Cycle with Stimulus-Response Compatibility," in *Currents in Alcoholism: Volume II*, ed. Frank A. Seixas (New York: Grune & Stratton, 1977).

*Always ask your doctor or pharmacist about the possible side effects of a medication and its interaction with other drugs you are taking, including alcohol and foods.

TYPE OF DRUG + ALCOHOL = POSSIBLE SIDE EFFECT

DIURETIC *(used to increase kidney function)*	Lasix	Enhances diuretic effect. Otherwise, there appears to be no interaction.
DRAMAMINE *(used in motion sickness)*		Same as for antihistamines.
INSULIN		Enhanced hypoglycemic effect (lower blood glucose). With large quantities of alcohol, coma and death could result.
PAINKILLERS	aspirin	Enhanced effects of drug, particularly inflammation of the stomach and intestine. This may lead to an increase in bleeding of the digestive tract.
	codeine	Enhanced side effects resulting in increased drowsiness and reduced coordination.
	Midol	Same as for aspirin.
	substitute aspirin (Tylenol)	None reported with recommended doses.
SEDATIVES	Nembutal phenobarbital Seconal	Greatly enhanced effects of these drugs. With large amounts of alcohol, cessation of breathing and death could ensue.
TRANQUILIZERS	Librium Valium	Impaired coordination and reaction times. Possible decrease in cardiac and respiratory function.
WEIGHT REDUCERS *(used as stimulants which depress appetite)*	amphetamines (Dexedrine) nonamphetamines (Ionamin, Tenuate)	Central nervous system stimulants decrease depressant effects of alcohol, but do not counteract its impairment of coordination.

It's also a good idea to do the mixing yourself rather than rely on the heavy-handed services of your host. And keep your cocktails on the weak side. Always use a shot glass. Be stingy with the spirits and generous with the ice, water and mixer. To get more mileage out of a glass of wine, try a spritzer. That's a combination of wine and carbonated water.

Then, don't rush it. Sip and savor your drinks. Remember: the faster you gulp, the quicker you get drunk. And the sooner you empty your glass, the greater the chance your host will notice that you need a refill.

Drinking on an empty stomach is also a no-no. Your best bet is to make mealtime a prerequisite to party time. If you can't arrange to eat within a half hour of the party, make a beeline for the hors d'oeuvres. Now, nibble on the cheese and chicken wings—not the chips. It's the fat and protein that ease the absorption of alcohol into your bloodstream. Carbohydrates do little. And the salt that clings like dandruff to those party snacks is liable to leave you itching for more margaritas.

If you can afford the calories, drinks with food in them, such as eggnog (which contains eggs, milk and cream) are probably better than a double Scotch when you start on an empty stomach.

One last thing: the time to start thinking about a hangover is before you get one. Once you've downed your drinks, there's nothing short of a stomach pump that's going to get that alcohol out of your system. And the more popular hangover hints are worthless at best; harmful at worst.

Aspirin on top of alcohol, for example, is one way to create a Bloody Mary in your stomach without tomato juice. It seems that alcohol is notorious for irritating the stomach lining. And so is aspirin. Put the two together and you double your chances of gastric hemorrhage.

Coffee's not much help either. It might wake you up. But it won't stimulate slowed reflexes or clear dulled senses. Actually, you'd probably be smarter sleeping it off than rousing yourself enough to get behind a steering wheel.

Better yet, remember abstinence is better for your health, better for your waistline, and better for your baby.

ALCOHOLISM

Do you drink *before* going to parties? Or to prime yourself before picking the kids up at school?

Do you drink to "get through the day"?

Do you fly to functions when the punch is spiked but drag your feet when it isn't?

Do you have a tendency to gulp drinks and beat everyone to seconds?

Did you ever tie one on till 2 A.M. but couldn't remember one thing about the party past 11?

Do you always drink to drunkenness?

Do you find hangover relief in yet another bottle of booze?

Do your drinking habits interfere with your life? In other words, have you missed work, lost friends, or really come down on your kids without cause? All because of alcohol?

If you find yourself nodding yes to any one of these questions, you may have a drinking problem, and that disease we call alcoholism could be just a couple of gulps away. If your nods outnumber your nays, then there's no question about it—you're already there.

According to Judy Wicks of the Office on Women, National Council on Alcoholism, the development of alcoholism is as closely entwined with patterns of drinking (that is, when you drink and for what reasons) as with the amounts of alcohol consumed. The woman who insists that she doesn't drink much—"Only on weekends," or "Only when I *need* it,"—may be kidding herself about a drinking problem that could lead to serious disease, she told us.

Just how many American women are kidding themselves or creeping out of the closet with serious drinking problems is not known. Various estimates place the figure at anywhere from one to four million. That's still somewhat behind our male population of alcoholics. But many authorities believe that the gap is closing. And it's not just the women's libbers that are filling it. Women from all walks of life—secretaries, schoolteachers, nurses, physicians, executives, housewives—are coming to crave the "hard stuff."

Actually, the start of alcoholism is exactly the same for men and women. In every case, it begins quite innocently—with a drink.

The One Reason for Heavy Drinking

"Almost all persons who drink, drink for exactly the same reason. To cope," says Jean Kirkpatrick, Ph.D., a recovered alcoholic and founding director of Women for Sobriety, a national organization of women for women alcoholics (see *Appendix*). "Even the social drinkers drink to cope. They might say they do it because it makes them feel more loose,

more sociable, more confident or charming. But, in essence, what they're doing is trying to cope with a faltering sense of self."

Dr. Kirkpatrick knows. She's been through it herself. And her story is just like those she hears every day in her treatment program.

"I began drinking when I was 17 because I grew up with alcohol at home. Nothing heavy, actually. My father drank very little and my mother, not at all. But it was just normal that when friends dropped by to see my parents, they'd offer them a mixed drink," Dr. Kirkpatrick recalled during our visit to her headquarters in Quakertown, Pennsylvania. "Later, when I went away to college, I looked forward to weekend parties and drinking. Alcohol was part of the socialization I had. And I found that I loved it. Not the taste. But I loved what it did to me. It made me feel confident, alluring, charming—all that sense of personality that I didn't feel I had.

"In time, alcohol became just as much a part of my life as smoking. It wasn't unusual to have a drink at four o'clock in the afternoon. Or with lunch and again at dinner. Pretty soon I fell into the pattern. Oh, of course, I didn't realize then what was happening. But, in retrospect, the pattern of alcoholism was clearly taking form. For one thing, I had several periods of severe blackouts, one before I was even 21 years old. This isn't a 'pass out' as most people think. It's a form of amnesia. The brain cells become anesthetized by the alcohol. The funny thing is, the person drinking is acting, talking and walking just fine. She doesn't appear drunk. But the next morning she can't remember a thing she said or did. It's frightening. And if you've ever had one, you should consider it a red flag to danger.

"Also, I would always drink to drunkenness (which is another warning sign of alcoholism). After a time, I came to crave alcohol. I'd do practically anything for a drink. And when I got one, I'd have it down so fast. There was no such thing as 'nursing' a drink in my book.

"It wasn't until I was in my early thirties that I realized I had a problem. I needed alcohol to get through the day. It was like medicine to me. My body craved it. So I'd have a shot. Then two hours later, I'd break out in perspiration and get this splitting headache. The only way to relieve it was with another drink. Two hours later, I'd need another one. Pretty soon I found that I was going through a fifth a day, and feeling terrible. I was having liver attacks, gallbladder attacks. My system could no longer tolerate the alcohol."

Dr. Kirkpatrick admits that in certain instances a life crisis—such as divorce, death of a child or spouse, or midlife with its frequently accompanying "empty nest syndrome"—can jolt a woman into a drinking pattern that leads to alcoholism. But in most cases, the pattern is already set long before the crisis occurs, she says. What happens is that the event pushes the susceptible woman over the brink into alcoholism. You'd practically never see a teetotaler picking up a bottle to cope with some catastrophe and drinking herself into cirrhosis of the liver. It doesn't happen that way.

Women and Vulnerability to Alcohol

The disease of alcoholism takes many years to develop—10 to 15 at least. And that goes for both men and women.

That is not to say there are no differences between the male and female alcoholic. There are. For starters, it may take less alcohol to create a physical dependency in women. This aspect is described more fully in the section Alcohol: Social Drinking. But briefly, if a man and a woman are given comparable doses of alcohol (adjusted for their given body weights), the woman's blood will reach a higher level of alcohol concentration than the man's. She becomes intoxicated sooner. The implication of this is, of course, that the female body metabolizes alcohol faster. Possibly, then, she may face a quicker progression of alcoholism.

The female body also seems more sensitive to alcohol damage. Possibly for the same reason that they become drunker faster, women also beat men to the debilitating ailments associated with alcoholism. Fatty liver disease, anemia, malnutrition, and gastrointestinal hemorrhage occur in women after a shorter period of heavy drinking (*Lancet*, November 12, 1977).

And, not only do they get hit faster, women get hit harder in their bout with the bottle. In a survey of 293 patients with alcoholic liver disease, women—particularly those under age 45—had a significantly higher incidence of alcoholic hepatitis, with or without cirrhosis, than men. Also, their long-term prognosis was poorer—even after having sworn off the bottle for good (*British Medical Journal*, June 11, 1977).

Besides all that, a woman sometimes has more than herself to consider. Suppose she's pregnant. Recently disclosed studies have made it clear: children born to alcoholic women run an incredibly high risk of suffering from Down's syndrome (mongolism), mental retardation, growth abnormalities and liver disease. All the more reason to see women on the wagon.

Unfortunately, their recovery records show them to be somewhat short of the male mark. Women drink longer than men before seeking help. They are less likely to stop drinking. And when they do stop, they stand a better chance of starting up all over again.

Why?

Many people believe that the one factor with the most profoundly negative impact on the female alcoholic is society. Dr. Kirkpatrick, for one, is very vocal on this point.

"Society denounces women alcoholics as being morally loose, emotionally weak. The stigma is still there. They do not see alcoholism as a physical illness," she says. "It's a little different for men. When a man has a drinking problem, it's 'Well, poor old Charlie can't handle his booze.' His employer may take him aside and tell him to shape up or leave. So he does something about it. He goes to Alcoholics Anonymous (AA). Or to a counselor. Or if he works for some large corporation, he may even sign up for a 28-day drying out program away from home at a company cost of $4,000 to $5,000. A woman, on the other hand, who's caught with a drinking problem is fired. This compounds her problem. She becomes depressed and drinks more."

Where Do Women Turn for Help?

Instead of speeding her recovery, society has succeeded in postponing it. What's worse, it can withdraw help entirely. It seems that society's mores are not only reflected, they're often magnified in the people she'd most likely turn to for assistance:

Her clergyman. In deciding to come out of the closet, 42 percent of women alcoholics confess first to their clergy-

men. Yet according to Dr. Kirkpatrick, it isn't unusual for a priest to insist that a person do penance for what he considers a moral weakness.

Her physician. Knowing women's affinity for the physician's office, this could be the female alcoholic's most frequent outlet for her fears of alcoholism. Often, however, since she may have trouble voicing her ultimate fear—that she is an alcoholic—she will instead harp on the symptoms. Anxiety. Insomnia. Depression. It takes a perceptive doctor with a real understanding of alcoholism to come up with the right diagnosis. More often than not, however, physicians are either too busy to spend the time needed to thrash out the real problem, too disinterested to care whether there's more to it than meets the eye, or too ignorant of the symptoms of the disease to recognize it. It's much easier to jot out a prescription for Valium or some other tranquilizer. According to the National Institute on Drug Abuse, doctors are twice as likely to prescribe tranquilizers to women as to men, which explains why 79 percent of all female alcoholics have at one time or another been dually addicted (to alcohol and drugs such as Valium), while male alcoholics rarely have dual addictions. Betty Ford's case brought this out into public view.

Her husband. If you had a serious problem, who would you confide in first? Most women, we would guess, would tell their husbands. But a shocking study in Canada has disclosed that while only 1 in 10 women would abandon her alcoholic husband, 9 out of 10 men would wiggle out of a marriage to an alcoholic woman. Doesn't say much for their staying power!

Where does that leave the woman with a drinking problem who wants to quit? According to critics, it leaves them high but not too dry. Most studies report that women in therapy for alcohol problems do not do well. In their book, *Alcoholism Problems in Women and Children* (Grune & Stratton, 1976), Milton Greenblatt, M.D., and Marc A. Schuckit, M.D., cite evidence that women alcoholics often prefer individual therapy while men like the group sessions common to many alcoholic treatment programs. They also quote Linda Beckman, Ph.D., as saying that mixed male and female therapies do not work well because women need time to build up their feminine identity.

Dr. Kirkpatrick agrees. "Almost all female alcoholics have two things in common, besides their drinking. They are depressed beyond belief and you can't even measure their self-esteem—it's so low. What they need is a program designed to help build their self-confidence and self-worth, not one that continually reinforces their shortcomings.

"For example, an integral part of the old AA meetings was the telling of drinking histories. The person gets up in front of the group, identifies himself or 'I was born in ＿＿＿＿ ＿＿＿＿, I took my first drink at ＿＿＿＿ ＿＿＿＿', and so on. This might work for men. But in my opinion, it is the most deterrent factor for women alcoholics to recover. Women have got to close the door of that past and move on.

"Another part of AA is the humility factor. 'In all humility, I turn myself over.' Feminists throughout the world know that the last thing any woman needs is another dose of humility."

Unfortunately, very few alcoholic treatment programs are geared to women. For example, the National Institute on Alcohol Abuse and Alcoholism, a branch of the U.S. Department of Health and Human Services (formerly HEW), funds about 400 alcoholic rehabilitation programs for the general public but only 28 specially designed for women.

Many women therefore have no recourse but to join male-oriented groups. AA, for example, reports that female membership has grown by one-third over the last five years. Some women, however, have been treated quite successfully in the AA program, which is slowly being revised to accommodate the female alcoholic.

Other women have found abstinence much easier in the atmosphere of an exclusively female group. One private nonprofit organization for women only is Women for Sobriety, mentioned earlier, which now boasts over 300 chapters in the United States and Canada.

Any woman who has a drinking problem or thinks she might should contact one of these chapters. This is not to say that a determined woman can't overcome alcoholism on her own. But generally speaking, getting on the wagon is much less traumatic when you don't have to go it alone.

A Four-Part Recovery Program

Whatever route you decide on, you'd do well to incorporate the following into your daily routine.

1. Make the decision to quit. Take a long critical look at yourself and your life. How do you look? How do you feel? How do you behave with others? Is alcohol changing your life? Be honest. Do you like yourself? If you can admit that alcohol is the villain in your life, you're already on the road to recovery. But, you've really got to want to quit—more than anything else in the world—in or-

THE WOMEN FOR SOBRIETY ACCEPTANCE PROGRAM

1. I have a drinking problem that once had me.
2. Negative emotions destroy only myself.
3. Happiness is a habit I will develop.
4. Problems bother me only to the degree I permit them to.
5. I am what I think.
6. Life can be ordinary or it can be great.
7. Love can change the course of my world.
8. The fundamental object of life is emotional and spiritual growth.
9. The past is gone forever.
10. All love given returns twofold.
11. Enthusiasm is my daily exercise.
12. I am a competent woman and have much to give others.
13. I am responsible for myself and my sisters.

SOURCE: Jean Kirkpatrick, *A Year of Sobering Thoughts* (Women for Sobriety Books, vol. 1, March, 1976–March, 1977).

der for any recovery program to work. You've got to make a commitment. Then do it. Empty your liquor bottles into the kitchen sink. Swear off alcohol for good. Then every time you have the urge for a drink, think back to the most distasteful memory you have of yourself during your drinking. The worst hangover, perhaps. Or the most painful liver attack. Or an especially embarrassing situation. Relive your feelings at that time in every painful detail. Chances are, 5 to 10 minutes of unpleasant reminiscences will make the taste of alcohol absolutely repugnant to your senses.

2. Step up your nutritional program. Half of the problems associated with alcoholism stem not so much from the alcohol as from the malnutrition that results from heavy drinking. When you drink substantial amounts of alcohol you dilute your diet. Each ounce of whiskey contains about 66 calories and dilutes the diet about 2½ percent. Eight ounces a day, which isn't at all unusual for an alcoholic, dilutes the diet by 20 percent. As a result, essential vitamins, minerals and amino acids are crowded out, setting the stage for severe dietary deficiencies.

Not only does alcohol crowd out essential nutrients, it destroys some very important vitamins and minerals that do manage to get into your body. Abram Hoffer, Ph.D., M.D., of British Columbia, pioneer in the studies of alcoholics and vitamin deficiencies, says, "Alcohol is a derivative of sugar and both are metabolized in the body in an analogous manner. Both require vitamins and minerals before they can be turned to energy and since they are devoid of these essential nutrients, they produce more and more deficiency in the body. The more that is consumed, the greater is the deficiency."

To make matters worse, many alcoholic treatment programs push candy and black coffee complete with a teaspoon or two of sugar on the recovering alcoholic as a sort of substitute for alcoholic cravings. That is absolutely the worst thing that they can eat. In fact, says Dr. Kirkpatrick, the "dry drunk" experience of extreme nervousness and anxiety in the early days of sobriety, which many people believe is a normal physical response to abstinence, is actually induced by candy and coffee.

Women especially are devastated by the effects. The B vitamins—that family of nutrients necessary for cheerful, healthy emotions—are among the most vulnerable to the onslaught of alcohol. And we all know how depressed the female alcoholic is!

What's more, women also face a greater risk of anemia—the result of diminishing folate (one of the B vitamins).

So for the recovering alcoholic, even a good diet may not be adequate. But it is a start. Begin by cutting out sugar, white flour and coffee. Instead, eat high-quality protein (lean meat, fish, eggs and cheese), vegetables and fruits.

Then, to help you over the hump of early sobriety, Dr. Hoffer suggests the following supplements:

- Niacin (B₃)—3 to 6 grams a day.
- Vitamin B₆—1 gram a day.
- Vitamin C—3 to 10 grams a day (vitamin C has been shown to aid liver function).
- Folate—according to your individual requirements.
- Brewer's yeast—at least one tablespoon a day.

Proof that it works: a study conducted with AA members in 1972 showed that many were unable to stay sober until they were placed on a sugar-free diet with megavitamins. And from an alcoholic rest home in Michigan which uses high-dosage megavitamins and sugar-free diets as part of their treatment program come reports of an overall recovery rate of 80 percent.

3. Get into a positive frame of mind. "The place to begin and maintain sobriety is in the mind," says Dr. Kirkpatrick. "You are what you think. If you think you are nobody, a drunk, that is what you will be. But if you think you are sober, competent, compassionate, that is precisely what you will be."

To charge our thoughts positively,

Dr. Kirkpatrick suggests 15 minutes of uninterrupted contemplation every morning. It's what she calls "getting square with yourself for the day."

After rising in the morning, take a few minutes away from the breakfast clamor to be by yourself. Carefully read through The Women for Sobriety Acceptance Program, see previous page, stopping briefly after each message to weigh its meaning in terms of your life. When you're through, think about the new day that's just unfolding. How will you spend it? Make a list of your priorities—things you want to accomplish today. Then get at it. Don't let the day manipulate you. You're in charge.

4. Take up a physical activity. While you're working out your schedule for the day, make time for exercise. Not just the calisthenic type, but any kind of physical activity that you enjoy. Tennis. Swimming. Aerobic dancing. Jogging. Walking. Then, whenever you feel like a drink, take an exercise break instead. How about a stop off at the tennis court or pool instead of the corner bar after work? Or what about a jog or brisk walk to prep your appetite for lunch? It's got to be a whole lot better than a Bloody Mary.

Not only does physical activity provide a healthful substitute for ingrained drinking habits, it actually discourages the craving of alcohol. "Physical activity is a positive addiction that is incompatible with heavy drinking," says Peter M. Miller, Ph.D., director of the Sea Pines Behavioral Institute at Hilton Head Hospital in South Carolina. In fact, according to his experiences, at least one-third of all heavy drinkers can reduce alcohol intake by embarking on a program of physical conditioning.

Alcohol reduces oxygen uptake, muscle response, coordination, and cardiovascular functioning—four things that are necessary for physical activity. Simply stated, alcohol and exercise do not mix. So a person must choose between them. And as anyone who's ever taken up jogging will tell you, exercise

can be as addictive as alcohol. The difference is, you'll feel about yourself. In fact, the conse increase in self-esteem and self-w may be just what the doctor ordere the female alcoholic.

Doctors rarely hit the nail on the head when it comes to diagnosing an iron deficiency.

They'll nod knowledgeably that women—especially menstruating women—face a greater risk of depleting their iron stores than men. They readily admit that an iron deficiency is sometimes the cause of vague and misleading symptoms. And they're the first to recognize anemia as the last deadly straw in iron deficiency.

Yet how many women suffering from fatigue, irritability, heartburn, heart palpitations, dizziness, headaches, weakness, overall itching, hair loss and brittle, ridged fingernails (all possible symptoms of iron deficiency), drag themselves to their doctors and slouch away with little more than an "it's-all-in-your-head" diagnosis and possibly a catchall prescription for tranquilizers? Probably quite a few.

As a matter of fact, in a recent survey of 252 physicians and medical students, researchers at the University of Southern California School of Medicine in Los Angeles were shocked to learn just how frequently anemia is ignored. To give you an idea of how ill-equipped physicians can be at diagnosing this problem, the investigators, headed by Ralph Carmel, M.D., found that half of all those questioned did not even know the standard textbook definition of anemia for women. What's worse, mild

anemias were often ignored, Dr. Carmel said, because the physicians set the bottom limit on hemoglobin values below textbook specifications—even when their own perception of the textbook lower limit was too low to begin with (*Journal of the American Medical Association*, November 23, 1979).

Why? "One obvious factor seems to be lack of knowledge of the facts," the researchers conclude, but they go on to say that the sheer commonness of anemia may have something to do with the fact that it just isn't taken too seriously anymore. "Physicians may choose to ignore mild anemia to avoid being overwhelmed by its frequency. . . ." they say. "Moreover, some physicians may have become desensitized in the process. They may 'expect' older patients, poor patients, and others to be anemic . . . and erroneously redefine normality to fit their skewed experience."

What Doctors Should Know about Anemia

But that doesn't help us much. As a matter of fact, in light of that and more current research, it looks as though many M.D.'s should brush up on their hematology homework. Truth is:

• Just because iron deficiency is common, there's no reason it should be ignored. And it is common—even in this iron-rich nation of ours. According to one specialist, one-third to one-half of apparently healthy young women have depleted iron stores.

- A typical woman's diet doesn't always provide enough iron to cover her iron losses.
- Even if your doctor is right on when it comes to reading your blood or hemoglobin test, the fact is, the standard blood test designed to detect anemia isn't always an accurate gauge.
- You don't have to be at the point of a severe iron deficiency to feel the effects.

There are several reasons why women are at high risk. For one thing, we require more iron if we menstruate. Since iron combines with molecules in the red blood cells, any blood loss also involves an iron loss. In the course of an average menstrual period, this amounts to an iron loss of about 18 milligrams. That boils down to a daily average loss of 0.6 milligrams over a month. As a result, a woman's body requires almost twice as much iron as a man's, whose iron loss is limited to exits through the skin, urinary tract and gastrointestinal tract.

And that doesn't take into account special circumstances, such as the excessive blood loss of menorrhagia (heavy or prolonged menstrual bleeding) caused by physiological problems or the use of certain intrauterine devices for contraception. (About 10 percent of women have menstrual iron losses that exceed a daily average of 1.4 milligrams.) Or the regular use of aspirin, which tends to cause irritation and bleeding of the stomach lining. Or the drain of maternal nutrient stores during pregnancy.

But the major reason why women more frequently suffer from iron deficiency is that we're just not getting enough of it in our diet. Preliminary data from the nationwide survey by the U.S. Department of Health, Education and Welfare in 1974 revealed that 95 percent of American women aged 18 to 44 are not getting enough iron—only a little more than one-half of the Recommended Dietary Allowance (*Ob. Gyn. News*, April 15, 1974).

Why So Many Women Are Anemic

To begin with, a woman generally eats less than a man—which means less iron. And if she's trimming her waistline by cutting down on iron-rich foods such as meat, potatoes and beans and substituting such poor iron sources as skim milk, yogurt and cottage cheese, then her iron intake is sure to fall short.

And, as if it weren't enough that a woman needs more but eats less iron than a man, her body's iron stores are considerably slimmer. On the average, a woman has a total iron store of only 250 to 350 milligrams as opposed to 800 to 1,000 milligrams for a man.

Put it all together—the menstrual losses, the reduced daily intake, and the paltry reserves—and it adds up to almost certain deficiency. In fact, a 1977 gynecology textbook advises physicians that "the majority of women enter pregnancy with partial or complete depletion of their iron reserves" (*Obstetrics and Gynecology*, Harper & Row, 1977). And that can set the stage for double disaster. The developing fetus coupled with the dramatic increase in blood volume during pregnancy puts even further strain on a woman's iron supply—which is why every obstetrician should prescribe iron supplements for pregnant patients.

Many more women could also do well with the boost of iron supplements. But for one reason or another, their physicians often overlook the real nature of their problem.

First of all, the symptoms of an iron deficiency are vague and misleading. In fact, every symptom can and has been linked to some other disorder—not uncommonly to nervous tension.

Second, it isn't true that you have to be at the point of severe anemia to feel the effects. "I've seen patients with marked anemia who didn't seem to have any symptoms and others with only slightly depressed iron levels who came to my office complaining of any number of related problems," says James D. Cook, M.D., professor of medicine and director of hematology at the University of Kansas Medical Center.

Even Mild Anemia Can Hurt

An excellent review of nutritional anemia, published in the *American Journal of Clinical Nutrition* (February, 1979), also cites several studies in which even mild anemia limited a person's work performance. One paper mentioned in the review explained that mild to moderate anemia handicapped people to the extent that they could not adequately perform their jobs.

But perhaps the primary reason many physicians overlook iron deficiencies in their diagnoses is that the standard blood test designed to detect anemia isn't always an accurate gauge.

"I know of cases where people suffering from appreciable fatigue responded to iron therapy even though initial blood tests did not show an abnormally low level in their blood," Dr. Cook told us. "This is not of course to say that some people feign improvement. It's just that what is considered a normal iron level for one person may represent an iron deficiency in another. The key is individualized hemoglobin levels."

Hemoglobin is the most essential component of red blood cells. A pigmented protein, it's what makes red blood cells red. But most importantly, it's what gets life-sustaining oxygen from the lungs to every cell and tissue of the body.

Every time we take a breath, oxygen molecules are sucked through the membranes of the lung walls into the microscopic pouches of hemoglobin and whisked off by the bloodstream to nourish all the body cells.

Since iron is necessary for hemoglobin production and is the hub of the hemoglobin molecules, a measure of circulating hemoglobin is considered a good indicator of circulating iron.

But the standard interpretation of this blood test isn't as useful or accurate a diagnostic measure as was once thought. For one thing, old reference points for "normal" hemoglobin levels assume that all people are alike. We know that this isn't so. A "normal" reading for one person may be low for someone else.

Sometimes, the only way of knowing whether you're deficient in iron is to have a blood test before and after a three-month course of iron supplementation. If hemoglobin levels show an increase at the time of the second test, you were deficient. If they don't, you probably weren't.

Notice we said "probably." It seems that there are cases in which supplemental iron has no effect on hemoglobin level even though it does benefit body function.

At University Hospital in Uppsala, Sweden, researchers tested the effect of

HOW MUCH IRON IS IN YOUR DIET?

		Iron (milligrams)	Vitamin C (milligrams)	Protein (grams)
FAST-FOOD MEAL (from Gino's, including salad bar)[a]				
Bac-O-Bits	¼ ounce	0.7	values not	2.8
Bean sprouts	1 ounce	0.3	available	0.9
Beets	1 ounce	0.2		0.3
Carrots	¼ ounce	0.1		0.1
Celery	½ ounce	(NA)		0.1
Cucumbers	½ ounce	0.2		0.1
Grated cheese	¼ ounce	(NA)		2.6
Green beans	1 ounce	0.4		0.4
Italian dressing	1 tablespoon	(NA)		(NA)
Kentucky Fried Chicken	1 leg	0.9		14.1
Lettuce	2 ounces	0.3		0.5
Onions	1 ounce	0.1		0.4
Peppers	¾ ounce	0.1		0.2
Radishes	¾ ounce	0.2		0.2
Tomato	2 ounces	0.3		0.6
Total intake:		3.8		23.3

SOURCES: [a] Information provided by Gino's, 1979.
[b] Catherine F. Adams, *Nutritive Value of American Food in Common Units*, Agriculture Handbook No. 456 (Washington, D.C.: Agricultural Research Service, U.S. Department of Agriculture, 1975).

NOTE: (NA) Information not available.

high doses of iron on a group of healthy *nonanemic* men and women. The volunteers, aged 58 to 71, were divided into two groups. One group received a three-month supply of iron supplements with instructions to take 60 milligrams twice daily, while the other group received the same amount of placebo or dummy pills with identical instructions. Several times throughout the test period the participants were tested on a bicycle ergometer to see if their work performances changed in any way. By the end of the test period, the increased pedal power was 4 percent higher for the iron-treated men and 12 percent higher for the iron-treated women than for those men and women in the placebo group. Yet, hemoglobin levels remained essentially the same as they were before the trial (*Acta Medica Scandinavica*, vol. 188, 1970).

So far, no one has been able to explain this finding. But recent studies on rats suggest that the amount of *total* body iron may affect enzyme activity

		Iron (milligrams)	Vitamin C (milligrams)	Protein (grams)
MEAT MEAL[b]				
Carrots	¼ *cup*	0.2	2.0	0.4
Liver, beef	3 *ounces*	7.5	23.0	22.4
Onions (on liver)	¼ *cup*	0.2	4.0	0.6
Peas	¼ *cup*	0.8	5.1	2.1
Potato, baked	1	1.1	31.0	4.0
Total intake:		9.8	65.1	29.5
VEGETARIAN MEAL[b]				
Brown rice	½ *cup*	0.5	0	2.5
Garbanzo beans	½ *cup*	6.9	(NA)	20.5
Green pepper	½ *cup*	0.2	35.0	0.4
Onions	½ *cup*	0.4	8.5	1.3
Tamari (soy sauce)	1 *tablespoon*	0.9	0	1.0
Tomatoes	2	1.0	42.0	2.0
Total intake:		9.9	85.5	27.7

and alter muscle function even in the absence of true anemia (as demonstrated by standard blood tests).

In other words, for some people, including postmenopausal women, iron has the ability to take a good body and make it better.

Putting Iron in Your Diet

Keeping that in mind, there's probably no woman whose diet couldn't use some remodeling. Actually, it's quite easy to increase your iron intake so long as you realize that how much you eat isn't the only consideration. You should also ask yourself what type of iron it is and what foods should be eaten in combination with it. These factors profoundly affect absorption.

For example, you might be patting yourself on the back because you happened to breakfast on a bowl of iron-fortified flakes. Well, it might surprise you to learn that the iron contained in that product didn't do you one iota of good. In a study conducted by Dr. Cook and associates, 15 of 21 infants eating iron-fortified cereals were found to be iron-deficient. Their research showed that the infants were absorbing *less than one percent* of the cereals' iron (*Pediatrics*, May, 1975). And it wasn't due to something lacking in a child's digestive system. In another study, over 100 iron-deficient elderly people ate iron-fortified grain products for six months or longer. The products did nothing to boost their iron levels either (*American Journal of Clinical Nutrition*, February, 1977).

Apparently, as Dr. Cook explained to us, there are different types of iron. One type, called "heme" iron, is readily available to the body. Another, called "nonheme" iron, is pretty much unavailable except when it is eaten in conjunction with certain other foods which unleash it. And a third type—such as the kind used by food processors to "fortify" their products—is often bound up and useless to the body. The cereal manufacturers use this last type because in doing so they meet the letter of the law for mandatory iron fortification without discoloring or reducing the shelf life of their products, which the other types of iron would do.

"So as you can see, the nature of the diet is more important than the amount of iron it contains," says Dr. Cook. "You can't just look at your total iron intake and say, 'Wow, I'm getting 5, 10 or even the 18 milligrams of iron that's the Recommended Dietary Allowance for menstruating women.' If it's not the right type of iron, it isn't going to do you any good."

For that "right" type look first to liver—especially calves'—but also to beef, chicken and fish. Meat is practically the only source of heme iron. With so many of us struggling to cut back on red meat, however, it's important to recognize and make the most of alternative iron sources. And there are many. Apricots. Prunes. Raisins. Cooked lima beans and kidney beans. Broccoli and spinach. Nuts. Whole wheat products and especially wheat germ. And let's not forget our super iron supplier, blackstrap molasses. Just one tablespoon of this black gold offers us 3.2 milligrams of iron.

But there's a catch. The iron in grains, vegetables and fruits isn't as eager to enter your bloodstream as the heme iron found in meat. What it needs is a little coaxing.

There are two things that can unleash nonheme iron. One is a "meat factor" found in meat, poultry, and fish (but not in eggs or dairy products). The other is vitamin C. By combining nonheme iron sources with one or both of these enhancers, you can increase your iron absorption by as much as fourfold, says Dr. Cook. To illustrate this he cites a scientific study in which the addition of 60 milligrams of vitamin C to a meal of rice more than tripled iron absorption. In another study, adding papaya containing 66 milligrams of vitamin C to a meal of corn boosted iron absorption by more than 500 percent!

To make the most of the nonheme iron in your meal, Dr. Cook recommends that you include *one* of the following with each meal: three ounces of meat, 75 milligrams of vitamin C, or one to three ounces of meat *plus* 25 to 75 milligrams of vitamin C.

Another way to *increase* your iron intake is to *decrease* the amount of tea and processed foods you have with your meal. The tannic acid in tea and the phosphate food additives found in soft drinks, ice cream, baked goods, candy,

MAXIMIZE YOUR IRON INTAKE

Food	Iron (milligrams)	Vitamin C (milligrams)
VEGETABLES (1 cup cooked unless specified)		
Amaranth[a]	3.2	22
Artichoke (*1 bud*)	1.7	12
Asparagus	1.1	47
Beans—lima	4.3	29
—mung	1.1	8
—mung, sprouted	1.4	20
—navy	5.1	0
—red kidney	4.4	(NA)
—soybeans	4.9	0
Beet greens	2.8	22
Broccoli	1.2	140
Brussels sprouts	1.7	135
Cauliflower	0.9	69
Lentils	4.2	0
Peas	2.9	32
Spinach	4.0	50
Tofu (*piece less than 1 cup*)	2.3	0
FRUIT (1 cup)		
Apricots—canned	0.8	10
—dried	7.2	16
—fresh	0.8	16
Bananas	1.1	15
Peaches—canned	0.7	7
—dried	9.6	29
—raw	0.9	12
Strawberries	1.5	88

Food	Iron (milligrams)	Vitamin C (milligrams)
GRAINS		
Corn (*1 ear*)	0.5	7
Oatmeal (*1 cup*)	1.4	0
Wheat, rolled (*1 cup*)	1.7	0
Wheat germ (*1 tablespoon*)	0.5	1
NUTS AND SEEDS (½ cup)		
Almonds	3.4	trace
Brazils	2.4	(NA)
Cashews	2.7	(NA)
Coconut, shredded	0.7	2
Sunflower seeds	5.2	(NA)
MEAT (3 ounces)		
Beef—flank steak	3.2	(NA)
—ground (*1 patty*)	2.6	(NA)
—liver	7.5	23
—liver, calves'	12.1	31
Chicken—dark meat	1.4	(NA)
—light meat	1.1	(NA)
—liver	7.2	13.7
Pork—ham	2.6	(NA)
—liver	24.7	19
MISCELLANEOUS		
Brewer's yeast (*1 tablespoon*)	1.4	trace
Egg (*1 medium*)	1.0	0
Molasses, blackstrap (*1 tablespoon*)	3.2	(NA)

SOURCES: Food values were adapted from *Nutritive Value of American Foods in Common Units*, Agriculture Handbook No. 456, by Catherine F. Adams (Washington, D.C.: Agricultural Research Service, U.S. Department of Agriculture, 1975) except:
[a] *Food Composition Table for Use in East Asia*, DHEW Publication No. (NIH) 79–465 (Bethesda, Md.: Department of Health, Education and Welfare, 1972).

NOTE: (NA) Information not available.

GETTING THE MOST IRON OUT OF YOUR MEALS

Absorption

LOW-AVAILABILITY MEAL
Any combination of iron-rich grains, vegetables, fruits and eggs with: 4%

less than 1 ounce meat, poultry or fish
or
less than 25 milligrams vitamin C

MEDIUM-AVAILABILITY MEAL
Any combination of iron-rich grains, vegetables, fruits and eggs with: 7%

1–3 ounces meat, poultry or fish
or
25–75 milligrams vitamin C

HIGH-AVAILABILITY MEAL
Any combination of iron-rich grains, vegetables, fruits and eggs with: 12%

more than 3 ounces meat, poultry or fish
or
more than 75 milligrams vitamin C
or
1–3 ounces meat, poultry or fish plus
25–75 milligrams vitamin C

Source: Adapted from "Estimation of Available Dietary Iron" by Elaine R. Monsen, *American Journal of Clinical Nutrition*, January, 1978.

Note: Figures given for an average woman whose iron stores are about 300 milligrams. (This will vary depending on your nutritional state.)

beer and a lot of other processed foods, as well as the preservative EDTA which is practically everywhere you look, actually cut down on the amount of iron you absorb. Antacids also block iron intake.

And by the way, don't worry that by increasing your absorption of dietary iron, you'll overdose on the mineral. The percentage of iron you absorb from food is regulated by the amount of iron you have in your body stores. If your reserves are low, you'll absorb more. If you've already got a good supply, then you'll absorb less. Your body knows how much it needs to function best. But it's up to you to provide an ample available supply—and that, as we've mentioned, depends not only on the amount of iron in your diet, but also on the type of iron you eat and the other foods with which it is eaten.

If you really want to steer away from the doldrums of iron deficiency, your best bet is iron supplements. Look for the word "ferrous" on the label, Dr. Cook suggests. "Ferrous" compounds contain appreciably more absorbable iron than "ferric" supplements. For example, two tablets of ferrous gluconate contain 70 milligrams of iron, of which about 25 milligrams will be utilized by the body. And that, Dr. Cook says, amounts to more available iron than you could get from eating 14 steaks.

Iron deficiency is, of course, caused by a lack of iron. But anemia—too little hemoglobin—has other nutritional causes as well.

B Vitamins May Be the Missing Link

"The commonest cause [of anemia] is iron deficiency, but folate deficiency . . . can also be a cause," says a report in *Lancet* (February 21, 1976).

The report goes on to cite a study in which women received either iron alone, folate alone, or iron and folate together. Only 26 percent of those who received a single nutrient had a rise in hemoglobin, while 96 percent of those who received iron and folate had a rise.

The B complex vitamin folate is a must for the creation of normal red blood cells. Without enough of this nutrient, red blood cells are too large, strangely shaped and have a shortened life span. A lack of healthy red blood cells means less hemoglobin, which in turn means less oxygen is delivered to the body. The result is lethargy, weakness, fatigue. Fatigue, perhaps, for pregnant women and women who use oral contraceptives, for teenage girls and the elderly, all of whom, studies show, run a high risk of folate deficiency. An easily corrected deficiency.

A psychiatrist found that four of his patients with "easy fatigability" and other symptoms had low levels of folate. He supplemented their diet with the nutrient. As folate levels rose, fatigue disappeared (*Clinical Psychiatry News*, April, 1976).

But all the folate in the world won't do any good unless you get enough vitamin B_{12}. Folate stays trapped in a metabolically useless form until B_{12} releases it. B_{12}, however, is more than folate's understudy. It plays an important role of its own. It can relieve tiredness.

Twenty-eight men and women who complained of tiredness but who had no physical problems were given B_{12} and then asked to evaluate its effect. For many of the 28, the vitamin not only made them less fatigued, but also improved their appetite, sleep and general well-being (*British Journal of Nutrition*, September 6, 1973).

This creates some confusion in diagnosing anemia, since a lack of either of these vitamins can cause anemia and it's difficult to tell which one's missing. Meat, poultry, fish and eggs all supply B_{12}. Fruits, vegetables, grains and grain products do not contain it.

The complex mechanism of blood production also relies partly on riboflavin (vitamin B_2). In a study of pregnant women in Germany, supplementation with both iron and riboflavin was much more effective in raising the red blood cell count than iron alone (*Nutrition and Metabolism*, vol. 21, suppl. 1, 1977). Researchers in London also found recently that even a marginal deficiency of riboflavin can shorten the life span of red blood cells (*Proceedings of the Nutrition Society*, February, 1980). Foods rich in riboflavin are brewer's yeast, liver and beef heart, followed by milk, cheese, eggs, leafy green vegetables and grains.

ANOREXIA NERVOSA

When was the last time you bared your body before a full-length mirror and declared with forthright determination that a diet definitely was in order? We've all done it—most of us more than once! After all, if there's one thing the American woman is in constant pursuit of, it's thinness.

Today, crash dieting has become as popular as social drinking. But unfortunately, like the social drinker who turns alcoholic, there are some women who can't quit dieting. They become obsessed with weight loss and reduce themselves to an empty encasement of skin and bones. Some eventually starve themselves to death.

The problem was named "anorexia nervosa," meaning loss of appetite due to anxiety, back at a time when the condition was misunderstood. In true anorexia nervosa there is no loss of appetite, only a deliberate avoidance of food—a sort of self-induced hunger strike. The object is to become thin at all costs. And the results pitifully demonstrate the severity of the problem. A 15-year-old girl weighing 65 pounds refuses more than three tablespoons of cottage cheese a day. A 13-year-old is threatened into eating a meal, only to slip away afterwards and stick her finger down her throat until she vomits every last trace of food.

Like alcoholism, anorexia nervosa is a disease. It primarily strikes attractive, perfection-oriented females aged 11 to 24 from upper- or upper-middle-class backgrounds. An off-the-cuff estimate is that 1 in 300 adolescent girls is affected. And thousands of young women may be afflicted with a sister syndrome, bulimarexia, a term coined by two Cornell University psychologists to describe a seesaw form of anorexia. "Women suffering from bulimarexia alternately gorge themselves with food and then empty themselves, whether by fasting, vomiting, or through self-induced diarrhea," says Marlene Boskind-Lodahl, Ph.D. "In most cases it leaves its victims little time or energy for any sort of life beyond its own binges and purges" (*Psychology Today*, March, 1977).

Understandably, both diseases were considered rarities 50 years ago—before Twiggy ushered in the era of the envied toothpick physique. It's also easy to understand why 98 percent of their victims are women (especially impressionable adolescent girls), since they are the primary targets of Madison Avenue advertising ploys.

But how do otherwise sensible young women become bent on self-destruction? "When they begin to diet, they seem to be doing nothing different from what thousands of other women are doing," says Hilde Bruch, M.D., professor of psychiatry at Baylor College of Medicine in Texas and author of numerous articles and books on this topic. "Not one of the patients I have known had intended to pursue the frightening road of life-threatening emaciation—and to sacrifice the years of youth to this bizarre goal. They had expected that being slimmer would improve not only their appearance but their way of living." Isn't that how we all feel?

Strange Self-Perception

Yes, but there are recognizable peculiarities in their logic. For one thing, only about two percent of these young women are overweight to begin with. Most are slender, attractive girls. But for some unknown reason, they perceive themselves as "too fat"—even after severe starvation has reduced them to a faded image of what they once were. "I have stood in front of a mirror with an anorexic girl who at 65 pounds was so thin you could pick her up by her pelvic bones," Steven Levenkron, M.S., a New York City psychotherapist and author of *The Best Little Girl in the World* (Contemporary, 1978), a book on anorexia nervosa, told us. "No matter how I'd try to point out that it isn't pretty to have protruding ribs or a concave abdomen, she'd insist that she looked just fine. It was as if we were seeing two distinctly different images in the mirror."

Also, according to Dr. Bruch, the *way* the girls experience hunger will determine whether dieting remains what it was intended to be—a means of losing a few extra pounds—or whether it becomes a compulsive force that dominates their whole life. "The fact that they are able to tolerate the sensation of hunger (and thus achieve the miracle of losing weight rapidly) seems to induce these girls to go on and on," says Dr. Bruch.

Truth is, however, that all that worry over dieting and losing weight, the obsession with thinness, and the twisted perspective of self-image are not causes of anorexia nervosa. They are symptoms—early warning signs of the drastic weight loss that will follow. The actual cause is much more deeply rooted.

"The real illness has to do with the way you feel about yourself," Dr. Bruch explains to a young patient. "There is a peculiar contradiction—everybody thinks you're doing so well and everybody thinks you're great, but your real problem is that you think you're not good enough. . . . This peculiar dieting begins with such anxiety. You want to prove that you have control, that you can do it. The peculiar part of it is that it makes you feel 'I can do something nobody else can do.' There is only one problem with this feeling of superiority. It doesn't solve your problem because what you really want is to feel good about yourself while feeling happy and healthy. The paradox is that you have started to feel good for being unhealthy."

The Symptoms . . . and Real Danger

Along with the weight loss comes a whole host of unhealthful and not-so-pretty symptoms. Menstrual periods stop. Hair falls out. The skin becomes very dry. Constipation becomes a problem. Heartbeat drops to 50 to 55 (72 is average for normal women) and blood pressure to 80/50 (120/70 is normal for a young woman). The sensation of cold is always present.

But the real danger is the upset of water balance in the body caused by bouts of vomiting combined with the repeated ingestion of laxatives and diuretics. It is often this and not the weight loss per se that causes death.

Until recently, standard treatment wasn't too successful. Drugs administered to improve appetite or tranquilize the senses have been outright failures. Psychoanalysis proved to be a meaningless and time-consuming exercise. And behavior modification techniques—in which an anorexic is put in a sparsely furnished hospital room without TV, books or visitors and forced to earn privileges by gaining weight—have successfully fattened up the patient, but not for long. Soon after release from the hospital, most girls get on with their dietary regimen all over again. Some are even worse off for the experience, feeling bitter about being coerced and attempting suicide afterward.

Anorexia nervosa is a psychological as well as a nutritional problem. Both are equally important in treatment. And both demand professional assistance.

Current trends in psychological counseling for anorexia nervosa involve the whole family. "In every anorexic's family, there is always somebody else who is the problem," says Steven Levenkron. Usually it's another child, perhaps a slow learner or a hyperactive child who demands and gets all the parents' attention. The anorexic child, on the other hand, is usually the model child—a docile girl, straight-A student, active in sports, and fairly sociable. She doesn't appear to need any special attention. As a result, she is all but ignored by her parents. "This is a mistake," the psychotherapist explains. "To avoid anorexia nervosa, parents should make sure their well-behaved children get as much attention as the poorly behaved ones. The family must move closer. And there must be trust."

In her book *The Golden Cage: The Enigma of Anorexia Nervosa* (Harvard University Press, 1978), Dr. Bruch points out that parents who place excessively high expectations on their children may be setting them up for anorexic tendencies. A child who is forever obliging to please others may have a more difficult time developing a sense of self. The weight loss becomes another achievement—a way of pleasing others, of doing what's expected (in this case by society), and of being accepted.

"Anorexic persons need parenting," says Steven Levenkron, who describes this as "an assertive kind of nurturing." But ironically, the more ingrained they become in this bizarre behavior, the less their parents are able to cope. First they become frightened, then angry. It's important that a psychologist step in and act as a sort of substitute parent.

How One Therapist Helps

Steven Levenkron's first step in his psychotherapy is to gain the anorexic's trust, "to convince her that my judgment is good, to get her to learn to relate to me as she would to her healthy mother.

"They [anorexics] want someone to take care of them, someone who's assertive, who knows what they are doing, and who's sensitive and understanding to what they're going through," he said. "They need direction. And they will accept your advice if you've succeeded in gaining their trust."

The roughest time is just getting over the first obstacle—when they begin to eat again. They become terrified. They think they're going to get fat, and that's the worst thing they can imagine. "For the first three or four weeks they call me every night after their meal," the therapist told us. "But I don't mind. The wonderful thing is that they get better."

Of course, the correction of the weight must also be an integrated part of the treatment. In severe cases, it requires forced feeding. But in most instances, it's a matter of reeducating the young woman. "The patient is usually terror-stricken at the thought of having to gain weight, "says Dr. Bruch, "so it's important to give her a meaningful explanation why better nutrition is an essential precondition for coming to an understanding of her psychological problems."

Chances are she won't be alien to a discussion of nutrition, since most anorexics have already demonstrated a basic interest (albeit with a twisted perspective) in what good nutrition is all about. Usually, they began their diet with some nutrition knowledge. Many decide to cut down on—and eventually are compelled to cut out—carbohydrates. But a low-carbohydrate, high-protein diet can be disastrous, not to mention extremely dangerous when undertaken for an extended period of time. Combine this with the fact that, for an anorexic, protein intake may not exceed a daily ration of two chicken livers, and you've got certain trouble.

She must be convinced that carbohydrates are not all bad, and whole foods such as whole wheat bread, baked potatoes (without the butter and sour cream) and fresh fruit are not "fattening." "She also needs reassurance that a good diet will be served in amounts that will protect her from gaining too fast and becoming fat," says Dr. Bruch.

Although, as we mentioned earlier, anorexia nervosa is not a result of loss of appetite, it's possible that in the course of severe dieting, the appetite can become somewhat depressed. To perk it up, some researchers look to zinc. According to Robert I. Henkin, M.D., Ph.D., director of the Center for Molecular Nutrition and Sensory Disorders at Georgetown University Medical Center, adding zinc to the diet may help stimulate taste, smell and appetite. Fresh air and exercise are also thought to stimulate appetite.

For anorexia specialists, see *Appendix*.

ANXIETY

Women are better able to tolerate stress than men, says professor Marianne Frankenhauser of Stockholm University in Sweden, whose research has shown that women's adrenaline levels do not rise as rapidly as men's in conflict situations. Trouble is, it may not do us much good anymore, now that the average woman is under a good deal more stress than the average man. Sorry, it looks like we're right back where we started: anxious, worried, tense—and with less time for relaxation than ever before.

Think about it. Today women have opportunities—career choices—they never had before. The "get married, get settled, get pregnant" syndrome doesn't appeal to everyone anymore. Those who opt for a career find themselves under a kind of stress their mothers never knew: the stress of competing on a man's level but being judged on another level that often demands bettering the best male in the department just to prove their equality. Those who think they can mix marriage with corporate responsibilities have yet more conflicts to contend with. And those with husband, children, and career . . . well, it's no wonder more women are losing their hair. As a matter of fact, no woman is immune from this kind of stress and anxiety. Even the woman with no other aspiration than to make her family a comfortable home comes under pressure from society and feels terribly guilty that she *doesn't* have a job. For her, the anxiety is in believing that she's not doing *enough*. And life becomes one big excuse after another.

So how do we cope?

Well, the first step is to recognize the stress before it calls out with problems so serious that you have no choice but to stand up and take notice. Stress, anxiety, tension—call it what you will—is a real threat to health. In fact, according to many doctors, between 50 and 80 percent of all illnesses—everything from cancer to dandruff—may be somehow related to stress. But nobody gets there overnight. Serious problems are usually preceded by years of warning symptoms—warnings that you've overshot your stress tolerance and it's time to turn back. Fatigue. Insomnia. Periods of rapid heartbeat and sweaty hands. Loss of appetite. Headaches. Possible stomach upsets. Perhaps an increased susceptibility to colds or viruses.

Of course, we all have different stress thresholds. And what may seem stressful to one woman—say, giving a presentation at work—may not faze someone else. Similarly, how we react, whether with fretful migraine headaches or just butterflies in the stomach, depends to a certain extent on genetic programming. But whatever the case, the key is to recognize early signs of stress, and to do something about what's causing them.

Notice we say strike out at the *cause*. In other words, don't think that by covering up the consequences you can find solace. Cigarette smoking, drinking alcohol or popping tranquilizers like Valium may lure you into thinking that they've eased you over the crisis when, in fact, they've provided little more than a temporary cover-up. And when repeatedly relied on, they could bring on some permanent problems (see Alcohol: Social Drinking, Alcoholism, Smoking, and Valium).

Instead, see what you can do about eliminating the cause of your stress, altering your reaction to the stress, or finding sensible habits that serve as outlets.

Eliminating the cause of your stress may not be easy. Then again, it may be very easy, once you convince yourself just how important such a change could be for your health. Suppose, for example, the stress is related to a bad marriage. Coming to grips with that problem doesn't necessarily mean packing your bags and finding yourself a Philadelphia lawyer. It could, however, mean fessing up to whatever troubles the marriage, openly communicating your feelings with your spouse and possibly seeking professional counseling might be in order. Similarly, relief from a stressful job doesn't have to be synonymous with the unemployment line. It could, however, suggest a transfer to another department or a heart-to-heart talk with whoever it is that's making you tense.

On the other hand, the stress in a situation can stem from your own perception of it. For example, one woman we spoke with—who is married, works full time in a very responsible position where she has a reputation for being extremely productive and efficient, and attends graduate school at night—complained because she "had no pep." She was also distressed because a medical exam complete with blood and glucose tolerance tests did not reveal that she was anemic or hypoglycemic. "I just can't understand why I'm so tired all the time," she told us. We, on the other hand, can see how much she pushes herself to perfection and so can understand it perfectly!

Ease Up on That Load

Actually, the problem is more common than you'd think. You know the woman. She wants to do everything—to be the Supermom; the best in the business world; the gourmet cook; the "gold-dust gal" with the cleanest house in town. And that's all just one woman! Women like this may not readily admit it, but they are essentially creating their own tension, compelled by who-knows-what to keep up with who-knows-whom. But whatever their motivation, the problem is, it's darn hard for them to slow down.

It takes a concerted effort and a strong will to admit that you don't have to do everything; that no one expects you to be perfect; and, yes, that you can take off a day now and then and not feel guilty. Having a dinner party? Don't be afraid to ask each guest to bring a dish. Up against a tight deadline at work? Why not ask others to help pull part of the load? We know it's tough, but if you cherish your health as much as your independence, you'll learn the joy (and relief) of sharing responsibility.

Finding outlets for stress is another

positive move you can make. And perhaps a most important outlet is one you never thought of that way: your friends. People who have strong personal ties with other people at home, at work and in church have been found to be especially resistant to the effects of stress.

A study of pregnant women found that those who experienced a high number of stressful events during pregnancy were not necessarily more prone to complications than women who were not stressed. But when the stress was combined with a lack of social ties, things were different. Ninety percent of the women scoring high in stress and low in social support suffered one or more complications of their pregnancies. Only 33 percent of the highly stressed women with a strong supportive network of family or friends developed complications (*American Journal of Epidemiology,* May, 1972).

And this may be one area where women have the edge. In an interview in the *Female Patient* (May, 1979), Frederic F. Flach, M.D., clinical associate professor of psychiatry at Cornell University Medical College explains, "I find that women are more likely to have friends to talk to. Many women maintain relationships with friends whom they met in high school or college, or when they were young mothers with small children," he says. In contrast, in the past 50 years men have tended to withdraw from close friendships, and men's clubs are a thing of the past for most men. Today a man's social contacts often consist mainly of his wife's friends. Consequently, a man caught up in despair is often unable to find someone in whom he can confide. When he has a marriage problem, he cannot talk to joint friends, and he usually cannot discuss it with his friends at work. A woman, however, can

pick up the telephone, call a friend and tell her what has happened, and feel better, because she has gotten support."

There's plenty you can do for yourself as well—most notably get into a regularly scheduled exercise program (perhaps an organized dancercise class or a daily walk), and put aside a few minutes each day for meditation and solitude. Much has been written on the stress-alleviating value of both exercise and meditation, but a recently published study comparing their benefits reveals that each works in its own way to attack anxiety and stress from two differing directions.

In that study, three psychology researchers at Yale University found that persons who meditated for at least six months tended to have a much-reduced level of "perceived" stress. That is, they were less likely to complain of such anxious psychological states as, "I find it difficult to concentrate"; "I worry too much over something that doesn't really matter"; "I feel like I am losing out on things because I can't make up my mind soon enough"; "I can't keep anxiety-provoking thoughts out of my mind." On the other hand, those who exercised regularly for six months or more were less likely to complain of such physical symptoms as "My heart beats faster"; "I feel jittery in my body"; "I get diarrhea"; "I feel tense in my stomach"; "I nervously pace"; or "I perspire" (*Psychosomatic Medicine,* June, 1978).

It's difficult to interpret these findings and the researchers readily admit that there are many outside factors that could enter into the conclusions. For example, they suggest, it may just be that people who are attracted to the practice of meditation as opposed to physical exercise differ in their usual response to anxiety.

Nevertheless, we don't feel that it would be too presumptuous to suggest that a double-barreled approach—that is, a combination of exercise and meditation—is your most assured way of getting the better of your jittery emotions before they get the better of you.

Don't worry, you don't have to belong to some bizarre cult to meditate. Herbert Benson, M.D., of the Harvard School of Public Health and Harvard Medical School (you can't get closer to the establishment than that!) has been working with relaxation techniques—which include meditation, for the most part—for more than 10 years. And not only do they work, but some of the results of his research suggest that regular practice of relaxation techniques might be used as a tool for combating high blood pressure and other illnesses as well.

The relaxation technique Dr. Benson used does not take the dedication of a Zen master to put in practice. He told us, "The specific technique used is not as important as the common response that all the different relaxation techniques evoke. That's what we're after. I try to . . . bring into play the innate capability we all have to use the mind to influence the body."

Four Steps to Relaxation

Dr. Benson calls the physical response that all these techniques evoke the "relaxation response." He believes this temporary slowdown of bodily processes, repeated twice a day, was responsible for the improved health of the persons he studied. All the different meditative practices of both Eastern and Western cultural traditions, he says, have been grounded in four basic components which are needed to evoke the

relaxation response in the body:

- The first is a quiet environment free of distractions. A quiet room is suitable.
- The second requirement is a mental device, a word or object you can keep in your mind, much like the dangling watch used by movie hypnotists. The trick is to focus all your attention on the mental device, by repeating the same word over and over to yourself, for example.
- The third requirement flows from this. You need to assume a passive attitude. Distracting thoughts are simply disregarded, and you redirect your attention to the mental device. You do not worry about how well you are performing the technique. If your mind wanders, let it go, then gently coax it back. The object is to relax, after all.
- The fourth requirement is simply to assume a comfortable position, so that there is no distracting muscle tension.

In his book *The Relaxation Response* (William Morrow, 1975), Dr. Benson describes how some people work relaxation breaks into their lives. One businessman tells his secretary he's "in conference" late in the morning and takes no calls. When he travels, he uses the relaxation response in airplanes. A housewife takes a relaxation break in the morning after her husband has left for work and her children have gone to school. A college student arrives at the lecture hall 15 minutes early and practices the response before class begins.

None of those people consider themselves hair-shirt mystics. They are just ordinary people, interested in their health, who have discovered one of the many ways the mind can heal the body.

They know the relaxation breaks make them feel better. For them, that's reason enough.

In addition, many people have found help and relief from tension and anxiety in biofeedback. Biofeedback is a method by which you can train yourself to consciously relax. The only drawback is that this treatment does require some professional services—perhaps 10 or so 30-minute sessions. But after that, you're on your own.

In a typical treatment, sensors are attached to the forehead to measure muscle tension and then you are told to concentrate on relaxing images—say, lying on the beach and listening to the waves roll up to shore. You can repeat the words "I am totally relaxed" but because the part of the brain that controls these "unconscious" processes doesn't understand language, it's important to translate that phrase into an image. When you've concentrated long enough on that image you should get a response: that is, the muscles in your forehead should ease up. And when they do, these changes will be transferred from the sensor on your forehead to a meter in front of you. After several training sessions like this, you'll become a pro at relaxation—where the initial visit might have met with a 30-minute wait for meter response, you're now able to muster up just the right image to ease those muscles in less than 10 minutes. And after all your sessions are said and done, relaxation will be no more than a soothing image away.

If it's muscle tension more so than emotional stress that's got you in its grip, try massage. Most health clubs and some YWCAs have their own licensed masseuses who can massage your neck and shoulder muscles where tension tends to accumulate in no time flat (well, in an hour or so). It's also very nice to precede massage with a short stint in the sauna, and best—according to Deborah Szekely Mazzanti, founding director of the famed Golden Door Spa—when preceded by a good physical workout.

And finally, don't forget healthy nerves that can stand up to stress depend on good nutrition—especially the B vitamins, vitamin C and magnesium. They don't call them the "stress supplements" for nothing!

BACKACHE

Sometime during the course of our lives, an estimated 80 percent of us will experience low back pain. Back problems are responsible for more "sick days" than the common cold and are the most common cause of doctor visits in this country.

Why are backs so troublesome? Aside from the rare inherited abnormality or damage done by accidental injury, the fault lies with human anatomy, posture and habits that aggravate the weaknesses of both. The spine, though a masterpiece of structural engineering, has weak spots—most notably the lower back, or lumbosacral area, where the spinal "S" terminates in five fused vertebrae. And unfortunately, this is one spot where women in particular have a weakened link.

Women, we are told, suffer more from back problems due to a more pronounced lumbar curve (inward curve sometimes known as a swayback) and the stresses of childbearing. Low back pain is common during pregnancy, particularly in the last few months. The pain is believed to be caused by the added weight and the softening of the ligaments surrounding the pelvis and lumbar (lower) area.

But lower back pain needn't be a problem during pregnancy or at any other time for that matter, so long as we keep our backs in good shape.

"Most of us don't take care of our backs," says Robert Lowe, M.D., an orthopedic surgeon who founded the Cabell–Huntington Hospital's Low Back School in West Virginia to teach people how to prevent back trouble. "Over time, we allow certain things to happen: our abdominal muscles weaken, the normal curve of our lower back increases, and we get back pain."

Sometimes, just a change in poor sedentary habits is enough to get you on the track of a better back condition. Sitting all day or lounging your leisure time away instead of lunging into more active and physically demanding pursuits is the quickest way to muscle deterioration. In addition, sitting puts an enormous stress on the lumbar region. The soft, shock-absorbing vertebrae are compressed and the muscles weakened.

Ideally, strong stomach and buttock muscles will keep this part of the spine aligned.

What do our abdominal muscles have to do with our backs, you may ask. Well, what happens is, as muscles up front become weak and sag due to inactivity, our posture compensates somewhat by shifting our weight to the back. The pelvis tilts forward, the hips stick out in the rear and the last joints in the spine require a lot of muscle to hold them up. Eventually, the muscles in the lower back tire of carrying the load and begin to hurt.

For that reason, a good overall fitness program with some emphasis on abdominal muscle tone is step one toward a pain-free back. Swimming and walking are terrific. So is yoga, which helps by improving the flexibility and strength of the spine. Calisthenics, however, are definite no-nos—with push-ups and sit-ups done in a straight-leg position being particularly stressful. For stomach strengthening exercises do the partial curl-up exercise illustrated.

Straighten Your Posture with the Pelvic Tilt

The pelvic tilt is an exercise designed to help reverse the curve temporarily, easing pressure on the disks and strengthening the supporting muscles. It is incredibly effective, considering its simplicity.

If it's easy, you're in pretty good shape and will be able to keep your back near to or on the floor without straining. If you find it difficult, your back needs work. "For some people, the pelvic tilt becomes an automatic part of their posture with little training," Dr. Lowe tells us. "For others, it requires a great deal of effort."

Inside your back, the benefits from this simple exercise are great: the pressure on the rear part of the lumbar disks is eased, the stretched muscles and ligaments are relaxed, and the supportive muscles of the stomach, buttocks and pelvis are toned and exercised.

You can perform the pelvic tilt while standing. Stand with your lower back against a wall and your feet six inches from the wall. Keeping the lower back tight against the wall, gradually bring your heels in, eventually touching the wall with your heels, buttocks, lower back and shoulders. Again, neck, shoulders and legs are relaxed, and stomach and buttock muscles are taut. In time, you should be able to assume the pelvic tilt posture without a supporting wall.

Can such a simple exercise really help? If faithfully practiced, the answer is yes. The benefits of the pelvic tilt have been documented by precise measurements of the pressure inside the spine. When you sit upright, 300 pounds of pressure per square inch are bearing on your lumbar disks (if you are of average weight); when standing, 200 pounds; and when lying flat on your back, 100 pounds. But lying in the pelvic tilt position reduces the force to 60 pounds per square inch! Another thing Dr. Lowe explains, "Most people think that when they lie down, no matter what position they're in, they are resting their backs. But that isn't so. Some positions relax the back, but some aggravate. Healing can occur only with rest, and maximum rest occurs when you're lying down on a firm surface with your knees elevated."

Get the Right Sleeping Position

Low back pain sufferers should sleep like children: either on their backs with knees raised, or curled into a semifetal position on their sides. Lying face down or lying on your back with your legs straight out is bad for your lower back.

Pillows can be used to help relieve pressure on the spine. While lying in the fetal position, place a pillow between your knees to ease tension on the lower back muscles. Hugging a pillow to your chest or placing one behind your back can give needed support. Your head should always be supported with a feather or down pillow—which won't "fight back" like a synthetic one—and

your mattress should be firm enough for good support, but also comfortable.

What you do while awake affects your back, too. Standing while working usually involves bending over, especially if you're standing over a sink of dishes or a pastry board for an hour or more. And a forward bend of as little as 20 degrees can increase pressure on the lumbar region by 50 percent. If you bend over that far the pressure on the fifth lumbar disk is increased from 200 pounds per square inch to 300 pounds. That increase can be particularly harmful, and many people find that their backs suddenly "go out" while they perform such a simple task.

Everyday Habits Can Help or Hurt

Standing work needn't be stressful. Raising the work surface to waist height can help; so can working with one leg elevated on a chair rung or a footstool. If you are at the sink, for example, open the cabinet door below it and rest your foot on the lower shelf. That flattens the back and eliminates the curve, which in turn eases pressure on the spinal column. Shoes, of course, should have low or flat heels, because high heels tend to throw the body's center of gravity forward, increasing the low back curve and bringing added force to bear on the lumbar region. Whenever you stand, try to maintain a flat back.

Prolonged sitting is very bad for your back, but there are techniques that can help. Always try to maintain the pelvic tilt by sitting well forward and elevating your knees higher than your hips with a footstool. A low chair with a straight back and a footrest is ideal for your back.

Human beings just aren't designed for prolonged riding in automobiles, but keeping your knees flexed as much as

Exercises for Your Back

PELVIC TILT

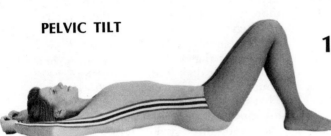

1 While lying on your back, bend your knees and place your feet flat on the floor near your buttocks.

2 Raise your pelvis and "tuck" it under, concentrating on pushing your lower back gently to the floor. Your shoulders, legs, neck and upper back should be relaxed. As you gently push your lower back to the floor, three things begin to happen: your pelvis rotates forward (reversing the curve of your lower back), your buttock muscles tighten, and your stomach muscles are exercised.

PARTIAL CURL-UP

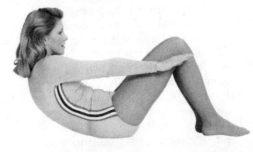

This exercise differs from a sit-up. Sit partially up, as shown, as if attempting to bring one vertebra at a time off the floor. Contract abdominal muscles and hold a few seconds.

possible can alleviate some of the stress on your back. If you're driving, sit close to the pedals and use a wedge-shaped cushion under your thighs. While riding, a traveling case can serve as a footstool. Think "pelvic tilt" while riding.

Two rules apply when lifting an object: keep it close, and bend your knees. Lift a 40-pound object at your feet and you're lifting 40 pounds. Move it three feet away and you're lifting the equivalent of 400 pounds.

The correct way to lift is to get as close to the object as you can, squat with your back straight, and let your large thigh muscles do the work. If you begin to lose balance while lifting or carrying, don't struggle to maintain it. It's better to let your load fall than to strain your back trying to hold it. Turning and lifting at the same time—loading groceries into a car, for instance—is particularly stressful, so learn to turn your feet, not twist your body. Furniture and other heavy objects that need slight rearrang-

ing should be pushed, not pulled. Again, a flat back fights strain.

We should mention here that aging can also bring with it back problems as a result of a decrease in bone density, called osteoporosis (see Osteoporosis). Hormonal changes in postmenopausal women, calcium deficiency and prolonged use of cortisone can contribute to the actual shrinkage of the spine. And for that reason special attention should be paid to improving nutrition for the muscles and surrounding tissue. That can be achieved by making sure that you get enough calcium, magnesium, vitamin C and the B vitamins.

Many back specialists believe that a significant percentage of back pain is tension-produced. It therefore seems appropriate to look into the various relaxation techniques, such as meditation, that will help to reduce stress, and massage which alleviates muscle tightness and tension across the back.

KNEE TO CHEST

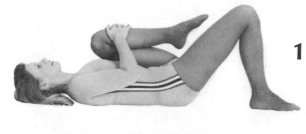

1 Best done on a thickly carpeted floor. This exercise flexes the lower back. (Use folded towels or a pillow for head support.) First bring one leg at a time up to chest. Repeat five times with each leg.

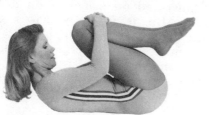

2 Then do both legs together.

BIRTH CONTROL

Everybody knows that if you don't want to become pregnant, you'd better use some form of birth control. That, or say goodbye to sex. Now, abstaining from intercourse may be 100 percent effective and completely safe, but it definitely lacks sex appeal and is low in the fun department, too.

Still, an unwanted pregnancy is no fun either. But that's what you'll get 9 times out of 10, if you indulge in unprotected intercourse.

So the object is to find a method of birth control that is totally effective and safe, one that has no side effects, is instantly reversible, and easy to use. Of course, it shouldn't interfere with lovemaking in any way and it should be inexpensive and require only the briefest of medical advice and care.

While all those qualities do exist in the contraceptive marketplace, no one method has them all. Instead, the ones with the highest effectiveness have the poorest track record for safety, while the methods with the least side effects can be inconvenient to use and have a higher rate of failure.

Sorry about that. We don't mean to paint such a gloomy picture of the state of the art, only a realistic one.

Most people searching for a birth control method they can live with would place effectiveness at or near the top of the list in importance. Yet, try to get realistic effectiveness ratings. Unless you are aware that there are two distinct sets of data that physicians quote from, you could be completely misled.

Specifically, *theoretical* effectiveness refers to the rate of pregnancy that would occur if the method were used absolutely perfectly each time according to the manufacturer's or doctor's instructions. But when you consider that people can goof once in a while, then you get a different set of numbers—the *user* effectiveness rates (see chart).

Where you might get confused is if a doctor provides theoretical effectiveness rates for a favorite method and user rates (which are lower) for the methods that he's not so crazy about. For example, it's not uncommon for a doctor to say, "The Pill is 99.7 percent effective, but the diaphragm is only 83 percent effective and foam, 78 percent effective." In other words, if 100 women used the Pill for one year, not even 1 would become pregnant, while 17 would conceive if they used the diaphragm and 22 if their method was foam.

Yet one look at the accompanying chart tells you that, given the same standards of comparison, the diaphragm or foam can be nearly as good as the Pill or intrauterine device (IUD). And what they lack in convenience they more than make up for in safety.

Clearly, it's important for you to be familiar with both types of effectiveness ratings if you're to make a decision based on accurate information.

Remember, too, if one method is good then two are better. Doubling up can raise the effectiveness to over 99 percent, so if you're especially fearful of an unwanted pregnancy, keep that in mind. Also, it generally makes good sense to have a backup method that you can turn to in an emergency. What if you're snowed in and run out of diaphragm jelly—or your can of foam suddenly runs dry?

Intentions Can Change Your Results

Of special importance is the fact that almost every method of birth control will actually work more effectively if you *really* want it to. It's true! According to a spokesperson for the National Center for Health Statistics in Hyattsville, Maryland, that's due primarily to motivation. At least that's what it appears to be for the 9,800 women who were surveyed by the government to determine the effectiveness of various contraceptives. In that study the women used birth control from 22 to 67 percent more effectively (depending on the method)

when their intent was to prevent pregnancy altogether rather than as a means to *delay* having children.

But whatever the reason, the point is that you can have personal control over the success of your particular method without necessarily sacrificing safety.

Speaking of safety, as far as we're concerned, it's just as important as effectiveness. Besides, it's not as though there are no safe methods to choose from. For starters, the good old condom shouldn't be overlooked. Improvements in materials have made them more acceptable now as a primary method and certainly as a secondary or backup method. Even rhythm can work quite effectively for some women, especially

HOW EFFECTIVE ARE THEY?

Birth Control Method	Theoretical Effectiveness (%)	User Effectiveness (%)
Condom	97	90
Condom and spermicidal foam	99+	95
Diaphragm	97	83
Intrauterine device (IUD)	97–99	95
Natural (basal temperature and cervical mucus)	99	90–95
Oral contraceptives (the Pill)	99.7	96
Rhythm	87	79
Spermicide (foam)	97	78
Sterilization	99.8	99.8
Withdrawal	91	75

SOURCES: Information provided by U.S. Public Health Service, Planned Parenthood Federation of America, Inc. and International Federation for Family Life Promotion, 1980.

those who definitely don't want any more children. Again, motivation or dedication to a particular method makes the difference between success and failure. And that goes for the newest of the natural birth control methods: taking basal body temperature and observing cervical mucus consistency (see Natural Birth Control). This combination has been shown to be as effective as the Pill and IUD in some women (see chart).

And, as a last resort, there's always withdrawal. It's one method that's always available, but we don't hold much hope for it since not many have the control (or desire) to pull it off.

Still, we must be realistic, and accept the fact that some women may choose the methods that don't exactly turn us on—namely, the Pill and the IUD.

However, before you make any choice we hope you'll scan the following list of questions we've compiled. It's one way to help you determine your particular birth control needs at any given time during your reproductive years.

- What is your personal health history?
- How old are you?
- Have you had any children yet?
- Do you ever want children?
- How much do you want to avoid pregnancy?
- How important is convenience to you?
- Can you count on cooperation from your partner?
- Do you mind if you have to touch your genitals?
- How often do you have intercourse?
- Are you afraid of any of the methods?
- How close are you to medical care?

To relate your answers to the specific methods, see Diaphragm, Intrauterine Device (IUD), Natural Birth Control, Oral Contraceptives, Spermicides, and Sterilization. By comparing the different methods and taking into consideration your own needs, you will have a head start on making an intelligent decision which you can live with safely, effectively and comfortably.

BREAST CANCER

The statistics are frightening: breast cancer is the single largest cause of cancer death among women in the United States. It will strike 1 out of every 13 women sometime in her life. The question is, what can you do to protect yourself?

Actually, what causes breast cancer is complicated and not fully understood. But theories abound. There is general agreement on a few main risk factors, based primarily on known links between estrogen metabolism in the body and breast abnormalities. Those risk factors do not say "you will get cancer" but

are helpful in identifying women who should be especially alert.

The main risk factors seem to stem from continuous production of estrogen in the body, without pause. Such a long menstrual life may result from early start of menstruation, no childbirth, first childbirth after age 30, or late onset of menopause.

Another recognized risk factor is breast cancer in a mother or sister, or prior cancer in one breast. There is only a one percent chance of cancer developing in both breasts at once, but a five to eight percent chance of later occurrence in the second breast. That is not surprising in light of the fact that both breasts are subject to the same influences that cause cancer in the first place, whatever they may be.

Other risks that have been blamed are obesity, use of oral contraceptives, cigarette smoking, estrogen replacement therapy in menopause, high-fat diets, and use of hair dyes. At this point it doesn't appear that large breasts or injury to the breasts increase the chance of breast cancer.

Suppose you do not have breast cancer in your immediate family but you do have a long history of benign breast problems yourself. Does that make you a more likely candidate for breast cancer? Not necessarily. While women with benign breast disease share some of the reproductive risk factors for breast cancer, the large number of cases of benign breast disease are not a prelude to breast cancer itself.

Obviously, you can't do a thing about how early you started your periods. And it's not practical to start a family just for the sake of staving off possible cancer. (However, if your mother or sister has had breast cancer and you definitely plan to have a family, getting one started in your twenties may not be a bad idea.)

If you are using oral contraceptives for birth control, an effective alternative should seriously be considered. Although not as convenient as the Pill, barrier contraceptives (diaphragm or condoms) used along with spermicidal foam approach the Pill in effectiveness when used correctly, with no risk at all to either partner (see Birth Control).

Taking estrogen for symptoms of menopause? There are so many alternatives that have worked for other women that you owe it to yourself to try them before you consent to oral or injected estrogen. Even then, ask yourself if it's worth the risk for the 18 to 24 months or longer that menopause lasts (see Estrogen Replacement Therapy).

Several studies have also underlined the link between high-fat diets, hormone production and metabolism, and women at high risk for breast cancer. Research from the Naylor Dana Institute for Disease Prevention in Valhalla, New York, shows that the breast duct fluids of high-risk women contain more hormones and circulating blood fats (lipids) than those of low-risk women. The researchers conclude the study by saying, "We propose that high fat intake, typical of the Western diet . . . promotes the growth of precancerous tumors by specifically altering the concentration of the hormones prolactin and estrogen in the breast duct fluids" (*Lancet*, October 22, 1977).

Lowering Your Risks

That delicate relationship between the fatty nature of breast tissues and circulating hormones makes the breasts more vulnerable to the harmful influence of cancer-causing substances (carcinogens) that enter and circulate throughout the body. Fat-soluble carcinogens are easily stored and recycled not only by breast fat but also by total body fat in general. So the fatter you are, the more prone you are toward developing breast cancer.

Consequently, reducing the amount of fat in your diet helps protect you against breast cancer in two ways. It reduces the blood fats that end up in breast ducts, and it probably will result in overall weight loss, since the fat in foods contains more calories than protein or carbohydrates. When you consider that obesity also directly increases your chances of dying from heart disease, hypertension, diabetes or stroke, the link between overweight and breast cancer is just one more convincing reason to get serious about controlling your weight—starting today.

In other words, keeping your weight down by exercising more and cutting down on calories will place you at less risk for breast cancer, and reducing calories by cutting down on fats will help even more. Primary offenders to be avoided are bacon, sausage, butter, cream, ice cream, sour cream, cheesecake, cream cheese, well-marbled steaks, doughnuts and french fries. You will notice that except for those last two, the culprits are all derived from animals. Even major sources of protein that come from animals—except for fish—are higher in fat than vegetable sources (grains and legumes).

So if you must eat meat, trim the fat off that chuck roast and take the skin off that chicken. Get into the habit of choosing broiled or poached fish instead of roast beef. Spread cottage cheese on your crackers instead of Brie. Dollop yogurt onto that baked potato instead of sour cream or butter. Poach—don't fry—your eggs. Make salads your main course and meat your side dish: pile lots of fresh greens, sprouts and raw vegetables into a deep bowl, and sprinkle with fat-free tarragon herb vinegar or lemon juice instead of creamy dressings. Scour your cookbooks for reduced-fat recipes. Drink your coffee without cream.

Better yet, don't drink coffee at all. Or tea. John P. Minton, M.D., Ph.D., the physician at Ohio State University College of Medicine who reported complete disappearance of benign breast lumps in women who eliminated methylxanthine-containing beverages and chocolate from their diets, feels it may take some time to definitely determine whether those chemicals contained in coffee, tea, cola and chocolate influence the development of cancer. But he says, "I tell women who have a family history of breast cancer to cut out methylxanthines completely." Smart thinking! (See Breast Lumps: Benign or Malignant?)

When it comes to diet, there is one further step you can take to back yourself away from breast cancer—and even other types of cancer. Adding to the growing body of evidence in favor of dietary protection against cancer is some very encouraging news of the role of the trace mineral selenium in prevention of breast tumors. Gerhard N. Schrauzer, Ph.D., at the University of California at San Diego, added selenium to the drinking water of specially bred mice that normally develop spontaneous breast tumors. Instead of the usual cancer incidence of 80 to 100 percent, only 10 percent developed tumors.

You might think, "So what? I'm not a specially bred mouse." But the fact that breast cancer is a familial trait makes the high-risk woman very much like a specially bred mouse.

Dr. Schrauzer's experiment was inspired by population data from 17 countries which showed that as levels of selenium in the blood rise, breast cancer death rates fall. In Western industrialized countries, including the United States, selenium was low and breast cancer mortality high.

Dr. Schrauzer feels that the daily selenium intake in American diets should be doubled, and to do that supplements of 150 to 250 micrograms should be added to a diet high in selenium-rich foods. Yeast supplements specially cultured to contain higher amounts of biologically active selenium are also available.

Selenium content of soils and of foods grown in them vary, but whole, unrefined grains are a rich source of the mineral. Dr. Schrauzer specifically recommends whole wheat over white bread, wheat cereals over corn cereals, asparagus over corn and peas, and seafood and fish over beef. Garlic and mushrooms are also high on his list. He warns that "the daughter whose mother developed breast cancer, or any individual subsisting on the typical American diet, should increase their consumption of cereals and seafood at the expense of meat, fat, sugar and potatoes." Those foods not only boost your selenium intake, but they coincide with your low-fat, low-risk diet.

Of course, to protect yourself from the ravages that advanced breast cancer can bring, your best insurance is still in monthly breast self-examination and a regular breast medical exam. Early detection is the only *proven* way to tip the scales in your favor (see Breast Medical Exam and Breast Self-Exam).

BREASTFEEDING

The simplest way to give a child the best possible start is something that came so naturally to our long-ago ancestress that she never even gave it a second thought. Breastfeeding. Unfortunately, though, early in this century technological advances and misguided ideas of propriety took mother's milk out of the mouths of most babes, replacing it with "modern" alternatives like formula and cow's milk.

Only in recent years has the pendulum swung back. Thanks to scores of scientific studies, doctors and nutritionists have come to accept what should have been obvious all along: human milk is the ideal food for human babies. Their opinion, apparently, is shared by growing numbers of mothers: since the early 60s, the proportion of women who breastfeed their infants has risen from about 15 percent to nearly 50 percent.

What makes breast milk so good for babies? Quite simply, it seems to provide, naturally, everything that a baby needs.

Not only does breast milk have all the vitamins and minerals that an infant requires, it also contains substances (which cow's milk lacks) that promote their absorption.

Of even greater interest is the recent discovery that mother's milk contains a powerful factor that stimulates the baby's growth. This "growth factor" seems to be most plentiful in the colostrum, or first breast milk, but continues to be available to the baby for at least six months. Also, researchers believe that this same substance may be absorbed through the child's digestive tract and somehow enhances his or her resistance to gastrointestinal disease.

Likewise, breast milk is known to transfer antibodies from mother to child so that babies, who are born with little or no resistance to the bacteria and viruses of the outside world, may find immediate immunization in this natural drink.

And viruses aren't the only thing babies gain immunity from. According to scientists at the University of Helsinki, Finland, babies who are solely breastfed for at least six months may be less likely to inherit any family problem such as allergic asthma, skin rashes or food allergies. Compared with formula feeding, they said, prolonged breast-feeding resulted in a lower incidence of severe or obvious allergic diseases, particularly in babies with a family history of them.

The researchers suggested that babies from families with a history of allergic diseases should be breastfed for at least six months or longer when possible. The most potent or most common allergenic foods also should be avoided during the first year of life and probably longer, they added (*Lancet*, June 28, 1979).

Of course, mother's milk does contain a hefty dose of cholesterol. But here again, there appears to be a very good reason for it. According to some studies, the high levels of cholesterol in human milk help develop a natural enzyme system in the infant's body, which will enable better handling of cholesterol throughout life.

Breast milk even changes in composition during each feeding, it seems, to perform a special function. The milk that is secreted early in a meal is rather thin, and it gets thicker and creamier toward the end. This, it has been suggested, helps the baby develop a natural appetite control mechanism. The rich, creamy milk tells the baby when it's time to feel full (a lesson that may prevent obesity later in life).

Physical advantages may not be the only ones that breastfeeding confers. Studies have suggested that breastfed babies develop faster intellectually and have fewer learning problems than bottle-fed infants. If an infant is born with deficiencies of thyroid hormone, he or she can suffer severe brain damage and retardation. But breast milk, observations show, provides substantial amounts of the needed hormones—enough, quite possibly, to allow normal brain development at this crucial stage in life.

There's also no question that breast-feeding with its intimate involvement of all the human senses—touch, taste, sight, smell, hearing and warmth—contributes to a very special bond of closeness between a mother and her child (see Childbirth).

How Mother Benefits, Too

Mother benefits in physical ways as well. For one thing, the sucking action of the baby on the breast stimulates your body's production of oxytocin, a pituitary hormone which causes the uterus to contract. This will help get you back to your prepregnancy shape faster. Hormones released during breastfeeding may also delay your menstrual period for several months.

The condition of your breasts may also improve as a result of the experience. Women with fibrocystic breast disease may find the lumps and bumps disappear, says Gideon G. Panter, M.D., a prominent New York City gynecologist. And if you want to maintain breast tone and minimize sagging, he says, you can't beat breastfeeding—provided, of course, you wear a good support bra

Lying down to nurse at least once a day is a great way to catch up on some much-needed rest. In addition, lying on your side with one arm under your head and the other free to assist your little one, is one of the most comfortable nursing positions you'll find.

during the nursing period, even while you're sleeping.

Of course, to breastfeed or not to breastfeed is a personal decision. Most women come to terms with their feeling on this long before the birth takes place. But there are so many considerations, and so many unexpected questions that come up in the course of breastfeeding that it may not be an easy choice to make. This decision may be further complicated if you work. Obviously, for some women, lunchtime commutes home to feed junior may not be practical. But there are plenty of working mothers who have worked out the details satisfactorily: either they have someone bring the baby to them, they keep the baby with them through the day, or they use a breast pump and bottle their milk for those feeding times that they'll miss.

Whatever the case, should you decide to breastfeed (and we would hope that you do), it's a good idea to begin preparing your breasts in the last half of your pregnancy. Nipples need to be conditioned. Otherwise, you're liable to feel some discomfort and even pain in the early weeks of breastfeeding.

Sandra C. Wallace

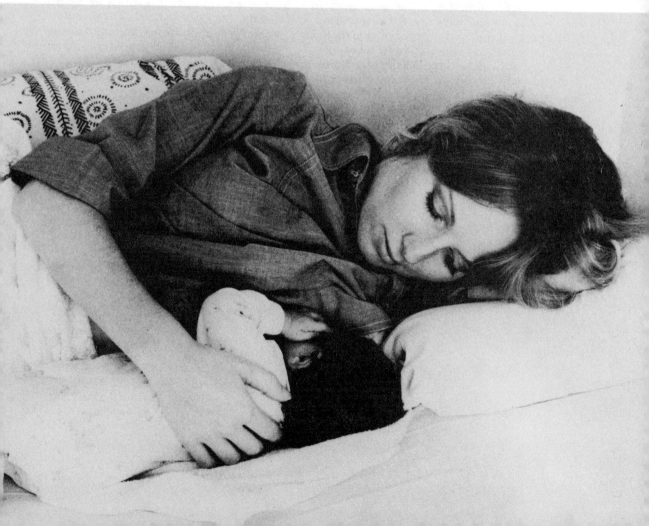

Actually, conditioning is no big deal. At home, turn down the flaps of your nursing bra so air circulates to the nipples. Don't use soap on your breasts during pregnancy (only water) since they secrete their own protective film which keeps them supple and elastic. After bathing, find a private sunny spot, if you can, and expose your breasts for just a few minutes each day. Dab lanolin on the nipple and work it in by supporting the breast with one hand and repeatedly pulling the nipple outward with the other hand until the lanolin is absorbed. It's also helpful to massage your breasts—or better yet—have your partner do it.

It's important, too, that you check to see if your nipples are flat or inverted; that is, if they pull inward or remain flat during sexual stimulation or when covered with an icy-cold washcloth. If they do, you could have some difficulty breastfeeding, so your predelivery conditioning program during the last three months should include the exercises illustrated. These exercises are designed to break the adhesions that prevent nipple erection.

Of course, even after you're long into breastfeeding, problems and questions are bound to come up. Ralph I. Fried, M.D., associate pediatrician, Pediatric Clinical Faculty, Babies' and Children's Hospital, Cleveland, offers the following advice to ease your mind:

- The human being is one of the few mammals that does not lactate on the first day postpartum. So don't get discouraged if your baby doesn't suck vigorously until the third or fourth day.
- The two main factors in maintaining lactation are complete draining of the breast and a serene attitude. Anxiety and tension will soon cause milk production to decrease.

EXERCISE FOR INVERTED NIPPLES

The exercise should be done for 10 to 15 minutes twice a day, and generally should be started as soon as you know you are pregnant. The exercise does cause some discomfort so if your breasts are tender during the early part of the pregnancy, wait until the tenderness lessens before starting the exercise.

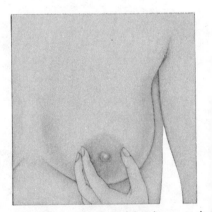

Place your thumb and forefinger at the edge of the right and left of the areola (the outer rim of color around the nipple).

- Whether to nurse from both breasts at each feeding or alternate breasts from one feeding to the next is an individual decision. One advantage of nursing one breast at a time is that it allows the opposite nipple up to an eight-hour rest. Also, the baby may drain the breast more completely if only one is offered. Still, many mothers find that they are more successful if they offer both breasts at each feeding.

- If there is some concern by either the mother or the pediatrician that the baby is not gaining weight satisfactorily, the problem can be solved by weighing the baby before and after a feeding once a day or, as an alternative, weighing the baby naked once a week. A well-fed baby will gain about four ounces immediately after a feeding, or four to seven ounces per week.

Dorothy Patricia Brewster, author of *You Can Breastfeed Your Baby* (Rodale Press, 1979), and a leader in La Leche League, an international organization that guides and encourages nursing mothers, adds a few more important bits of advice. Namely:

- Feed your baby frequently. Breast-fed newborns usually need to nurse about every two to three hours. Demand feeding usually works best. Though your baby may be nursing about every two to three hours, he or she may have one longer stretch, perhaps during the night. Also, you may find that there are some days when the baby seems to need to nurse more frequently than usual.

- Drink lots of liquids—water, juice, milk or soup—to replace the fluids used in making milk, as well as for your own needs. One to two quarts a day is usually a good amount.

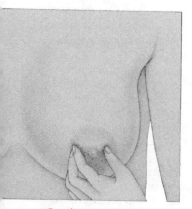

Gently press back toward your ribs,

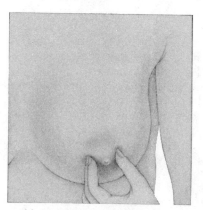

and bring your thumb and finger together behind the nipple.

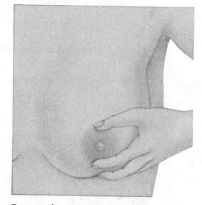

Repeat the exercise, working around the edge of the areola. This helps to gently force the nipple out as the adhesions at the base of the nipple are stretched.

Nutrition for Breastfeeding

Of course, everyone we talked to agreed that the best advice anyone can give a nursing mother is to be extra careful about her diet. For one thing, during this breastfeeding period a woman will need an additional 500 calories and 20 grams of protein a day just to maintain her weight and keep up her energy. You'll know right away when you haven't been eating enough!

Also, what comes out in breast milk reflects what goes into the mother's body—food, drugs and environmental chemicals. To make sure your infant gets "nothing but the best," put solid, sensible principles of good health into practice.

There is probably no time when nutrition is more important—for a baby or its mother. After nine months of pregnancy, a new mother's nutritional needs are still well above those of the average woman. And a failure to meet these needs may mean low nutrient levels in the breast milk, with consequences to both mother and child.

Such dietary inadequacies apparently are not uncommon. A study performed in Texas, for example, found intakes of vitamins B_{12}, B_6, folate and ascorbic acid (vitamin C) below two-thirds of the Recommended Dietary Allowance in nearly half of a group of low-income women. Tests revealed low levels of those nutrients in their milk, too (*Federation Proceedings*, March 1, 1979).

And don't think this is just a problem of the poor. A small sampling of middle-class, well-educated nursing mothers who did not take supplements found nearly half consuming inadequate amounts of calcium and iron.

One place where well-nourished nursing mothers can be found is the Childbirth Center of Daytona, in Florida, where a birthing center starts nutritional counseling even before conception. "We give detailed lectures about good nutrition, and we have a lending library, so mothers can become quite knowledgeable on the subject," says Maryann Malecki, R.N., nutritional counselor at the center. "We put mothers on a specific diet during pregnancy, and we continue it during lactation. And we recommend that nursing mothers continue to take their prenatal vitamin supplements."

Supplements can, in fact, make a measurable difference in the quality of breast milk, according to the Texas study. When milk levels of vitamins B_6, B_{12} or folate were low due to dietary deficiencies, supplementation brought them up, investigators reported.

What Not to Eat

Important as it is for a nursing mother to make sure enough nutrients are in her milk, it is just as essential to keep other substances out. She should realize, for example, that when she takes a drug, her baby will get it, too.

"Just about everything gets across into the breast milk," says Cheston M. Berlin, M.D., of the department of pediatrics and pharmacology at Pennsylvania State University. And, he says, we know very little about the process, or its potential effects.

Recently, Dr. Berlin and a colleague studied the breast milk of a patient who (after her baby had been weaned) received isoniazid, an antitubercular drug. They measured concentrations of the drug in the patient's blood, saliva and breast milk at various times up to 24 hours after a single dose. The amount of the drug excreted through breast milk, they found, added up to a dosage high enough to cause possible damage to cell functions and to the infant liver.

Research on the subject shows that a wide variety of drugs taken by a mother may cause undesirable effects in her nursing infant. Valium and similar tranquilizers can make a baby lethargic and cause weight loss. Antibiotics may produce diarrhea. The baby boy of a mother who took birth control pills while she nursed developed gynecomastia—an abnormal swelling of the breasts.

Just because a drug is available without prescription doesn't mean that it is safe for a nursing mother to take. The California Department of Health Services, citing evidence that over-the-counter drugs may pose real dangers to nursing infants, is considering an order forcing manufacturers to label their products potentially hazardous to unborn and nursing children.

Certain drugs are so dangerous that if a mother must take them, she just should not nurse, says Dr. Berlin. These include lithium (used to treat depression), anticancer drugs, chloramphenicol (an antibiotic) and isoniazid. "If a mother must take any radioactive diagnostic substances, her breast milk should be monitored until traces of the radioactivity are gone," he adds.

"In general, nursing mothers should not take any medication unless they really need it," Dr. Berlin says. "The hazard from small amounts of aspirin, Tylenol or such things, taken occasionally, is probably very small—but unknown. There's a more serious hazard in exposure on a daily basis, if the mother is on chronic medication."

When a nursing mother *must* take some medication, it should be timed to minimize its effect on the infant. "Take it right after nursing, and if possible wait four to six hours before nursing again, to give the substance a chance to be eliminated."

Those cautionary words, Dr. Berlin insists, should not discourage women from nursing. "I want to emphasize the great virtues of breastfeeding. There's absolutely no reason why most women can't nurse. If they have to take aspirin once in a while, it's nothing to get upset about."

Restricting drugs for the baby's benefit may bring a hidden benefit to the mother, too, Dr. Berlin adds: "Once they cut out drugs, a lot of women find out they don't really need them at all!"

An especially cautious attitude should be brought to the use of "leisure drugs" such as coffee, cigarettes and alcohol. They all release chemicals that find their way into breast milk (see Alcohol: Social Drinking; Coffee, Tea and Caffeine; and Smoking).

Here, too, Dr. Berlin says, a sense of proportion is in order. "It's okay to have a cup of coffee or two a day. If a mother does have an alcoholic drink or some coffee, though, she should ideally time it for least effect—wait four to six hours before nursing, if she can."

What about Chemicals?

Some chemicals, of course, cannot be avoided completely. Insecticides and industrial pollutants such as PCBs (polychlorinated biphenyls) are everywhere—in our air, water and food. Because these compounds are fat-soluble, they are stored in fatty tissue and readily find their way into breast milk.

Very high levels of insecticides have been found in mother's milk in Central

America and Japan, and significant amounts have been reported in such places as Israel and Scandinavia. When the Environmental Protection Agency conducted a survey of breast milk samples in the United States, they found sizable quantities of pesticide residues. In many, levels were higher than the Acceptable Daily Intake *for adults,* as determined by the World Health Organization. In one sample, the levels were 100 times higher than the amount considered safe.

"Most of these chemicals are laboratory carcinogens," says Marcia Silcox, science associate with the Environmental Defense Fund. "If a child ingests too much, the effect later may be carcinogenic." While the harmful effects of PCBs are not fully understood, low levels have been found to cause behavior problems and learning disabilities in monkeys, "and the average nursing infant in the United States gets one-sixth of this amount."

An infant may be particularly vulnerable to the effects of those toxic substances, she warns. "His immune system is immature, and his liver can't detoxify chemicals as well as an adult's."

While it's impossible to avoid all exposure to environmental contaminants, their hazard may be minimized by sensible precautions. Animals are on top of the food chain—they eat plants that contain pesticides, and concentrate those chemicals in their bodies—so eating meat means taking in a heavy dose. One study found that vegetarian mothers (who eat no meat) have about *half* as much pesticide residue in their milk as meat-eating mothers.

This doesn't mean that a nursing mother must be a vegetarian (if she is, in fact, she must take special care to pro-

vide enough protein and vitamin B_{12} for her infant). But it suggests real advantages in cutting down on meat. "In particular, avoid animal fats," Marcia Silcox suggests. "Fat is where these chemicals are stored. Choose leaner cuts of meat, and remove fat before and during cooking. As for dairy products, eat low-fat things like skim milk, low-fat cheese and yogurt. Instead of ice cream, have ice milk."

When you eat fruits and vegetables, make sure they are thoroughly washed or peeled (or grow them yourself, organically).

To minimize the danger of PCB exposure, the Environmental Defense Fund recommends avoiding fatty fish and fish from inland waters that may be contaminated, "especially from places like the Hudson River or the eastern Great Lakes." Ocean fish, which are not subject to this kind of pollution, are preferable for that reason.

La Leche League suggests other steps to reduce the danger of milk contamination. Nursing, says the League, is the wrong time to lose a lot of weight through a crash diet program: this may release into the breast milk PCBs and other chemicals stored in body fat. "Try to cut down on pollutants at home, like pesticides and other sprays," adds spokesperson Carolyn Hayes. "Avoid clothes that have been treated to resist weather, water or wrinkling. And don't wear permanently mothproofed garments—they may contain dieldrin, which can be absorbed through the skin."

And as Maryann Malecki of the Childbirth Center points out, any nursing mother can and should avoid personal sources of pollution by cleaning up her diet. "That means staying away from additives, chemical-laden processed foods, things like that."

A woman who feels she may have been exposed to very high levels of contaminants may want to have her milk tested (state departments of health may provide information on how and where this can be done). By and large, though, most experts agree: while sensible precautions are worth taking, the risk of

chemical contamination should not deter most women from nursing.

"Here's what we tell mothers," says Maryann Malecki. "Avoid what you can avoid. Don't be hysterical about what you can't avoid—like environmental contaminants. And remember: the milk of a nursing mother is still superior to any other infant food."

BREAST LUMPS: Benign or Malignant?

From prenatal life through maturity, the growth and development of the female breasts depend on their response to levels of hormones circulating in the blood. When an error occurs in those normal processes of growth and development, disease results. The cause could be too little or too much of a hormone in the blood or too little or too much response by the breast. The problem can be harmless but annoying (benign, noncancerous), acute and life-threatening (malignant, cancerous) or somewhere in between.

Remember, if you or your doctor should discover a lump, that does not automatically mean you have cancer. For example, if your exam falls just before your period, the harmless nodes (lumps) that develop premenstrually may incorrectly suggest a malignant tumor. In addition, there are many more types of lumps and cysts that occur independent of your menstrual cycle that are just as harmless.

Eighty percent of all lumps confirmed by doctors are benign. That is, they are not cancerous. But only your physician can diagnose the difference. Although there is no need to panic, it is just as unwise to "wait and see," hoping the lump will disappear.

Besides, no matter how much you've heard or read, there's no way that you'll be able to differentiate between a harmless and a not-so-harmless lump. Certain symptoms of cancer—including redness, nipple puckering or discharge, and skin dimpling, as well as lumps and pain—can also characterize a variety of benign breast diseases.

The most common cause of benign breast lumps is fibrocystic disease, also called chronic cystic mastitis or mammary dysplasia. There is no one distinct fibrocystic disease. Rather, that term covers a range of abnormal conditions that develop in the breast, sometimes simultaneously. It is the most common type of breast disease, usually showing up between the ages of 18 and 50, while the ovaries are still functioning. After menopause, it subsides. Half of the women in the United States will be diagnosed as having fibrocystic disease sometime in their lives.

What Is Fibrocystic Disease?

"Fibrocystic" is a tag that explains what has happened to a previously healthy breast, possibly due to the slight rise in estrogen that is normally secreted by the ovaries about midpoint in the menstrual cycle. A deviation from the normal process of manufacturing new cells in glands, ducts and connective tissues may result in two types of symptoms. Either long, threadlike fibers aberrantly grow to form a solid, scarlike mass, or a small pocket among the tissues fills with fluid or semisolid material to form a cyst. Both result in unwelcome lumps the size of a grape or larger that cling to healthy breast tissues. And they can hurt!

Immediate relief is gained by minor surgery—either in the doctor's office for needle aspiration (a technique of draining fluid from the cyst) or surgical removal of a lump as an outpatient in a hospital. Either way, you feel better. However, the disease tends to be chronic. After a few months, the system goes out of kilter again, and you may find yourself returning for repeated removal of lumps or fluid. Repeated aspirations call for removal of the cyst itself. Like lump removal, that is done as an outpatient procedure under local anesthesia. Recurring discomfort may be somewhat relieved by a support bra.

But recurrence may be preventable. Vitamin E can often reduce not only the discomfort but also the size and number of breast cysts. The vitamin seems to work by reversing the abnormal ratio of estrogen and progesterone circulating in the body during the menstrual cycle. That change in hormone levels is an antidote for estrogen's disturbing effect of cyst formation in the breasts.

Success with vitamin E for fibrocystic disease is very real. Robert London, M.D., director of the Ob. Gyn. Endocrinology Research Lab at Sinai Hospital in Baltimore has seen promising results from daily oral doses of 600 international units (I.U.) of vitamin E in 80 percent of one group of women studied.

"Some women respond better than others," Dr. London reports. "But relief usually follows within two months at most. That's very encouraging, because there is so little attention paid to the effective treatment of fibrocystic disease other than surgical removal of the cysts."

Benign breast lumps may also regress after a change in dietary habits. John P. Minton, M.D., Ph.D., department of surgery at Ohio State University College of Medicine, has seen benign lumps completely disappear within two to six months in 13 out of 20 women who completely eliminated coffee, tea, chocolate and cola from their diets. And relief eventually came to 3 others within 18 months after the change. Those beverages contain chemical stimulants called methylxanthines, which hinder the work of enzymes in cells (*Journal of the American Medical Association*, March 23, 1979).

Dr. Minton has also found that nicotine stimulates abnormal breast tissue growth and suggests that cigarette smoking be discontinued by women with breast lumps. After only eight weeks of avoiding smoking and methylxanthine-containing foods, some patients had total regression of their disease. Two-thirds of his patients were lump-free after two years of total abstention. The remaining third, whose lumps did not disappear and were consequently biopsied, were nevertheless advised to avoid nicotine and methylxanthine-containing foods as an extra precaution. Again, be sure to have any lump evaluated by a competent physician.

Another lumpy pest goes by the name of fibroadenoma. These firm, round, nontender lumps range from about the size of a large pea to that of a golf ball and are somewhat mobile.

They usually occur singly, make their appearance within 20 years after puberty, and are removed surgically.

The most frequent cause of clear or bloody nipple discharge is small, warty, usually unpalpable growths blocking the ducts underneath the nipple and areola (area surrounding the nipple). Your doctor may opt to have the discharge smeared onto a glass slide and examined at a lab, but that is not totally reliable. More than likely the growth—papilloma—or the duct itself will be cut out and studied to determine if it is cancerous or benign.

Pain, tenderness and redness are sometimes caused by an inflammation of the milk ducts (mammary duct ectasia). About half of its victims will suffer inverted or cracked nipples, or have difficulty nursing. It may also produce a lump, sometimes with pulling in of skin or the nipple. Suspicions can only be overruled by surgical removal and biopsy.

An occasional incident of drawing in of a nipple or dimpling of skin may be due to death of a small area of fatty tissue below the surface. That condition sometimes follows a slight injury, perhaps from a fall or a blow to the breast.

What Happens When a Lump Is Found

Whatever the case, if a lump is present, your doctor may order a breast x-ray called a mammogram, not only to help determine whether it may be cancerous but also to discover any other unpalpable masses and their location—in either breast (see Breast Medical Exam).

Once mammography has told your physician exactly where any problems are located, he may remove some of the suspicious tissue for further study. That is usually done in the office by fine-needle aspiration and/or needle core biopsy. Either procedure is simple and takes about 15 minutes.

For fine-needle aspiration, the physician will insert a long, thin, hollow needle through the fatty breast tissue into the growth and drain it of any fluid. Lumps are often just pockets of innocuous fluid, called cysts. If the fluid is clear, it generally means the cyst is non-cancerous, and the fluid is discarded. If the fluid is bloody or aspiration doesn't completely eradicate the cyst, it may be sent to the lab for study.

If the mass does not completely disappear, recurs, or turns out to be solid rather than fluid-filled, some physicians may proceed with a needle core biopsy. First the breast will be numbed with a local anesthetic, much as you get a "local" for tooth extraction. By inserting a slightly larger needle through a tiny incision on the breast surface, a core sample of the problem tissue will be pulled out. That leaves a small scar.

The smear of suspicious aspirated fluid or biopsied material is sent to a pathologist for examination under a laboratory microscope. Although truly benign cells do not become malignant, they often mimic the cancerous kind—and can coexist in the same breast—so sampled cells are always examined by a pathologist. Based on the size, formation and other characteristics of the cells, the pathologist will tell your doctor if the disease appears to be benign, malignant, or questionable. Benign means the abnormal cells have neither gone berserk nor invaded healthy tissue. Besides cysts, benign lumps may be merely masses of scarlike tissue among the fat. Malignant cells are a threat to life because after first invading the ducts and fatty tissues of the breast, they eventually penetrate the lymph glands and blood vessels, by which they are spread to bones and vital organs, especially the liver and lungs.

The lab test itself takes just a few minutes to process, and your physician will have the results in a few days at the most.

If the pathologist and your doctor are certain that your symptoms are due to one of those benign conditions, the growth will be removed on an outpatient basis and that's that.

However, some abnormal cells are neither clearly benign nor clearly malignant. Some growths are too small to yield enough tissue for an accurate office biopsy diagnosis. Fine-needle aspirations are only 92 percent accurate for diagnosis, and a benign reading is not to be trusted in a woman aged 50 or older, who is more likely to have cancer. A cyst may refuse to disappear, even when repeatedly aspirated. In any of these cases, your doctor may very likely want to take a closer look at the tissue by means of an open biopsy.

That is now widely performed as an outpatient procedure, in an operating room under either general—or, preferably, local—anesthesia. Using a mammogram of the breast as a guide to the location of the mass, a small incision is made in the breast. If the incision is made parallel to the natural skin contours that surround the areola, scars tend to eventually fade, minimizing unsightly marks. That should be a consideration especially in a woman who undergoes repeated surgical biopsies.

Analyzing the Suspicious Lump

Removing only what is necessary, a chunk of tissue containing the suspicious cells is cut out for immediate study by a pathologist. A section of the soft tissue is quickly frozen and stained so that it can be examined under a microscope. The test itself takes about 5 minutes and the surgeon can have the results in 20 minutes.

The trouble is, diagnosing cancer in five minutes using that quick-set method isn't always easy or clear-cut. And yet many surgeons require women to sign a consent form prior to the biopsy allowing the surgeon to proceed with radical breast surgery (mastectomy) on the basis of that instant report.

The scenario of such a one-step procedure can go like this:

Your physician may skip the fine-needle aspiration and you are admitted to the hospital for open biopsy. The surgeon asks you to sign a paper giving permission to go ahead with any treatment deemed appropriate based on the pathology test done while you are on the operating table, unconscious. What that means is that the surgeon goes into the open biopsy all suited up to do a mastectomy based on results of the frozen section. The pathologist announces that the verdict is "malignant," and you wake up without a breast.

An alternative to that—and we believe a better alternative—is to have the biopsy done in one procedure and, if necessary, additional surgery performed during a separately scheduled procedure.

Why wait?

Well, while it's true that most cell samples are readily distinguishable as cancer on frozen section—some say as many as 85 percent are—others fall into a gray area between the extremes of benign and malignant. Some, for instance, that lurk midway between are so sluggish they never become malignant. It takes a very well-qualified and experienced pathologist to recognize the difference. And even the most experienced one will admit there are some that are impossible to call on the basis of the frozen section alone.

In addition to the difficulty in determining whether a lump is benign or malignant, the frozen section does not differentiate too well among the different types of cancer. Cancers vary from very isolated growths to those more likely to spread, or metastasize. Also, while it is logical to assume that all large cancer tumors were once small, there is no evidence that all small growths become large. Those noninvasive cancers less than the size of a large pea or confined to a local spot are tricky to diagnose and not well understood. Again, it's chancy to undertake a mastectomy before all the facts are in.

To get a better reading, then, the surgeon should make what is known as a "permanent section" from the tissue samples taken from the tumor. Sometimes a surgeon will take one sample from the most suspicious area of the tumor, other times he or she may take several samples from different locations. In either case, the sample or samples are then fixed in formaldehyde, dehydrated, set in paraffin, stained and read. The whole process takes from 12 to 24 hours, so your surgeon won't have the results until at least the next day.

About half of the samples that were questionable on the frozen section can be diagnosed by permanent section. The remaining half (or 1 in 25 biopsies) may require the consulting opinion of a second pathologist. All the more reason to wait on mastectomy till a few days after biopsy.

Delay in treatment after open biopsy does not affect the course of the disease one way or the other. It was once believed that after cancer was exposed during surgery, it spread like wildfire. Today, we know that isn't so, and a couple of days or a week more shouldn't make any difference in the success of treatment. Besides, the advantages of the two-step procedure over the one-step are many.

Just to recap, agreeing first to a "biopsy only" better insures an accurate diagnosis, allows for tailoring the treatment to the type and extent of the disease, enables the woman to prepare herself emotionally for the second part of the surgery, and affords her the option of getting a second opinion.

Actually, only about 1 in every 15 or 20 women who require open biopsy for cancer diagnosis actually has cancer confirmed. For the majority, then, the two-step approach eliminates the fear of waking up without a breast. It also avoids unnecessary hospitalization and expensive preoperative tests not needed in those who do not require further surgery. A simple open biopsy can be done on an outpatient arrangement.

There are personal considerations, too, as pointed out by Morton Comess, M.D., a surgeon in Phoenix, Arizona. "If you are a working woman, the boss will want to know if you'll be out for a day or a month. If you have children, you have to arrange for babysitters. So scheduling the major surgery apart from the outpatient biopsy makes sense that way, too."

Discuss the possibility of minimal cancer, should it be found, with your surgeon before open biopsy. He can remove the breast later, if he feels that the presence of unseen microscopic cancer cells is likely elsewhere in the breast. Amputation of a breast—or anything else—is serious enough to warrant close observation of those worrisome cells rather than automatic removal.

BREAST MEDICAL EXAM

Self-examination is very similar to but not a substitute for the breast medical exam (be sure to read Breast Self-Exam). For one thing, it is possible for you to miss lumps, even when you have been very thorough. Like the story of the princess and the pea, it takes a sensitive hand to feel a lump buried under layers of fatty tissue, and it takes professionally trained hands to detect more elusive, hard-to-feel lumps. That is particularly true if you are older or have large breasts. In a small breast, even a very small lump can be felt. As the breasts become larger, fattier or more pendulous after childbirth or weight gain, even a large growth may be difficult to detect. Tumors developing in the milk ducts are often missed.

Because hormonal swings during the menstrual cycle can change the character of the breasts and create abnormal—though benign—conditions, which can either mimic or obscure a serious problem, the timing of your breast exam is extremely important. According to Sven Kister, M.D., associate professor of surgery at Columbia University College of Physicians and Surgeons, the best time to schedule a breast exam is between the 7th and 14th day of your menstrual cycle (day one is the first day of menstrual flow), which is just after menstruation but before ovulation. This will better your chances of an accurate diagnosis.

Once in the examining room of your physician, insist on a complete exam—it should take more than just a minute or two—and have the physician or nurse practitioner review the self-exam with you to be sure that you are performing it

correctly and to point out the normal ridges, muscles and bumps in the breasts.

The physician or nurse practitioner may record the location, size and consistency of any lumps or thickenings on a sketch of the breasts, for future reference. At that time, he or she should also record or update your complete medical history, including your age, previous benign breast problems, childbearing and menstrual history, and any breast cancer in your mother or a sister (also, the age at which these family members had the cancer).

Physicians estimate that breast cancer mortality might be reduced by nearly 20 percent through widespread self-examination and up to 48 percent when combined with yearly physician's exams (*New England Journal of Medicine*, August 10, 1978).

The Breast Checkup Gets Its Own Exam

The "yearly exam" is one guideline in breast cancer screening that has never been questioned. Most physicians have, and still do, consider the annual breast medical exam the best safeguard against cancer for all women. But interesting new data suggests that not every woman benefits equally from the yearly exam and that perhaps, for some women who are at low risk and who practice breast self-examination monthly, a breast exam by a physician need only be performed every three years.

Several bits of evidence have led to this reevaluation of breast medical exams. First, more breast cancers are detected by women themselves (at least 95 percent) than by doctors during an annual exam. Second, says Dr. Kister, a woman's age is directly related to her risk of breast cancer: the older she is, the greater her risk. For women under age 30, breast cancer is so rare it's practically nonexistent; between 35 and 45, the risk doubles; and from 55 to 64, the risk increases by 50 times.

Third, the recently published results of a long-term study by the Health Insurance Plan of Greater New York (HIP) have disclosed that while the annual breast medical exam, including mammography (breast x-ray), can decrease the number of deaths due to cancer by about 40 percent in women over age 50, mammography does not appear to have such a benefit in women younger than 50.

All things considered, the American Cancer Society announced amended guidelines on March 21, 1980. Basically, the new recommendations are as follows:

- Every woman between 20 and 40 years of age (who practices breast self-examination monthly and is not considered at risk of breast cancer) should have a breast exam performed by a physician every three years.
- Every woman over 40 should have such an exam every year.
- Every woman over 20 who is considered at higher risk of breast cancer— because she has either a family history of the disease (especially if a mother or sister had both breasts removed before menopause), or a personal history of the disease—should consult her physician about the value of more frequent examinations. In such cases, the annual breast medical exam may still be advisable.

Of course, these are just recommen-

dations—nothing more. If you or your physician still feels that the annual breast exam is a good idea no matter how old you are and how slim your risks, then follow your better judgment. Also, any time you find a lump or notice an abnormality in the breast, it is wiser to check with your doctor right away rather than wait for a scheduled appointment in the distant future.

The Controversial Mammogram

We can't discuss breast exam without discussing another diagnostic procedure—and one that's even more controversial. Mammography—the infamous breast x-ray. Some physicians believe that every annual breast exam should include a routine mammography. There's no question, these x-rays are the most reliable way to detect whether or not unpalpable masses (ones that can't be felt during self- or medical examination) are present. In fact, 90 to 95 percent of breast lumps can be detected by mammography while only 60 percent are felt during physical examination. What's more, studies have shown that combining mammography with physical examination reduces death from breast cancer by one-third over chance finding of lumps, because mammography can detect localized tumors before they spread to the armpit glands or beyond (*Mayo Clinic Proceedings*, March, 1977). If a cancerous mass is caught while small and confined to just the breast, there is an 85 to 95 percent chance for survival, compared to only 50 percent if the cancer has invaded the lymph nodes or beyond.

Sounds like the ideal diagnostic tool for breast cancer—except for one thing. Mammography exposes the breast to radiation, which is itself another risk factor in the disease. At present, there is great controversy over the use of routine mammography to screen young, symptom-free women because of the theoretical possibility that repeated mammography may in itself *cause* cancer, especially in those already at high risk. And those are precisely the ones who are recommended for screening.

On the other hand, these hazards may be offset by the potential value of mammography. Estimates state that only about 120 malignancies will be produced for every million women exposed to one rad (meaning "radiation absorbed dose") to each breast in one year and that is after a latent period of anywhere from 10 to 20 years (not too consoling if you're one of the victims). But, say its advocates, when you compare it to the nearly 10,000 early cancers that would be missed if mammography were not done at all, the slim radiation risk seems worth it (*Journal of the American Medical Association*, August 22, 1977).

Besides that, newer, higher-quality x-ray films are now being used which permit faster mammography and consequently less radiation exposure—0.2 rads to 0.6 rads for a two-view examination (*Postgraduate Medicine*, June, 1980). As yet, no study that we're aware of has projected the risk based on that much-lowered dosage—although some specialists maintain that no dose, no matter how low, is safe.

Obviously, there is no question about the use of mammography in women who show any of the suspicious signs of breast cancer. But when expert opinions on use of mammography for regular screening of symptomless women range from the view that it will save many lives to the belief that the practice will produce potentially fatal illness in those same women, where

does that leave you?

Again, the 1980 guidelines offered by the American Cancer Society should help. They are as follows:

- At any age, mammography can be valuable in detecting a suspicious mass in the breast, even if it is a recurring symptom of benign breast disease. A clinically suspicious lump should be removed even if mammography is negative.
- Every woman age 50 or older should have a mammogram every year. After age 50, the benefit of detecting an unpalpable cancer outweighs the potential risk. That is due to both the increased likelihood of cancer showing up at that age and the reduced exposure to radiation by beginning mammograms at that time. Also, the breasts of women over 50 are less glandular and dense than those of younger women, making mammography more accurate.

The National Cancer Institute has added two guidelines:

- Routine mammography for women under 40 years of age should be limited to those women having a personal history of breast cancer.
- Routine mammography for women between the ages of 40 and 49 should be restricted to women with a personal history of breast cancer or with a mother or sister with a history of breast cancer.

What to Expect from a Mammogram

You will be asked to disrobe to the waist and given a dressing gown to wear into the closed-off examination room. You will either stand or sit against the mammography equipment, depending on the type of machine used. One breast at a time is exposed, and the chest itself is not involved. (A chest x-ray is a low-dosage shot of the whole chest and should not be confused with a mammogram.) To protect your ovaries from radiation exposure, ask to be shielded with a lead apron.

Each breast is slightly compressed between a small shelf projecting from the machine and a cone lowered from above. Two exposures are made of each breast, to view the breast from the side and the front. Mammographic equipment is calibrated to indicate exposure time and consequently the amount of radiation delivered to the breast, measured in rads, and the amount will vary depending on the size of your breasts. Larger breasts require slightly more exposure time. Ask the x-ray technician or radiologist (a physician specializing in the use of x-rays) how many rads will be absorbed. It should be about one-half rad for a two-view exposure. If your radiologist won't say or if the rad dose is too high (some clinics and hospitals operate with outdated x-ray equipment, which delivers unnecessarily high radiation on exposures), ask your doctor to suggest an alternative exam site.

Mammography itself takes only five or six minutes altogether. The result will be images of the interior of your breasts, recorded on film. These images are studied by the radiologist and interpreted to your physician.

Incidentally, mammography for diagnosis of a suspicious sign is covered by major insurance plans and Medicare; breast x-rays as part of a *routine* exam are not. An alternative method to mammography is Xeromammography (also called Xeroradiography) in which the images of the breasts are projected onto a Xerox plate. From that, the images are transferred to special paper, much like that of the photocopier system you may use in your office. Xeromammography yields better-quality images, but the dosage is not quite as low as in mammography.

Under evaluation is another technique, thermography, which uses no radiation at all, but rather measures the heat radiated by various masses in the breast. Approximately 45 to 70 percent of breast cancers cause an abnormal heat pattern on the skin surface. But so do some noncancerous masses. Although it is safe, the high false-positive rate (indicating cancer when there is none) makes thermography valuable only when combined with physical examination, in order to determine if a woman should have mammography, or to help clear up a questionable abnormality on a mammogram.

BREAST PAIN

Breast pain and tenderness (with or without a lump) may send you to your doctor not so much out of fear of cancer but sheer discomfort.

It's true, breast pain is rarely a symptom of a serious problem. But it's no longer considered the sure sign of non-cancerous disease it once was, according to nursing researchers at the State University of New York at Buffalo and California State University (Long Beach). Bonnie Bullough, R.N., Ph.D., a nurse practitioner and dean of Buffalo's School of Nursing, explains that pain was a primary symptom of breast cancer in 13 percent of 139 California women surveyed. The pain, she adds, wasn't severe but rather a "pulling" or "funny feeling" caused by the tumor's displacement of tissue (*Modern Medicine*, June 15, 1980). So, despite previous thinking, this is another symptom you shouldn't ignore.

Still, the majority of breast pain complaints are innocuous—the result of water buildup in the fatty tissues just before or during the menstrual period. In some women, fluid buildup is a habitual response to the natural rise in the hormone estrogen which occurs between ovulation and menstruation. The waterlogged tissues swell, nudge against nerves, and you feel pain (see Cramps and Other Premenstrual Miseries).

Diuretics are the common medical prescription for that. But diuretics are drugs capable of causing toxic reactions such as dizziness, headache, ringing in the ears or nausea—not to mention depleting your body of much needed potassium. Another conventional approach involves the use of small doses of the hormone progesterone to counteract estrogen's effect on water retention.

But unless your pain becomes unbearable you might want to try some less drastic measures first. To reduce water retention, decrease your salt intake and try some of the natural diuretics mentioned in our section on cramps.

In addition, physicians ranging from a country doctor in Indiana to a Park Avenue gynecologist in New York report that supplemental doses of vitamin B_6 soothe tender breasts. Backed up with lesser amounts of other B complex vitamins, B_6 has a natural diuretic effect on water buildup. Vitamin B_6 also seems to regulate out-of-proportion hormone levels in some women. Kenneth I. Sheek, M.D., a practitioner in Greenwood, Indiana, sees excellent results in women who take just 40 milligrams of pyridoxine (vitamin B_6) a day in B complex tablets. Other women need much more. A New Jersey gynecologist gives his patients up to 600 milligrams a day, beginning at ovulation (about midpoint in the menstrual cycle). Sore breasts are usually only a memory by the second month of supplementation. While your needs for B_6 will not be exactly the same as your neighbor's, a baseline dose is a daily total of about 100 milligrams, according to Gideon G. Panter, M.D., a New York City gynecologist and a faculty member at New York Hospital–Cornell Medical Center.

You might also try enlisting the support of your bra for relief. For many women, wearing a bra to bed during the problem period is the answer. The elastic support of the bra acts as a second skin, counteracting the pressure within the breast tissues.

Even for daytime wear, and especially if your bosom is a somewhat generous 36C or larger, an inadequate brassiere can aggravate either premenstrual pain or pain due to benign disease. Just choosing a pretty bra from among the underwire push-ups and lacy styles on the rack does not insure that you've chosen the right bra for you.

Bulges over the bra top mean either the cup is too small or you have the back and shoulder straps adjusted too tightly. The bra style you choose should distribute most of the weight of your breasts across your back.

HOW TO FIND YOUR BRA SIZE

1 Body size equals rib cage measurement plus 5 inches (32, 34, 36, etc.)

2 Cup size equals chest measurement minus body size

If 1-inch difference, A cup
2-inch difference, B cup
3-inch difference, C cup
4-inch difference, D cup

BREAST SELF-EXAM

The breast, for all its functional and ornamental attributes, is vulnerable to some very uncomfortable and worrisome ailments, the most alarming of which is cancer. Confusion over risk factors and mass screening for breast cancer, combined with blazing headlines that 1 out of every 13 women faces breast cancer each year, can prompt you to react in either of two ways: you nervously devour all the facts and theories and pray that you never have trouble, or you throw up your hands in utter hopelessness.

Those same hands of yours, however, can easily be educated to steer you through the maze of breast abnormalities with confidence, and at the same time help to minimize your chances of becoming a cancer statistic.

While a lump is occasionally found during a routine medical checkup, 95 percent of breast lumps are found by women themselves, often during habitual breast self-examination. And because better cure rates generally result from treatment of smaller cancers than of larger ones, routine breast self-examination could save your life. Relying on accidental discovery of a lump is very risky.

Frequent examinations—monthly self-exams plus regular physician's exams—are more likely to result in diagnosis of cancer in its earlier stages, with less likelihood of spread to the lymph glands under the arm. In a National Cancer Institute-supported study of the self-exam habits of 246 newly diagnosed breast cancer patients, over one-third of the patients who never practiced breast self-examination had advanced stages of cancer, compared to only five percent of those who had routinely done self-exam. Furthermore, patients who never practiced self-examination showed up with significantly larger tumors than those who practiced it at least monthly (*New England Journal of Medicine*, August 10, 1978). And the larger the tumors, the more lymph nodes that were cancerous.

Only one-fourth of American women practice self-examination. If all took the time for regular, thorough home and office exams, early detection would result in a more favorable picture for cure. Breast cancer cannot yet be prevented, but the woman who does her homework greatly improves her chances of catching it in its most treatable stages. According to Roger S. Foster, Jr., M.D., and his co-researchers in the above study, each woman "destined to develop breast cancer has in her own hands the possibility of increasing her chance of survival through performance of breast self-examination."

Many women do not examine their

breasts because of fear of what they might find, when actually what they might find may save their lives. Others are not confident enough or just don't bother.

When and How to Examine Your Breasts

Not only must self-examination be done regularly, it must be done properly. It's simple and takes only a few minutes. A woman should ideally begin routine exams in her late teens or early twenties—not because of the possibility of cancer but because the unlikelihood of cancer at that time helps her to learn the unique consistency of her own breasts without anxiety over cancer. Self-examination should be continued throughout life, even during pregnancy. Once you get into the habit, you will become familiar with the natural thickenings, bumps and irregularities that occur in the normal, healthy breast, and your hands and eyes will become trained to detect any abnormalities that may develop. That is one reason that self-examination should be performed between your doctor's exams. Another is that it can be done frequently, at no expense or time spent in a waiting room. There are certainly no side effects or risks, and, at worst, it is only slightly uncomfortable.

SELF-EXAM

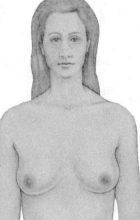

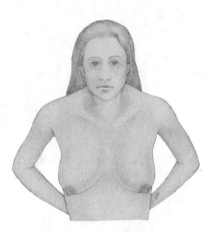

Disrobe to the waist and stand or sit before a mirror in a well-lit room, with arms down at your sides. Look for changes from one exam to the next, such as dimpling of the skin or pulling in of an otherwise turned-out nipple. Observe any crustiness or scaling on the nipple. Watery, yellow, pink or bloody discharge from the nipple should also be noted at any time. (Milky discharges are not uncommon, and are caused by benign changes in the breast.)

Still sitting or standing, lean forward slightly, watching for those same changes.

It is best to choose a specific time of the month, preferably right after your period if you are still menstruating. That allows for cyclic changes in the breast which normally occur between periods. If you are past menopause, the first day of each month is a good reminder.

Breasts may vary in many ways even when disease-free. On the same woman, one breast may be somewhat larger, shaped differently or more sensitive than the other. Both may be very tender all over or only in certain areas, or tender only at certain times of the month or year. They may be lumpy, or free of any nodules at all. They may be firm, full, small, a little saggy or very saggy.

They may change slightly from one year to the next. The nipples may be flat, erect, inverted, large or small, and the surrounding areola (or ring surrounding the nipple) may be dark brown or pale pink. The purpose of regular self-examination is to keep in touch with *any changes* that might suddenly occur. That requires both looking and feeling.

It may be easier to feel for lumps with the skin of the hands and breast wet and soapy. The soap allows the hands to glide very lightly over the skin's surface, as you would stroke a length of fabric to determine the nap or grain. That will help you to detect any small changes underneath the breast surface. You may

Raise your arms slowly and evenly overhead and press your hands together behind your head— then just in front of your forehead— observing any changes in contour of one breast, puckering or dimpling of the skin, or "pulling" in the skin (that is, tendency of the breast tissues to not easily slip over the underlying muscles). Raising the arms in this way may accentuate changes that may not otherwise be obvious.

Next, place your hands on your hips and tighten your chest and arm muscles by pressing firmly inward. Again, observe the breast for changes.
(continued on page 74)

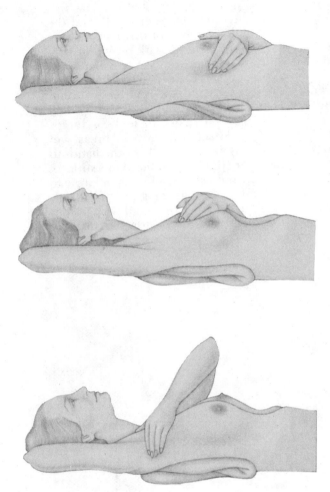

To palpate (feel) the breast, lie flat on your back with a small pillow or folded towel under your right shoulder. Raise the right arm overhead. With the left hand slightly cupped and the fingers together, feel for any unusual lumps or change in the texture of the breast skin. Use the flat of the fingers, not the tips. Lumps are palpable at about the size of a pea or larger. Avoid compressing the breast tissue between the thumb and fingers, as that may give the impression of a lump that is not actually present.

Begin either at the nipple, proceeding in a rotary direction toward the outer regions of the breast, or palpate half of the breast at a time. If you prefer the latter method, start with the inner half of the right breast, examining the areas from the collarbone to the underportion and from the nipple to the breastbone (sternum) in the center of your chest.

Then pay special attention to the outer area between the nipple and the armpit, including the armpit itself. That is where the majority of breast cancers occur. A ridge of firm tissue in the lower curve of each breast, however, is normal.

Transfer the towel or pillow to the left shoulder and repeat, using the right hand to feel the left breast.

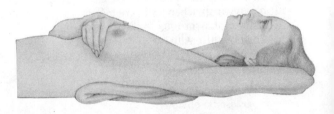

find it convenient to practice this in the shower, either before or after the rest of the exam.

Other signs to be alert to are itching of the nipple, noticeable enlargement or shrinking of both breasts and generalized hardness or redness. Also, contrary to previous beliefs, new evidence indicates that breast pain—or more specifically, a "pulling" or "funny feeling"—may be a symptom of breast cancer in a small but significant number of women.

BREECH BIRTH

Bottoms up. That is the way nature intended children to dive headfirst into the world. But for many, labor day catches them unprepared in a feet-first, heads-up position. It's called a breech birth—either a "footling" breech (feet-first) or "full" breech (bottom-first). And according to an article in the *British Medical Journal*, few problems in the delivery room demand finer judgment, more experience or greater skills on the part of the obstetrician (June 30, 1979).

Despite rumors, a breech birth is not necessarily synonymous with a cesarean section. In fact, the decision to go for a vaginal or a cesarean delivery is anything but straightforward. Sometimes—particularly if the baby is approaching the birth canal buttocks-first with the legs either flexed or extended—a vaginal delivery can be safely carried out. In one small study, 48 women whose children were in the buttocks-first presentation were permitted to continue labor and 47 delivered by the vaginal route—with no damage to their babies.

However, there are many other instances when a cesarean is essential to the safety and well-being of both mother and child. For example, a baby who is approaching delivery feetfirst is up against many dangerous obstacles. "The major complication—and one which occurs in 20 to 25 percent of footling births—is a cord prolapse, which is a premature expulsion of the umbilical cord from the uterus," says Albert Haverkamp, M.D., director of perinatal research at Denver General Hospital in Colorado. This usually results in brain damage or death. The other danger of a feetfirst delivery, he explains, is that the head can become trapped because the cervix isn't dilated enough. This is due to the fact that the cervix dilates to the size of whatever is pushing against it. If a foot is pressing on the cervix, it may dilate only to that size—which obviously is a far cry smaller than the head.

This same problem of inadequate cervical dilation is even more critical in premature babies because the head is even larger in proportion to the rest of the body. Consequently, it is generally agreed that the risks of footling and premature breech are too great to attempt vaginal delivery.

Unfortunately, when your time comes to deliver and your child is in a breech position, the decision to go cesarean or vaginal isn't yours. Nor should it be, since as we said, this can be an extremely dangerous and risk-ridden delivery. This is strictly a case for a qualified obstetrician—which is just another reason why a trusted and qualified M.D. is of the utmost importance.

We're not saying that you should relinquish responsibility entirely. A breech birth isn't usually something that

This simple, effortless posture practiced just 10 minutes twice a day can often save a pregnant woman from the complications of a breech birth.

surfaces mysteriously on delivery day. Most, if not all, women are warned ahead of time of a potential problem with the baby's positioning. And this is the time that she should voice any fears and questions she may have. Ask your obstetrician how he or she intends to handle it. Some physicians opt for cesarean in all breech cases in the belief that it's best for baby. Only problem is, this could open up the possibility of immediate or long-term problems for mom (see Cesarean Birth), and you should know about all the risks and/or any options beforehand.

There is also a chance that if you are aware of a breech position early enough, a simple, effortless exercise practiced for 10 minutes twice a day will change the position of the fetus and lead the way to a normal delivery.

Juliet DeSa Souza, M.D., originator of the postural treatment and retired professor of obstetrics and gynecology at Grant Medical College, Bombay, India, told the World Congress of Gynecology and Obstetrics that exercise or posture corrected the breech presentation to a headfirst presentation in 89 percent of 744 patients studied. She also reported that in her private hospital, 70 of 73 cases were corrected (*Ob. Gyn. News,* January 1, 1977).

The posture involves lying for 10 minutes on a hard surface with the pelvis raised by pillows to a level 9 to 12 inches above the head. This position should be practiced twice a day on an empty stomach. To be effective, the treatment should be started at the 30th week of pregnancy and continued for at least 4 to 6 weeks.

BUST DEVELOPERS

"The bigger the better"—that's the way many women feel about their breasts. And if nature doesn't smile on them, they're prepared to go to all ends of the cosmetic counter and figure salon to find happiness.

We decided to follow them—in a manner of speaking.

We began our investigation by checking a well-stocked newsstand and sifting through an assortment of popular women's and movie magazines. In the seven magazines we selected, there were 13 ads promising bigger, better bosoms—yours for the clipping of a coupon. And a check, of course.

So we clipped and mailed our money (prices ranged from $3.00 to $20.98) to 10 nationally advertised companies. Then we waited . . . and waited . . . and waited.

According to the Federal Trade Commission's rulings on mail-order merchandise transactions, a seller "must ship within 30 days of receipt of an order or, if unable to do so, provide the buyer with a notice and an option to cancel."

Yet after a month's time, we had received items from only 3 companies and not one notice of the delay from the remaining 7. What's worse, all 10 companies cashed our checks!

Tracer letters—including a Xerox copy of the cancelled check as proof of purchase—were sent out a month and a week after the original orders were placed.

The Sara Micheals company responded that the item had been mailed (we found out later that it wasn't properly addressed, so the people in our mailroom opened it, passed it around, had a few laughs and tossed it in the trash can). Precious Pounds returned our money—no explanation, just a check. Enjoy Enterprises didn't respond at all—we're still waiting for word of our money or merchandise.

And Starburst not only neglected to send the item, but actually cashed the Xerox copy of the check we enclosed in the follow-up letter!

The remaining three filtered in. But it took up to 60 days from the day we mailed our money to receive some of them—that's twice as long as the law permits.

Mail-order maneuvers aside—the real question here is whether or not these things work. Well, what better way to find out than by trying one out firsthand?

The obvious choice for testing purposes was the Mark Eden Bust Developer. For one thing, Mark Eden looks pretty safe and we felt that it was enough to evaluate the benefits of a device without worrying about whether it's going to do you any harm. Second, the rationale behind the exercisers made slightly more sense than that for the creams or massagers.

Besides, Mark Eden has been around for a long time. They're the ones with the "doctor's test," the scores of supposedly satisfied customers, the money-back guarantee, and just the right disclaimer—"Results may vary due to individual response and application"—to keep the postal authorities from getting to them.

What it is, is an exercising device that resembles a pink plastic clamshell held open by a heavy-duty spring. The idea is to take it in your hands (with your arms extended and flexed in a series of exercise positions) and press against the resistance of the spring to close the shell.

To see the busty, bikini-clad blonde in the instruction manual perform the exercise, it looks like effortless grace. But any weakling like me will tell you that you almost need Arnold Schwarzenegger to carry it off picture perfect!

I could barely budge it. And my husband only managed to clamp it shut after several seconds of grunts and groans. Egos shattered, we concluded that the model in the manual must have been using a modified exerciser—minus the spring.

Anyway, I persisted. I huffed and puffed and put in my 10 or 20 repetitions of each exercise just like you're told in the instructions.

I must admit that the exercises do seem to work on the chest muscles. If you place the palms of your hands together in front of your chest, elbows out to the sides, and press together hard, you'll actually feel the muscles across your chest tighten. And if you're somewhat out of shape, 10 minutes of Mark Eden is liable to leave your chest muscles feeling like your stomach muscles do after 100 sit-ups. My aches and pains can vouch for that!

Yet, after three weeks—the same amount of time that it took "Diane C." to increase her bustline from "29½ inches to 35 inches," according to the Mark Eden ad—my tape measure read about the same as when I started, give or take a half inch for breathing.

Interestingly enough, in an ad for a new and improved Mark Eden device called the Mark II developer with "Infinitely Variable Resistance" (from the ad copy, I would guess that means the clamshell now comes equipped with a gadget to adjust the resistance of the spring), a busty blonde makes the even more outrageous claim that "Between Monday and Friday I gained three beautiful inches on my bust."

How do these companies get away with it?

Clyde Ross, inspector in the Medical Fraud Unit of the U.S. Postal Service, is in charge of investigating fraudulent advertising claims for bust developers and bust-developing programs. "There isn't any actual evidence that these things work," he told us. "The purported 'medical evidence' is usually a lot of hot air and contriving. And as far as the testimonial evidence—someone saying, 'It worked for me'—that means nothing."

I can certainly vouch for that! Besides, $25 (the amount offered by one company for juicy testimonials) can buy a lot of "dream bosoms"—even if they are imaginary.

How Do They Get Away with It?

We're being bamboozled. But, according to Clyde Ross, companies are wise to the law and it's not that easy to convict them.

"There's fine line between what's actually said and what may be implied by the ads," he told us. "It's what we call 'puffery.' They take a product such as a cream that may soften the skin, and build it up in the copy so that you think it will make you more alluring. But they don't exactly say so. They're staying within the bounds of the law—technically."

Thomas A. Ziebarth, attorney for the Consumer Protection Branch of the U.S. Postal Service and prosecuting attorney for many of these cases, agrees. "There are a lot of technicalities involved. And some of these cases are vigorously contested," he said.

The attorney sent us some decisions from the trials involving a few of these offenders. He was absolutely right. The defendants supplied affidavits from medical doctors and prominent fitness authorities. In addition, they brought witnesses who testified that they had benefited from the device or program.

To find out more, we divided our items into five basic categories—exercisers and exercises, nutritional supplements, massagers, creams, hormone preparations—and consulted leading authorities on physical education, anatomy, gynecology and drugs.

Does Exercise Enlarge or Lift the Bosom?

We expected to hear the most legitimate backing for the exercisers. But surprisingly, Dorothy V. Harris, Ph.D., a professor of physical education and the director of the Research Center for Women in Sports at Pennsylvania State University, gave us the "thumbs down."

"There's no way exercise will increase mammary tissue," she told us. "In fact, it's a misnomer to say that anything will increase the size of the actual breast."

That's because exercise tends to strengthen and enlarge muscle mass. Since the breasts consist of fatty and glandular tissue—no muscle—there's nothing there to build up.

The chest muscles, or pectorals, on the other hand, may benefit from a daily workout, but not to the extent that most women would hope, Dr. Harris explained.

"Thanks to mother nature and hormone levels, females just do not have the same predisposition to muscle bulking that males do," she insists. "A high testosterone [male hormone] level is needed to increase muscle girth. That's why the average woman can pump iron regularly and experience only a minimal increase in chest size."

Proof of this comes to us from Jack H. Wilmore, Ph.D., professor and head of the department of physical education at the University of Arizona, Tucson.

In *Journal of Sports Medicine* (January/February, 1975), Dr. Wilmore writes that he put 47 women and 26 men through an identical weight training program. The group worked out twice a week, 40 minutes a day, for a total of 10 weeks. During that time, both the men and the women increased the strength of their upper bodies. But, he reports, there was very little increase in the muscle bulk of the women participants.

Well then, what about firming and toning sagging breast tissue?

"No exercise in the world will regain the elasticity of the breast once it's lost," Dr. Harris sighs. That's because there are no muscles in the breasts, only two ligaments—called Cooper's ligaments—which keep the breasts tilted upward. But once they've stretched, you've got "Cooper's droop" and there's not too much you can do to reverse it. "Better to prevent it before it happens by providing adequate support—especially during physical activity," Dr. Harris suggests.

Protein for the bust is another advertising ploy that seems to have little merit. Granted, good nutrition is essential to a healthy body. And when your body is alive with good health, it radiates in the way you look.

But as Gideon G. Panter, M.D., a prominent New York City gynecologist and a faculty member at New York Hospital–Cornell Medical Center, indicated to us, "to suggest that there is one food that goes directly to the breast is absolutely ridiculous!

"The only thing that determines the size of a woman's breasts is genetics. That and the amount of weight she carries. Certainly, if she eats more, she will eventually increase the fat deposits in her breasts. But then she'll be getting heavier all over, not just in one area."

Dr. Panter also disagreed with the idea that a flat-chested woman may be protein-deficient and need a protein supplement to increase muscle and body tone. "Protein deficiency indicates malnutrition," he said. "And that's going to show up with more serious symptons than a flat chest."

But by their own admission, malnutrition is what these companies aim to treat. Although they don't say so in their ads, a witness for Sara Micheals testified during a recent court hearing that many people are obsessed with junk food and fad diets. And for $10.95, they offer a way to supplement a potato-chips-and-soda-pop diet.

What they didn't mention—but which the attorney for the Postal Service did—is that the daily allowance of protein in this supplement is equal to the amount in two eggs. And, not only are eggs cheaper, they're a higher-quality source of protein than the supplement.

What about Massage and Hormones?

Massage has also been touted as an aid to bust development. We sent for two massage devices. One was described as a "power-packed electric bust-builder" and promised to "melt away fat as it builds up your bust"—can't imagine how they intend to do that!

The other was called a "Hydro-Stimulator," which turned out to be a rather bizarre contraption that hooks up to your water faucet at one end and encases your breast in a blue cup (size 52D) at the other. By producing a whirl of water pressure around the breast, this device supposedly increases circulation and stimulates breast growth.

We asked Dr. Panter if there is anything to this notion. "For sure, stimulation does increase the size of the breasts," he conceded. "Masters and Johnson monitored the breast during preorgasmic stimulation and found that it enlarges by 20 percent."

But don't get your hopes up. It's not what you think. Dr. Panter further explained that the effect does not involve permanent growth but rather temporary swelling. The breasts return to their original size shortly after stimulation.

Can creams increase the size or improve the appearance of the breasts? "That's a Madison Avenue concept!"

says Dr. Panter. "You can't change the composition of the skin by smearing it with a greasy cream. Any alteration in skin texture must come from within." For example, estrogen levels seem to be an important influence on a woman's skin—and breast size, for that matter.

Every authority we consulted agreed that estrogen can increase breast size when taken by mouth—as was the case a few years ago with women on the Pill, before the dosage was decreased. But there was quite a bit of discrepancy over its effectiveness when mingled with a cream base and rubbed into the skin.

We asked four medical doctors—one gynecologist, two medical consultants for the Food and Drug Administration, and an officer in public health at the Centers for Disease Control (CDC) in Atlanta, Georgia—whether estrogen can penetrate the skin and enter the bloodstream.

The first M.D. said no. "Only mucous membranes such as those found in the vagina are capable of absorbing an estrogen cream." The second physician conceded that a small amount may seep through the skin, "but not enough to cause any biological changes." The third warned us that the skin absorbs "a lot more than you'd think." And the last candidly stated, "Yes, it is absorbed. Estrogens can pass through lipid or fat membranes more readily than water."

Doctor number four is Gary Stein, M.D., epidemiology intelligence service officer for the CDC. And he has good reason to believe that you don't necessarily have to *swallow* the Pill to send estrogen into your bloodstream.

Dr. Stein took part in a study in Puerto Rico where employees of an Ortho Pharmaceutical plant were developing high blood levels of estrogen. The employees affected were involved with the manufacture of birth control pills.

Five out of 25 men who worked in this division showed symptoms of an increase in the female sex hormone and 3 actually developed enlarged breasts. Among the women employees, 2 of the 5 who came in contact with the powdered birth control substance and 10 of 18 in the production line working with the finished product experienced unusual vaginal bleeding.

How can this phenomenon be explained? "I doubt very much whether there was any direct ingestion of the substance," Dr. Stein explained. "But there's a good possibility that skin contact and breathing the airborne particles caused the high estrogen levels in these workers."

Of course, some physicians may argue that there's a difference between powdered estrogen and the estrogen tied up in a cream. So we again asked Dr. Stein if he thought that mattered. "Not really," he replied. "It is still a lipid-soluble-type compound. It can still be absorbed as a cream."

At best, it seems, estrogen creams will produce no results. At worst, they could expose their users to all the possible risks of oral estrogen. In case you've forgotten, those risks include breast tumors, menstrual bleeding, blood clots, gallbladder disease and cancer.

So what's a woman genuinely concerned about her breast size to do? "There's always plastic surgery," Dr. Panter says lightly. "But," he adds, "that's not without considerable risk. It's safer—and cheaper—to pick up a copy of *Vogue* magazine and realize that it's very fashionable these days to be small-chested. Otherwise the only thing that will increase actual breast size is pregnancy. And to minimize sagging and improve tone try breastfeeding."

Unfortunately, many modern women deny themselves the satisfaction of breastfeeding their children for fear of losing what some consider their "feminine charms." Actually, it may improve their figure.

"Even if you haven't breastfed the first child, breastfeeding the second will help you regain the tone you may have lost during the first pregnancy," Dr. Panter explains. Just be sure to wear a good support bra during the nursing period—even while you're sleeping.

And if you're too old—or too young—for that, remember that body *proportion* is a hundred times more important to your total image than the size and shape of your breasts. So keep in shape with a good physical activity like swimming or jogging. It will improve your posture and get your whole body glowing.

CELLULITE

You can try rubbing it off or beating it off but you've still got it—ripples round the rump. Maybe you've seen it, those wings of fat that protrude just outside the hip joint and pucker up along the back of the thighs. It's what the French call cellulite (pronounced SELL-u-leet). And leave it to the French to come up

with a fancy name for fat. Of course, they won't admit to such a simplified, mundane description. To them, it's "fat-gone-wrong"; it's "fat, water, and toxic residues bound up in a gel-like mass." And they've got their own recipe for reducing it, which combines a special bland diet with massage and yoga.

But Maria Simonson, Sc.D., Ph.D., M.D., director of the Health and Weight Program at the Johns Hopkins Hospital and Medical Institute, laughs. Having once wrestled with a serious weight problem and been saddled with fatty hips that resembled "riding breeches," she decided to put the cellulite solution to test. The end result, she told us, was far from flattering. In fact, she says, "this whole cellulite concept is nothing but window dressing. It's a sales pitch. Of course, there is water and perhaps some toxins in it. There is in all fat. But there is no evidence that cellulite is anything but ordinary fatty tissue and there is no point in treating it differently than any other kind of fat."

To get the inside story on cellulite, we contacted Gerald Imber, M.D., a plastic surgeon affiliated with the New York Hospital–Cornell Medical Center. As a surgeon, Dr. Imber has seen first-hand the fat called cellulite. He told us it looks the same as fat that is deposited elsewhere in the body. The only difference is that in some locations, fat can develop in little pockets.

With women, he explains, there is a hormonal predisposition to accumulate fat on the breasts, buttocks, hips and thighs. Heredity dictates where the greatest concentrations will be (not all of us can be a perfect figure eight, we're afraid). But in some women, the fat can build up in areas to the point where it outstrips the blood supply. This poor circulation, he believes, is the reason why fibrous bands develop between the fatty pockets and the skin, creating that cottage cheese appearance.

So what do you do if you're troubled by these lumps and bumps of fat? Well, first off, ask yourself if perhaps you need to lose some weight. A good diet and exercise program will cut into those excess fat deposits. And usually the first fat deposits to go are those at the site of greatest accumulation.

According to Dr. Simonson, the best type of exercise for reducing the girth of hips and thighs without overly increasing muscle mass is aerobic exercise. That is, walking, running, cycling and swimming (see Fitness for more on aerobic activities).

Theoretically at least, massage might also help to smooth out those patches of unsightly smocking by breaking up the fibrous bands that hold the fat pockets in place. In any case, it's not a good idea to do anything that might cut down on the circulation to your buttocks and thighs. Says Dr. Simonson, "The woman who squeezes into a girdle week after week shouldn't be surprised if she emerges one day with a tail end that resembles a cocker spaniel's ear."

CERVICAL CANCER

Each year, invasive cervical cancer singles out 16,000 women—most of them younger women between the ages of 35 and 55—and kills 7,400 of them. Sound bleak? Actually, when you consider that 50,000 people die each year in traffic accidents and 300,000 of heart attacks, cervical cancer is mildly destructive by comparison.

The frustrating thing about it, though, is that *anyone* dies from it. Invasive cervical cancer is preceded by a long (8 to 30 years) period of "precancerous" cervical abnormalities. And, through the Pap smear, nearly 90 percent of all those potential cancers can be detected early enough to insure 100 percent cure—a cure which, by the way, rarely hinges on hysterectomy.

The cervix is the lower section of the uterus. If you envision the uterus as an upside-down pear, the cervix would be its neck projecting an inch or so into the vagina.

Actually, the sheer location of the cervix—somewhere between the outside world and the inner sanctum of the womb—probably makes it more vulnerable to disease. Bacterial, viral and fungal organisms attack it, causing infections. And a penile battering ram periodically pounds it.

Of course, it's not known for sure what provokes cancer in the cervix. But since promiscuous women or women who've begun sexual activity early and had their first baby in their teens face the highest risk, while nuns are virtually immune, sexual intercourse seems to be the common denominator in its development. Several factors, including herpes (a sexually transmitted virus; see Herpes), poor hygiene, and even the protein makeup of sperm have been suggested as possible causes.

Presumably, then, prevention could mean living the life of a celibate. But for those of us not willing to sacrifice sex, the next best solution may be switching contraceptives. According to a group of Oxford University researchers, the incidence of cervical abnormalities including dysplasia (an alteration in cells, possibly an early stage in cancer development) and invasive cancer in diaphragm users was only about one-quarter that in Pill or intrauterine device (IUD) users. Why that is, no one knows for certain. But these researchers suggest that it could have something to do

with the fact that the diaphragm, like the condom, protects the cervix from direct contact with sperm (*British Journal of Cancer*, August, 1978).

Evidence that the hormones in the Pill may be contributing to cervical cancer comes to us from the University of California. There researchers have discovered a close correlation between use of the Pill and the conversion of cervical abnormalities, or dysplasia, to cancer. Apparently, cervical dysplasia can go either way: it can shrink to the point where it actually disappears or it can grow into a cancer. Based on this study, women who continue taking the Pill after a dysplasia has been diagnosed stand a greater chance of falling victim to the "Big C" (*Science*, June 24, 1977).

Another estrogen compound, diethylstilbestrol or, more simply, DES, has also been associated with an increased risk of cervical cancer. But the strange thing here is that the woman who develops the disease as a result of DES exposure probably didn't take the drug: her mother did. DES is a hormone prescribed to pregnant women to prevent miscarriages. Now evidence suggests that women who came in contact with the drug while in the womb may face a fivefold increase in their risk of developing cervical cancer up to 30 years later (*British Medical Journal*, July 28, 1979).

Your Best Safeguard: the Pap Smear

But no matter what the case against hormones, your best safeguard against advanced disease is the Pap smear.

Based on the little we know of cervical cancer, it looks like the Pap smear may be able to detect abnormal cell changes in the cervix at least eight years before a full-fledged cancer develops. With prompt treatment, then, advanced life-threatening cancers can be prevented (see Pap Test).

Of course, the Pap smear is only a preliminary test in the screening for cervical cancer. So, if word of suspicious cells calls you back to the examination table and stirrups, here's what to expect from further diagnostic tests:

- *Colposcopy.* That may sound frighteningly invasive, but it's no more hassle than a Pap smear. After a speculum is inserted and the vaginal walls swabbed with a vinegarlike solution to remove mucus, the exposed cervix is viewed through a binocular instrument called a colposcope, which magnifies the surface features. The instrument is held outside the body, so don't freeze up in anticipation of pain. It won't hurt and, in fact, may save you additional and perhaps unnecessary follow-up.

- *Biopsy.* And preferably a colposcope-directed biopsy. Once the problem is located, and evaluated through colposcopy, the physician can take a tissue sample from the suspicious area. That can be done in the office. At most you might feel a little pinch, but it isn't enough to require anesthesia or hospitalization. *No treatment—and least of all, hysterectomy—should be undertaken without a biopsy.*

- *Conization.* If, on colposcopic examination, the physician discovers that the suspicious area reaches into the cervical canal, or if the biopsy results return from the lab labeled moderate to severe dysplasia, it may be necessary to evaluate the extent of disease further by cutting a cone-shaped wedge out of the cervix. Since half of the volume of the cervix is actually

removed during this procedure, hospitalization and anesthesia are required. Immediate complications including hemorrhaging and long-term complications such as infertility can result. Obviously, this is not your basic biopsy. Yet, it remains an invaluable diagnostic tool which could save you from a hysterectomy. And, by comparison, the risks are small.

Treatment is then tailored according to the extent of the trouble and the stage of cancer development. As mentioned earlier, it usually takes many years for a full-fledged cervical cancer to take hold. And it isn't even known for fact whether every problem labeled "precancerous" would develop into a cancer. But most are removed as a precautionary measure. Other minuscule lesions diagnosed as "mild dysplasia" may disappear on their own, perhaps a result of some kind of body defense mechanism. But generally speaking, the earlier the diagnosis, the less drastic the treatment and the more effective the cure. It's rare for any diagnosed mild to moderate dysplasia or lesion to require hysterectomy.

Nonradical Treatments

Sometimes the method of diagnosis doubles as treatment. In a small lesion, for example, a biopsy might whisk away every last trace of trouble. Similarly, conization can clear up certain larger but still localized dysplasias with no need for further surgery, depending on their location. In fact, there is a growing body of American physicians who consider conization adequate treatment for cancer *in situ* (a definite cancerous condition that has not yet spread to underlying tissues), particularly in younger women. Myron Melamed, M.D., chief pathologist at Memorial Sloan-Kettering

Hospital in New York City, is among those physicians. And John Mikuta, M.D., director of gynecologic oncology at the Hospital of the University of Pennsylvania, points out that the high hysterectomy rates in the United States relative to foreign countries may reflect the fact that here hysterectomy is still considered routine for cancer *in situ,* whereas conization is the treatment of choice in other countries.

With smaller, less advanced abnormalities, hysterectomy is never an acceptable option. If they cannot be removed entirely at the time of biopsy, and the results of the biopsy show no further invasion, they can be quickly eradicated in another office visit.

Cauterization, which uses a heated wire to burn away abnormal tissues, is the longstanding treatment of choice. Years ago, it was customary to cauterize women after childbirth. That cleaned up any abnormal coating left behind by the pregnancy and gave the uterus and cervix a nice, shiny covering. Today, you'd be hard pressed to find an obstetrician who still practices cauterization routinely, but according to Dr. Mikuta, there are some papers suggesting that women who have had routine cauterization after delivery have a lower incidence of cancer of the cervix. Whatever the case, it does seem to destroy diseased tissue and promote new growth of healthy cells.

Another procedure elbowing its way into the gynecology suite is cryosurgery. That procedure, which destroys the abnormal cells by freezing rather than burning them, is preferred by some physicians because it is easier and less painful than cauterization. However, one physician we spoke with regarded it as still an experimental procedure.

Both cauterization and cryosurgery can be performed in the doctor's office with no anesthetic. Possible side effects include bleeding and discharge—nothing that a vinegar and water douche can't clear up—and minor cramping.

Treatment for More Serious Cases

A biopsy that verifies a more serious dysplasia or cancer *in situ,* however, is more likely to lead to hysterectomy than to conization in this country. And much hinges on the age and emotional maturity of the woman. But at this stage, surgery is still relatively limited. For noninvasive cervical cancers, only the uterus, including the cervix, is removed. The ovaries and the fallopian tubes may be left intact.

Once the cancer has invaded the underlying cervical tissues, however, you're talking about much more extensive surgery. Dr. Mikuta explains, "You can't solve this problem with just a simple removal of the uterus and the cervix. This requires taking out the uterus and cervix plus three additional things: the tissues at the side of the uterus all the way over to the pelvic wall; the pelvic lymph nodes; and the upper third of the vagina. Along with this, we usually remove both tubes and ovaries. This is called a radical hysterectomy. You can treat cancer of the cervix by radiation just as well in terms of survival. But I feel that you get a better result with surgery, particularly in younger women where you might be able to preserve an ovary or two. Radiation wipes everything out. Plus you have to deal with possible damage to the bowel, bladder or to the vaginal tract itself. There can be some fairly significant shrinkage to the vaginal tissues with the radiation therapy."

That kind of surgery requires the

skill of a gynecology specialist known as a gynecologic oncologist. It is an extremely complicated and risk-ridden procedure which should be undertaken only by persons with adequate training, with fully certified anesthesiologists and in hospitals that can supply good backup facilities. Don't expect your G.P. or even your obstetrician to take care of this problem in a smalltown community hospital. Invasive cervical cancer is definitely a case for the "big boys." Check yourself into a comprehensive cancer center or at least contact one for a referral to the closest hospital that's capable of handling this type of problem (see *Appendix* under Cancer Information Service).

CESAREAN BIRTH

At a time when more and more couples are gearing up for "natural" childbirth experiences, the delivery mode that's making the most dramatic rise in popularity among obstetricians is probably the least natural of all—cesarean section. Twenty years ago, c-sections accounted for 1 in every 25 deliveries. Today, in some U.S. hospitals, as many as one in four women will have their babies delivered via a surgical incision through the abdomen.

The obvious question is, why? Why the sudden upswing?

In the past, it seems, the cesarean delivery was primarily reserved as a last resort in a life-threatening situation. Today, obstetricians tell us, because much of the risk has been removed from the procedure—thanks to improved surgical and anesthetic techniques, the development of safe blood transfusions, and the discovery of antibiotics—c-sections are undertaken with greater frequency in less dire, though subtly dangerous situations. The rationale now is that cesarean sections can *prevent* complications of a difficult delivery rather than just remedy an impossible one.

In accordance with that, acceptable indications for the procedure have expanded to include almost any situation where there exists even a slight possibility that a problem might arise during labor or delivery. Specifically, in cases where:

- The baby is presenting in a full breech, feetfirst, or transverse (sideways) position.
- Labor does not appear to progress as it should.
- The mother is diabetic.
- The mother is suffering from toxemia of pregnancy (preeclampsia), which is characterized by high blood pressure and serious water retention.
- It appears that the mother's pelvis might be too small to accommodate the baby's head.
- Active genital herpes sores have erupted at the time of labor.
- The baby is premature.
- There is an Rh blood factor involved.
- The mother has a heart condition or high blood pressure.
- The birth involves twins or triplets.
- The umbilical cord or placenta prolapses from the uterus before the baby is delivered.
- There is any indication of fetal distress.
- The woman has had a previous child delivered via a cesarean section.

Depending on the individual circumstances, a cesarean section for any one of those reasons is perfectly justifiable according to today's obstetrical standards. And there's no question that precautionary surgical deliveries have indeed saved more than a few lives and prevented serious damage to countless newborns. Nevertheless, there is a growing concern among women, women's health organizations, and even physicians, that obstetricians are perhaps a little too eager to cut on the basis of potential rather than actual risks.

Are Some Cesareans Needless?

For example, one modern obstetrical practice that seems to have a direct influence on the escalating c-section rates is fetal monitoring. By way of a belt wrapped around mom's belly and a probe threaded through the birth canal and attached to baby's head, physicians can now monitor fetal heartbeat and other vital signs so they are immediately alerted to even the slightest indication of fetal distress. Electronic fetal monitoring can, of course, be a lifesaver. But the information it provides can also be misinterpreted. And since physicians are sometimes unable to distinguish between real and imaginary distress signals, it's no wonder women who labor amidst sophisticated electronic monitoring equipment are more likely to make a last-minute trip from the delivery room to the operating room.

According to one investigation, 16.5 percent of the women who were monitored during labor subsequently delivered via cesarean section compared to only 6.8 percent of the women whose labors were not monitored (*American Journal of Obstetrics and Gynecology,* June 1, 1976). What's more, none of the women in the second group were any worse off for *not* undergoing the operation—which brings to mind the distinct possibility that for approximately 10 percent of the monitored mothers, surgery was performed unnecessarily.

The "once a cesarean, always a cesarean" dictum is likewise coming up against some stiff opposition recently. And the conclusions drawn after the next few years of evaluation are bound to have tremendous consequences. At the present time, past cesarean delivery is a major reason for performing a cesarean section—at least one-fourth of all abdominal births in this country are done for this reason alone. But every study on this indicates that if these women are given the chance to go into labor, at least 50 percent—and as many as 65 percent—will successfully deliver the second time around.

Those who adamantly oppose vaginal deliveries for mothers who previously delivered surgically argue that the risk of uterine rupture is too great and its consequences far too serious to take any chances. In uterine rupture the scar from the previous c-section ruptures— usually under the stress of labor. In a "catastrophic" rupture the fetus is expelled from the uterus into the abdominal cavity, a fatal move for baby and sometimes mother.

Those who favor vaginal deliveries for some c-section women, however, explain that while uterine rupture is possible, it's extremely rare. Bertold Salzmann, M.D., clinical professor of obstetrics and gynecology at New Jersey College of Medicine found in an analysis of 110,000 deliveries that half of the 4,000 women who had previous cesarean sections delivered vaginally with only one case of uterine rupture (*Female Patient,* June, 1979).

The placement of the original c-section incision is critical in calculating the risk involved in a subsequent vaginal delivery. Women with a "classical," or vertical, incision through the uterus face a two percent risk of rupture while those with a low transverse or horizontal incision face a risk no greater than one-half of one percent.

For that reason, physicians who do permit their former c-section patients to go into labor and try for a natural delivery before deciding whether another cesarean will be necessary, strictly limit this "trial of labor" to women whose previous child was delivered through a low horizontal incision through the abdomen and uterus. Incidentally, the scar on the abdomen is usually but not always indicative of the scar on the uterus; only your physician knows the exact placement of that hidden one.

"Trial of Labor"—Both Sides

There are other factors to consider as well before attempting a trial of labor. For example, many doctors exclude women who have had more than one cesarean or whose cesarean was necessary because of a chronic problem such as diabetes or heart disease. Also, to be considered for a trial of labor you must be committed to the concept of natural childbirth with little or no medication. That's because during labor it's extremely important that you are able to detect any unusual pain or tenderness in the area of your old scar, which could be a warning that it may rupture.

Otherwise, if you have a low transverse scar, had your first and *only* other cesarean because of fetal distress, breech birth or some other one-time complication, and have taken natural childbirth preparation classes, there's a good possibility that your next child can be born naturally.

Nancy Wainer Cohen, co-founder of C/SEC Inc. (Cesareans/Support Education and Concern), with headquarters in Boston, is very optimistic about that. "Individually or in my classes, I've counseled well over 100 women. All but 3 of them have had vaginal births," she says. She has personally gone through with two VBACs—a term she coined which stands for vaginal birth after cesarean (pronounced vee-back). "This country has an attitude that women aren't capable of giving birth without tools, tubes and machines. Women are frightened, tense and tight. Then, many of the routine medical procedures—monitoring, intravenous tubes, no food, drugs, induction, restricted mobility—increase their chances of cesarean. I believe most cesareans can be prevented, and certainly most repeats aren't necessary."

Actually, though, the women Nancy Cohen counsels are luckier than most. Many Boston city doctors are open to the concept of VBAC. But the truth is, except in a few caring hospitals—usually in big cities like Boston or New York—very few vaginal deliveries are attempted in women who had previous c-sections. And even if you manage to find a physician who seems open to the idea, be careful that he's not just giving your request lip service.

Monitoring a mother with a previous cesarean takes time. She must be admitted to the hospital the minute she begins labor and from that point on she must be closely supervised. This can entail many hours' worth of watching and waiting, something that the average doctor in a smalltown hospital may not be able to take. Also, for some physicians, time means money—and they may feel that it's too impractical (if not impossible) to spend that much time with one woman.

Besides, the "better safe than sorry" argument that physicians frequently use to defend their decision to operate may, according to the critics, describe the obstetrician's gamble more accurately than it does the mother's or her child's. After all, a physician who attempts a natural birth in the face of a well-recognized risk may be held responsible if anything goes wrong. But one who performs a cesarean delivery for any of the indications mentioned earlier—even if the surgery is of questionable necessity—covers himself in the event of a malpractice suit. For the physician, then, cesarean section is the safe way out. But unfortunately, that's not necessarily so for the two on the table.

Despite medical claims that the cesarean section is now as safe a surgical procedure as the appendectomy, there's still a great deal more risk involved in a c-section than in a normal vaginal delivery. Given ideal situations for both, the natural vaginal delivery is still considered far and away the safest and most advantageous delivery method for mother and child.

Risks in a Cesarean

For baby, the biggest risk associated with c-section—especially repeat sections—is that the due date will be miscalculated and the operation undertaken prematurely before he or she comes of age for a normal delivery. What's more, studies have shown that babies delivered surgically are twice as likely to die as those delivered normally. For mother, the complications of a cesarean section are likewise far from innocuous.

Generally, however, physicians insist the higher risk associated with surgical deliveries is a result of the initial problem that leads to the c-section in the first place. The truth is, however, studies undertaken to evaluate complication rates from c-section specifically refer to problems encountered due to the surgery or the actual birthing process. Anesthetic mishaps, excessive blood loss, urinary tract infections, wound infections, thrombophlebitis and pulmonary embolism (blood clot in the lung) occur in 25 to 50 percent of the patients.

The risk of maternal death during a cesarean procedure varies, of course, according to the hospital. But in the course of an 11-year study, John R. Evrard, M.D., and Edwin M. Gold, M.D., from the department of obstetrics and gynecology of Brown University Medical Program and the Women and Infants Hospital of Rhode Island, found that in their state a woman's risk of death at delivery was 26 times higher if she had a cesarean section than if she was allowed to deliver vaginally (*Obstetrics and Gynecology*, November, 1977). The national death rate, however, is 4 to 10 times higher than for vaginal birth. Better, but not terrific.

Those who make it through the surgery with flying colors, however, may not be home free. Serious complications directly related to a cesarean are known to surface years later. The dense scar tissue left in the wake of a c-section has been responsible for deaths years later from intestinal obstruction or from hemorrhage or bladder complications in the course of a hysterectomy. Vertical cesarean incisions have also been known to rupture during subsequent pregnancies.

The Emotional Impact

Of course, the psychological impact of a cesarean delivery is nothing to be scoffed at either. With the big push toward natural and husband-coached childbirth, women who are rushed off to surgery at the last minute, and who are unconscious and alone during the birth of their children, are often overcome with emotion-charged feelings of inadequacy, violation and lack of control. They may be depressed because they feel that they have failed somehow, or angry because they believe that the physician has cheated them out of a very important personal experience. These feelings are not unusual.

In *Birth and the Family Journal* (Fall, 1977), Nancy Cohen, of C/SEC, writes: "Judging from 13,000 letters, and several thousand personal interviews, we have observed that a significant number of cesarean couples are devastated by the experience. An unexpected cesarean delivery, often following a long, arduous labor or a terrifying alarm for the baby's well-being during labor, can be a shattering emotional experience."

When a C-Section Is Really Needed

Obviously, the best way to avoid the pitfalls of cesarean is to avoid the procedure altogether—or at least avoid it except in those cases when it's absolutely, positively necessary. But unfortunately, that's not always practical. If your doctor recommends that you have a cesarean because your child's life will be threatened otherwise, or your condition absolutely warrants it, you'd better take his advice despite whatever misgivings you

may have. It would be pretty hard to live with the guilt later if you ignored his warning and something went wrong.

Of course, if you know ahead of time that your doctor plans to do a cesarean, it's not a bad idea to get a second or third opinion. But if you're on the delivery table when the decision is made, it's not going to be easy to defy him—and it probably wouldn't be too wise, either.

Support groups like C/SEC as well as concerned physicians and psychologists generally agree that the best way to minimize at least the emotional devastation following cesarean section is to better inform and prepare yourself for the experience. That goes for every pregnant woman, whether or not she expects to have a c-section—because you never know. Remember, as many as 25 percent of all delivering mothers in the United States do have cesareans. And according to a study by an assistant professor of nursing at the University of Arizona at Tucson and a head nurse at Tucson Medical Center, 41 percent of the women interviewed had less than two hours to prepare for the reality of it (*Birth and the Family Journal*, Summer, 1978).

Two hours, they say, may be insufficient time to grasp all the events occurring and to rally one's resources for coping. The result: anxiety. "Some women," the nurse-researchers add, "actually experience near-panic."

The first thing you should arm yourself with is the knowledge of why cesarean sections are performed. That way, should an unforeseen situation arise in the course of your labor and delivery, you'll know whether or not surgery is justified. Second, you should be well informed about what happens during a cesarean delivery. Some prepared-childbirth classes now include a session on cesarean section, including a film of the procedure and a tour of the operating room. Of course, if you do expect to have a cesarean, there are special preparatory classes just for you. C/SEC's classes, for example, discuss common concerns and feelings, as well as explanations of why and what will happen. (see *Appendix*).

The Bright Side of C-Sections

It's also a good idea to educate yourself and to discuss with your doctor both his practices and the hospital's policies regarding cesarean birth. You might be surprised at some of the options you do have. For example, an approach that is gaining wide acceptance is the family-centered cesarean childbirth experience. What it does is allow both mother and father to become participants in the birthing process—at least to the extent that both are present during the birth and are able to touch, hold and bond with their infant immediately after birth. Mother is sedated with spinal or epidural anesthesia, which numbs her from the waist down but allows her to be awake to greet her newborn.

For years hospitals and physicians have resisted couples' desire to participate in cesarean deliveries. Many still do, for all the kinds of reasons you'd suspect. Fathers will faint, opponents insist. They'll interfere with the surgical procedure and contaminate the sterile surroundings.

But in the book *Having a Cesarean*

Baby (E. P. Dutton, 1978), Richard Hausknecht, M.D., and Joan Rattner Heilman strongly disagree with that kind of rationale. They cite a recent study by a group of obstetricians at the University of Michigan School of Medicine, in which "there was no increase in the incidence of infection when fathers, gowned, masked, and scrubbed, were allowed to attend cesarean births. Nor were there any significant interferences in the surgical procedure." Even more importantly, they add, "the women whose husbands were there for the delivery showed a more positive feeling toward the birth than the usual cesarean mother; they felt less lonely, less inadequate, and less helpless."

In Nancy Cohen's paper on "Minimizing the Emotional Sequellae of Cesarean Childbirth," she, too, reports that husband-supported cesarean childbirth benefits both partners. "For a great many cesarean couples, the single most important factor influencing feelings about the birth is whether the father was present at the delivery," she says. "The most intense feelings are those of separation, occasionally desertion, on the part of both parents" (*Birth and the Family Journal*, Fall, 1977).

Of course, any couple who is interested in sharing the cesarean childbirth experience should be sure to get the full cooperation of their obstetrician, anesthesiologist and hospital. In addition, both parents must attend a prepared-childbirth class that includes illustrated sessions on cesarean birth.

CHILDBIRTH

If there's one word that typifies today's childbirth experience, it's "choices." Choices in delivery methods, birthing locations, attendants, procedure, you name it—even choices in painkilling drugs if that's the route you choose. There's no longer one absolute way of doing things. Each case is different. And since this is your special day—and how this day comes off could have some definite long-range implications for you and your child—you're the one who should be helping to make these decisions . . . very carefully.

Actually, we shouldn't give the impression here that childbirth choices automatically fall into your lap. Much depends on the community you live in, the hospital policies that exist there, and of course, the attitudes of your physician. Some women still have to fight for every birthing belief they hold. Others may find an attentive obstetrician who agrees 100 percent with their ideals, only to face some unforeseen problem in the final hours of labor that preempts all that careful planning. It happens. But the point is, the better informed you are of all your options, the better prepared you'll be to deal with decisions when they come up—even those that pop up unexpectedly in the delivery room. And with all that good sense and know-how behind you, you've got no choice but to have a better (safer and more satisfying) childbirth experience.

Where Should You Give Birth?

For the longest time, home births were routine. When a woman's time came, she took to her own bed, and with a little help from her family and friends, gritted her teeth and bore down until her baby came crying into the world. Then all that changed (for the better, we thought) and the hospital became The Place to have your baby. A laboring mother was whisked off to a white-washed delivery room where a crew of scrubbed and masked strangers stood by to "deliver" her. And often that first impression of the delivery room was the last recollection she'd have of giving birth. If she wasn't knocked completely unconscious by an injection or inhalation of some potent anesthetic, she was reduced to an incoherent, restless, mumbling mom through the use of another anesthetizing technique referred to in almost rock-a-bye-baby terms as "twilight sleep."

Surely nobody thought for a minute that such a state could be considered tranquil. But the practice persisted. It wasn't until women really woke up to the depressing reality of such dehumanizing treatment that things began to change and women began to have choices. Many couples are no longer satisfied by simply having a good baby. They're looking for a good experience, too.

For many women, a good experience means having a natural childbirth at home without all the drugs, hassles or family separation that a hospital birth often entails. For assistance, these women are turning away from the typical ob-gyn and putting their faith in a new breed of age-old birthing professionals—midwives. Today, we've got "certified nurse-midwives," which means that they are registered nurses with special obstetrical training (see

Gynecologists and Their Alternatives).

One woman who had it both ways (a hospital birth and a home birth) explains the difference this way: "At home with a nurse-midwife and my husband I was able to endure the waiting and contractions in comfort and dignity. In the hospital, I just endured.

"I remember when they wheeled me into the delivery room for my first baby, I was annoyed to see three interns standing off to one side of the room. They were there, I suppose, to observe the procedure, but this particular 'procedure' was my private experience. No one had thought to ask my permission before issuing invitations. I felt helpless. I was lifted and placed on a cold delivery table and covered with what seemed like a dozen surgical drapes. My feet were fitted into stirrups and my legs and arms were strapped to the table.

"By contrast, my second very different childbirth experience began with my husband and I going calmly into the bedroom to do the Lamaze breathing exercises. As we worked together, I heard my son outside laughing as he played on his swings. Hearing his voice gave me comfort. And I thought—how many women are fortunate enough to give birth to their second child as the sound of their first child's laughter fills the air?

"By 1:00 the midwives had arrived. We all got in our positions. I was sitting up, my hands locked behind my knees, in the position I'd learned in the Lamaze class. My husband was with me. The midwives at my head and feet. I pushed, hard . . . I gasped. I sobbed. I laughed. All the waiting, the pain, the work—all the discomfort vanished in that one fantastic moment."

You may be wondering, however, whether home births are safe. And un-fortunately, the answer to that question depends on which study you read or which expert you choose to listen to.

Lori Breslow, editor of *How to Get the Best Health Care for Your Money* (Rodale Press, 1979) thoroughly investigated the pros and cons of home vs. hospital births. The following discussion has been excerpted from her research.

Lewis Mehl, M.D., and his associates at the Center for Research on Birth and Human Development have done probably the most thorough testing to date on the safety of home birth, she explains. In a 1977 study conducted by Dr. Mehl, Lewis Leavitt, Gail Peterson and Don Creevy, 1,046 hospital births in Madison, Wisconsin, were compared to 1,046 home births in northern California. Each hospital patient was matched with a home birth patient for age of the mother, number of previous children, income, education, state of health, and medical history. One hundred percent of the hospital births had physicians in attendance; two-thirds of the home births were attended by the family doctor, the rest by midwives. According to *NAPSAC News* (put out by the National Association of Parents and Professionals for Safe Alternatives in Childbirth):

> The results were astonishing: In the hospital, the fetus had a 6 times greater incidence of distress in labor, babies were caught in the birth canal 8 times more frequently, and mothers were 3 times more likely to hemorrhage in the hospital than at home. Furthermore, 4 times as many babies in the hospital needed resuscitation, infection rates were 4 times higher, and chances of permanent injury at birth were over 30 times greater in the hospital. . . .

This and similar studies led NAP-SAC to conclude, "Birth at home with a competent attendant and hospital back-up is safer than the hospital for healthy mothers."

Their conclusion is countered, however, by the American College of Obstetricians and Gynecologists (ACOG). In its official statement on home deliveries, ACOG maintained, "Labor and delivery, while a physiological process, clearly present potential hazards to both mother and fetus before and after birth. These hazards require standards of safety which are provided in the hospital setting and cannot be matched in the home situation."

While it may be impossible to draw definite conclusions about the safety of home birth at this time, there are several things that can be said with relative certainty. First, not even the most ardent home-birth supporters believe that every birth should be a home birth. NAPSAC itself recognizes that hospitals are necessary for mothers who have serious medical problems.

If, for instance, you have any of the following, you should not plan on having your baby at home: diabetes; previous cesarean birth or other serious uterine surgery; toxemia symptoms; previous history of hard-to-control hemorrhage; a first baby that is in the breech position; a baby of less than 36 weeks gestation; the possibility of Rh factor incompatibility; generally poor health including severe anemia or malnutrition; extreme overweight; and twins (sometimes). Check with your doctor or midwife about other possible problems that could make you a poor home-birth risk. And remember that no one can guarantee that your birth will be problem-free—all they can do is give you the odds.

Home births take an enormous amount of preparation, so another factor to take into consideration is whether or not you're willing to put in the necessary time and effort.

As in all pregnancies, prenatal care is extremely important. That includes a preliminary and thorough examination within the first trimester, periodic checkups, a good nutrition program, and regular exercise. In addition, classes in prepared childbirth, which train the woman and her coach to deal with the hard work of labor and delivery, should also be taken, and you can enroll in classes in other areas relating to pregnancy, birth, breastfeeding and child-rearing, as well. The Association for Childbirth at Home, International (ACHI), for instance, offers a series of six classes covering advantages of home birth, the normal birth, psychological issues, medical considerations, preparation for birth, and the newborn. Finally, you would no doubt benefit from the advice of one pregnant woman who simply said, "I read everything I can get my hands on," for, as another mother expressed it, "the more we learned the better we felt."

Along with your own knowledge of what to do in an emergency, you must also have a plan for easy access to a cooperative hospital should the need arise. (The word "cooperative" needs to be stressed here, since there have been horror stories of women in need of prompt medical attention who were turned away from a hospital because they had attempted a home birth.) It's your responsibility to prepare both emotionally and physically for the possibility of going to the hospital by attending the tour for expectant parents at the backup hospital, obtaining and filling out preregistration forms and checking in advance to find out what kinds of financial arrangements may be necessary. Some attendants will not take families who live more than 30 miles from a hospital.

A Compromise Many Are Choosing

Again, it needs to be emphasized that deciding for or against home birth is often not an easy matter. The primary tradeoff seems to be access to emergency equipment and facilities at a hospital vs. the psychological benefits of being in one's own home. For some, the perfect compromise seems to be a maternity center.

Most simply, a maternity or childbearing center is a place where couples can come to have their babies in a homelike atmosphere. But since nurse-midwives are in attendance and some medical equipment is available, it is also a place that is more medically oriented than a private home. You might call it a "halfway house," for it combines many of the advantages of both home and hospital.

Unlike home-birth families, parents who choose maternity centers tend to have some reservations about giving birth at home. They may want to be closer to medical equipment or a backup hospital. Or they may want to have the continued contact with and support of medical professionals. Whatever the reason might be, the maternity or childbearing center provides the perfect alternative for people caught in the home-or-hospital dilemma.

Maternity centers may combine the best of hospital and home birth, but, as with all compromises, they have their drawbacks, too. Just as maternity centers do not have the sophisticated

medical equipment found in hospitals, they also are not as comfortable or familiar as your own home. Considering these disadvantages against the advantages will help you decide if a maternity center birth is for you.

For some women—even those with no apparent problems—having sophisticated medical care and equipment close at hand "just in case" provides a certain amount of emotional reassurance that they need. For them, a hospital birth is a must. But there's no reason that that experience must be anything less than fulfilling. Today, many options in hospital birthing experiences exist, depending, of course, on your community.

For example, in Reading, Pennsylvania, and other areas, certified nurse-midwives function as independent health care practitioners. There a woman can have a hassle-free, home-style birth experience in the sanctuary of a hospital delivery room. In other areas, hospitals have set aside birthing rooms which are decorated very much like a bedroom so a woman can deliver in a comfortable "at home" atmosphere even though she isn't in her own home—and best of all, know that emergency care is just down the hall, if she needs it.

Hospitals are sensitive to consumer demands and criticisms—especially from an economic point of view. According to one nurse-midwife who is responsible for many innovations at her hospital (many changes have been made through the efforts of hospital personnel), "Consumers have to take the initiative. They have to say, 'Look, I want X, Y, Z in maternity care.'"

Aiming for a Drug-Free Delivery

One area where women have really begun to put their foot down is in the anesthesiology department. It's not that they relish pain. It's just that they're beginning to realize that childbirth can be a rewarding, enriching and satisfying experience. Ask anyone who's been there. To watch as the fruit of your labor makes its way from your body to the outside world has got to rank as one of the most thrilling experiences of all time. But, in order to be a participant and observer in the delivery room, you obviously can't be out cold.

Beyond the psychological benefits, of course, a drug-free delivery means a better start for your baby.

Unfortunately—and unbelievable as it may sound—research into the after-effects of birthing anesthesia on the infant remains somewhat scant. But those studies that have been carried out do indicate that newborns of anesthetized mothers fare worse than the newborns of nonmedicated mothers in many important ways, including strength, coordination, sucking ability, heart rate, breathing, response to stimuli, and electroencephalograph (brain wave) readings. Whether these immediate difficulties hold any long-term implications is not clear. But there are many who are voicing serious concern.

In particular, they point to the fact that at birth the human baby is still at a tender stage of ongoing physical and mental development. Not only may this rapidly developing body be more vulnerable to damage by potent drugs, but those organs most susceptible to drugs (brain and central nervous system) or most needed for drug detoxification (liver) and excretion (kidneys) are the least well developed at the time of birth. In short, the newborn is poorly equipped to handle potent drugs.

Furthermore, most if not all drugs used in labor and delivery cross the placenta readily, and once they enter baby's circulation, there is the tendency for them to accumulate in the most susceptible organs—brain, liver, and kidneys—to a much greater extent (proportionately) than in the mother. For example, within two minutes of lidocaine administration to pregnant guinea pigs, lidocaine concentration is three times as great in the fetal liver as in the maternal liver and remains that high (*Anesthesiology*, February, 1972).

Of course, there are many types of drugs and anesthetic agents administered to laboring women and not all of them, obviously, are responsible for the same type or degree of side effects. Generally, however, the less anesthesia you require, the better the outcome for your offspring.

Seven studies have shown that the use of general anesthesia (which causes total loss of sensation as well as loss of consciousness) is associated with poorer infant performance than the use of regional anesthetics (which cause a loss of sensation to just one region of the body, as is the case with an epidural or saddle block). In addition, one study suggests that a regional anesthetic is still worse, in terms of infant outcome, than a local anesthetic which numbs an even smaller area of the body (*Anesthesiology*, February, 1974).

Again, what long-term effects any of these painkillers have on the infant is still unclear. But according to the preliminary analysis of an important study now awaiting approval by the National Institutes of Health (NIH), babies born to anesthetized mothers are likely to experience physical and mental disorders for a longer time after birth than was previously believed.

In what may be the first large-scale, long-term study of its kind, over 3,000 infants born in several teaching hospitals (95 percent of them to anesthetized mothers) were tested at 4, 8 and 12 months of age. The results were then correlated to each drug or drug combination given to their mothers.

The researchers concluded, among other things, that the inhaled anesthetics were by far the worst and that meperidine, the synthetic narcotic that "has been for many years the most popular painkiller in obstetrical practice" also appeared to leave its mark on the offspring even after four months' time.

Unfortunately the specific results of this study are being held up by NIH officials, who are reevaluating the data and who may very well draw conclusions that vary widely from those stated above. But whatever the case, we should consider this at least a red flag to potential problems that may result.

For that reason, many childbirth preparation classes advocate several methods of natural pain relief. The Lamaze technique, for example, stresses breathing exercises and deep concentration by focusing on an intricate painting or your partner's face to distract from the painful contractions. The Bradley method, on the other hand, emphasizes body relaxation and "going with" the contraction.

Studies have confirmed that women who take these preparatory programs before giving birth are better able to deal with the experience. In one such study, it was shown that mothers who were prepared to participate in the birth process tended to experience significantly shorter labors, and require less

medication and obstetrical intervention. And consequently they remembered the childbirth experience more favorably than did those mothers who did not attend these classes beforehand (Third Institutional Congress of Psychosomatic Medicine in Obstetrics and Gynecology in London, April, 1971).

Have a Labor Partner with You

If ever there was a family affair, giving birth to a new member of the family certainly qualifies. Yet until relatively recently, all family members (barring the one who obviously had to be there) were refused admission to hospital delivery rooms. Today, some hospitals have relaxed their guidelines and invite fathers-to-be to attend the birth of their children—even if it means allowing them in the operating room during a cesarean section. Others, however, resist the idea of a dad standing by, citing not only the prospect of his losing control and interfering with the work of the delivery personnel, but the added liability for the hospital, if, for example, he should faint and fall to the delivery room floor. Unbelievable, but true. One criticism that is no longer valid is that this extra stand-in will contaminate the sterile environment of the delivery room. Studies have shown and most physicians will readily agree that that's just not so if the father is appropriately gowned and masked (which is usually a prerequisite in most delivery room situations). In addition, most if not all hospitals require that the expectant couple complete a prepared childbirth education course such as Lamaze or Bradley.

Then, unless some unforeseen emergency arises or your particular hospital has some unique rules and regulations, there's no reason that you can't have your husband or partner near at hand to share the experience. That is, if you choose to. And, not surprisingly, most women do. In fact, according to a recent survey on maternity options, the number one priority involves the father. "Mothers want their husbands with them in labor and delivery, and they want them to have unrestricted visiting privileges after the birth," the researchers conclude (*Birth and the Family Journal*, Spring, 1978).

Actually, there's more than one advantage to having him there. Mates offer comforting moral support. They look out for a woman's better interest at a time when she may not be able to do it herself. And they actually aid the process of labor and delivery by participating in the experience, coaching the woman through her contractions. Their familiarity of presence is likely to add to a laboring woman's sense of calm. And calmness and cooperation during labor are now recognized as the key elements in a successful and satisfying birth experience for all involved.

For women who do not have a husband or partner to accompany them to the labor and delivery room, a mother, sister or close friend may provide the same kind of support. Researchers from Case Western Reserve University in Cleveland, Ohio, recently conducted a study in Guatemala on the effects of a supportive lay woman on women in labor and delivery. Their findings were pretty encouraging. Those women who were assisted by a caring person had much shorter labors than those who had no one to turn to besides the attending doctor and nurses—on the average, less than 9 hours compared to almost 20 hours for those in a control group who did not have that supportive person at hand. Also, when the mothers in the two groups were later observed alone with their newborns, there were some marked differences in their behaviors. The supported women resisted sleep longer so that they could fondle the babies. What's more, they smiled, talked to and stroked their babies more than the other women (*New England Journal of Medicine*, September 11, 1980).

Eat, Drink, and Be Mobile during Labor

Doris Haire, president of the American Foundation for Maternal and Child Health, reports that in practically every country except the United States, women are encouraged to get up and walk around during the first stage of labor. In those countries it is commonly believed that such activity facilitates labor by distracting the mother's attention from the discomfort or pain of her contractions and also by encouraging a more rapid descent of the baby's head into the birth canal.

At an annual meeting of the ACOG a few years ago, Dr. Roberto Caldeyro-Barcia, former president of the International Federation of Gynecologists and Obstetricians, presented information (obtained with accurate, modern methods of recording) that supports that concept. Uterine contractions are less frequent but considerably stronger when a woman is upright than when she is lying flat on her back, he said. This greater efficiency of contractions, combined with the natural pull of gravity, results in a significant shortening of the first stage of labor (*Family Practice News*, June 1, 1978).

In a cooperative effort at the Latin American Center of Perinatology and Human Development, over 250 laboring women were divided into two study groups. One group was told that they could walk around at will; the other was confined to bed. Women who walked through their first stage of labor (and 95 percent of those who were given that option did so) progressed from 4.5 centimeters to the full 10 centimeters of cervical dilation in 25 percent less time than those confined to bed. All told, Dr. Caldeyro-Barcia reports, the first stage of labor was reduced on the average by almost an hour and a half just by having the women up and around. In addition, forceps were required for the delivery in only 1 woman among the 181 who remained upright during the first stage of labor, compared to 11 women among the 143 who were in bed.

In another study—this one across the globe in England—68 women were similarly divided into two groups to determine what, if any, effects walking had in the first stage of labor. Here again, the length of labor was shorter for women who were allowed to move about—over two hours shorter, this time! In addition, some other very important benefits were noted.

For one thing, the mobile mothers needed significantly less drugs—either to speed the delivery along or to deaden the pain—than the mothers tucked away in bed. Benefits for baby were likewise recorded. According to Dr. Anna Marie Flynn and her associates at the Birmingham Maternity Hospital, there were 17 cases of reduced fetal heartbeat during the delivery of the recumbent women, compared to only 4 such fetal distress signals among the babies of those on the go. Apgar scores—the rating of a newborn based on assessments of heart rate, respiratory effort, muscle tone, reflexes, and color—were also lower for the babies of the bedridden group (*British Medical Journal*, August 26, 1978).

As for eating and drinking during the early stage of labor, evidence for *or* against is just not available. Doris Haire suggests that there's something unnatural if not unhealthy about depriving a woman of food and water during this very difficult and physically draining experience. Nevertheless, most obstetricians draw the line at ice chips, their argument being that in the event general anesthesia or major surgery becomes necessary, there shouldn't be anything in the woman's stomach.

"In the hospital, we're only allowed to give the woman in labor ice chips to eat," a nurse-midwife who assists both home and hospital deliveries told us. "At home we tell her to drink and drink and drink. She can even eat if she wants to. We haven't had any problem or complications resulting from that."

To Have and to Hold the Baby Immediately after Birth

Something very special takes place between a mother and her child—and a father and his child—in those first tender moments after birth. It's a time for greeting, touching, holding; a time for an intimate exchange of feelings and messages. It's called "bonding" and it's during this time, many experts now agree, that an attachment develops that may have long-lasting effects on the parent-child relationship. Studies have shown that the more contact a mother and child have with each other after birth, the stronger the ties between them seem to be.

Hospitals routinely present the new mother with her baby for only a short time after delivery, before the child is whisked off to the nursery. Parents are often not allowed to pick up crying infants in the nursery, fathers are barred or discouraged from being present in delivery rooms, brothers and sisters are kept from seeing their mother or the new baby. It's hygienic, mechanical birth for a hygienic, mechanical age.

When departures are made from this sterile routine, however, the results are significant. In one early study at Case Western Reserve University, mothers and babies who received routine treatment were compared with mothers who were given an hour of skin-to-skin contact with their babies at birth and five hours of extra contact each day they were in the hospital. At one month after birth, the mothers who had extra contact with their babies showed much more affectionate behavior toward them, and were more likely to enjoy gazing into their eyes. At one year, the extra-contact mothers spent more time at their children's side during a visit to the doctor, and more time soothing their children when they cried during the examination. At two years, these mothers used fewer commands and more questions whan talking to their children. Even at five years, their children had higher IQs and scored better on language tests than the children who had routine births.

Scientists at the University of Umea in Sweden found that even a slight increase in skin-to-skin contact between mother and child at birth can have important consequences later on. Mothers and infants who spent just 15 to 20 minutes together immediately after birth were compared with those who went through the routine procedure. Except for those 15 minutes, the two groups had identical experiences. At 36 hours after the birth, first-time mothers who had extra contact with their babies held their babies more often than first-time mothers without the extra contact, and their babies cried only half as much. After three months, the effects of those 15 minutes were still apparent. The extra-contact mothers continued to show more affection for their children, and their infants laughed or smiled more frequently. Fifteen minutes of touching had established an emotional bond so apparent it could be scientifically measured (*Acta Paediatrica Scandinavica*, March, 1977).

Even before research proved such things could happen, people were calling for restoration of the human touch to human birth. The French obstetrician Frederick Leboyer developed a system of birth to eliminate the gleaming-porcelain, bright-lights, slap-on-the-rump shock tactics of most hospital delivery teams. Leboyer birth takes place in a silent, darkened room. The baby rests quietly on the mother's stomach after birth, still attached to her by the umbilical cord, and is gently massaged for four or five minutes. The umbilical cord is cut only after it has stopped pulsing, and the baby is then immersed in a warm-water bath.

Again, the benefits of touching at birth are evident in later years. Leboyer babies observed in France at ages one, two and three showed advanced development. They were particularly adroit with both hands, started walking earlier, and had less trouble with toilet training.

Avoiding Unnecessary Medical Intervention

With all the tests, tubes, and monitoring equipment that surround even a problem-free birth these days, it makes you wonder if there is such a thing as a "normal" delivery. "The electronic fetal monitor (EFM), oxytocin challenge test (OCT), a cesarean section for breech presentation are now common practices, and amniocentesis is following the same pattern," writes Frederick M. Ettner, M.D., in *Women and Health* (September/October, 1977). "All are replacing the natural practice of birth."

Of course, there are those who would cite, for example, study after study that applauds fetal monitoring for its life-saving record. They wouldn't be wrong. EFM is credited with saving an untold number of newborns by alerting the attending physician of fetal distress early enough so that he or she has time to act and prevent a disastrous situation.

Understandably, however—and this is where the critics have their say—the biggest benefits of EFM occur in women who face the biggest risks—that is, in cases of a low birth weight and/or premature baby; induced labor; premature detachment of the placenta; or a maternal medical problem such as diabetes, high blood pressure, or toxemia of pregnancy. For women who face no unusual risk, the benefits of fetal monitoring are debatable—at best. In one study, for example, it was suggested EFM use in high-risk deliveries would save approximately 109 lives per 1,000 births. For women at low risk—76 percent of the mothers who took part in this study—there was no indication that being monitored made any difference in the outcome (*Journal of the American Medical Association*, April 27, 1979).

What's more, other studies suggest that the risk of fetal monitoring may well overshadow whatever slim benefit this procedure affords the low-risk mother. In order to monitor a fetus as it lies in the uterus, an electrode-containing probe is passed through the birth canal, its spiral tip embedded in the baby's scalp. As you can imagine, this procedure is not without some risk. For one

thing, scalp infections develop in 4.5 percent of the monitored infants. Other problems such as minor vaginal and cervical lacerations and fetal scalp bleeding occur during insertion. Once in place, the probe also provides a possible pathway for bacteria to move from the vagina into the amniotic fluid.

But perhaps the worst possible complication of fetal monitoring for the low-risk mother is that of cesarean section. In a landmark study by Albert D. Haverkamp, M.D., of Denver General Hospital in Colorado, 16.5 percent of monitored mothers were subsequently delivered via cesarean section compared to only 6.8 percent of those whose labors went by unrecorded. Most interesting of all, Dr. Haverkamp reports that there was no difference in infant outcome in either group, which makes you at least wonder: were 10 percent of the cesareans performed on monitored mothers done unnecessarily? (*American Journal of Obstetrics and Gynecology*, June 1, 1976). (See Cesarean Birth.)

Also, the whole experience of childbirth is notably hampered by electronic monitoring. Several studies have shown that as many as 30 to 40 percent of all women monitored have a negative reaction to the experience. This, these same studies indicate, can be softened somewhat by educating women to EFM in the course of their prepared-childbirth classes. Also, despite some obstetricians' insistence that monitored mothers must remain flat on their backs, these researchers contend that a woman with a monitor may move in bed, sit elsewhere in the room, and walk short distances. In fact, based on overwhelming evidence that mobility aids delivery, we would say that any movement you can manage in spite of the monitoring equipment would be to your advantage.

Another area of medical intervention in childbirth is labor induction. In order to get on with delivery, doctors often administer an I.V. drip containing Pitocin (a synthetic derivative of the hormone oxytocin which is naturally secreted by the pituitary gland and stimulates uterine contractions). Sometimes just a small amount of the drug is administered so contractions stop short of a full labor—just enough to test baby's stamina to go through with a full delivery. This is called the oxytocin challenge test, or OCT. And again, where once this test was prescribed for high-risk pregnancies, it has now become almost routine in some settings.

Trouble is, there is some question concerning the interpretation of the OCT—and worse, there may be complications created by the procedure of artificially inducing labor.

Studies have shown that about 25 percent of the patients who "fail" the OCT are nevertheless able to complete a normal labor and delivery with no complications. Meanwhile, cesarean sections continue unabated.

The process of labor induction—whether as a method of testing or an artificial start-up of the delivery which is usually undertaken when a pregnancy appears to be overdue (at least according to doctors' calculations, which are notoriously unreliable)—has definite drawbacks. Dr. Caldeyro-Barcia has demonstrated that uterine contractions stimulated with Pitocin put tremendous pressure on the fetal head. Contractions tend to be stronger, longer, and with shorter relaxation time in between. With each contraction, blood supply to the uterus is temporarily shunted, presenting the possibility that blood supply to the baby is likewise hampered.

When it comes to childbirth, there's new evidence that nature really does know best. The process of labor, for example, is not just a meaningless ordeal, researchers at Yale University's department of pediatrics and Lung Research Center have discovered. Instead, they report, natural labor somehow stimulates the formation of a critically important substance, called "surfactant," in the infant's lungs.

Without adequate surfactant, Seamus A. Rooney, Ph.D., and his colleagues note, the baby's lungs can't expand fully and respiratory distress—even serious illness and death—can result.

The Yale team found that in newborn rabbits, delivered by cesarean section prior to labor, lung surfactant levels were substantially lower than in newborns delivered after labor. Their research was published in the September, 1977, *Journal of Clinical Investigation*.

Another recent study, from the infant intensive care unit at Milton S. Hershey Medical Center, Hershey, Pennsylvania, also points to advantages in letting nature take its course. The study suggests that *elective* deliveries—deliveries performed at the scheduling convenience of either doctor or mother via cesarean section or drug-induced contractions—can lead to unnecessary and dangerous consequences. Eighteen of 38 infants admitted to the center following elective delivery suffered from hyaline membrane disease (HMD), a serious breathing problem which was clearly related to their premature arrival. One infant died (*Journal of the American Medical Association*, November 7, 1977).

Noting that other studies conclude that from 15 to 33 percent of HMD cases result from "inappropriate obstetrical management," the Hershey team concludes that "these observations are awesome when one considers the amount of time and effort that must be expended in the management of this condition in neonatal units, the potentially devastating (sometimes fatal) short- and long-term effects . . . and the enormous monetary investment.

"It has been estimated conservatively that there are about 40,000 cases of HMD in the United States annually. We have seen why it is possible that 6,000 (15 percent) and perhaps double that number are preventable."

COFFEE, TEA AND CAFFEINE

What do you get out of a cup of coffee? A morning morale booster? A late afternoon pick-me-up? That, plus maybe a whole lot you *didn't* bargain for.

My case in point: there was a time, several years ago, when I couldn't eat, sleep, or remember where I dropped my house keys five minutes after I pulled the front door shut behind me. I was nauseated and had indigestion after each meal. And I was so anxious and fidgety that I couldn't finish a cup of coffee before reaching for a refill.

So I did what any persevering and self-preserving person would do—I dragged my tired, vaguely aching body to no less than three physicians.

The first promptly diagnosed my condition as a simple stomach virus of elusive origin and sent me away with a week's prescription for antibiotics.

Doctor number two proclaimed me a nervous wreck. No bug this time—only a bad case of "acid stomach," which, he explained, may be brought on by stress. The cure: two tablespoons of antacid and one blue tranquilizer with each meal.

Still no change. But before committing myself to an early retirement, I decided to give one more M.D. a whirl. This time, the examination revealed a very low blood pressure reading and extremely rapid pulse rate.

"Do you like coffee?" he asked.

"Uh-huh," I nodded skeptically, though, in fact, during the past month or so—while I'd cut out food for the sake of a few pounds—coffee had been sustaining me. Eight cups a day were not unusual. I had coffee for breakfast, an apple and coffee for lunch and coffee breaks straight through the afternoon.

He concluded that I was having a severe reaction to caffeine. My only alternative was to give up my long love affair with coffee and my short-lived fling with weight control.

Some prescription, huh?! Well, there must have been something to it, because within two weeks of giving up coffee and digging into a balanced diet supplemented with plenty of B complex vitamins (caffeine is known to destroy the B vitamin thiamine which is essential to nerve function), I felt the frustrations of forgetfulness flee. I regained my appetite and that long-lost ability to sleep.

Actually, I was lucky to find a physician with the foresight to link my kaleidoscope of crazy symptoms with diet. Truth is, just because Robert Young booms across our TV tube with reminders that "caffeine can make you nervous," few Dr. Welbys out here in the real world think to inquire about coffee and tea habits.

Anxiety by the Cupful

For example, in 1974, John F. Greden, M.D., reported the case of a 27-year-old army nurse who visited a base clinic complaining of lightheadedness, headache, breathlessness, irregular heartbeat and a sense of anxiety that had developed over a three-week period. After a number of laboratory tests turned out negative, she was referred to the psychiatric clinic. The diagnosis: "anxiety reaction (probably secondary to the fear that her husband would be transferred to Vietnam)."

The nurse thought this was nonsense, and decided to take a closer look at her diet, something the clinic doctors had ignored completely. She realized that since the purchase of a drip coffeepot that produced much better-tasting coffee, she had been drinking 10 to 12 cups a day. Her anxiety had started just after she bought the pot. Putting two and two together, she quit drinking coffee, and her symptoms disappeared within 36 hours.

In another case reported by Dr. Greden, a 34-year-old army personnel sergeant was driving the base medical staff "crazy with frequent clinic visits." He complained of severe headaches and anxiety. Three thorough medical exams in two years turned up nothing. The exams, of course, were not so thorough that they included questions about the sergeant's diet.

It was not until he was referred to the psychiatric clinic that someone thought to ask him about his caffeine intake.

The sergeant was a heavy coffee drinker, and had been taking 8 to 10 caffeine-containing headache pills a day. When he cut back on caffeine, the headaches and anxiety disappeared.

These cases and others Dr. Greden discovered, led him to conclude that "high doses of caffeine—or 'caffeinism'—can produce pharmacological actions that cause symptoms essentially indistinguishable from those of anxiety neurosis" (*American Journal of Psychiatry*, October, 1974).

Bad as this sounds, it's not all of it. Edwin J. Mikkelsen, M.D., a psychiatrist at Yale University, reports two cases of psychotic reactions triggered by caffeine in patients with an underlying schizophrenia (*Journal of Clinical Psychiatry*, September, 1978). In one case, a 28-year-old woman suffered from delusions and hallucinations. Before her first psychotic episode, she recalled later, she felt "a mounting sense of anxiety" and greatly increased her coffee drinking above her usual four to five cups a day. After she was released from the hospital she found "that if she drank coffee she would 'feel strange' and begin to think in a paranoid manner." She stopped drinking coffee.

Caffeine and its sister drug, theobromine, may also be at the root of restless legs syndrome—a creeping crawling sensation in the legs which we discuss more fully later under its own heading.

What Coffee Can Do to Women

Actually, caffeine and theobromine have recently been implicated in problems that specifically affect women. At the University of Washington in Seattle, for example, researchers have discovered that drinking six to eight cups of coffee a day during pregnancy may cause babies to have lower birth weights and poorer-than-average muscle tone sometimes resulting in breech births. In a separate study of 16 heavy coffee-drinking mothers-to-be (eight or more cups a day), only 1 came through labor and delivery without complications. The other 15 pregnancies ended in spontaneous abortion, stillbirth or premature birth (*Postgraduate Medicine*, September, 1977).

And, finally, an Ohio State University scientist, John P. Minton, M.D., Ph.D., reports that in two-thirds of all the women tested, benign breast lumps disappeared when they eliminated coffee, tea, chocolate and cola from their diets (*Journal of the American Medical Association*, March 23, 1979).

Clearly, caffeine presents a greater potential for harm in the hands of women than of men. Yet according to studies of coffee-drinking habits in the United States, women are right up there with men in their average consumption of slightly more than two cups a day. What most people fail to realize is that it takes just two cups of strong, black coffee to deliver 300 milligrams of caffeine. That's 50 milligrams more than the minimum dosage cited by the American Pharmaceutical Association's *Handbook of Nonprescription Drugs* (Fifth Edition, 1977) as capable of causing "insomnia, restlessness, irritability, nervousness, tremor, headaches, and in rare cases, a mild form of delirium manifested as perceived noises and flashes of light."

Caffeine—which occurs naturally in the coffee bean, as well as the leaves of tea, cola (kola) nuts, and the maté plant—is a powerful drug that acts directly on the central nervous system. Initially, it peps you up, gives you a lift, and makes you feel more energetic. What could be wrong with that?

Well, the trouble is, caffeine creates an artificial high and, as the effects wear off, it dumps you in a very real pit. Now you know why, in the aftermath of the afternoon coffee klatch, you feel lethargic, lazy, drowsy, and occasionally depressed. The only way to get back up is by reinforcing this stimulation throughout the day with more coffee, cokes or tea. No wonder caffeine is addictive. And chances are, if you drink two or more cups a day every day, you're hooked.

A Warning about Coffee Withdrawal

Don't believe us? Think you can quit—cold turkey—tomorrow? Let me warn you, giving up coffee can be as difficult as kicking a cigarette habit or swearing off alcohol. Depending on the severity of your addiction, withdrawal can be a headache—literally. One recent study describes caffeine withdrawal symptoms as follows: "The subjects experienced lethargy in the morning of the day of withdrawal. By noon, there was fullness in the head. Headache usually began early in the afternoon and reached a peak three to six hours later. Nausea occurred in some and vomiting was also reported. Mental depression, drowsiness, yawning, and disinclination to work were also noted" (*New York State Journal of Medicine*, February, 1977).

So as not to burden your head with withdrawal, try eliminating caffeine gradually. An easy first step would be to quit drinking cola soft drinks. At this point the colas make up only one-quarter of the total American caffeine diet, and eliminating them won't put you too much on edge. As a bonus, you'll be cutting a lot of refined sugar (that's empty calories) from your diet. There are plenty of natural fruit juices to substitute and there's always water.

CAFFEINE CONTENT IN EVERYDAY BEVERAGES, CHOCOLATE AND MEDICATIONS

BEVERAGE	Milligrams per cup (about 5 fluid ounces)
COFFEE[a]	
instant	40–108
instant decaffeinated	2–8
percolated	64–124
roast and ground decaffeinated	2–5
TEA, BLACK[a]	
bagged	48–78
instant	24–31
loose leaf	30–48
TEA, MATÉ[b*]	35–45
HOT COCOA[c]	0.5

CHOCOLATE[c]	Milligrams per 2-ounce bar
bittersweet	17
milk	17

MEDICATION[d]	Milligrams per tablet
STIMULANTS	
Nodoz tablets	100.0
Vivarin	200.0
WEIGHT CONTROL DRUGS (reduce appetite)	
Appedrine	100.0
Dexatrim	200.0
PAINKILLERS	
Anacin	32.5
Bromo-Seltzer	32.5/capful
Excedrin	64.8
COLD AND ALLERGY DRUGS	
Dristan	16.2
Midran Decongestant	32.5
Sinarest	30.0
MENSTRUAL AIDS	
Femicin	65.0
Midol	32.4
Pre-Mens Forte	100.0

SOURCES: [a] Alan W. Burg, "Effects of Caffeine on the Human System," *Tea and Coffee Trade Journal*, January 1975.
[b] Information provided by Celestial Seasonings, 1979.
[c] Information provided by Wisconsin Alumni Research Foundation, 1976.
[d] *Handbook of Nonprescription Drugs*, 5th ed. (Washington, D.C.: American Pharmaceutical Association, 1977).

NOTE: Caffeine belongs to a group of chemicals called xanthines, which includes theophylline (found in tea) and theobromine (found in chocolate). All act on the central nervous system as stimulants and while caffeine has been studied more extensively, all potentially have the same side effects.

*Maté is also used in some herb teas.

A second step is to exercise great caution when using cold and allergy tablets. These pills represent an invisible dose of caffeine; when you drink coffee you know what you're getting into, whereas with cold remedies, you want relief, and are generally less inclined to worry about how the pill does it. You should worry, because these pills, taken with coffee or tea, can boost your caffeine intake to dangerous levels.

The big question, of course, is what to do about the coffee. Perhaps the best way to handle this problem is to do some downshifting—and by that, we don't necessarily mean switching to decaffeinated coffee.

The solvent commonly used to extract caffeine from coffee beans is methylene chloride, a chemical suspected of causing cancer. A water solvent extraction method has been developed, but this still uses methylene chloride as part of the process. Also, despite its name, decaffeinated coffee *does* contain caffeine—from 2 to 15 milligrams per cup.

So even if you do decide to switch over, make it a temporary substitute. Keep cutting down slowly on the number of regular or decaf cups you drink each day. When you've reached a reasonable level, the leap from coffee to strong tea is not that far. And once you've switched to tea, you can take a number of further steps down the caffeine ladder. As our table shows, there is a significant variation in caffeine strength among the different brands of tea, and significant differences between tea brewed strong and tea brewed weak. You can move all the way down the scale from a strong cup of English Breakfast, with 107 milligrams of caffeine, to a weak cup of Tetley's, with only 18 milligrams.

Coffee . . . Tea . . . and Free

Researchers have also found that brewing tea from a bag or using a porous metal container cuts back on the caffeine content of the tea. Tea brewed loose for the same amount of time or to the same degree of color will have more caffeine than tea brewed from a bag.

So when you're drinking weak Tetley's brewed from a bag, you can make the final step to caffeine-free herbal teas (a few "herbal" teas contain maté, so be sure to read the label), and you're home free. Sounds easy, doesn't it? We know it isn't.

Just don't start feeling sorry for yourself before you have to. The words "herbal tea" weren't exactly designed to set off rockets in a caffeine junkie's brain, but there's more natural excitement lurking in a subtly blended herbal brew than could ever be found in that umpteenth coffee fix of the day.

For example, do you remember what it was like to taste what you were drinking? Well, your neglected palate won't know what hit it when you start experimenting with the myriad herbal blends.

The possibilities are endless. The blends can include as many as 20 ingredients such as camomile, spearmint, tilia flowers, lemongrass, raspberry leaves, passionflowers, orange blossoms, hawthorn berries, skullcap and rose petals. There is a whole spectrum of shadings of taste and emphasis possible. You'll find that certain combinations bring out the taste of a particular herb, while others serve to moderate the more blatant flavors in just the right way. One blend will be the perfect thirst quencher, while another will soothe a head cold like nothing else. You can even come up with your own concoctions if you feel like it.

This is the good old decaffeinated real world, where you're in charge of what you drink, rather than the other way around. It's not that bad, actually.

For more on the risks of caffeine, see Breastfeeding, Breast Lumps: Benign or Malignant? and Pregnancy and Nutrition.

CAFFEINE IN SOME BRANDS OF COFFEE AND TEA
(milligrams per cup)

COFFEE[a]	Drip Filter	Percolated	Instant
Brim (decaffeinated)	3	3	2
Maxim	(NA)	(NA)	55
Maxwell House	92	97	57
Sanka (decaffeinated)	5	3	2
Yuban	81	75	50

TEA[b]	Weak	Medium	Strong
Darjeeling (Twinings)	39	74	91
English Breakfast (Twinings)	26	78	107
Lipton	25	53	70
Red Rose	45	62	90
Tetley	18	48	70

SOURCES: [a]Information provided by General Foods Corporation, 1979.
[b]Daniel S. Groisser, "A Study of Caffeine in Tea," *American Journal of Clinical Nutrition*, October, 1978.

NOTE: (NA) Information not available.

While today's woman understandably resents comments like "a woman's place is in the kitchen," that's one place where many women still feel at home. And it's one place where what we do can affect not only our health, but the health of our whole family.

Actually, the first lesson in healthful cooking doesn't take place in the kitchen. Good kitchen sense begins in the supermarket.

Meandering from aisle to aisle on the heels of a shopping cart can leave you mesmerized by the colorful packages and towering merchandising displays. If you don't have a "plan" or haven't eaten dinner yet, there's no telling what you'll come home with. But chances are good that it will be a pretty bad selection—nutritionally. The odds are against you.

In your typical supermarket, for instance, you will probably find—as we did—more varieties of soda than you will of all the fresh fruits and vegetables put together. You might easily find 30 or 40 different kinds of cookies and 20 different kinds of crackers; if you find one kind of whole wheat flour, you're lucky. And the supermarkets further encourage the sale of soda, cookies, crackers and marshmallows with large end-of-aisle or last-minute, before-the-cash-register displays. With willpower faltering, you won't have much of a chance. In fact, according to one report I've seen, most people have no intention whatsoever of buying a lot of snack foods when they visit a supermarket; 78 percent of shoppers said their snack food purchases were made strictly on impulse.

This doesn't mean you *shouldn't* shop in a supermarket—but it does mean you should shop sensibly. One way to fight the urge to splurge on junk food is to eat first, then shop. There's no question that a full stomach can bolster your resistance to junk food. A good shopping list is another marketing must.

Let's look at your list now. It won't take us more than a few minutes to sort out the best nutritional bets from the worst ones. Just check off every item that is fresh, unprocessed, free of chemical additives, and low in fat. The fresh fruit and vegetables. Salad greens. The skim milk, yogurt and cottage cheese. The fish and poultry. The brown rice and whole grains. Don't be too discouraged if what you have left is practically your whole week's menu. Sunday's pot roast. Monday's bottled spaghetti sauce. Tuesday's canned tomato soup, white bread and processed American cheese spread. And so forth. This virtual smorgasbord of fat, sugar, salt, chemical preservatives and flavorings, and empty calories is the kind of diet that made America famous. And poor eating habits, like traditions, don't change overnight.

Nor should you expect them to. The key to successful kitchen metamorphosis is in the word "gradual." So don't automatically scratch the remaining items off your list. But do consider healthful and acceptable alternatives—say, brown rice for white; fresh vegetables for canned; mineral water or unsweetened fruit juice for sugary soda pop; and maybe roasted, unsalted peanuts for your usual potato chip snack fare. Also, try limiting your intake of red meat somewhat by substituting poultry and fish whenever possible. Or roast a fresh turkey breast or chicken for use in sandwiches instead of the usual lunch-meat items, which are often loaded with cancer-causing nitrites.

Now's the time to think about trying out some new recipes—maybe a healthful substitute for Wednesday night's pork roast with scalloped potatoes. If you don't already have a good natural foods cookbook, get one. Some suggestions: *Recipes for a Small Planet* (Ballantine, 1973); *The Vegetarian Epicure,* (Alfred A. Knopf, 1972) and *The Vegetarian Epicure: Book Two* (Alfred A. Knopf, 1978); *Laurel's Kitchen* (Nilgiri Press, 1976); *The Deaf Smith Country Cookbook* (Macmillan, 1973); *The New York Times Natural Foods Cookbook* (Quadrangle, 1971); and *The Natural Healing Cookbook* (Rodale Press, 1981). To get you started on your natural foods adventure, why not designate one dinner a week as vegetarian night? And don't be surprised by the subsequent deluge of requests coming in for *more* meatless meals!

You might also want to consider vegetables and fruits with more nutritional punch. For example, pink grapefruit has more than 40 times the vitamin A of white grapefruit and is usually sweeter—so you won't be tempted to sprinkle sugar over the top. Substituting romaine lettuce for iceberg could give you more than three times as much calcium, iron and vitamin C, and nearly six times the vitamin A.

Or maybe it's time to introduce your family to some altogether new vegetable flavors. A study done by a University of California scientist listed 39 of America's favorite fruits and vegetables in order of their popularity, and then ranked them again according to nutritive value. It was a shock to see that some of the most nutritious vegetables were at the bottom of the popularity poll.

Super-Nutritious Vegetables

Number one on the nutritional list, absolutely head and leaves above all others, is broccoli. Rather astonishingly, this green giant scores in the top 10 for every single one of the vitamins and minerals tested in the study—including vitamins C, A, and the B vitamins riboflavin, thiamine and niacin, as well as the minerals calcium, iron and potassium.

Second on the list is spinach. Third is brussels sprouts. Fourth belongs to the lima beans. Peas are listed as fifth. Asparagus is next, followed by artichokes, cauliflower, sweet potatoes and, yes, carrots (*Nutritional Qualities of Fresh Fruits and Vegetables*, Futura, 1974).

It's a good idea to buy your vegetables fresh rather than frozen or canned. And the fresher the better. Although it's a wonderful treat to indulge in strawberries or tomatoes in the middle of February, these pale vestiges of summer's harvest are nutritionally inferior. Produce shipped long distances is usually picked green and allowed to ripen en route. And therein lies the catch. In 10 tomato varieties tested, for example, Alley Watada, Ph.D., research food technologist with the U.S. Department of Agriculture (USDA) found that those picked green and ripened off the vine contained an average of 1,343 international units (I.U.) of vitamin A. Those plucked at the first blush of color contained 1,687 I.U. And those left on the vine until the optimum stage of ripeness, a whopping 1,960 I.U. That's quite a difference! And other studies suggest that vitamin C content may be likewise affected.

For optimum nutrition, then, rely on

fresh-picked produce preferably purchased from a local farmer's market or country produce stand. If fresh is out of season, buy frozen, but beware of added salt and sugar, not to mention those gooey cream sauces. Read labels carefully. *Canned* fruit and vegetables are at the bottom of the list nutritionally—but if you're in a pinch, canned fruit packed in water (usually available in the dietetic section of the supermarket) is a perfectly acceptable substitute for the real thing.

Be more aware of what's in the food you choose to eat. Comparison shopping should involve an ingredients check as well as a price evaluation. So read labels and avoid foods containing chemical additives and preservatives. Don't take headliners like "all natural" or "100% pure" for granted. The fine print may reveal otherwise. For example, a popular spaghetti sauce mix touts itself as an "all-natural blend of Italian flavors." Careful scrutiny of the box, however, discloses that the number one ingredient is sugar. Number two is salt. And further along in the list of ingredients you'll find monosodium glutamate and artificial color. Beware of different names given to the same ingredient. Sugar, for example, is disguised as dextrose, fructose, glucose, molasses, honey, brown sugar, sorbitol and so forth.

Draw the line at the obvious processed and convenience foods such as TV dinners, whipped toppings and frozen desserts found usually along one aisle in the supermarket. Paul J. Dunn, M.D., a Chicago nutrition-oriented pediatrician and father of 10, recommends that all his new mothers eliminate the obvious sugar-laden foods: cakes, pies, jelly rolls, sugarcoated cereals and so on. So don't stock your kitchen with these empty-calorie "foods"—their presence will only serve to haunt you.

"It isn't easy to find unchemicalized products," you're thinking. Well, you're right. But you can beat the system in some cases by making your own. Many of us, for example, use salad dressings every day that are full of chemicals. One popular commercial oil and vinegar dressing contains soybean oil, wine vinegar, water, sugar, salt, onion, flavoring, oxystearin, polysorbate 60, calcium disodium EDTA and artificial color.

A much more delicious dressing can be made quickly for only a few pennies a day—minus the chemicals. Just mingle some of your favorite herbs—garlic, basil, chives, parsley, mustard seed, even mint—in a delicate blend of oil and vinegar. Generally, the proportion of oil to vinegar is two to one—that is, two tablespoons of oil for every tablespoon of vinegar. But if you like a dressing with more zing, try a one-to-one combination. The great thing about homemade vinaigrette is that, in addition to being more healthful and tasting better, it's easy to make and fun because you can create a new and different combination every night.

Shopping for Healthful Meals

If you're lucky enough to have a fresh herb selection at arm's reach on the windowsill or just outside the kitchen door, you're set. If not, the herb and spice rack in your local supermarket offers an absolutely mind-boggling array of possibilities. You can also experiment with the various types of vinegar. Try apple cider vinegar or red wine vinegar, or a delightfully subtle vinegar infusion with fresh tarragon sprigs. For another twist, use a half-and-half combination of fresh lemon juice and vinegar.

Oils, too, provide an unexpected health and taste treat—at least they should. Unfortunately, some supermarket varieties fall short. They may contain chemical preservatives, and some, like soybean oil, are partially hydrogenated (a process that destroys the essential fatty acids).

Again, read the labels carefully. Or better yet, use vegetable oils as the perfect excuse to check out the stock in your local health food store. You'll be amazed at the selection. Sunflower, walnut and sesame oils—all low in saturated fat and high on flavor—are guaranteed to lend your salad the distinction it deserves. And, if your taste buds are bored by supermarket corn oils, treat them to the rich corn flavor of the "pressed" variety found in health food stores. Just remember, because these oils are less refined and contain no chemical preservatives, they should be stored in the refrigerator. It's not a lot to ask when you consider that good-quality fresh vegetable oils are not only more nutritious (with vitamin E and essential fatty acids) but help the body better absorb fat-soluble vitamins like E, A and D.

While wandering through the aisles of a health food store, check out the pasta rack. Whole wheat pasta products like macaroni, noodles and spaghetti add fiber and good nutrition to an otherwise ho-hum meal. But don't add them too quickly. "They look and taste different," cautions Bonnie Lappin, one of the owners of The Natural Grocer in Framingham, Massachusetts. She recommends a whole wheat and soy pasta for newcomers. "It looks similar to the white, but is more nutritious and easier to substitute than the completely whole wheat variety." Later you can add some whole wheat pastry flour (from soft wheat) for use in light pie crusts, cookies and even pancakes. One pound should start you off. Try making cornmeal bread, too. It's easy and takes only a few minutes. About a pound of whole grain cornmeal would be more than enough.

Eventually, you may want to add other whole grains, such as millet, buckwheat, barley, triticale (a cross between wheat and rye grain), and bulgur. But remember not to overbuy! Introduce one new grain at a time to your family and give them some time to adjust.

When snacking times come around, shun the pretzels and potato chips in favor of more healthful goodies. Almonds and walnuts are good for beginners, as are raisins. Buy one-half pound of each, then gradually add more when needed. Dried pineapple is great for a sweet tooth. Or sprinkle fresh coconut over fruit. Later you might like to add pumpkin seeds, sesame seeds and sunflower seeds. Nuts and seeds are great protein complements to legumes (beans and peanuts) and milk.

When you get into the natural swing of things, you can use nuts and seeds in muffins, salad dressings, dips and pastries. But beware! Nuts and seeds are high in calories, so if you're watching your weight, you had better limit your intake.

Legumes are another natural food important to the natural foods cook. Many people impulsively try soybeans when they first begin to change their diet. Don't make that mistake. True, soybeans are great alternatives to meat, but you have to grow used to their taste. So don't start with them. There are many other beans you can try first.

Stock up on lentils, kidney beans, chick-peas and limas at first. About a pound of each should start the ball rolling. Later you might want to try soybeans, black beans and pinto beans. Just remember to buy small quantities at first. One cup of raw beans usually makes 2½ to 3 cups of cooked beans.

Don't be afraid to try beans because you're uncertain how to cook them. We can suggest two excellent sources of information on cooking beans: *Diet for a Small Planet* (Ballantine, 1975) and a book by Nancy Albright called *Rodale's Naturally Great Foods Cookbook* (Rodale Press, 1977).

Probably the closest things to a boost-nutrition-quick scheme are sprouts. Ounce for ounce (based on dry weights) these concentrated powerhouses of goodness have less fat and 100 percent more protein than the seeds from which they sprang. Riboflavin, niacin and vitamin C content also take a leap when liberated from the lowly seed. Best, of all, sprouts taste good and make a delightful addition to salads and stir-fried dishes. For starters, try alfalfa, mung, garbanzo or lentils. Just follow our easy directions. Once you sample this delicately crunchy flavor, you'll want to start a jar every other day to insure a continual supply of fresh sprouts.

Keeping All That Good Food Fresh

After you do your shopping, *don't* get sidetracked and leave your groceries in the car while you run an errand. Make a beeline to your kitchen. Fresh fruits and vegetables contribute vitamins A and C and minerals like iron and calcium, so we should try hard to preserve what we can. Green leafy vegetables like spinach, Swiss chard and beet greens if allowed to wilt can lose nearly half of their vitamin C (*Journal of Agricultural and Food Chemistry*, March/April, 1976). Storing vegetables at room temperature for three days will cost you up to 70 percent of their folate.

SPROUTING SEEDS FOR SUPER NUTRITION

1. Toss about one tablespoon of alfalfa (or other) seeds into a glass jar. Cover with lukewarm water. Then top the jar with a doubled piece of cheesecloth and a rubber band or a special sprouting lid available in health food stores.

2. Soak seeds overnight.

3. In the morning, pour off the water, rinse seeds and drain with the jar turned upside down.

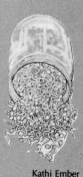

4. Set the jar aside (preferably in a dark cupboard) for three to four days. But don't forget it—you've got to remember to rinse the seeds with water and drain them three to four times each day.

5. On the third to fifth day the seeds should have sprouted sufficiently so you can transfer them to a sunny windowsill and watch those tender white morsels turn a delicate green.

Kathi Ember

Store your foods carefully as soon as you enter your kitchen. Refrigerate greens like kale, spinach, broccoli and turnip greens properly in the vegetable crisper to cut down on air circulation and loss of nutrients. Or store them in plastic bags, but be sure to punch holes to prevent sogginess. Exceptions to this rule are cucumbers, eggplants and peppers, which tend to go soft in bags. Don't wash your vegetables before storing. Leave green peas and lima beans in the pod until you're ready to cook them, and avoid bruising, cutting or crushing berries. They're excellent sources of vitamin C but if capped, cut or mashed, they lose much of it within a few hours.

In fact, don't prepare any fruits or vegetables in advance of your meal. You may save time, but you lose nutrients in the bargain. As much as half of the vitamin C in boiled, peeled potatoes may be lost if not used until a second day. If you must, cook potatoes in their peels and peel just before using.

Keep foods whole whenever possible or cut in large pieces. Different parts of plants vary in their nutrient content. Collard greens and kale, for example, have more vitamin A in their leaves than in their stems. The outer green leaves of lettuce, although coarser than the inner ones, have more calcium, iron and vitamin A. Broccoli leaves have more vitamin A than stalks or flower buds. Don't discard nature's treasures! Prepare them at the time you're cooking the vegetables or use them for soup stocks.

Trim fruits and vegetables only when absolutely necessary. Don't cut lettuce—it causes browning very quickly. Pull the leaves off and tear gently with your fingers. And never buy any precut vegetables like the "tossed salad" varieties if you want to preserve nutrients. Any crushing, chopping and shredding of foods increases surface area and sets free enzymes that cause loss of water-soluble nutrients. Because there is more loss with bruising, a sharp-bladed knife is usually recommended for paring and cutting produce. If you're nutrition-wise, you won't cut vegetables into small pieces before cooking them. French-cutting green beans increases loss of vitamin C, and cutting carrots crosswise results in greater loss of vitamin C than cutting them lengthwise into quarters.

Scrub but never peel potatoes—that's right, red skins in the potato salad make for better nutrition plus good looks! Experiments on commercial processing of potatoes done by two researchers associated with the University of Idaho and Washington State University found that peeling caused losses in all vitamins, but most severely in folate (*American Potato Journal*, October 1976). Potatoes boiled in their skins retain 90 percent of their thiamine compared to 75 percent in boiled, peeled potatoes. And a sweet potato boiled in its skin can retain close to 100 percent of its vitamin C. Washing and soaking add to the problem by leaching out vitamin C and the B vitamins especially.

Although fresh vegetables are always the best, there are times when they are not available. When using frozen vegetables, keep them frozen until you're ready to cook them to prevent nutrient losses.

Meats, too, are affected by various preparation methods. Most home economists and nutritionists recommend defrosting meat in the refrigerator immediately before you know you're ready to use it. Paul A. Lachance, Ph.D., and John W. Erdman, Jr., Ph.D., in *Nutritional Evaluation of Food Processing*

(Avi, 1975), report greater losses in nutrition and quality from thawing in water and at room temperature. And remember—nutrients are contained in the drip. The drip from thawed frozen beef contained 33 percent of the B vitamin pantothenate, 15 percent of the niacin and 8 percent of the folate that the meat had before thawing. And never wash or soak meats and poultry—just pat dry with a damp paper towel. Don't salt your meat, either, before you broil it—otherwise you'll be drawing nutrients and juices out.

How to Make Civilized Beans

Beans like soybeans, black beans and lima beans are a great part of a natural foods kitchen. They're an excellent source of B vitamins, high-quality protein and unsaturated fat. But many people avoid them primarily because they cause flatulence—gas. Joseph Rackis, Ph.D., a research chemist at the Northern Regional Research Center of the USDA, Peoria, Illinois, discovered that the flatulence factor can be completely removed by proper preparing and cooking beans.

Dr. Rackis explained to us that the gas is created because we cannot break down certain carbohydrates normally found in beans into simple sugar. These undigested carbohydrates move into our lower intestine and provide a banquet for the bacterial flora. During this process of intestinal digestion, carbon dioxide, hydrogen and methane are produced and result in gas.

As a result of his research, Dr. Rackis found that these hard-to-digest carbohydrates are water-soluble and can be completely eliminated by soaking beans for three to four hours, discarding the soaking water, cooking the beans in

boiling water for one-half hour, and discarding that cooking water. Then complete cooking in fresh water. "This procedure will get rid of the flatulence factor and keep nutrient loss to a minimum."

It is true that discarding the soaking and cooking water does destroy some nutrients, but if you are troubled by flatulence, that would be your best alternative. Dr. Rackis recommends that we add back to the beans vitamins and minerals that were lost in the soaking. To do this, he recommends the addition of about a teaspoon of brewer's yeast for every half cup of dried beans.

Whole grains also lose nutrients if washed before they're cooked. Brown rice, for example, loses 10 percent of its thiamine value if it's prewashed. So unless you're directed to do otherwise, don't wash your grains before you cook them.

Cooking with Nutrition in Mind

Did you know that the best cookery method could mean all of a 50 percent savings in lost nutrients? And a big boost in flavor, too.

The first rule is—don't waterlog your food. Flavor as well as important water-soluble nutrients like vitamins B and C and minerals like phosphorus, potassium and iron will be lost or leached into the cooking water.

"Quickly" is a word that offers an important clue to the mystery of lost nutrients. The shorter the cooking time, the greater the savings. Brian A. Fox and Allan G. Cameron, in their book *Food Science—A Chemical Approach* (Hodder & Stoughton, 1976), write that potatoes cooked for half an hour retain 66 percent of their vitamin C value. Cooked for an hour, they retain 50 percent. After 90 minutes, only 17 percent of the vitamin C is left.

One way to shorten cooking time is by adding vegetables directly to boiling water. Starting them in cold water causes the loss of additional vitamin C even before the water has a chance to boil. The loss is due to the continued activity of enzymes, which does not stop until the heat reaches a high enough temperature.

Eating your vegetables at the just-barely-tender stage rather than the soggy stage is another way to save time—and vitamins.

Still another good idea is an investment in plenty of pots with matching tops. Cooking with a tight-fitting lid eliminates continuous exposure to air, prevents steam and vapor from escaping, and makes possible the use of a small amount of water.

If you're in the habit of perking up those bright green vegetable colors by using baking soda—break it fast! Baking soda, because of its alkaline nature, changes the chlorophyll in green vegetables and creates a brighter green color. But water-soluble nutrients, especially vitamin C and thiamine (and to some degree riboflavin) are destroyed by it. Your best bet is to take it from your cabinet and store it in the refrigerator where it can eat up odors instead of nutrients.

Cooking liquid is a valuable reservoir of soluble vitamins and minerals. Serve it at the same meal with vegetables and meats as a sauce or gravy. And if you're watching calories, it's delicious on baked potatoes instead of butter. Or save it to add to your homemade soups. Since nutrients, especially vitamin C, are lost during refrigeration, keep a special container in your freezer and continue to layer all leftover vegetables and their liquids until it's filled. Then add it to your soups.

On the top of your things-to-remember list be sure to include steam cooking for vegetables. It requires very little water, so there's not much opportunity for snatching water-soluble nutrients.

In a review of scientific studies measuring cooking methods and nutrient loss, Dr. Lachance and Dr. Erdman in *Nutritional Evaluation of Food Processing* (mentioned earlier), refer to the work of Gordon and Noble, who measured the loss of vitamin C—the most sensitive—in vegetables cooked by boiling water, pressure cooker, tightly covered saucepan and steamer methods. Asparagus cooked in boiling water retained only 43 percent of its vitamin C compared to 80 percent when pressure cooked, 78 percent when steamed and 71 percent when prepared in a tightly covered saucepan.

So the next time you buy fresh raw spinach, spend a little more and drop a foldout steamer into your shopping cart. Just make sure it fits into your favorite pot, the one with the tight-fitting lid. When dinnertime rolls around, drop your steamer into the pot, cover the bottom of the pot with a small amount of water, bring it to a boil, add your spinach, cover and within a minute or two you'll have the best spinach you ever tasted!

Try a Pressure Cooker

And if you have a mind to—and the pocketbook—you might invest in a four- or six-quart pressure saucepan. It's an airtight utensil which heats food fast with steam under pressure. It's usually available wherever cooking appliances are sold, but is relatively expensive (about $35). A pressure cooker picks up where the steamer leaves off. Like the steamer, foods are cooked in a minimum amount of water, but much faster.

Pressure cooking does make use of higher temperatures and can influence nutrient losses. Georgene Barte, an associate professor in the department of nutrition at Oregon State University, Corvallis, told us that because of the high heat, pressure cooking may destroy heat-sensitive nutrients like folate, thiamine and vitamin A. However, regarding vitamin C, Fox and Cameron conclude that "...the amount of ascorbic acid [vitamin C] lost because of the increased temperature is more than compensated by the amount conserved due to the shorter cooking time. The use of pressure cookers is valuable, therefore, in conserving the ascorbic acid in fruits and vegetables as well as reducing cooking time."

Pressure cooking offers an important advantage to busy cooks or last-minute decision makers. "It's especially great for cooking potatoes, beets and beans," one natural foods cook told us. It can add a variety of foods to the diet, like beans, for example, that may not usually be included if slower methods are used. It isn't very good for leafy vegetables such as spinach—excessive heat affects the bright green colors. It's also not very good for strong-flavored vegetables like broccoli, cauliflower and cabbage, concentrating the flavor too much.

The "waterless" method also makes use of steam. Cooking is done in heavy saucepans with tight-fitting lids using only the water that remains on foods after rinsing, and the natural juices. Although it is preferred to boiling, it does not permit quick cooking, which may cancel the advantage of using little or no extra water. Nutrient loss is comparable to cooking quickly in a small amount of water.

Stir-frying is yet another way to bring deliciously interesting variety to your table. It is an oriental technique of quick-frying small pieces of vegetables or meats in a small amount of hot oil. Usually a special bowl-shaped pan with high-slanted sides called a wok is used, but a regular frying pan can be used as well.

There have been few scientific studies measuring nutrient loss during stir-frying and those that have been done report inconsistent results.

Most nutritionists and home economists we contacted agreed that stir-frying is a nutritious method because food is cooked quickly for a short period of time without using a lot of water. Therefore, soluble nutrients like minerals and B and C vitamins are sealed in, as are flavor and color.

The health hazards of conventional frying are also minimized in stir-frying. For example, frying methods which use a panful or, worse, a potful of oil dramatically increase the caloric content of foods. Stir-frying uses only a tablespoon or two of oil so any increase in calories is nominal. Even more important, stir-frying cooks quickly so the oil shouldn't get too hot for too long, which can cause polyunsaturated oil to break down into saturated fats and form potentially cancer-causing by-products in the process. Incidentally, this is the trouble with deep frying and commercially fried foods, which *reuse* oil (a definite no-no in a natural foods kitchen).

To be on the safe side, keep the oil below the smoking point. Consider smoke a signal that the oil is undergoing a transformation. Throw it out and start fresh. Or, if you prefer to stay away from heated oil entirely, try "steam-stirring."

Better Than Frying

In *The Natural Healing Cookbook*, Mark Bricklin and Sharon Claessens describe this ingenious technique, which is essentially stir-frying without oil. Basically, it calls for the substitution of a small amount of liquid—orange juice, broth, tamari (natural soy sauce) or lemon juice in water—for the cooking oil. About two or three tablespoons of the liquid are placed in a wok and brought to a boil. The vegetables and meat are then added and shuffled around (just like stir-frying) to a just-tender stage of doneness. And remember, what's good for the wok is good for the frying pan, too. All you need is a little bit of liquid to keep foods from sticking.

Slow cooking in an electric crockery cooker has become very popular and with good reason. For busy people on the go, dinner can be prepared in the morning, cook all day and be waiting at mealtime. Studies have already been done on the possible dangers of cooking foods at low temperatures, but no problems of food spoiling have been found when directions are followed.

There has been little scientific literature comparing slow cooking and conventional methods in regard to nutrient loss, however. Jane Bowers, Ph.D., head of the department of foods and nutrition at Kansas State University, Manhattan, and a colleague cooked turkey breast in a slow cooker and by conventional roasting methods. They found a greater loss of thiamine in slow cooking but a greater tenderness and less shrinkage (*Home Economics Research Journal*, September, 1975).

Meats supply both protein and vitamins, so cooking methods that best preserve them are important. Roasting, braising and broiling are the preferred methods. In general, protein loss is minimal during cooking except under extreme heat. The loss of B vitamins varies from one-third for thiamine, biotin and B_{12} to less than one-tenth for riboflavin and niacin.

Cooking your meats slowly will cause less shrinkage and save more juices. Braising at low heat and roasting at low temperatures (about 300°F) are best. To tenderize your meats, marinate them in vinegar or lemon juice—never use commercial tenderizers.

Don't salt your meat. Salting adds to the loss of juices.

Be sure to add a meat thermometer to your kitchen necessities list and take the guesswork out of cooking meats. Well-done roasts appear to lose more thiamine than those done rare or medium.

And if you have a poor cut of meat or a problem chewing meat, braising—which is frying in a shallow pan followed by stewing—might be the best method for you.

Fresh fish is practically a staple among natural foods enthusiasts because of its high protein, rich mineral content and low fat. Broiling and baking it will save on flavor, nutrients and calories. Just remember not to overcook it! Cooking only until the flesh flakes easily with a fork is best.

And what about those leftovers? Storing and reheating foods does tell its tale of lost vitamins. Keeping vegetables in the refrigerator for two or three days can wreck half their vitamin C. Freezing leftover vegetables in their cooking liquid is a good solution. The thiamine levels in leftover meats, too, are affected by holding and reheating. Serving cold slices at a second meal might be a good alternative.

To be on the safe side, however,

wrap leftovers in waxed paper rather than plastic wrap, which may contain polyvinyl chloride, a dangerous chemical. Aluminum foil is another good alternative except for tomatoes or other acidic foods, which draw the aluminum out of the paper.

One of the best ways to eat leftovers is by making them into soups. But letting them simmer all day like grandma used to is not a good idea. To make the most out of your soups, cook meat off a bone that has been sawed open to ex-pose the marrow. Add a little acid substance like lemon juice or tomatoes to the broth to pull out the calcium from the bone. Legumes or pasta will improve protein quality, as will adding vegetables just *at the end* of the cooking period. Spiking with a teaspoon of brewer's yeast is a good idea. If you're a vegetarian, there are recipes for garlic and potato peel broths which are absolutely delicious joined with leftover vegetables—or fresh garden vegetables, for that matter.

NO-KNEAD WHOLE WHEAT BREAD

Yield: 1 generous loaf

4	teaspoons dry yeast		⅔	cup lukewarm water
⅔	cup lukewarm water		⅓	cup wheat germ
2	teaspoons honey		1⅓	cups lukewarm water
5	cups whole wheat flour		½	tablespoon butter
3	tablespoons unsulfured molasses		1	tablespoon sesame seeds

Sprinkle yeast over lukewarm water. Add honey. Leave to "work" while preparing the dough.

Warm whole wheat flour by placing it in a 250°F oven for about 20 minutes.

Combine molasses with lukewarm water.

Combine yeast mixture with molasses mixture. Stir this into the warmed flour, then add the wheat germ and lukewarm water. Mix well, but don't knead. The dough will be sticky.

Butter a 9¼ × 5¼-inch loaf pan (measured across the top) taking care to grease the corners of the pan well. Turn the dough into the pan. Smooth the dough with a spatula that has been rinsed under cold water to prevent sticking. Sprinkle sesame seeds over top of loaf. Leave to rise to top of pan in warm, draft-free place.

Bake at 400°F for 30 to 40 minutes or until crust is brown and sides of loaf are firm and crusty. Set pan on rack to cool for about 10 minutes, then remove loaf from pan and cool completely on rack before slicing.

Note: *We believe bread is best without added salt. But if you feel the need for some, add 1½ teaspoons of salt along with the wheat germ.*

CRAMPS AND OTHER PREMENSTRUAL MISERIES

It doesn't have to hurt. But, according to most gynecology textbooks, for 30 to 50 percent of all menstruating women, their monthly periods come complete with pain—backache, headache, leg pain, cramps, breast tenderness, depression, bloating, constipation, diarrhea, and sometimes even nausea and vomiting. So what's a woman to do?

Well, the problem is that menstrual discomfort is to women what the common cold is to the general population. Practically everyone gets it at one time or another but modern medicine has yet to get a handle on how to effectively treat it.

Some physicians have a neat way of dealing with this common female complaint. They don't. Instead, they insist it's just mind over matter. And, in fact, gynecological conferences still host an occasional speaker who tries to psych out the most susceptible female personality; women who have menstrual pain are high-strung, nervous or neurotic, or are unsure about their role as wives or mothers, they say. Other gynecologists put women off with a "wait and see" solution, citing the theory that menstrual cramps are caused by a tight cervical opening and the inevitable stretching during childbirth will bring everlasting relief. Gideon G. Panter, M.D., a prominent New York City gynecologist and faculty member at New York Hospital–Cornell Medical Center, takes issue with that. "That's just an old-fashioned misconception," he told us. "It's very rare that cervical narrowing is a cause of menstrual cramps." We spoke with women who would agree—women who gave birth to one, two and even three children with little subsequent relief from cramps. So much for that theory!

It's also a good idea to guard against physicians who push the Pill for menstrual problems. Menstrual miseries usually plague only women who ovulate and oral contraceptives suspend ovulation, they explain. In other words, no egg, no ouch. The only trouble is, you could get an awful lot you didn't bargain for (see Oral Contraceptives). In our opinion, the trade-off of monthly pain for the potential misery of cancer doesn't make sense.

Diuretics don't fill the bill either. Oh, they'll reduce bloating all right. But they can also deplete your body of potassium in a hurry—and that's just the beginning. In most cases, close medical supervision is needed to insure that the body's salt and water balance doesn't go completely out of check.

Tranquilizers such as Valium are also commonly prescribed for premenstrual tension. And we don't have to remind you that they're not a good idea, either. They may ease a few superficial symptoms but they won't touch the root of the problem—which is, in fact, excessive uterine contraction. Plus they bring with them a whole host of dangerous side effects (see Valium).

You can draw your own conclusions on the new prostaglandin-inhibiting drugs—indomethacin, ibuprofen and mefenamic acid. In case you haven't heard, prostaglandins are hormonelike fatty acids which are produced throughout the body. And within recent years, scientists have shown that some women with severe cramps have higher levels of uterine prostaglandins which, they say, may be responsible for strong, painful uterine contractions.

The only trouble is, prostaglandins aren't altogether bad. In fact, the more we learn about them, the greater our respect for their role in our health. They aid digestion, heart, lung and kidney function, reproduction and other bodily processes. And a study published in the *Journal of the American Medical Association* (June 22, 1979), adds a word of caution to women with rheumatoid arthritis, Bartter's syndrome, lupus and assorted kidney disorders. Prostaglandin-inhibiting drugs, the researchers say, may subject this group to kidney failure. Nevertheless, the drug company ads assure us that, for normal healthy persons, "side effects [from any one of these prostaglandin-inhibiting drugs] are minimal and dose-related"—which, we guess, implies that the drug is safe when taken in the prescribed two-day doses.

There are two interesting sidelights to the prostaglandin story, however. One is that aspirin—an old standby for menstrual relief and one that is particularly effective when taken before the cramps take hold—is, in fact, a weak prostaglandin inhibitor. The other is that while gynecology textbooks and women's self-help groups maintain that orgasm will alleviate cramps, Dr. Panter informed us that because prostaglandins are released during orgasm, the tendency is for the opposite to hold true. Orgasm at the time of menstrual cramping can make matters worse. Sorry about that.

So where do we go from here?

Cramps Usually Lessen with Age

Well, before we go anywhere, it's important to understand that these monthly misadventures occur with greater frequency and intensity during adolescence while hormones are adjusting to new levels. Most women experience a gradual lessening of symptoms through the years. Also, because hormones take their instructions from the brain, which, among other functions, serves as the seat of our emotions, any undue stress or emotional upset can have a profound effect on menstrual function. Don't worry, though, the physical pain should subside with the psychological turmoil.

We should also point out here that while cramps are as common as rainy Mondays—and usually as innocuous—they can occasionally be indicative of more serious problems. Endometriosis. Fibroid tumors. Pelvic inflammatory disease. Even an ill-fitting or perforating intrauterine device (IUD). For those reasons, severe cramplike symptoms should be discussed with your gynecologist—especially if these symptoms strike after several years of relatively painless periods.

For those who come through the exam with a shrug and a "don't worry" pat on the shoulder, there are several safe and effective steps you can take to avert those monthly misadventures.

Tops on the list are the B vitamins and especially vitamin B_6.

As we mentioned earlier, there are many possible causes of premenstrual and menstrual discomfort. Lucienne Lanson, M.D., a San Francisco gynecologist and author of *From Woman to Woman* (Alfred A. Knopf, 1975), maintains that excessively high estrogen levels are at least partially to blame for premenstrual bloating. The more estrogen in your system, she says, the less sodium and water pass through the kidneys. The result: you pass less urine. And the water that bypassed your kidneys is redistributed back into your tissues. What's more, many physicians and researchers now believe that those premenstrual headaches and emotional upheavals—irritability, nervous tension, insomnia, depression and so on—may well be caused by water retention within the brain tissues.

How B Vitamins Can Help

Here's how B vitamins can help: according to Leon Zussman, M.D., diplomate of the American Board of Gynecologists and Obstetricians, and affiliated with the Long Island Jewish–Hillside Medical Center, "B complex is essential to the health of the liver. And the liver plays a key role in neutralizing the excessive amounts of estrogen produced by the ovaries during the course of the normal menstrual cycle." What this means to you is that B vitamins could protect against the bloating and bristling nervousness that occurs premenstrually.

In fact, in his book *Vitamin B₆: the Doctor's Report* (Harper & Row, 1973), John M. Ellis, M.D., describes how vitamin B₆ in particular can relieve that heavy, bloated, puffy feeling so many women experience a week or so before "that time of the month."

For example, a nurse complained to Dr. Ellis that her fingers swelled so badly midway in her menstrual cycle that she couldn't wear rings or use a typewriter comfortably. Dr. Ellis prescribed two 50-milligram tablets of B₆ daily for five days. After only two days on the regimen she was noticing improvements. By the third day, she reported that she was able to wear rings, type and sleep much better. For the next 12 months she took one 50-milligram tablet daily and had no pain or swelling.

Actually, so much research has been done on the relationship of vitamin B₆ to women's "cyclic" health problems that it can and has filled volumes. For example:

- Dermatologists in Erie, Pennsylvania, have reported that vitamin B₆ alleviates flareups of acne before menstrual periods.
- Medical journals, including the *Lancet*, have reported that vitamin B₆ can relieve depression and anxiety associated with estrogen therapy. While this estrogen was synthetic, and given for therapeutic reasons, its biochemical effects are similar to those of internal estrogen.
- A report from New York Medical College points out that pyridoxine (vitamin B₆) corrects estrogen-caused biochemical abnormalities.
- Unpublished work done at the Northwest Health Foundation in Seattle, Washington, shows that B₆ will eliminate nearly all cases of premenstrual fluid retention and some cases of chronic fluid retention in nonmenopausal women.

Following *Prevention* magazine's mention of the role of B vitamins in preventing premenstrual problems, quite a few letters came in from grateful women. This is typical of the response:

"I am a 26-year-old woman who has been suffering with menstrual cramps, premenstrual tensions, irritability, water retention, breast tenderness, low back pain, headache and dull aching legs each and every month for the past 15 years. I would dread this 'curse' and I was even starting to resent my femininity, when I happened to read in

Prevention that vitamin B$_6$ might help eliminate premenstrual tension and cramps as well as reduce water retention and breast tenderness.

"I thought it was worth a try, so four months ago I started taking 50 milligrams per day of B$_6$. One week before expecting my period, I would increase the dosage to 100 milligrams. In addition to taking B$_6$, I take three dolomite tablets every day between meals during this week.

"The results were astonishing. Not only were my symptoms reduced, they were completely eliminated! For the first time in 15 years, I can get through my monthly cycle without so much as a flinch in my tummy."

More Help from Vitamin E and Calcium

Vitamin E is another supplement worth careful consideration here. G. E. Desaulniers, M.D., of the Shute Institute in London, Ontario, Canada, told us that the various properties of vitamin E make it an excellent weapon against menstrual pain and swelling. For starters, vitamin E is a mild prostaglandin inhibitor similar to aspirin but without the unwanted side effects. Vitamin E is also widely recognized for its ability to improve circulation and there is some speculation that menstrual cramps are perhaps caused by a constriction of blood supply when the uterine muscle forcefully contracts. "Where this is the problem," says Dr. Desaulniers, "vitamin E, by promoting better vascular supply, reducing spasm as it does in other muscle groups throughout the body and by reducing the uterus' need for oxygen, will also reduce the pain resulting from this."

Calcium, too, has brought relief to many women suffering from painful menstrual symptoms. Unfortunately, we have no scientific evidence to back this up. But when you think about it, it's easy to understand how calcium could have such an effect.

For one thing, calcium is an integral part of muscle fiber, where it plays a key role in normal muscle contraction. In fact, persons prone to muscle cramps or spasms in their calves often find that a good calcium supplement such as bone meal or dolomite can prevent these nocturnal annoyances. Menstrual cramps may be caused by a similar mechanism. After all, the uterus, like the calf, is muscle. And menstrual cramps are commonly attributed to excessive contractions of the uterine muscle.

What makes calcium even more plausible as a treatment for female complaints is its link with estrogen. Estrogen apparently helps the body retain calcium and also use it more efficiently. We know this because the dwindling estrogen supply of postmenopausal women leaves them significantly more susceptible to the calcium-robbing bone condition, osteoporosis. The interesting thing is that a menstruating woman's estrogen level fluctuates cyclically each month—with the highest level occurring at midcycle (which, as you recall, is the time that water retention begins) and the lowest level immediately prior to her period (which is the time when menstrual cramps are usually the most debilitating).

A few years ago when *Prevention* magazine surveyed a cross section of its readers on their personal experiences with calcium, 293 respondents (about 10 percent of the total) reported improvement or total relief of menstrual cramping and distress. An Arizona woman remarked, for example, that "For 10 years I took birth control pills to avoid the terrible menstrual cramps that sent me to bed every month since I began menstruating. But I was afraid of the Pill, so I tried calcium. Now I have absolutely no incapacitating menstrual cramps." She reports taking 1,000 milligrams a day in the form of calcium carbonate, along with moderate amounts of other vitamins and 500 milligrams of magnesium a day.

Another letter suggests that muscle cramping and menstrual cramping may indeed be connected. "I had hard menstrual cramps, lasting two or three days.... Also I had arm cramps sometimes going from my little finger up to my shoulder and all the way down my spine. These arm cramps awakened me almost every night." After taking 1,800 milligrams of calcium daily in the form of bone meal, however, the writer reports that "all conditions have been completely eliminated."

Of course, supplements are probably the best way to get concentrated nutrients when you need them. But these vitamins and minerals are also readily available from a well-planned diet. And if your daily diet adequately covers all your womanly needs, there's a good chance you'll be able to ward off monthly distress before it takes hold.

Foods That Will Help

Obviously, getting plenty of foods with vitamins B and E as well as calcium should be top priority. For the B vitamins look to lean meats, whole grains, dark green, leafy vegetables and brewer's yeast; for vitamin E, count on wheat germ; and for calcium stick to the low-fat varieties of milk, yogurt and cottage cheese. One way to insure all of these essential food vitamins is by whipping up a morning breakfast drink with a half cup of yogurt, a tablespoon of brewer's yeast (ask your nutrition center sales person about good-tasting varieties), a tablespoon of wheat germ, a banana (which is a superior source of potassium), and a half cup of skim milk. Whirl briefly in a blender and drink. You'll be surprised how delicious and satisfying a breakfast that can be!

It's also a good idea to eat liver about once a week since this B-rich food is also an excellent source of iron—something that silently slips out of the body along with the blood flow (see Anemia). And try to steer clear of coffee, tea, chocolate and alcohol—the infamous B vitamin destroyers.

While we're on the topic of foods to avoid, we should mention that salt is another potential contributor to menstrual woes. Namely, it encourages the water retention responsible for bloated abdomens and painfully swollen breasts. Salt draws water out of the digestive tract and bloodstream, where it belongs, and pours it into the fatty and muscle tissue where it creates saturated bogs. As a result you may feel waterlogged when in fact you're water-deficient in the places that count. For that reason, a good diet contains a minimum amount of salt and a good, healthy supply of water. That's right, you may not be able to fight fire with fire, but one way to fight water retention is with more water because water helps flush salt from the system. If, in spite of a healthful diet, you still experience any unwanted water or bloating, try some natural diuretic foods such as cranberry juice, watercress, parsley and kelp as well as those foods rich in vitamin B_6—which include muscle meats, liver, vegetables, whole grains and egg yolks.

If your periods are preceded by a few days of constipation, water retention may also be the cause. With water diverted to the tissues, your digestive tract may be too dry to flush itself clean. Again, more water and less salt will help. Also you may need more fiber in your diet. Concentrate on whole grain foods and fresh fruits and vegetables, and sprinkle your morning cereal with a tablespoon or two of bran. Prunes can serve two functions here. Not only do they boost bowel function, but they are also excellent sources of iron.

Relief Can Come from Exercise

That brings us to exercise, and the big question: should I or shouldn't I exercise to relieve menstrual discomfort? Our reply: a resounding yes! In fact, exercise not only can ease the pain of menstruation while it's got you in its grip, but when performed as a daily routine it also can help prevent cramps and other common menstrual complaints in the first place. According to the President's Council on Fitness, 70 to 80 percent of the women who suffer menstrual discomfort are guilty of poor living habits—with bad posture and lack of exercise leading the list.

That's no surprise to us. Exercise works in many ways to relieve symptoms commonly associated with menstruation. It relieves constipation by increasing intestinal contractions. It helps curb that waterlogged feeling by getting you to work up a good sweat.

It requires healthy deep breathing and, after all, deep breathing brings more oxygen to the blood, which helps relax the uterus to ease even the painful contractions of childbirth. It's been known to alleviate depression. With irritability and tension vying for your heart

and soul, exercise, with its potential for being as good for the spirits as it is for the spine, would seem the ideal medicine.

So, get thee into a good training program. Anything that exercises the major muscle groups and gets you breathing good and hard is great for preventing cramps. Jogging. Swimming. Cycling. Even a regular fast-paced walking regimen will do.

If you belong to a health club or prefer the mat-and-music type of exercises, think "aerobics." Dancercise is perfect. You might also want to concentrate on stretching exercises for the hips and lower back. Sit-ups, too, are good. Eight weeks of the bent-knee variety done on a daily basis were found to make life a lot easier once a month for 36 college women tested by a team of doctors recently (*Physical Fitness Research Digest*, July, 1978).

There's also something to be said for the trusty heating pad. Heat is a wonderful soother as well as a promoter of blood flow. So any type of warmth—from sipping herbal tea to soaking in a hot tub—may be beneficial during painful periods (see Saunas and Other Hot Baths). Massage can be of help at this time as well—to soothe aching back muscles, to aid relaxation, and also to promote the flow of blood.

Menstrual Relaxercises

When menstrual cramps become unbearable, your natural instinct is probably to double up or curl up on your
side. When you think about it, it is the
fetal position that you assume when you
need to quell the pain. And if exercising
in this position can bring you more relief
than just lying still, why not try it?
Exercise in general is good for cramps,
but these exercises in particular should
help when the going gets rough.

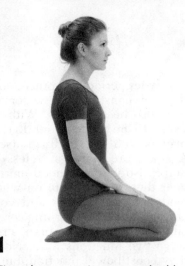

1

First, choose a quiet spot, preferably
with carpeting. Kneel on the floor,
sitting back on your heels with the tops
of your feet flat against the floor, knees
together.

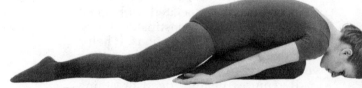

7

While shifting your weight, extend the
right leg back,

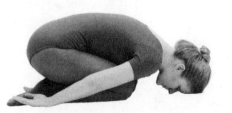

8

and then bring it forward again.
Alternate extending your legs according
to your own pace with pauses in
between.

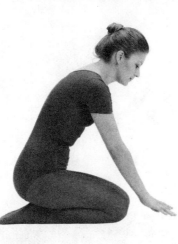

2

Slowly bend forward, sliding your arms and hands—palms flat—straight out in front of you until your back is rounded and your chest is resting on your legs.

3

Touch your forehead to the floor. Hold there for as long as you like, breathing normally and with your eyes closed.

4

When you feel relaxed, open your eyes and pull your arms straight back along your sides, bringing them to rest with the palms up.

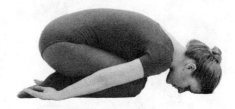

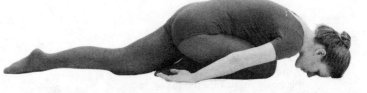

5 Shift your body so that the heel of the right foot is under the pelvis. (This helps you to balance.) At the same time, slowly slide the left leg straight back as far as it will go. Again hold this position for a few minutes.

6

Then pull it back up and tuck it under—knee under chest, heel under pelvis.

1

Next, pull back to the original crouched position and roll over onto your back.

2

Slowly release the legs into a bent-knee position until your feet are flat on the floor, about a foot or so away from your buttocks. Let your arms relax at your sides, palms down.

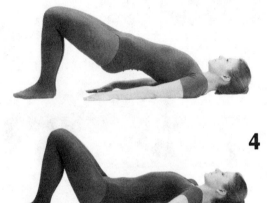

3

Tighten the stomach muscles and lift your hips off the floor in a "bridge" so that your trunk and legs form a straight line to the knees.

4

Slowly lower your hips and back to the floor, and when you are fully down, push down toward the floor with the small of your back. (Just to be sure you are working the right area, place one hand under the arch of your back and try to make your back press against your hand.)

5

Then release and pull your knees up, clasping them to your chest. Relax in this position, just holding your legs gently but firmly against your abdomen. Keep breathing nice, deep, steady breaths. When you are ready, lower your knees and raise your hips off the floor in a "bridge" as you did before. Lower them, flatten the arch in your back, then release. Draw your knees back up to your chest. Close your eyes and imagine yourself in a peaceful setting—a meadow perhaps, or the bank of a stream. Simply rest.

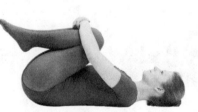

After a few minutes, you may wish to repeat the whole sequence in reverse. Just remember to keep breathing normally and follow your body's rhythm. Don't rush it. You'll be amazed at how these natural relaxing movements can ease the pain out of menstrual cramps.

If all else fails, consider biofeedback. Biofeedback is a method by which you can train yourself to consciously alter body functions that are generally carried out unconsciously. You've probably already heard of it as an effective method of stress reduction—people learning to consciously calm themselves. But biofeedback is being used for many physical ills. Hypertensive persons are learning how to consciously lower their blood pressure. Migraine sufferers can train themselves to avert an attack. And now, according to Keith W. Sedlacek, M.D., chief of Biofeedback Services at St. Lukes–Roosevelt Hospital in New York City, women with severe menstrual cramps are able to sidestep their usual symptoms using this same technique.

The treatment plan does involve some professional services—usually about 10 to 15 30-minute sessions. During those training sessions, a banjo-shaped thermometer which is hooked up to a digital readout machine is self-inserted into the vagina like a tampon. The woman is then taught how to consciously raise her vaginal temperature, which brings relief from the cramping. After the initial training sessions, the woman should be able to raise her temperature at will, Dr. Sedlacek told us.

And in 60 to 70 percent of the women tested, relief was but a moment's concentration away.

Dr. Sedlacek describes two 25-year-old women with such severe cramps that it kept them out of work and home in bed for at least one day each month. Both had received a gynecological exam to rule out more serious causes. During the training sessions, the patients were taught to close their eyes and concentrate on feelings of relaxation. The therapist would tell them to open their eyes whenever the digital unit recorded a change.

As the patients learned voluntary control, they began to open their eyes automatically just before a change in temperature registered on the machine, Dr. Sedlacek explains. And, by the end of the 10 or so sessions, both women had learned to increase their vaginal temperature by at least $0.2°F$. More importantly, both showed a significant decrease of symptoms. They reported only slight cramps by their second period and no longer considered interrupting their work because of slight pain. Interestingly, both women also reported a feeling of control over their cramps, less nervousness and a less bloated feeling. Who could ask for more?

DANCE

If you haven't caught the fever already, maybe you should. Dancing, as Arthur Murray has been telling us for years, can be darned good exercise.

Physiologists at the University of Akron recently studied a recreational class of 17 female belly dancers and found that they were burning calories at the rate of 6.2 a minute—372 an hour. That's more than tennis, and nearly twice as much as golf.

Of course, not every type of dance is as demanding as disco or belly dancing. But all burn calories. And if you really stick with the two-step, you'll find those excess pounds slipping away with ease. Let's face it, have you ever seen a ballerina who *wasn't* lean?

Besides burning calories and fat, dance improves posture, flexibility, strength, endurance, breathing patterns and agility. It quickens reflexes, increases heart efficiency, reduces blood pressure, and improves muscle tone by the squeezing action of the muscles on the veins.

And you thought Ginger Rogers was just gliding decoratively along under that diaphanous gown! Little did you know that she was strengthening her pelvic muscles, speeding her metabolic rate and probably soaking that sequined chiffon with a hearty sweat.

"Cutting a rug" is also a great way to release that tension and stress you've been sweeping under the carpet.

But best of all, dancing is just plain fun.

"I just can't wait for Sunday afternoons and Monday evenings. Why? Folk dancing!" says Shirley Mokren of Rolling Hills, California.

"About four years ago, a friend told me she went folk dancing twice a week and both she and her husband really enjoyed it. I remember thinking at the time, I guess that's just some weird thing about her that doesn't show otherwise. Folk dancing? How ridiculous!

"Then one day I stayed after services at the church and thought I'd watch and see what folk dancing really looked like. It looked like fun. Also, the ages ran from about 7 to 70. There are very few things people of all ages can do and enjoy together. Our teacher is fantastic. He's so very patient, and he seems to be having the time of his life. It's the best and most fun exercise I do all week. The night I dance, I know will be the night I have no trouble falling asleep.

"There is a special feeling about folk dancers—when we dance, we are in another realm. There is really no way to explain what one feels. The only way to feel it is to dance."

Dance throughout the ages has had specific therapeutic uses. As part of the wedding celebration in Turkey, for example, brides were taught a belly dance to help them enjoy painless childbirth and avoid stretch marks after delivery.

And today, dance therapists in private practice and on the staffs of institutions work with neurotics, psychotics, alcoholics, the retarded and brain-damaged to help them integrate themselves physically, mentally and emotionally through dance. Ballet is used by some mastectomy patients (that is, women who've had a breast removed) to restore confidence and movement after breast cancer operations. Children with learning disabilities dance to overcome lack of coordination.

In some cultures, dance is considered so vital that those who can't dance themselves can *be* danced. Babies, the elderly, the sick or those too weary from the rigors of initiation and other ceremonies can all be danced on the shoulders of their friends and relatives.

In a long career as a dance instructor, John Conrad of Allentown, Pennsylvania, has taught blind, deaf and retarded people to dance, as well as students with partial loss of limb movement and other problems.

Everyone Can Dance

"People with handicaps have something very important going for them—the desire to learn," says John Conrad. "They can often do just as well as the nonhandicapped person who has more natural ability but isn't as motivated. For them, we emphasize not competition, but enjoyment.

"One of our students now," says the instructor, who now directs an Arthur Murray school, "is a lady who learned to dance rather late in life and got a tremendous amount of enjoyment from it. Now she is going deaf and she worries about how it will affect her dancing. We are trying to prepare her to enjoy dance without hearing music."

John Conrad added that it is never too late to take up dance for the first time or to rediscover it.

"We want the best for our children. We want to give them a good start in life, so we encourage their interests and send them to lessons," he says. "But what about adulthood? Adults lose sight of what they started. Adulthood is when you should be reaping the benefits of that early training."

Learning about people who enjoy dance despite profound problems makes the healthy person's claim that he has "two left feet" sound slightly hollow.

A ballet teacher and dance school administrator tells us, "I doubt that there are many people who really are too uncoordinated to dance. There's some grace in all of us." Susan Gottlieb, who trained for many years to be a professional ballerina, is now an administrative assistant at the Philadelphia College of Performing Arts. "I've gotten calls from people who are 45 and haven't danced since their twenties," she tells us, "but really want to learn to dance again. Some people are terribly out of shape and just want to regain some grace. Of course, there will be self-consciousness involved in the first class or two. But even in beginner adult classes, I've seen so much beauty. Some people are so naturally graceful, without ever having formally learned a dance step."

When embarrassment overcomes the beginning dancer as she attempts her first leap or glide, it's easy for her to overlook the fact that her body is effortlessly expressive most of the time. Think of the differences in the way she stands at a party and when she's being fitted by a seamstress, when she hails a taxi or is introduced to a group. What about the differences in the way she holds her head to look at the horizon, fine print or an attractive man across the room? Even watching dance stimulates the body's expressiveness, with the spectator's muscles sympathetically tensing and relaxing along with the dancer's.

Susan Gottlieb suggests that a stiff beginner may benefit from doing yoga exercises along with dance. "It's ideal because yoga moves with the body, not against it," she notes. "It increases the flexibility you need for dance."

Choose Your Favorite Style

Nothing says your dancing has to be restricted to the discotheque, or that it has to follow in the footsteps of *Saturday Night Fever*, for that matter.

Aerobic dance is a fancy name for getting in shape to music, and if you think anything goes with disco, you can enjoy out-and-out *anarchy* with this.

What it amounts to is 15 to 20 minutes of constant movement—everything from running in place to the rumba.

"We try to incorporate *some* legitimate steps," says Beverly Smith, dance instructor at the Wyomissing Institute of Fine Arts in Reading, Pennsylvania, "but our goal, really, is just to get you breathing. And you'd be amazed. Folks good for a couple of miles of jogging have found it can be pretty tough."

Movements involve every part of the body, and in combinations that make running look easy.

Feeling tense? "Rock out" to the Rolling Stones. Serene? Slow things down with a serenade. The nice thing about aerobic dancing is that you can choose the music to suit your mood.

Warm-ups, says Beverly Smith, should take 5 or 10 minutes. Start out easy, maybe to something classical.

Once warm, you're pretty much on your own. You can do leg kicks, arm flings, shoulder rolls, hip pushes and head circles. Leave no limb unturned, and give prime time to areas where you're weak.

The important thing is to *keep moving*. Fifteen to 20 minutes a day, three to five times a week. That's the formula for fitness. And the nice thing is, you can do it anyplace, anytime. All you need is music.

"One of the most frustrating aspects of having small children for me," says Mrs. Nancy Hetherington of Decatur, Georgia, "is the difficulty of maintaining a regular exercise program. When I try yoga and floor exercises, they climb all over me, and my husband works late hours, so jogging or cycling before dinner is out. Mornings are too hectic, and by the time the children are in bed, I'm too pooped to really work out.

"I am very interested in the aerobics principle, and have applied it to a very fun, exciting and creative form of exercise—aerobic dancing. Sometime before lunch each day I put on some very lively music (the waltz just won't do) and begin running around, hopping, skipping, kicking, jumping or whatever creative way my body wants to move. I keep moving (and grooving) for 20 minutes (my goal is 30). My children love it. Either they participate or sit back, clap and let me entertain them.

"I do a few yoga and stretching exercises before I begin and some toning exercises at night, but basically the aerobics dancing is my total program. I have also cycled and walked whenever possible, but have never felt so good, and enjoyed exercising so much since I began this program."

How to Get Moving

Opportunities for taking dance lessons abound. Lessons in aerobic, folk, jazz, ballet, ethnic, ballroom and other types of dancing are available in most communities. Check the community calendar in your newspaper, schools offering adult education classes, YWCAs, YMCAs, nonprofit social and cultural organizations, and commercial studios. A career can even be spawned from a casual interest in dance.

Two professional belly dancers we interviewed said they happened on their careers quite by accident. Marie started taking belly dance lessons five years ago after the birth of her first child.

"I saw a demonstration at the Y and decided it would be a good way to get back in shape," she told us.

The dancer with whom Marie rehearses, Beverly, had to laugh when we asked how she got started.

"I was at a party when I heard that a belly dancer had been brought in to entertain. I told my date I wouldn't stay because I didn't want to see some girl gyrate around. He persuaded me to stay and I found it really elegant and graceful, not suggestive at all. I hadn't known that belly dancing is really a Mideastern folk dance, a form of art."

The dancers' teacher, Marika Skoufalos, told us, "I get three kinds of students in my classes—those who are looking for an unboring way to exercise, those who are just plain curious, and those who think they might want to be professionals.

"I've had students of all ages, shapes and sizes. Some in their seventies do remarkably well. No matter why they come, in all of them I try to put the love for the dance. If I can do that, they're hooked," she said.

Like the other teachers and dancers interviewed, Marika Skoufalos agreed that dance—even for amateurs—requires much more hard work and concentration than the beginning dancer might bargain for.

Yet despite the sore muscles, self-consciousness, sweat and discipline, all of them agreed that the payoffs are worth the hard work.

After a few weeks, the teachers say they see a new sparkle in the students' eyes, a new erectness in their carriage, a new sleekness to their bodies, sometimes even new hairstyles and wardrobes.

But maybe more important than the tangible self-improvement teachers note is a feeling from dancing that amateurs and professionals share. They call it joy, ecstasy, pure motion and freedom, but it all boils down to a single theme: dance allows them the luxury of forgetting themselves.

After the beginner is able to quit whispering "one, two, three, step" to herself, after she can quit reminding herself to keep her shoulders high and her back relaxed, comes the point where she can wholeheartedly enjoy. She is momentarily swept away from the rigidities of her earthbound daily life. Leaping feels like flying, gliding like floating, the rhythm of the drum like the beat of her heart.

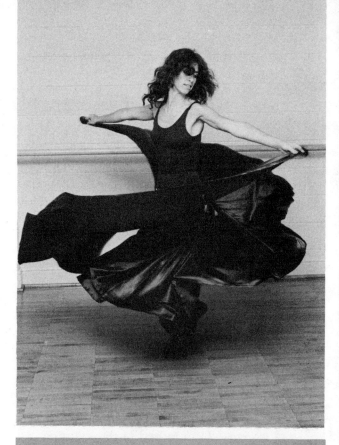

DANCE AWAY YOUR CALORIES

Dance	Calories Burned per Hour	
	110–125 pounds	150 pounds
Aerobic (low)	215	275
(medium)	350	445
(high)	515	655
Ballet	470	600
Belly dance	195	250
Jazz (traditional)	350	445
(vigorous)	515	655
Modern dance	470	600
Rock	195	250
Rumba	235	300
Square	330	350–420
Waltz	195	250

DEPRESSION

Happiness hinges on a certain amount of depression dodging. That doesn't mean we should ban the blues from our repertoire of emotions and sail through life on a perpetual high. Obviously, there are times when feeling depressed is perfectly natural, perhaps even healthful if you allow yourself to outwardly express that emotion. Besides, an occasional dash of this negative emotion can help intensify the flavor of more positive and pleasant feelings.

The trouble is, no one can exist on a steady diet of feeling down. And when a simple bout with the blues becomes a battle against the black siege of overwhelming gloom, it no longer serves as a healthful growing experience. In fact, it can be downright health-robbing.

Maybe you have trouble dragging yourself out of bed in the morning? Or feel generally fatigued throughout the day? Lack initiative? Have you lost interest in projects that you once enjoyed? Do you cry without cause? Avoid friends? Have trouble sleeping?

If your answer is yes to all or most of those questions, you're probably suffering from the kind of depression we're talking about—the kind that often strikes for no apparent reason, robbing millions of women of health and happiness.

According to the latest surveys and hospital reports, American women are bogged down in depression more than twice as frequently as men. They're weary, weeping and worried. All too often, they turn to tranquilizers and alcohol in desperation.

Of course, there are times when you'll need more than moral support to get you over the hump—and times when professional counseling may be in order. But often simple, natural methods are your brightest ray of hope. And we've got at least five better ways to beat the blues naturally.

1. *Up your intake of B vitamins.*

A growing body of evidence suggests that, for one reason or another, women are more prone to B vitamin deficiencies than men. And since this family of vitamins is so closely related to nerve function, it's conceivable that a B deficiency may be at the core of many a rotten mood.

Take women on the Pill as an example. At last count, 10 million women in the United States were downing a daily dose of hormones to prevent pregnancy. And of those, about seven percent plummeted into the depths of depression as a direct result.

For years, physicians recognized that something in birth control pills triggers depression, irritability and anxiety in certain women. But they didn't know exactly what it was or how it worked. Now, more and more are convinced that it has to do with the Pill's depressing effect on the body's B vitamin stores—especially B_6, B_{12} and folate.

Writing in the British medical journal *Lancet* (April 28, 1973), Dr. P. W. Adams and others at St. Mary's Hospital Medical School in London reported that of 22 emotionally distraught women on the Pill, 11 were found to be severely deficient in pyridoxine (vitamin B_6). All the women were then treated with 20 milligrams of vitamin B_6 twice a day. And within two months' time, the dark moods of the vitamin-deficient women brightened significantly.

In a more recent report by Dr. Csaba Banki of the Regional Neuropsychiatric Institute in Nagykallo, Hungary, 120 milligrams of pyridoxine daily brought marked relief to many women on the Pill. By the end of the first week, 52 percent reported a lifting of depression and after three weeks, 65 percent were symptom-free (*Ob. Gyn. News*, March 15, 1978).

Jonathan V. Wright, M.D., of Kent, Washington, author of *Dr. Wright's Book of Nutritional Therapy* (Rodale Press, 1979), describes an exemplary case:

Gail Peters scarcely sat down in his consultation room when she burst into tears and sobs. She was an attractive young woman apparently in her mid-twenties, who had just recently gone off the Pill.

When she regained her composure, she apologized. "I'm sorry," she said, "I promised myself I wouldn't do that, but I couldn't help it. That's part of the problem—I get so depressed over nothing. I'm so cranky and irritable, even I can't stand it. It gets worse before my menstrual periods—much worse. I cry at the least thing; when I'm not crying, I'm screaming or yelling. Sometimes I don't realize I'm doing it until halfway through. Then I can't stop."

Dr. Wright suspected an imbalance in estrogen and B vitamins and prescribed 100 milligrams of B_6 and a B complex tablet (with at least 50 milligrams of B_6), three times a day. The result, he told us, was extremely satisfying. Mrs. Peters' depression subsided and she was able to keep the blues at bay on a somewhat modified intake of the B vitamins.

Depression, fatigue, irritability and forgetfulness have also been known to occur in people with a vitamin B_{12} deficiency. And here again, this could be a real concern for you Pill users.

According to Harold L. Rosenthal, Ph.D., of Washington University Medical Center, St. Louis, women on the Pill for six months or more average approximately 25 percent lower blood B_{12} levels than women using alternative methods of birth control. And if that doesn't sound serious enough, Dr. Rosenthal also mentions that in 7 out of 14 women tested, B_{12} levels fell in the range of women with pernicious anemia.

And that's not just a mild "down in the dumps" feeling. That's the pits!

"I'm too young for my life to be over," Mrs. Acton (one of Dr. Wright's patients) sobbed. "But that's exactly how I feel. Nothing interests me, I have no ambition. I'm depressed a lot. I'm tired all the time. And I can't control my moods; I cry with no reason, or get laughing fits that won't stop. I lose my temper much too quick. I'm tense nearly all the time.

"I know what you might be thinking, but I've already been to see two psychiatrists. In fact, I've been in therapy for 11 years. I've been tranquilized and antidepressed; I'm taking an antidepressant now. But it only helps a little. I don't want to be on drugs forever."

Mrs. Acton was suffering from a B_{12} deficiency—but she hadn't been taking the Pill. Her depression, it seems, was somehow tied up with another problem involving digestion. Her stomach wasn't producing enough acid and her pancreas fell behind on its secretion of digestive enzymes so that she couldn't digest and absorb her nutrients properly.

To remedy the digestive problem, Dr. Wright asked Mrs. Acton to take three betaine hydrochloride tablets, five grains each, before meals. (He also cautioned her to stop them immediately if she had any adverse symptoms and warned against taking any form of aspirin or anti-inflammatory medication with the acid because of the increased danger of ulcers.)

For the mental symptoms, Dr. Wright recommended an injection of vitamin B_{12}, 100 micrograms, twice a week to start. And because B_{12} and folate are "metabolic partners," he also asked her to use one milligram of folate twice daily.

Her response? Striking!

Both Mr. and Mrs. Acton reported that the effect of each B_{12} injection was obvious within 24 hours after taking it. (They also reported it wore off after just two to three days. Mrs. Acton quickly learned when she needed another one.)

Mrs. Acton's mental attitude was entirely different with the B_{12}. She reported she had "energy and ambition." She could control her emotions "for the first time in years." Her depression lifted, and tension dissipated. Her anger fits became a thing of the past. She reported she was interested in life again and that it felt like a second honeymoon.

Even more interesting, however, is a case described by a South Carolina physician in which "baby blues," or postpartum depression, responded to treatment with the B vitamin folate.

Will E. Thornton, M.D., of the department of psychiatry and family practice at the Medical University of South Carolina in Charleston, describes a 17-year-old woman who became noticeably withdrawn and depressed a few weeks following the birth of her first child—the typical "baby blues."

Her condition quickly deteriorated. She became disoriented and feared that some harm was going to come to her baby. In time, frightening visual hallucinations prompted her family to have her hospitalized.

After two stints in mental institutions—where she was treated with electroconvulsive shock therapy and a conglomeration of mind-boggling drugs—she made three suicide attempts. By the time Dr. Thornton got to see her, she was a frightened, whining young lady literally withdrawn into the corner of her room.

Blood tests didn't reveal anything abnormal—save for a depressed folate level. No one suspected that something so simple as a vitamin deficiency could be at the root of such a tremendous psychological problem. But she was nevertheless treated with five milligrams of folate twice a day for 10 days.

To the surprise of her family and physician, her mental attitude began to show signs of improvement after only 7 days of folate treatment. And by the 10th day, she was completely well.

She was released from the hospital on one milligram of folate daily. And today, Dr. Thornton reports, she is alive and well and excelling in her studies at nursing school (*American Journal of Obstetrics and Gynecology*, September 15, 1977).

2. *When depression and insomnia coexist, consider tryptophan therapy.*

Tryptophan is an essential amino acid—a building block of protein.

In a paper presented to the annual meeting of the American Psychiatric Association in 1977, a group of Canadian doctors reported significant improvement in the depressive symptoms of 11 patients when given 2 to 6 grams of tryptophan and 0.5 to 1.5 grams of another amino acid, nicotinamide, per day for a four-week period.

Dr. Wright also verifies that tryptophan works. In one case, one gram of tryptophan taken three times a day (with one dose taken right before bedtime) relieved a female patient of unexplained depression and severe insomnia which she had suffered for years.

Some foods are rich in tryptophan, but the therapeutic dose necessary to douse severe depression represents about 10 times as much of this amino acid as occurs in a 3½-ounce serving of soybeans, which are very rich in this protein component. Better to get a bottle of tryptophan tablets in your health food store or ask your physician's advice.

3. *Check your calcium and magnesium intake.*

Tryptophan and B$_6$ aren't the only nutrients involved in depression. Low levels of calcium may also cause it, says a London psychiatrist (*Lancet*, January 25, 1975).

"The possibility that some mental illness may be brought on in a metabolic setting of calcium loss or deficiency is intriguing," he writes. "It is known that many people's vitamin D intake [without which calcium can't be absorbed] is borderline deficient, especially at the end of winter (when affective illness [emotional illness] may also be commoner). Postmenopausal women, and the elderly generally, are more prone to calcium deficiency ... and so they are to depression. Postpartum depression occurs at a time when the mother has undergone a calcium drain and may be lactating."

Magnesium is another mineral that research links to depression. In one study, depressed patients had "significantly lower" blood levels of magnesium than healthy people (*Journal of Nervous and Mental Disease*, December, 1977).

In a second, depressed patients who took the drug lithium and improved had a rise in their magnesium levels, while the magnesium levels of those who took lithium and didn't improve stayed much the same (*Lancet*, December 14, 1974).

August F. Daro, M.D., a Chicago obstetrician and gynecologist, routinely gives all his depressed patients calcium and magnesium.

"Many depressed women are short on calcium and magnesium," he told us. "I put them on a combination of 400 milligrams calcium and 200 milligrams magnesium a day. These minerals sedate the nervous system, and most of the depressed patients feel much better while taking them. Calcium and magnesium especially take care of premenstrual depression."

4. *Double-check your diet.*

It amused us to read in a book written by a physician that diet has nothing to do with depression. "It doesn't matter at this time if your diet is balanced or not. Anything will do—Cokes, milkshakes, potatoes, bread and gravy, ice cream, anything."

That's not the way Dr. Daro sees it.

"The first thing I do when a depressed patient comes to see me is to have them take a glucose tolerance test, the laboratory test that measures blood sugar levels," he says. "Anyone who has depression, apprehension, anxiety, crying spells or loss of desire for sex should have this test. Low blood sugar is the most common cause of depression, though it's not commonly diagnosed."

To treat depressed patients who have hypoglycemia, Dr. Daro recommends a diet rich in protein and free of refined carbohydrates and coffee.

"A lot of depressed people don't eat well," he says. "Perhaps they'll have a cup of coffee and a sweet roll for breakfast. I make sure they eat three good meals every day. A good diet has to be the foundation of the nutritional treatment of depression."

And a poor diet can make depression worse.

"Depressed people generally don't eat well, which will make any nutritional deficiencies more severe and may aggravate their depression," Yasuo Ishida, M.D., of St. Louis, told us. There are many reasons why this is so.

Foods made up largely of refined sugar and flour are sadly lacking in B vitamins and other essential nutrients which, as we just mentioned, have a profound effect on moods. To make matters worse, some foods like coffee actually destroy thiamine (vitamin B_1). Don't believe us? Just check the medical literature. You will find clear evidence that emotional problems are very often linked to poor diet.

Here's something else you may not have considered as a source of your touchy temperament: food allergy. That's right, food allergies don't have to be the garden-variety strawberry intolerance that causes a breakout of hives. There are many more types of food reactions to many more types of foods.

In his book *Food Allergy* (PSG Publishing, 1978), Frederic Speer, M.D., includes a list of emotional problems that have been caused by food addiction (a craving for the very food[s] you are allergic to):

"Increase in temper; screaming attacks; patient is mean or sulky, irritable, whining, impatient, quarrelsome, sensitive, easily hurt, unhappy, morbid, depressed, restless, tense, nervous, jumpy, fearful, anxious, irresponsible, erratic, uncooperative, unpredictable, pugnacious, or cruel; can't be pleased; is not open to reason; cries without cause;

worries, feels terrible, contemplates suicide; is nervous and high-strung; has nightmares; loses pride in work, in clothing, and in cleanliness; doesn't care, can't make decisions; loses interest in the opposite sex; has childish compulsions."

You'd be hard pressed to think of a negative emotional response that isn't on the list. "Food addiction is like that," says William Philpott, M.D., an Oklahoma City specialist in food allergy. "It can cause any type of emotional problem.

"But usually," he says, "a food addiction causes either a heightened or a lessened response. A person becomes either manic or depressed, wildly excited or totally apathetic."

The reason for these ups and downs, Dr. Philpott explains, is that a food addiction abnormally increases or decreases the amount of neurotransmitters in the brain, the chemicals responsible for determining most behavior. Food addiction also causes emotional upset by swelling brain tissues, which irritate sensitive nerves. (This type of swelling, says Dr. Philpott, is responsible for 69 percent of all headaches!)

One way to tell if you have a food addiction, says Dr. Philpott, is to deliberately skip a meal. If, after a few hours, you begin to feel bad—not just hungry, but very irritable, tense, headachy, depressed, nauseous—chances are you're addicted to a food and have begun to experience withdrawal symptoms. Another sign of food addiction, he says, is overweight.

How can you begin to correct the problem? One step is to increase your intake of nutritional supplements.

Food addiction can lead to a deficiency of vitamin A, says Dr. Philpott, which causes the mucous membranes to overreact and clog the respiratory tract. It can also lead to a deficiency of the B complex vitamins, particularly B_6, and of vitamin C. A lack of these vitamins, he says, "produces unhealthy brain function."

Dr. Philpott believes that 80 percent of all Americans have a food addiction, and that the same number probably have suboptimal levels of vitamins B_6 and C. He suggests that a person with a food addiction supplement his diet with "supernutritional" levels of these vitamins.

But over and above nutritional supplementation, Dr. Philpott believes that eating a highly varied diet goes a long way toward either the cure or prevention of food addiction. And, if possible, the foods you eat should be organically grown.

5. *Exercise.*

According to John H. Greist, M.D., exercise may not cure everyone who is depressed, but some people with run-of-the-mill problems may find happiness in a daily jog. The University of Wisconsin psychiatrist conducted a study in which he randomly assigned 24 patients, 18 to 30 years old, to running or one of two types of psychotherapy. Those who ran did so three or more times a week with or without a therapist at their side. They never talked about their depression, but learned to focus on breathing and the sound of pounding feet to avoid thinking about problems. Interestingly enough, the jogging patients improved as well as those undergoing short-term psychotherapy, which involved simple problem solving. After 10 weeks, they all reported feeling "just a little bit" depressed and only occasionally so. Those on long-term psychotherapy (described by Dr. Greist as "deep psychoanalysis"), however, felt no better than they did at the start.

Robert S. Brown, Ph.D., M.D., a University of Virginia psychiatrist, has studied more than 800 students who worked out an hour a day, three days a week, for three months. He finds that exercise aimed at physical fitness alleviates depression better than competitive sports. Exercise, he says, improves self-image and instills a feeling of achievement as well as providing an outlet for anger and anxiety, which, when turned inward, can cause depression.

DIAPHRAGM

With the risk-studded intrauterine device (IUD) and the Pill falling out of favor, the diaphragm is emerging from its recent exile. The reason is obvious: its winning combination of safety and effectiveness.

The diaphragm, which must be used with spermicidal (sperm-killing) cream or jelly, is made of soft rubber in the shape of a shallow dome and has a flexible metal spring rim. When properly in place, it covers the cervix (opening of the uterus) and holds the spermicidal jelly directly against the cervix. The dome helps keep the sperm out. And the spermicide serves to zap any straggler that slips through.

But that's the only thing that does get

zapped. As far as we can tell, serious health drawbacks do not exist with the diaphragm. (See Editor's Note at the end of this section.) Occasionally a woman may be allergic to the rubber or the spermicide. That is rare, however, and can be corrected by switching to a plastic model or changing spermicide brands. Also, infections can occur if the diaphragm is left in for more than 24 hours because bacteria can be trapped and multiply. This should not pose a problem, though, since it can be removed 6 to 8 hours after intercourse, or the morning after, as the case may be.

If safety is important, then effectiveness is imperative. That's one reason why the Pill and IUD have been so popular. But according to recent studies, the diaphragm has proven to be more effective in preventing pregnancy than the IUD and almost on a par with medically dangerous oral contraceptives. In one report, 2,168 diaphragm users were studied for two years and their method had a 98 percent effectiveness rate. And this group consisted of young, unmarried women who had no previous diaphragm experience (*Family Planning Perspectives*, March/April, 1976). What's more, of the 2 percent (or 37 women) who became pregnant, 22 admitted that they had used the diaphragm inconsistently or not at all. Taking that into consideration, the effectiveness rate was actually better than 99 percent.

But the diaphragm's effectiveness goes beyond preventing pregnancy. Women who use the dome with spermicidal cream or jelly have less likelihood of developing infections such as vaginitis (inflammation of the vagina) and cervicitis (inflammation of the cervix), and in general enjoy better vaginal health (see Spermicides).

Also, as we explain more fully in the section Cervical Cancer, diaphragm users may even be less prone to this much-dreaded disease. A study of 17,032 women revealed that the incidence rate of cervical cancer among diaphragm users was 82 percent lower than among Pill users and 80 percent lower than among IUD users (*British Journal of Cancer*, August, 1978).

But a diaphragm can protect you from pregnancy (or disease) only if it fits perfectly and is used correctly. For that reason it is essential that you be fitted for your diaphragm by someone who is well experienced and has the time to do it right (see Gynecologists and Their Alternatives). It takes considerably longer to measure you for a diaphragm than it does to write a prescription for the Pill. And it requires a certain amount of patience to instruct you on the correct insertion technique. For example, since every cervix is in a slightly different position, your doctor or nurse practitioner should take the extra time and effort to show you your cervix. How else will you ever know if your diaphragm is in exactly the right place?! Also, a conscientious clinician will not let you leave the office until you have demonstrated that you can insert the diaphragm correctly and check its position yourself. Then he or she should have you come back in a week or two wearing the diaphragm in order to confirm the size and position after use. In the interim, use additional protection such as a condom during intercourse.

Diaphragms range in size from 50 to 105 millimeters in diameter (two to four inches). That's because vaginas vary in size, too. Variations can also be due to muscle tone, previous pregnancies and frequency of intercourse. A diaphragm that's too small will swim around, possibly becoming dislodged. Too large, and cramping may occur. When the fit is perfect neither you nor your partner should be able to feel it.

Incidentally, there are a few cases where the diaphragm is not recommended—that is, in the case of a prolapsed or severely tipped uterus, or when the bladder or rectum protrudes into the vagina. Otherwise, most women can be fitted easily for a diaphragm.

Inserting a Diaphragm

Most clinicians recommend inserting the diaphragm by hand. It's part of becoming comfortable with your own body. But you can also use a gadget called an "introducer" or "inserter." The diaphragm hooks onto the introducer, which is a slightly curved plastic stick with notches to accommodate diaphragms ranging in size from 60 to 90 millimeters. The spermicidal jelly or cream (one to two teaspoons) is added after the diaphragm is on the introducer. It is then inserted as far as possible into the vagina and released by giving the introducer a quarter-turn twist.

You must insert your diaphragm with jelly or cream *each time* you plan to have intercourse. (It won't prevent pregnancy if left in your lingerie drawer.) Most clinicians say to insert it no more than two hours ahead. But a recent study showed 98 percent effectiveness when women were encouraged to insert their diaphragms up to six hours before intercourse.

You can even use your diaphragm during your menstrual period. It makes for tidier lovemaking since the dome holds back the flow for several hours.

When properly in place, the diaphragm will not fall out. There are times, however, when it may bounce around or become dislodged. The woman-on-top position during initial penetration of the penis may be especially risky. Masters and Johnson, the famous sex therapists, also found that the diaphragm tends to move around when the woman reaches orgasm because of "vaginal ballooning" which occurs at that time. But judging from the diaphragm's high effectiveness rating, this apparently does not present a significant problem. Perhaps—as suggested in *The Hite Report* (Macmillan, 1976)—most women do not experience orgasm *during* intercourse anyway. Or, if they do, the spermicide must easily compensate for any slight shift of the dome.

After intercourse the diaphragm must remain in place for six to eight hours. That's because it takes the jelly or cream nearly that long to kill off all the sperm. If you plan to have sex again before that time is up, add an extra dollop of spermicide with an applicator or have your partner use a condom.

When it's time to remove the diaphragm, simply reach in, grasp the rim with your index finger, and pull. Sometimes after sleeping with it in place all night the dome's suction may increase, making it difficult to withdraw. If that happens just walk around for about 15 minutes. That's usually enough time to loosen the suction and allow for easy removal.

Caring for your diaphragm is even easier than using it. Just wash with plain soap and water, rinse and dry with a towel. You can dust it with cornstarch, but don't use talcum powder or perfumed powder. Talc may be a cancer-causing agent and perfume may deteriorate the rubber. Petroleum jelly (or any medicines containing it), cocoa butter, heat, bright lights, metals such as copper, zinc and silver all may damage the dome. So it's best to store it in its own plastic case.

It's also a good idea to check periodically for holes, especially around the rim. Carefully stretch the rubber to expose tiny tears, but watch that your fingernails don't create the holes you're trying to avoid. With just a little tender loving care your diaphragm should last from one to two years.

Old age (of the diaphragm, that is) is not the only reason you may need a new one. If your vagina changes size, after a delivery or a miscarriage or after pelvic surgery, your diaphragm size will probably change, too. Even a weight loss or gain of 15 pounds or more may necessitate a size check (although one woman told us that a loss of 5 pounds was enough to change her diaphragm size). And if for any reason you have doubts about its fit or insertion technique, or you have any discomfort or pain, it's time to visit your clinician.

Your diaphragm has the potential to protect you from an unwanted pregnancy with the effectiveness of the Pill and IUD but with virtually no health

WHEN INSERTING THE DIAPHRAGM WITHOUT THE INTRODUCER

1 Apply 1 to 2 teaspoons of jelly or cream to the inside of the dome. Spread it around the rim, too.

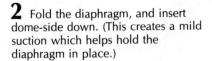

2 Fold the diaphragm, and insert dome-side down. (This creates a mild suction which helps hold the diaphragm in place.)

risk. Use it correctly and consistently, and your rate of success will be better than 99 percent. With the diaphragm, you are in control of the method; the method does not control you. It can be used year after year since it does not cause any physical, chemical or hormonal changes in your body. No wonder it's been called the "Queen of Contraception."

This is probably a good place to mention another contraceptive method that is similar to the diaphragm, the cervical cap.

The "cap," which is cup-shaped and made of rubber, polyethylene or lucite, is smaller than the diaphragm and when properly inserted fits snugly over the cervix, much as a thimble covers your fingertip. The strong suction which holds it in place also makes removal somewhat more difficult than for a diaphragm. It can be used with or without a spermicide and can be left in for a minimum of six to eight hours or for as long as two weeks.

To remove the diaphragm, grasp it with your index finger at the forwardmost part of the rim (the area wedged behind the pubic bone) and pull.

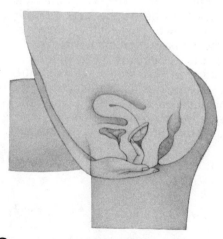

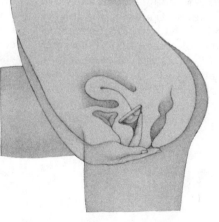

3 Then tuck the rim securely behind the pubic bone. Whether you use an introducer or not, always check with your finger to be sure the dome covers your cervix.

It's very important that you also check around the back of the rim to insure that the diaphragm is firmly looped over the entire cervix.

Be forewarned, however, the U.S. Food and Drug Administration has not yet approved the cervical cap for use, since there are no good studies to support either its safety or effectiveness. But it's been used for years in England, where some women swear by it.

Here, clinicians worry that the cap may promote infection since leaving it in for extended periods prevents the natural, free flow of cervical mucus, and creates a possible buildup of fluid and bacteria. At present doctors feel that anyone with preexisting cervical erosion or infections should not use the cap.

But the question of its inducing infection still must be answered.

On the positive side, the cap is even easier to fit than a diaphragm since the cervix apparently does not vary in size and shape as much as the vagina does. Also, the cervical cap can be worn by some of the people for whom the diaphragm is not recommended—women with a prolapsed uterus, for example.

The cervical cap seems worthy of further investigation. Check with your own doctor or nurse practitioner periodically for an update on the status of this old/new method.

Editor's Note: As this book goes to press, a preliminary study has just been published which raises some question about the safety of spermicides—at least for an unborn child in the event pregnancy should occur. The study, conducted by Hershel Jick, M.D., director of the Boston Collaborative Drug Surveillance Program, and his colleagues, found a higher incidence of certain birth defects (2.2 percent) among 763 infants whose mothers had used spermicides near the time of conception. That compared to a 1.0 percent incidence among 3,902 infants whose mothers did not use that method of birth control for several months prior to conception (*Journal of the American Medical Association,* April 3, 1981).

The large number of children in this study makes this association noteworthy. But because there was no distinct pattern to the abnormalities, it's very possible that other factors were involved. Therefore, Dr. Jick cautions that these results should be considered tentative until more data is published. Meanwhile, to be on the safe side, he says, women who suspect they are pregnant should have a pregnancy test to be certain, then stop using spermicides. He also suggests that women discontinue using spermicides for two months prior to a planned pregnancy. Otherwise, the key is to do what you can to insure your contraceptive's highest effectiveness.

"A man's activity would not permit him to be hindered by clothing. Not so with women! Vanity, conceit and extravagance of dress have smothered their reason."
—*The Wife as the Family Physician* by Anna Fischer-Dueckelmann, M.D. (1908)

So wrote a woman at the turn of the century—though for all our current fads in fashion, she might as well have written it today.

Just recently, for example, British doctors reported the case of a 20-year-old model suffering from numbness and pain in her groin area, diagnosed as genitofemoral neuropathy. Although her symptoms had appeared earlier, the doctors felt that modeling skintight jeans probably aggravated the problem. They explain as follows:

"A special technique is used to put on jeans that are several sizes too small. It requires the help of three assistants. The model wears nylon pants which extend from the waist to the knees to overcome friction. Two assistants, one on each side, help to pull on the jeans while the model lies on her back. The third assistant kneels at the head of the model holding a wooden coat hanger, whose hook is looped into the zip fastener ready to pull as soon as the special device to hold the front of the jeans together has been applied, and provided the material does not tear. Once encased it is impossible to stand up without help or to sit down" (*British Medical Journal*, April 21, 1979).

If ever there was a case of "smothered reason"—not to mention a smothered woman—this is it! Of course, you may counter, that is an exaggerated case; women in real life don't stoop to such atrocities in dress. Maybe not quite. But some of our frivolous fashions over the years have come pretty close. Jeans are one thing. What about girdles? Or "long-line" bras? Or the bra-and-girdle-all-in-one? And you thought you were above "genitofemoral neuropathy"!

Aside from being downright uncomfortable, clothing that is too tight restricts circulation, paving the way for such problems as varicose veins. What's more, if your choice of clothing is such that you can't move or breathe, then you're setting yourself up for even more hassles.

Modern fashion includes many items of clothing made from synthetic fibers. Synthetics don't breathe easily. Perspiration can't escape freely.

Women who wear nylon leotards, pantyhose and similar tight-fitting clothes are in effect humidifying the one part of their body that is most in need of coolness and continuous ventilation. It is almost as if they are walking around all day in a plastic bag. The result is that certain organisms can find exactly the environment they like in the vaginal area, and they thrive (see Vaginitis). There is no question that vaginal infections have become more of a problem since fashion began dictating that a woman's genital area should be almost hermetically sealed.

Natural vs. Synthetic Fibers

Natural fibers, such as cotton and wool, are cooler in the summer, warmer in the winter and just more comfortable all year round than many synthetics.

They permit circulation and are very absorbent.

Not so with synthetics. Nylon, polyester and acrylic are no more than plastic by-products of the petroleum industry. They've got about as much absorbency as plexiglass. Know that clammy, uncomfortable feeling you get in a polyester blouse or nylon stockings? That's because these fabrics trap the moisture on your skin so that the heat can't escape.

It's true, synthetics are easier to care for. They don't wrinkle as much as cotton. But you can look fresh and still feel comfortable by choosing a blend—say, 50 percent cotton and 50 percent polyester.

Also, if you must wear nylon pantyhose, choose those that have cotton sewn in at the crotch. And even so, wear socks, not tights or pantyhose, under slacks. The less restricted you are in your clothing, the more comfortable and healthy it is.

What's more, judging from the fashionable footgear many women are wearing today, common sense seems to have fallen from favor here, too. "If the shoe fits, wear it" doesn't fit our shoe-shopping habits anymore. For many women today, a more appropriate slogan might be, "If the shoe doesn't fit, wear it anyway . . . so long as it looks good." And that's where we can really be jeopardizing our health.

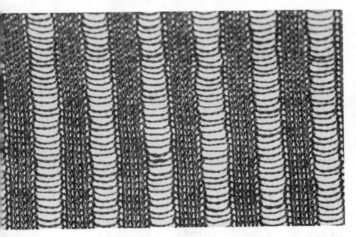
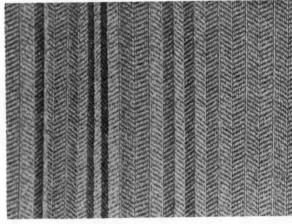

Cotton fabric (left) lets your skin breathe through thousands of "windows." Synthetics like nylon (right) trap moisture on your warm skin.

Why Women's Feet Hurt

"About 85 percent of the foot problems I see are in women," says Melvin Jahss, M.D., chief of the Orthopedic Foot Ser-

vice at New York City's Hospital for Joint Diseases and Medical Center, and founder and past president of the American Orthopedic Foot Society. "This is because of the style of women's shoes—they don't conform to the foot.

High heels make the whole foot slide forward; it jams in the front of the shoe. The higher the heel, the more weight is carried on the ball of the foot, which can cause a callus. If a woman has a wide forefoot, it will be especially jammed, and raise the danger of deformities like corns, bunions and hammertoes." High heels worn habitually can shorten the Achilles tendon, leaving the wearer open to injuries.

Other styles are associated with other problems. Platform shoes tie with high heels for causing the worst foot and ankle injuries. Wearing a shoe with a stiff wooden sole that hikes you one, two, even three inches off the ground is like walking on stilts. It throws your center of gravity off, and reduces the foot's flexibility so that a misstep could result in a seriously twisted ankle, or sprain, or worse.

Boots can present problems aplenty as well—at least those that are chosen for their all-day good looks rather than their bad-weather practicality. High heels, as we've already mentioned, have their built-in hazards—some of which can be further exaggerated by the bad weather conditions that boots are commonly subject to. But, in addition to that, a boot that is too tight around the calf can actually cut off circulation and contribute to or cause circulatory problems. And boots that are made of synthetic material or those that have been waterproofed with silicone don't allow the foot to breathe and should not be worn indoors for extended periods of time.

Your best bet, then, is to buy yourself a pair of warm, waterproof, skidproof boots for those wicked winter days but switch to comfortable shoes at home or at the office.

When buying shoes, you'd do well to follow the example of podiatrist Neal Kramer of Bethlehem, Pennsylvania: "I use style as the last criterion—after fit and sensible design." Whatever the style, make sure the shoe fits. That may sound obvious, but it's not always easy, podiatrists warn.

For starters, don't buy shoes in the morning. Wait until the afternoon or evening when your feet have swelled from a day's worth of walking. If they're comfortable then, there's a good chance they'll be comfortable in the long run. Even so, it's not a bad idea to wear the shoes at home, on carpeting for an hour or so (providing of course, that you take care not to damage or dirty the soles). If after that time you feel a pinch, don't be afraid to return them.

Also, don't be taken in by a fast-talking shoe salesman who's more interested in the sale than the fit. The old argument that you've got to "break them in" before they become comfortable just isn't so. If they don't fit on the floor of the shoe store, they're more than likely to be a pain down the road.

Another point is to buy a shoe based on fit, not size. One manufacturer's 7 medium may be another one's 7½ narrow. So rather than offer your size up front, have the shoe salesman measure your foot while standing.

But the real question is, how do they feel?

To give your toes a chance to spread out naturally, your shoes should be about a quarter of an inch longer than your longest toe. They should be high and wide enough not to squash your toes. The shank (the part of the shoe between the ball of the foot and the heel) should be wide enough to accommodate your foot. Ideally, there should be no more than a one-inch difference between the height of the heel and the sole. And the sole should be flexible enough to bend with your foot, and thick enough to absorb some of the shock of life on concrete.

"The shoe should conform to the foot, not the foot to the shoe," says Dr. Jahss. "Children's shoes conform to their feet, so we don't see children with the foot pains and complications that adults have. If adults wore kids' shoes, they'd be fine."

Give an eye to material when you buy shoes. Because they retain heat and moisture, some nonporous man-made materials are more likely to promote fungus and bacterial infections than naturally porous leather, or canvas.

DRUGS

The chart on the following pages is a guide to drugs frequently used by women, and it has some necessary limitations you should be aware of. It covers only a few of the side effects and interactions that may occur with the drugs listed. That's because how a drug affects you depends on your dose, your physical makeup, and your general well-being. What's more, anything else you swallow at the same time—food, drink, even over-the-counter drugs such as antacids—will alter its effect. You should also remember that practically *no* drug is a safe drug while you're pregnant. What affects you will affect your baby. That goes for breastfeeding, too. Most medicines cross the placenta and may harm the fetus in doing so. Likewise, many drugs will go on to appear in your breast milk and give a baby a bit more than she or he bargains for—or needs.

There's also the problem of the form of the drug itself. When a new drug is developed, it's given not one but *two* names—a common or "generic" name and its brand name. The company that discovers a drug may hold a patent on it for 17 years, during which time the discovery can be sold only under the brand name the company gives it. After this period the drug enters the public domain and may be sold by other firms under its generic name. For example, Tylenol is well known as a popular pain-killer, but few people would recognize its generic name, acetaminophen. Aspirin, on the other hand, is a generic drug sold on the open market under both its common name and several brand names such as Anacin and Bufferin. The tricks to this game are two: one is to learn which drugs are available generically, because they're cheaper that way, and the second is to make sure that the lab that produces a generic drug has been approved to do so by the Food and Drug Administration (FDA). You can check on this by asking your pharmacist. He'll tell you when you are buying a product quality-controlled by the government and when you're not.

Still another sticky spot is the fact that the FDA also approves drugs for specific uses. For example, clonidine has been officially approved *only* for the treatment of hypertension, but some physicians also prescribe it for migraine and symptoms of menopause. Most of the drug uses we've listed in the chart have been government-approved, but to make sure you're not becoming an unsuspecting guinea pig by taking a drug your doctor orders, ask him if *his* use is an approved use. If it isn't, ask him why he's sure about the use when the FDA is not.

Which brings us to this maxim: the key to taking medications safely is open communication with your physician or pharmacist. A few questions—like those in the last paragraph—will help take the magic out of *their* potion and prepare *you* to get the best results with the fewest complications.

When your doctor prescribes a particular drug, you should ask most of the following:

What's the name of the drug you're prescribing? What are its possible side effects? Are there any that warrant contacting you when they show up? Does the drug interact with any foods, drinks or other medicines, including common drugstore items, I might use? Which interactions should be avoided at all costs? How long can the drug be stored before it loses its potency? Is there anything I should know about storing it?

Finally—and you may balk at this—ask, "Is this drug absolutely necessary? What would happen if I didn't take it or stopped in the middle of the treatment for some reason?" Why? Look at it this way. You go to a doctor when something is really bothering you. You want him or her to give you a charm to eliminate that complaint. More often than not that something is a piece of paper that sends you directly to a pharmacist. The question is, is there some less medicinal, perhaps slower, way to get the job done? If your problem is only an annoyance, it may go away on its own, given a proper diet and plenty of rest. Ask. Your physician may be more willing to suggest alternative treatments if he or she knows that you'd like to avoid medication.

What about stopping a drug in the middle of a prescribed period? This is a particularly important question when you are taking an antibiotic, because its side effects may tempt you to quit before you should—and that could leave you with more problems, since it can allow your infection to return. True, some side effects do warrant stopping a medication, but you should always ask your doctor before you act.

Sounds like a mouthful for you and an earful for your doctor. But it just makes sense to know what you're putting in your body, why, and what it may do while there. If you don't feel comfortable interrogating your doctor, or he or she refuses to cooperate, maybe it's a sign to look for one who is more open and informative. And remember: if you forget to ask your doctor something, you can always grill your pharmacist.

How to Use The Drug Chart

In looking at the chart, you'll notice that some drug names begin with a small letter and others are capitalized. A drug name beginning with a small letter is generic, while a capital letter indicates a brand name. The side effects and interactions of a particular drug are always given under its generic name.

For example, your doctor may prescribe a drug called Marax for asthma. Consulting the chart, you will find that Marax is a brand name and that it contains ephedrine and theophylline, two generic compounds often used in the treatment of asthma. Both have specific and distinct side effects and interactions, and so, to get a complete picture of what may be in store for you, you must look up each of these ingredients and combine the results.

A WOMAN'S REFERENCE GUIDE TO DRUG SIDE

DRUG	USES	SIDE EFFECTS
acetaminophen **Tylenol**	Painkiller	Usually mild. May cause skin reaction. With high doses, vomiting, gastrointestinal hemorrhage, liver
Aldomet (*methyldopa*)	Treatment of hypertension	See methyldopa
Alka-Seltzer **Effervescent Pain** **Reliever and Antacid** (*aspirin, sodium* *bicarbonate and* *citric acid*)	Painkiller and antacid	See aspirin
aluminum hydroxide **Gelusil** **Maalox**	Antacid	Softening of the bones may occur if combined with a diet low in phosphate since the drug tends to deplete the body of phosphates. Constipation may also occur if not combined with
amitriptyline **Elavil**	Treatment of depression	See imipramine Side effects occur less frequently here.

*The information in this table was compiled by Takla Gardey and should be considered informative and not prescriptive or all-encompassing. It was reviewed for medical content by Stephen Paul, Ph.D., chairman of the department of pharmaceutical economics and health care delivery of Temple University in Philadelphia, Pennsylvania.

Effects & Interactions *

INTERACTIONS

and kidney damage. Use with caution with liver or kidney disorders.

Alcohol
May enhance activity of acetaminophen.
Barbiturates (including some sedatives)
May reduce effectiveness of acetaminophen due to increased breakdown.

See methyldopa

NOTE: Antacid (sodium bicarbonate) makes intestinal contents more alkaline. This inhibits the absorption of weak acids such as aspirin and sulfonamides, but enhances weak bases such as antihistamines and narcotic painkillers. See also aspirin.

magnesium hydroxide. Should not be taken during pregnancy since malformation of the fetus has been known to occur.

NOTE: Antacids containing aluminum salts tend to inhibit intestinal absorption of many drugs and vitamins, reducing their effectiveness. Also, absorption will vary since all antacids make intestinal contents more alkaline. This inhibits weak acids such as aspirin and sulfonamides, but enhances weak bases such as antihistamines.
Anticoagulants
Antacids further increase blood clotting time.

See imipramine
Side effects occur less frequently here.

SOURCES: Adapted from *Martindale, The Extra Pharmacopoeia*, 27th ed., ed. Ainley Wade (London: Pharmaceutical Press, 1977).
Hazards of Medication, 2d ed., by Eric W. Martin et al. (Philadelphia: J. B. Lippincott, 1978).
Physician's Desk Reference, 34th ed. (Oradell, N.J.: Medical Economics, 1980).
Physician's Desk Reference for Nonprescription Drugs, 1st ed. (Oradell, N.J.: Medical Economics, 1980).
Handbook of Nonprescription Drugs, 6th ed. (Washington, D.C.: American Pharmaceutical Association, 1979).
The People's Pharmacy, by Joe Graedon (New York: St. Martin's Press, 1976).

152

DRUG	USES	SIDE EFFECTS
amphotericin B Fungizone	Antifungal agent. Treatment of vaginitis.	Vein irritation resulting in pain and clotting of the blood if injected. Headache, nausea, vomiting, chills, fever, muscle and joint pains, lack of appetite, diarrhea and gastrointestinal cramps. Occasionally, changes in blood pressure, heart problems, blurred vision, and convulsions may occur. Changes in kidney function
ampicillin Totacillin	Antibiotic. Treatment of urinary tract infections.	See penicillin G Allergic reactions may occur in sensitized persons. Skin disorders—usually after 5 days, diarrhea, nausea, vomiting.
Amytal (amobarbital)	Barbiturate used as a sedative	See phenobarbital
Ancobon (flucytosine)	Antifungal agent used for severe urinary tract and Candida albicans infections	See flucytosine
Antivert (meclizine)	Antihistamine used to treat nausea of motion sickness and morning sickness and also some allergic reactions	See meclizine
Anusol-HC (hydrocortisone acetate, bismuth gallate and other compounds)	Treatment of hemorrhoids	Side effects will be minor due to poor absorption from the rectum. Safety during pregnancy has not been established so use with caution.
aspirin	Relief of headaches, muscular and rheumatic pain. In colds or flu, causes reduction of temperature.	Nausea, vomiting and stomach pain. High doses may cause dizziness, rapid breathing, mental confusion and fever. May lead to heart and breathing difficulties and coma. More important is the irritation of the stomach even in small doses,

INTERACTIONS

and blood disorders such as anemia and low blood potassium occur frequently. Application to the skin may produce a rash and discolor nails.

NOTE: If given orally or in the form of vaginal suppositories, the above side effects are unlikely to occur due to poor absorption through the mucous membrane.

Muscle relaxants
Low blood potassium has been reported to produce muscle weakness, so muscle relaxants may have enhanced effect with amphotericin.

See also griseofulvin

Should not be used with penicillin or cephalosporin sensitivity. Caution with kidney problems or infectious mononucleosis.

Other antibiotics
Ampicillin is incompatible with some (e.g., tetracycline and erythromycin) but may have enhanced activity with others against certain infections (e.g., streptomycin).

See phenobarbital

See flucytosine

See meclizine

None in available sources.

which may lead to ulceration. Slight blood loss may occur and cause iron deficiency anemia with prolonged dosage. Should be avoided during pregnancy as may cause bleeding problems in the newborn and delivery complications.

Alcohol
Enhances blood loss from irritation of the stomach.
Anticoagulants
Aspirin increases blood clotting time.
Corticosteroids (e.g., cortisone)
Enhances irritation of the stomach, leading to ulcertion.

Vitamin C
Aspirin increases rate of excretion of vitamin C in the urine which, in turn, decreases excretion of aspirin, enhancing its activity.

DRUG	USES	SIDE EFFECTS
Bactrim *(sulfamethoxazole and trimethoprim)*	Antibiotic. Used in urinary tract infections.	See Sulfonamides With prolonged doses may have blood complications due to interference with folate metabolism.
Benadryl *(diphenhydramine)*	Antihistamine used for allergic reactions, cold symptoms, and motion sickness	See diphenhydramine
Bendectin *(doxylamine succinate—an antihistamine—and pyridoxine)*	Treatment of nausea during pregnancy	Drowsiness, nervousness, headache, palpitations, diarrhea, disorientation and irritability. User should not drive or operate machinery. Has been
Benylin *(diphenhydramine and other ingredients)*	Treatment of cough and respiratory congestion	See diphenhydramine Should be avoided during pregnancy.
Bonine *(meclizine)*	Antihistamine used to treat nausea of motion sickness and morning sickness and also some allergic reactions	See meclizine
Cafergot *(ergotamine tartrate and caffeine)*	Relief of migraine. Also used to stimulate uterine contractions in the prevention of postpartum hemorrhage.	See ergotamine tartrate
Catapres *(clonidine)*	Treatment of hypertension, migraine, and menopausal symptoms	See clonidine
cephaloridine **Loridine**	Antibiotic. Used in treatment of urinary tract infections.	Allergic reactions including itchiness and skin rashes may occur, particularly in those hypersensitive to penicillin. Additional infections such as

INTERACTIONS

See Sulfonamides

See diphenhydramine

shown to produce fetal abnormalities in laboratory animals. Should not be used during pregnancy.

See diphenhydramine

See diphenhydramine

See meclizine

See ergotamine tartrate

See clonidine

Candida and *Pseudomonas* may ensue. May cause kidney complications which can be fatal.

Furosemide (Lasix)
Combination enhances kidney complications, which may be dangerous.
Gentamicin
Combination increases kidney complications, which may prove lethal in those with kidney problems, in the elderly, or in those taking large doses.

DRUG	USES	SIDE EFFECTS
chlordiazepoxide Librium	Tranquilizer	See diazepam
chlorpropamide Diabinese	Treatment of diabetes (antidiabetic)	Mild effects include nausea, vomiting, dizziness, weakness, and headache, depending on dose. If hypersensitive may cause fever, blood
Choloxin (*dextrothyroxine sodium*)	Lowers blood cholesterol	See thyroid Hair loss, skin rashes, visual disturbances and menstrual irregularities also occur. Should not be used with
cimetidine Tagamet	Treatment of stomach ulcers	Diarrhea, muscle pain, dizziness, mental confusion and skin rash occasionally occur.
Clomid (*clomiphene citrate*)	Treatment of infertility (to stimulate ovulation) and endometrial hyperplasia	See clomiphene citrate
clomiphene citrate Clomid	Treatment of infertility (to stimulate ovulation) and endometrial hyperplasia	Depending on dosage may cause hot flashes, blurring of vision, abdominal discomfort, nausea, vomiting, ovarian complications. (Check with your physician if these side effects persist.) Occasionally, skin and liver disorders may occur. Also depres-

INTERACTIONS

See diazepam

disorders and skin rashes. Can cause prolonged hypoglycemia (low blood sugar). Increases sun sensitivity. Should not be used during pregnancy.

Alcohol
In larger quantities, alcohol induces breakdown of anti-diabetics, leading to high blood sugar. Alcohol itself has hypoglycemic action, which interferes with the antidiabetic. May be lethal.

Antibiotics
Tetracycline and sulfon-amides both enhance anti-diabetic activity.

Anticoagulants
Enhance antidiabetic activity of drug.

Aspirin
Enhances antidiabetic activity. Coma may occur

Coffee
Coffee consumption by a mature onset diabetic may raise blood sugar levels (opposite to the nondiabetic).

Corticosteroids (e.g., cortisone) Raise blood sugar levels, antagonizing the drug.

Diuretics
Tend to produce high blood sugar levels and aggravate sugar intolerance. Insulin shock may occur.

Epinephrine (adrenaline) Raises blood sugar levels and may inhibit antidiabetic activity.

Marijuana
May decrease sugar tolerance and increase drug requirement.

Oral contraceptives
May increase blood sugar levels and decrease sugar tolerance. (Other forms of contraception may be preferable for diabetics.)

Thyroid drugs
May increase requirement for oral antidiabetic agents. Caution.

liver or kidney disease. Caution with hypertension or heart disease.

See thyroid

None in available sources.

See clomiphene citrate

sion, fatigue, dizziness, sleep diffi-culties, breast tenderness, weight gain, heavy menses or spotting.

Should not be taken with liver dis-ease or during pregnancy (Warning: multiple births possible, particularly at high doses.)

None in available sources.

DRUG	USES	SIDE EFFECTS
clonidine Catapres	Treatment of hypertension, migraine, and menopausal symptoms	Drowsiness and dryness of mouth frequently occur. Reduced heart rate, constipation, water retention, and weight gain are common. Also anxiety, pain near the ear, and itchiness. Depression, dizziness, nausea, head-
codeine	Relief of pain, insomnia, cough, nausea and anxiety	Difficulty in breathing, slow heartbeat, constipation, nausea, vomiting, dizziness and drowsiness with recommended doses. Prolonged use of
Colace (docusate sodium)	Treatment of constipation	See docusate sodium
cortisone	Used for replacement therapy with adrenal insufficiency. The dose is increased with infection, stress or trauma. Has been used for allergic disorders but synthetic forms such as prednisone are now preferred.	See prednisone
CoTylenol Cold Formula (acetaminophen, a decongestant and an antihistamine)	Relief from cold symptoms	Nervousness, sleeplessness, or possibly drowsiness. User should not drive or operate machinery. Not recommended with asthma, glaucoma,
Coumadin (warfarin)	Treatment to prevent blood clotting (anticoagulant)	See warfarin

INTERACTIONS

ache, eye irritation and sleeping difficulties. User should not drive or operate machinery. Withdrawal symptoms occur when the medication is discontinued suddenly.

Amphetamines
Clonidine incompatible with amphetamines. Disruption of blood pressure results.
Antidepressants
Inhibit lowering of blood pressure.
Central nervous system depressants (e.g., alcohol)
Clonidine may enhance depressant effect, leading to sedation and low blood pressure.
Diuretics
Clonidine enhanced by some diuretics.

Licorice (natural)
Antagonism with clonidine occurs, which may result in a rise in blood pressure. Avoid eating large quantities (over ¾ ounce).
Nasal decongestants
Inhibit lowering of blood pressure.
Oral contraceptives
Oral contraceptives tend to raise blood pressure, which is antagonistic to blood pressure drugs.

codeine may lead to dependence. If hypersensitive, may produce skin reactions. Take with food to avoid stomach distress.

Alcohol (and other central nervous system depressants)
Increases depressant activity of codeine.

See docusate sodium

See prednisone

high blood pressure, heart disease, diabetes or thyroid disease. Avoid if taking medication for high blood pressure or emotional disorders.

See acetaminophen and diphenhydramine

See warfarin

DRUG	USES	SIDE EFFECTS
Cytomel (*liothyronine*)	Treatment of thyroid deficiency by producing a general increase in metabolism	See thyroid
danazol **Danocrine**	Treatment of endometriosis and inflammation of the breast	Mainly symptoms of estrogen deficiency occur, because drug inhibits ovarian function. Weight gain is common partly due to water retention. Acne, hairiness, hot flashes, breast changes and menstrual disturbances may occur. Nausea, vomiting, headache, dizziness, skin rashes, nervous-
Danocrine (*danazol*)	Treatment of endometriosis and inflammation of the breast	See danazol
Demulen (*ethynodiol diacetate and ethinyl estradiol*)	Oral contraceptive	See Oral contraceptives
Dexedrine (*dextroamphetamine sulfate*)	Weight-reducing aid	See dextroamphetamine sulfate
dextroamphetamine sulfate **Dexedrine**	Weight-reducing aid	Dryness of mouth, nausea, difficult urination, restlessness, insomnia, headache, dizziness, tremor, constipation or diarrhea. Large doses may produce rapid heartbeat. Mental problems such as depression, fatigue, disorientation, convulsions and coma may occur.
Diabinese (*chlorpropamide*)	Treatment of diabetes	See chlorpropamide

INTERACTIONS

See thyroid

ness, backache, muscle pain and hair loss have been reported. (Check with your physician if male characteristics develop.)

Should not be used with heart, kidney or liver disorders, migraine or epilepsy. Also avoid taking during pregnancy and breastfeeding.

None in available sources.

See danazol

See Oral contraceptives

See dextroamphetamine sulfate

Prolonged use may produce dependence. Should only be used when alternatives have been ineffective. User should not drive or operate machinery. Avoid with even mild hypertension. Should not be taken during pregnancy or breastfeeding.

Alcohol
Central nervous system stimulants decrease depressant effects of alcohol, but do not counteract its impairment of coordination.
Antidepressants
Amphetamines increase antidepressant activity.
Bananas, pineapples and plums (containing serotonin, a derivative of tyramine: see Tyramine-rich foods at right)
Caffeine
(see Tyramine-rich foods at right)

Reserpine
Amphetamines inhibit lowering of blood pressure by reserpine.
Sodium bicarbonate
Enhances intestinal absorption, leading to increased effectiveness of drug.
Tyramine-rich foods
Fermented foods such as cheese and red wine, avocados, chocolate, meat extracts may cause severe high blood pressure.

See chlorpropamide

DRUG	USES	SIDE EFFECTS
diazepam Valium	Tranquilizer, sedative, muscle relaxant, and anti-convulsant	Usually mild and infrequent. Drowsiness, lack of coordination. Also low blood pressure, gastrointestinal dis-
Dietac (*phenylpropanolamine*)	Weight-reducing aid	See ephedrine
diethylstilbestrol (DES)	Treatment of menopausal symptoms, amenorrhea due to ovarian disorders and symptoms of breast cancer	See estradiol DES was the first estrogen shown to induce vaginal adenosis (formation of glandular tissue in the vagina where normally there is none) and adeno-carcinoma of the vagina and cervix (cancer of the glandular tissue) in daughters of women who took DES during pregnancy. Also there have
digitalis	Treatment of heart failure	Side effects usually result from the high doses required, which can be fatal. Nausea, vomiting, loss of appetite, diarrhea and abdominal pain are early symptoms of overdosage. Also headache, drowsiness, depression, confusion, tingling in hands and
dimenhydrinate Dramamine	Treatment of nausea, particularly motion sickness	Drowsiness. User should not drive or operate machinery.

INTERACTIONS

turbances, skin rashes, headache. Prolonged doses may lead to dependence (see Valium section).

Alcohol
Diazepam lowers tolerance to alcohol. Enhances sedation and low blood pressure.
Antacids and foods
Reduce absorption of drug.

Central nervous system depressants
Greatly increase depressant effect of diazepam, leading to deep sedation, possibly coma and death.

See ephedrine

been abnormalities noted in sons of DES mothers. Should not be taken during pregnancy. Lack of appetite, abdominal pain, diarrhea, painful urination and skin rashes may occur. Also may cause salt and water retention.

See estradiol

feet, blurring of vision or a disturbance in color vision. Irregular heartbeat may also occur. These effects may be enhanced with potassium deficiency. Caution with certain heart complications and kidney problems.

NOTE: Check with your pharmacist or physician before taking any other medications including weight loss aids, cold and allergy drugs, antacids, antiasthmatics and diarrhea drugs.

Amphotericin B
Often causes potassium deficiency which leads to enhanced side effects of digitalis.
Barbiturates
Reduce effectiveness of digitalis.
Calcium
Enhances side effects of digitalis, which can be fatal if calcium is injected. Irregular heartbeat may occur if digitalis is given with calcium or vitamin D supplements.

Corticosteroids (e.g., cortisone)
May cause potassium deficiency which leads to enhanced side effects of digitalis.
Diuretics
Some diuretics deplete the body of potassium and magnesium and increase calcium levels. This makes the heart more sensitive to digitalis which may cause irregular heartbeat, leading to death. Side effects may be increased.

Alcohol
Enhances side effects of dimenhydrinate.
Antibiotics
Dimenhydrinate may mask ear damage that can occur

with certain antibiotics. Combination should be avoided as the damage may reach an irreversible state before it is recognized.

DRUG	USES	SIDE EFFECTS
diphenhydramine Benadryl	Antihistamine used for allergic reactions, cold symptoms, and motion sickness	Sedation from drowsiness to deep sleep, inability to concentrate, lethargy, lowered blood pressure, muscular weakness, and reduced coordination. Also gastrointestinal disturbances, blurred vision, headache, mood changes, nightmares, irritability, loss of appetite. May also include insomnia, rapid heartbeat, tremors, and bring on fits in epileptics.
docusate sodium Colace Materna	Treatment of constipation	Rare. Bitter taste, sore throat and nausea may occur. May become habit-forming with continued usage.
Dramamine (dimenhydrinate)	Treatment of motion sickness	See dimenhydrinate
Dymelor (acetohexamide)	Treatment of diabetes	See chlorpropamide
Elixophyllin (theophylline)	Treatment of asthma	See theophylline
Emetrol (sugars and orthophosphoric acid)	Treatment of nausea and vomiting	None in available sources.
Enovid 5 (norethynodrel and mestranol)	Oral contraceptive	See Oral contraceptives
ephedrine	Treatment of asthma (to prevent bronchial spasm), and allergic disorders	Giddiness, headache, nausea, vomiting, thirst, rapid heartbeat, chest pain, muscular weakness, tremors,
Equanil (meprobamate)	Tranquilizer and muscle relaxant	See meprobamate

INTERACTIONS

Occasionally has produced allergic symptoms, particularly when applied to skin.

Caution: if affected by drowsiness, do not drive or operate machinery. Avoid drinking alcohol.

Should not be used when breast-feeding.

Alcohol and other central nervous system depressants
Enhance side effects of drug, particularly drowsiness.
Corticosteroids (e.g., cortisone)
Diphenhydramine reduces effectiveness of corticosteroids due to increased breakdown.
Estrogen (e.g., oral contraceptives)
Diphenhydramine reduces effectiveness of estrogen due to increased breakdown.

NOTE: Colace may decrease absorption of drugs and nutrients due to more rapid passage through the gastrointestinal tract.

See dimenhydrinate

See chlorpropamide

See theophylline

None in available sources.

See Oral contraceptives

anxiety, sleeping difficulties, hypertension, and irregular heartbeat may occur if injected.

Blood pressure drugs
Ephedrine and blood pressure drugs inhibit each other's activity.
Ergotrate
Ephedrine with ergotrate may induce a postpartum rise in blood pressure, sometimes extremely dangerous.
Tranquilizers
Severe high blood pressure can occur when taken with certain types of tranquilizers.

See meprobamate

DRUG	USES	SIDE EFFECTS
ergonovine maleate **Ergotrate maleate**	Treatment of postpartum hemorrhage	See ergotamine tartrate Usually not as severe.
ergotamine tartrate **Gynergen**	Relief of migraine. Also used to stimulate uterine contractions in the prevention of postpartum hemorrhage.	In high doses nausea, vomiting, diarrhea, thirst, chilliness, itchiness, numbness, rapid and weak pulse, and confusion may occur; and death may ensue with overdose. Should not be taken during pregnancy, during first and second stages of labor or when breastfeeding.
Ergotrate maleate (*ergonovine maleate*)	Treatment of postpartum hemorrhage	See ergotamine tartrate
erythromycin	Antibiotic. Treatment of urinary tract and respiratory infections.	Rare and usually mild. Large doses may produce nausea, vomiting, diarrhea and cramping. Hypersensitivity
Esidrix (*hydrochlorothiazide*)	Diuretic used for water retention, premenstrual tension, and hypertension	See hydrochlorothiazide
estradiol	Estradiol is the most active of naturally occurring estrogens. Used for primary amenorrhea, delayed onset of puberty; also given in combination with progestins for oral contraception (see Oral contraceptives). In estrogen replacement therapy and for menopausal symptoms other forms are now preferred.	May cause alterations in uterine function such as endometrial growth with withdrawal bleeding or amenorrhea. Sodium and water retention, weight gain, enlargement of the breasts, changes in liver function, jaundice, depression, headache, dizziness, nausea, vomiting, skin reactions. Low doses have been shown to stimulate breast cancer, but high doses may suppress cancer growth. Prolonged use in postmenopausal women has been associated with endometrial and breast cancer. Vaginal and cervical cancer has also been reported in daughters of women given estrogenic drugs during pregnancy (see diethylstilbestrol). Has been shown

INTERACTIONS

Avoid with severe infections, vascular disease, and liver or kidney disorders. Numbness or tingling of the arms and legs indicates the need to stop taking the medication and contact physician. Should not be taken in prolonged doses or in excess of prescribed dosage.

Propranolol
Propranolol with ergotamine causes severe peripheral constriction of the blood vessels which may lead to more severe migraine.

See ergotamine tartrate

and additional infection are rare. Liver toxicity may occur with estolate form of drug; check with your pharmacist.

Fruit juices and other acidic beverages
Reduced activity of erythromycin occurs with low pH (acid). As pH increases (becoming more alkaline) activity is enhanced (as with bicarbonate of soda).
Other antibiotics
Erythromycin incompatible with some (e.g., tetracycline) but may actually have enhanced activity with others (e.g., streptomycin) against certain infections.
Theophylline
May require reduced dose of theophylline due to decreased breakdown.

See hydrochlorothiazide

to increase the possibility of urinary tract infections. Also has effects on the eye which may require a change in contact lenses.

Should not be taken with history of cancer of the breast or sex organs, blood-clotting disorders or liver complaints. Caution if over 35 years of age, following an operative delivery, with epilepsy, heart or kidney disease. Also may aggravate diabetes and porphyria.

NOTE: Hormone pregnancy tests have been associated with fetal malformations.
(See also Oral Contraceptives section.)

Alcohol
Estrogens may lead to lowered tolerance for alcohol (see Alcohol: Social Drinking section).
Corticosteroids (e.g., cortisone) Estrogens enhance anti-inflammatory activity of corticosteroids.

Insulin
Estrogens can cause an increase in blood glucose, increasing insulin requirement.
Meprobamate
Meprobamate reduces effectiveness of estrogens.

DRUG	USES	SIDE EFFECTS
ethinyl estradiol	Treatment of menopausal symptoms either alone or combined with methyl-testosterone. Treatment of symptoms of breast cancer and menstrual disorders. Used as an oral contraceptive when combined with progestin.	See estradiol
ethynodiol diacetate	Used in combination with an estrogen for treatment of menstrual disorders and as an oral contraceptive	See progestin
Ex-Lax (*phenolphthalein*)	Treatment of constipation	See phenolphthalein
Fiorinal (*butalbital, aspirin, phenacetin and caffeine*)	Relief of headache	Drowsiness and dizziness. Also gastrointestinal disturbances including nausea, vomiting and flatulence. Prolonged use may lead to depend-
Flagyl (*metronidazole*)	Antibiotic used particularly in the treatment of *Trichomonas vaginalis* infections. Also used to treat other infections of the genitourinary tract, liver and intestine.	See metronidazole
flucytosine Ancobon	Antifungal agent used for severe urinary tract and *Candida* and *Cryptococcus* infections	Nausea, vomiting and diarrhea. Also skin rashes, confusion, headache, sedation and dizziness. Changes in liver function and blood disorders occasionally occur depending on dose. Should not be taken if with kid-
Fulvicin (*griseofulvin*)	Antifungal agent used particularly for ringworm of skin, hair or nails	See griseofulvin
Fungizone (*amphotericin B*)	Antifungal cream used in the treatment of severe vaginitis	See amphotericin B

INTERACTIONS

See estradiol

See progestin

See phenolphthalein

ence. Caution during pregnancy and
when breastfeeding.
　See also phenobarbital

See phenobarbital

See metronidazole

ney, liver or blood complications.
Caution during pregnancy.
　NOTE: Stomach symptoms may be
reduced or avoided by spreading
dosage over a 15-minute period.

See griseofulvin

See griseofulvin

See amphotericin B

DRUG	USES	SIDE EFFECTS
Furadantin (*nitrofurantoin*)	Antibiotic used in treatment of urinary tract infections	See nitrofurantoin
furosemide **Lasix**	Potent diuretic used in water retention, kidney failure and hypertension. (Should be taken with supplementary potassium.)	Nausea, diarrhea, skin rash, low blood pressure. Single large doses or prolonged treatment may cause profound diuresis leading to salt (notably sodium and potassium) and water loss, weakness, muscle cramps, thirst
Gantanol (*sulfamethoxazole*)	Antibiotic. Used in treatment of urinary tract infections.	See Sulfonamides
Gantrisin (*sulfisoxazole*)	Antibiotic. Used in treatment of urinary tract infections.	See Sulfonamides
Gelusil (*aluminum hydroxide*)	Antacid	See aluminum hydroxide
Grisactin (*griseofulvin*)	Antifungal agent used particularly for ringworm of skin, hair or nails	See griseofulvin
griseofulvin **Fulvicin** **Grisactin**	Antifungal agent used particularly for ringworm of skin, hair or nails	Reactions are usually mild. Headache, skin rashes, dryness of mouth, gastrointestinal disturbances. Occasionally allergic reactions may
Gynergen (*ergotamine tartrate*)	Relief of migraine. Also used to stimulate uterine contractions in the prevention of postpartum hemorrhage.	See ergotamine tartrate

INTERACTIONS

See nitrofurantoin

and loss of appetite. Possibly anemia and deafness when kidney disorder present. Should not be used by women of childbearing age. Has been shown to produce malformations of the fetus in laboratory animals.

Alcohol
Combination may cause fainting.
Antibiotics
Combination with kanamycin and other antibiotics that are toxic to the ears may result in irreversible deafness.
Aspirin
Aspirin toxicity may develop with high doses of furosemide.

Corticosteroids (e.g., cortisone) Combination may cause a potassium deficiency. This can have dangerous consequences especially if taken with some heart medications.
Licorice (natural; see Corticosteroids above.)

See Sulfonamides

See Sulfonamides

See aluminum hydroxide

See griseofulvin

occur. Should not be used with liver failure and porphyria. Sun sensitivity has been reported. Has been shown to cause cancer in laboratory animals.

Alcohol
Alcohol with griseofulvin may cause flushing and rapid heartbeat.
Anticoagulants
Griseofulvin increases breakdown of anticoagulants, reducing their effectiveness.

Barbiturates
Griseofulvin reduces effectiveness and enhances depressant activity.

See ergotamine tartrate

DRUG	USES	SIDE EFFECTS
hydrochlorothiazide **Esidrix** **HydroDIURIL**	Diuretic used for water retention, premenstrual tension, and hypertension. (Should be taken with supplemental potassium.)	Occasionally allergies, skin rashes, lack of appetite, irritation of the stomach, nausea, vomiting, diarrhea, constipation, sun sensitivity, dizziness, headache, and weakness. Also changes in salt content of the body
HydroDIURIL *(hydrochlorothiazide)*	Diuretic used for water retention, premenstrual tension and hypertension	See hydrochlorothiazide
ibuprofen **Motrin**	Treatment of rheumatoid arthritis and osteoarthritis. Also used for relief of menstrual cramps.	See indomethacin May have delayed side effects.
imipramine **Tofranil**	Treatment of depression	Drowsiness, dry mouth, constipation, urine retention, blurred vision, irregular heart rate. Also nausea, vomiting, dizziness, tremor, lack of coordination, fatigue, blood reactions, skin rash and itching, sun sensitivity, changes in libido, breast enlargement and release of milk from the nipples. Heart complications which may be
Inderal *(propranolol)*	Treatment of hypertension, migraine, irregular heartbeat, and overactive thyroid gland	See propranolol

INTERACTIONS

(notably sodium and potassium) and prolonged use may result in potassium deficiency.

Caution with diabetes, kidney or liver disorders. Also during pregnancy and when breastfeeding.

Antidiabetics
Diuretics may alter the dosage of antidiabetic required due to modification of blood sugar levels.
Blood pressure drugs
Diuretics enhance lowering of blood pressure.
Cold and allergy drugs
Caution: check with pharmacist or physician first.

Corticosteroids (e.g., cortisone) Combination may deplete the body's minerals.
Licorice (natural)
Combination may deplete the body's potassium, resulting in paralysis in extreme cases.
Muscle relaxants
Combination may result in paralysis of the muscles used in breathing.

See hydrochlorothiazide

See indomethacin

fatal also occur. Should not be taken with liver damage, kidney disorders or heart disease. Caution with epilepsy, diabetes, asthma, mental problems, or constipation. User should not drive or operate machinery. Check with your physician if eye pain develops.

Alcohol
Potentially lethal combination due to enhanced sedation and lowering of blood pressure.
Anticoagulants
Combination further increases blood clotting time by as much as four times.
Antidepressants
Two types of antidepressants should not be taken together due to enhanced effects.
Antihistamines
Combination enhances side effects. Imipramine has been associated with malformations of the fetus when taken with the antihistamine chloropyramine during the first trimester.

Aspirin
Potentially fatal combination due to enhanced activity of imipramine.
Blood pressure drugs
Caution when an antidepressant is discontinued: profound lowering of blood pressure may result.
Estrogen
Combination enhances activity of imipramine due to inhibition of breakdown, particularly with high doses of estrogen.
Reserpine
Imipramine inhibits reserpine activity.

See propranolol

DRUG	USES	SIDE EFFECTS
Indocin (*indomethacin*)	Treatment of rheumatoid arthritis and osteoarthritis	See indomethacin
indomethacin **Indocin**	Treatment of rheumatoid arthritis and osteoarthritis	Headache and dizziness, nausea, vomiting and stomach pain occur frequently. Loss of appetite, and diarrhea. Also stomach ulcers with possible bleeding, blood disorders, skin rashes, drowsiness and confusion.
insulin	Treatment of diabetes (lowers blood sugar)	Overdose causes hypoglycemia (low blood sugar), especially if too little carbohydrate is eaten or if patient exercises more than usual. Early symptoms are weakness, giddiness, pale skin, palpitations, nervousness, headache and tremor. Later there is an inability to concen-
Ionamin (*phentermine*)	Weight-reducing aid	See dextroamphetamine sulfate
kanamycin **Kantrex**	Antibiotic. Also used to treat urinary tract infections.	May cause irreversible partial or total deafness depending on dose, which is enhanced by liver or kidney impairment. Occurs less frequently when user is under 40 years of age. Caution especially in the event of previous treatment with streptomycin.
Kantrex (*kanamycin*)	Antibiotic. Also used to treat urinary tract infections.	See kanamycin
Lasix (*furosemide*)	Potent diuretic used in water retention, kidney failure and hypertension. (Should be taken with supplementary potassium.)	See furosemide

INTERACTIONS

See indomethacin

Caution with liver or kidney complaints, epilepsy or mental problems. Should not be taken with stomach ulcer, aspirin sensitivity, or during pregnancy.

Antacids
May reduce effectiveness of indomethacin by as much as 50 percent.
Anticoagulants
Extreme caution, since the combination changes the blood clotting time.
Aspirin
Combination enhances ulceration of the stomach, which may be fatal.

Corticosteroids (e.g., cortisone) Indomethacin enhances activity of corticosteroids, resulting in increased ulcer formation.
Probenecid
Increases blood levels of indomethacin, which increases its toxic potential.

trate, drowsiness and amnesia. May lead to convulsions and coma.
NOTE: Different immunological responses to beef and pork insulin have been reported, and changing from beef to pork insulin may result in hypoglycemia.

Alcohol
Alcohol enhances lowering of blood sugar.
Aspirin
Aspirin enhances lowering of blood sugar.
Diuretics
Diuretics may antagonize the hypoglycemic effect, possibly leading to hyper-

glycemia (high blood sugar).
Oral contraceptives
Oral contraceptives may increase blood sugar levels, which counteracts insulin activity.
Propranolol
Enhances insulin activity.

See dextroamphetamine sulfate

Nausea, vomiting, diarrhea and intestinal infections may occur. Should not be given for minor infections or with impaired hearing. If ringing in the ears or dizziness occurs, contact physician immediately.

Dimenhydrinate (Dramamine) May mask the loss of hearing due to kanamycin and delay its detection.
Diuretics
Combination with potent diuretics such as furosemide (Lasix) may result in

rapid and irreversible deafness.
Other antibiotics
With certain antibiotics, side effects of kanamycin may be increased, notably hearing loss and paralysis.

See kanamycin

See furosemide

DRUG	USES	SIDE EFFECTS
Librium (*chlordiazepoxide*)	Tranquilizer	See diazepam
Loestrin (*norethindrone acetate and ethinyl estradiol*)	Oral contraceptive	See Oral contraceptives
Loridine (*cephaloridine*)	Antibiotic. Used in treatment of urinary tract infections.	See cephaloridine
Maalox (*aluminum hydroxide and other ingredients*)	Antacid	See aluminum hydroxide
Marax (*ephedrine sulfate, theophylline and hydroxyzine*)	Treatment of asthma	See ephedrine and theophylline Should not be taken during pregnancy. Should be taken with food to minimize stomach distress.
Materna (*various vitamins, minerals, and docusate sodium, a stool softener*)	Supplement for use during pregnancy and breastfeeding	See docusate sodium
meclizine Antivert Bonine	Antihistamine used to treat nausea as in motion sickness, morning sickness and some allergic reactions	See diphenhydramine Should be avoided during pregnancy since meclizine has been associated with malformations of the
mefenamic acid Ponstel	Relief of pain, including menstrual cramps	See indomethacin May have delayed side effects.
meprobamate Equanil Miltown	Tranquilizer and muscle relaxant. Used in premenstrual tension.	Drowsiness, nausea, vomiting, diarrhea, weakness, headache, dizziness, lack of coordination, low blood pressure and rapid heart rate. Occasionally hypersensitivity reactions, notably skin disorders, may develop. Blood disorders have been reported. Large doses may result in convulsions and shock.

INTERACTIONS

See diazepam

See Oral contraceptives

See cephaloridine

See aluminum hydroxide

See ephedrine and theophylline

See docusate sodium

fetus in humans and in laboratory animals. Also should be avoided when breastfeeding. User should not drive or operate machinery.

See diphenhydramine

See indomethacin

Prolonged doses may lead to dependence. Should not be taken with porphyria, a history of hypersensitivity to meprobamate or epilepsy. User should not drive or operate machinery. Should not be taken during pregnancy or when breastfeeding.

Alcohol and other central nervous system depressants
Alcohol enhances and prolongs the tranquilizing effect. This may lead to overdosage resulting in drowsiness, coma, cessation of breathing, or death.

Barbiturates
(see Alcohol at left)
Estrogen
Meprobamate reduces effectiveness of estrogen therapy.

DRUG	USES	SIDE EFFECTS
mestranol	Used in combination with a progestin for treatment of menstrual disorders and as an oral contraceptive	See estradiol
Metamucil (*psyllium compound*)	Treatment of constipation, particularly with intestinal ulcer, diverticular disease, hemorrhoids and during pregnancy	See psyllium
methocarbamol	Muscle relaxant	Itching, skin rash, nasal stuffiness, red eyes. Also drowsiness and dizziness. Allergic reactions may occur,
methyldopa Aldomet	Treatment of hypertension	Drowsiness, dizziness upon standing suddenly, dryness of the mouth, nasal stuffiness, gastrointestinal disorders, diarrhea, constipation, fever, dizziness; and, more rarely, headache, water retention, joint and mus-
methysergide maleate Sansert	Treatment of severe migraine	See ergotamine tartrate Side effects severe. Should be used under supervision.
metronidazole Flagyl	Antibiotic used particularly in the treatment of *Trichomonas vaginitis* infections. Also used to treat other infections of the genitourinary tract, liver and intestine.	Gastrointestinal discomfort, dryness of mouth, headaches, skin rashes. Depression, drowsiness, urethral discomfort may also occur. Should not be taken during pregnancy as has been shown to produce birth defects.
Midol (*aspirin, cinnamedrine and caffeine*)	Used to relieve premenstrual tension	See aspirin
Miltown (*meprobamate*)	Tranquilizer and muscle relaxant	See meprobamate

INTERACTIONS

See estradiol

See psyllium

especially if sensitive to meprobamate.

Alcohol and other central nervous system depressants
Methocarbamol may enhance depressant effect, which is lethal in high doses due to breathing difficulties.

cular pain. Also reduced heart rate and blood disorders and may cause the urine to darken. Caution with liver or kidney complications or a history of mental depression. Contact physician if fever develops.

Amphetamines
Reduce effectiveness of methyldopa.
Antidepressants
Combination may result in headache, high blood pressure and related symptoms.
Cold and allergy drugs
Caution: check with pharmacist or physician first.

See ergotamine tartrate

Has been shown to cause cancer in laboratory animals and chromosome damage in patients following prolonged therapy at high dosage. Take with food to minimize stomach distress.
(See Vaginitis section.)

Alcohol
Drug slows breakdown of alcohol, resulting in severe intolerance. Headache, nausea, rapid heart rate, vomiting and faintness may ensue.
X-ray
Drug increases sensitivity to x-rays (has been used in radiation antitumor therapy).

See aspirin

See meprobamate

DRUG	USES	SIDE EFFECTS
Motrin (*ibuprofen*)	Treatment of rheumatoid arthritis and osteoarthritis. Also used for relief of menstrual cramps.	See indomethacin May have delayed side effects.
Mycostatin (*nystatin*)	Antifungal agent used in vaginitis, notably *Candida albicans* infections	See nystatin
Nembutal (*pentobarbital*)	Barbiturate used for treatment of insomnia and as a sedative	See phenobarbital
nitrofurantoin Furadantin	Antibiotic used in treatment of urinary tract infections	Occasionally nausea, vomiting, drowsiness, headache, and skin rashes. Allergic reactions with symptoms of lung and blood disorders have occurred. Should not
nitroglycerin	Lowers blood pressure by relaxing the blood vessels. Aids blood flow to the heart.	Dizziness, rapid heartbeat, throbbing headache. Large doses can cause vomiting, restlessness, syncope (respiratory and circulatory difficulties due to reduced blood flow in the
norethindrone	Treatment of menstrual disorders, delayed menstruation, and endometriosis. May be taken alone ("progestogen-only") or in combination with an estrogen as an oral contraceptive.	See progestin
norethindrone acetate	Treatment of menstrual disorders, endometriosis and breast cancer. Also combined with an estrogen for use as an oral contraceptive.	See progestin

INTERACTIONS

See indomethacin

See nystatin

See phenobarbital

be used with kidney problems. Should be avoided during pregnancy and when breastfeeding. Take with food to minimize stomach distress.

Acidic beverages (such as fruit juices)
Enhance activity of nitrofurantoin.
Alcohol
Drug slows breakdown of alcohol, resulting in severe intolerance. Headache, nausea, rapid heart rate, vomiting and fainting may ensue.

brain), and psychosis. Keep medication in original container and get fresh supply at least every three months.

Alcohol
Combination may cause low blood pressure and cardiovascular collapse.
Blood pressure drugs
Combination increases tendency to faint upon standing suddenly.
Licorice (natural)
If eaten in large quantities while taking drug, headache, high blood pressure and heart failure could result.

See progestin

See progestin

DRUG	USES	SIDE EFFECTS
norethynodrel	Used in combination with an estrogen for treatment of menstrual disorders and as an oral contraceptive. Also used to treat endometriosis.	See progestin
norgestrel	Used in combination with an estrogen for the treatment of menstrual disorders and endometriosis. Also may be taken alone ("progestogen-only") or in combination with an estrogen as an oral contraceptive.	See progestin
Norinyl (norethindrone and mestranol)	Oral contraceptive	See Oral contraceptives
Norlestrin (norethindrone acetate and ethinyl estradiol)	Oral contraceptive	See Oral contraceptives
nystatin Mycostatin	Antifungal agent used in vaginitis, notably Candida albicans infections	Usually mild and not likely to occur if applied via vaginal suppositories since drug is not absorbed through
Oral contraceptives Demulen Enovid 5 Loestrin Norinyl 1 + 50 Norlestrin Ortho-Novum Ovral Ovulen	There are four types: "combined," "sequential," "progestogen-only" and "post-coital." The "combined" is the most effective and consists of an orally active estrogen (ethinyl estradiol or mestranol) and an orally active progestogen (ethynodiol diacetate, norethindrone, norethindrone acetate, norethynodrel or norgestrel). For the specific side effects of these hormones see estradiol and progestin. For more information see also Oral Contraceptives section.	Generally the side effects of the "combined" depend on dosage, particularly the estrogen content (see Oral Contraceptives section). Hypertension and increased blood clotting, liver disorders, depression, and other mental changes occur. Also, gastrointestinal disorders, skin

INTERACTIONS

See progestin

See progestin

See Oral contraceptives

See Oral contraceptives

None in available sources.

the skin or mucous membranes. Orally, nausea, vomiting and diarrhea may occur with large doses.

or hair changes, headache, water retention, weight gain, increased breast size, and *Candida* infections in the vagina. Spotting or lack of periods may also occur. May have problems with contact lenses. Caution with diabetes.

Alcohol
Drug may lower alcohol tolerance.
Anticoagulants
Oral contraceptives decrease blood clotting time.
Antihistamines
May reduce effectiveness of oral contraceptives due to increased breakdown.
Barbiturates
Increased breakdown of oral contraceptives, reducing their effectiveness.
Insulin
Oral contraceptives cause an increase in blood sugar levels, antagonizing insulin activity.

DRUG	USES	SIDE EFFECTS
Orasone (*prednisone*)	Treatment of cystitis, breast cancer, rheumatoid arthritis, bronchial asthma, allergies and leukemia (acts as a corticosteroid)	See prednisone
Ortho-Novum (*norethindrone and mestranol*)	Oral contraceptive	See Oral contraceptives
Ovral (*norgestrel and ethinyl estradiol*)	Oral contraceptive	See Oral contraceptives
Ovulen (*ethynodiol diacetate and mestranol*)	Oral contraceptive	See Oral contraceptives
Pamprin (*acetaminophen, pamabrom—a mild diuretic—and pyrilamine maleate—an antihistamine*)	Treatment of premenstrual tension	See acetaminophen
Panwarfin (*warfarin*)	Treatment to prevent blood clotting (anticoagulant)	See warfarin
penicillin G	Antibiotic. Also used in urinary tract infections.	Diarrhea, nausea, heartburn and pruritis ani may occur. High doses may produce convulsions and other nervous disorders particularly with kidney failure. Most notably, hypersensitivity may occur which in extreme cases results in shock and collapse.
penicillin VK	Antibiotic	See penicillin G Sensitivity reactions may be less frequent.

INTERACTIONS

See prednisone

See Oral contraceptives

See Oral contraceptives

See Oral contraceptives

See acetaminophen

See warfarin

Death may ensue. A generalized sensitivity reaction can occur within 1–3 weeks with skin disorders, fever and painful joints, especially when applied to the skin by a patient 20 to 50 years of age. If you are allergic to other drugs, use with caution.

Anticoagulants
Enhance antibiotic activity.
Cheese
Blue cheese inhibits penicillin activity.
Other antibiotics
Certain antibiotics such as erythromycin and tetracycline may inhibit penicillin.
Painkilling drugs
Enhance antibiotic activity.

See penicillin G

DRUG	USES	SIDE EFFECTS
phenobarbital	Barbiturate used in treatment of insomnia as a sedative, and as an anticonvulsant	Central nervous system depression, particularly in the elderly. High doses will cause breathing difficulties, profound shock, low blood pressure, low body temperature, and prolonged coma. Prolonged use may lead to dependence. Because of drowsiness, user should not drive or operate machinery.
phenolphthalein Ex-Lax	Treatment of constipation (laxative)	Prolonged use of laxatives may result in dependence. This is due to a loss in sensitivity of the intestinal wall leading to the need for higher doses. Abdominal discomfort, gas, excessive loss of water and salts, notably
phenylpropanolamine Dietac	Used as a weight-reducing aid	See ephedrine
Phillips' Milk of Magnesia (*magnesium hydroxide*)	Antacid. Also acts as a mild laxative.	See aluminum hydroxide
Ponstel (*mefenamic acid*)	Relief of pain, including menstrual cramps	See indomethacin. May have delayed side effects
prednisone Orasone	Treatment of cystitis, breast cancer, rheumatoid arthritis, bronchial asthma, allergies and leukemia (acts as a corticosteroid)	Often large doses are necessary, and this results in salt and water imbalance in the body, leading to side effects such as water retention, hypertension, and loss of potassium in the urine. In extreme cases heart failure may occur (more common with cortisone than prednisone). These side effects may also occur if applied to the skin. Also loss of calcium and phosphorus from the bones resulting in osteoporosis and brittle bones may occur. High blood sugar develops, increasing the insulin requirement in diabetics. Corticosteroids may cause a delay

INTERACTIONS

Alcohol
Combination enhances depressant effects which are potentially lethal due to cessation of breathing.

Antibiotics
Combination with certain antibiotics may produce cessation of breathing and muscular weakness. However, tetracycline and griseofulvin both increase breakdown of phenobarbital, leading to reduced effectiveness.

Antihistamines
May inhibit phenobarbital and vice versa.

Aspirin and other pain-killing drugs
Drug reduces effectiveness of painkillers.

Vitamin C
Enhances sedative effect of phenobarbital through a reduction of discharge in the urine.

Vitamin D
Drug increases breakdown of vitamin D, resulting in deficiency, which in turn leads to reduced calcium levels in the blood.

potassium, muscular weakness and weight loss may occur. If hypersensitive, skin rash may develop. Should not be taken with abdominal pain of unknown cause.

NOTE: Due to the more rapid passage through the gut, laxatives may have an effect on drug absorption, reducing their effectiveness.

See ephedrine

See aluminum hydroxide

See indomethacin

in wound healing and increase vulnerability to infection. Also adrenal disorders may result, particularly if the corticosteroid is suddenly withdrawn. Muscle weakness, low blood pressure, hypoglycemia, headache, nausea, vomiting, restlessness, and muscle and joint pain may ensue.

Withdrawal should always be gradual. High doses for short periods of time appear to cause fewer side effects than prolonged treatment with lower doses. Should not be taken with stomach ulcer, osteoporosis or mental disorders. Caution with heart failure, diabetes, infectious diseases, kidney failure and in the elderly.

Amphotericin B
Combination may result in fungal infections.

Anticoagulants
Drug shortens blood clotting time. Severe hemorrhage has also been reported with the combination.

Antidepressants
Drug enhances antidepressant activity.

Antidiabetics
Drug increases blood sugar levels, resulting in the need for higher doses of antidiabetic.

Aspirin
Combination increases irritation of the stomach, leading to ulceration.

Barbiturates
Combination inhibits prednisone activity and enhances sedation effect of barbiturates.

Diuretics
Combination results in excessive potassium depletion.

Estrogen
Enhances anti-inflammatory effects of prednisone.

DRUG	USES	SIDE EFFECTS
prednisone *(continued)*		Also avoid with acute bacterial infections, herpes and other viral infections. (However, corticosteroids may be used with the appropriate antibiotics in treatment of some life-threatening infections.)
Premarin *(a mixture of estrogens from natural sources)*	Used primarily for treatment of menopausal symptoms. May be taken as tablets or used as vaginal cream.	See estradiol NOTE: Estrogens are absorbed directly via the mucous membranes of the genital tract into the body where
progestin	Progestin is a synthetic form of progesterone, a hormone which is produced from the ovaries and placenta. Used in treatment of menstrual disorders, uterine bleeding, breast cancer and endometrial cancer (other forms are now preferred).	Acne, water retention, weight gain, gastrointestinal disturbances, headache, depression, skin problems, vaginal infections (such as *Candida*), cramps, changes in libido, and menstrual patterns with unpredictable bleeding. Changes in liver function also may occur. Should not be used during preg-
propranolol **Inderal**	Treatment of hypertension, migraine, irregular heartbeat, and overactive thyroid gland	Nausea, vomiting, diarrhea, fatigue and dizziness. Circulatory depression with slow heart rate and low blood pressure occur. Also depression, sleep and vision disturbances, blood disorders, and skin rashes. Additional effects include constipation, water retention, weight gain,

INTERACTIONS

Indomethacin
Enhances prednisone activity, notably the severity of gastrointestinal ulcers.
Smoking
Nicotine increases the blood levels of body corticosteroids, resulting in an increased effect of drug.

Vaccines, live virus
(Measles, smallpox, rabies, yellow fever)
Serious and possibly fatal illness may develop. Corticosteroids may depress response to all vaccines. Discontinue 3 days before and until 14 days after vaccination.

they may produce the same side effects as if they had been taken by mouth.

See estradiol

nancy because of the risk of masculinization of the female fetus and other fetal abnormalities. Also may cause partial or complete vision loss. Caution with vaginal bleeding, breast cancer, heart or kidney disease, blood clotting, asthma or epilepsy.
See Oral contraceptives.

Antihistamines
Reduce effectiveness of progestin.
Barbiturates
Reduce effectiveness of progestin due to increased breakdown.

muscle cramps and dryness of the mouth.
Should not be taken with bronchial asthma, hypoglycemia, slow heart rate, or partial heart block.
Should not be taken during pregnancy or when breastfeeding.
Reduce the dose gradually when stopping medication.

Antidepressants
Combination should be avoided.
Antidiabetics
Combination may induce prolonged hypoglycemia. With hypertension it may also induce a hypertensive crisis.
Blood pressure drugs
Combination enhances lowering of blood pressure.
Epinephrine (adrenaline)

Combination enhances constriction of the blood vessels, which may result in raised blood pressure.
Ergot alkaloids (e.g., ergotamine)
Combination increases severity of migraine due to pronounced constriction of blood vessels.
Smoking
Combination may increase blood pressure considerably.

DRUG	USES	SIDE EFFECTS
Provera (*medroxyproges-terone acetate*)	Treatment of menstrual disorders, endometriosis, uterine cancer, and threatened miscarriage	See progestin
psyllium	Treatment of constipation	None with recommended doses. May become habit-forming with prolonged use.
pyrilamine maleate	Antihistamine	See diphenhydramine
Rau-Sed (*reserpine*)	Used as a sedative and in the treatment of hypertension	See reserpine
reserpine Rau-Sed Sandril	Treatment of hypertension	Drowsiness, nasal congestion, dryness of mouth, depression, lethargy, nightmares, diarrhea, gastrointestinal disorders; sometimes skin problems, and weight gain. High doses may cause irregular heartbeat and severe depression. Also anxiety, blurred vision and enlargement of the breasts may occur. Has been associated with the development of breast cancer, but is still unconfirmed. Should not be taken with
Rolaids (*dihydroxyaluminum sodium carbonate*)	Antacid	See aluminum hydroxide
S–P–T (*thyroid*)	Treatment of thyroid deficiency states producing a general increase in metabolism.	See thyroid
Sandril (*reserpine*)	Used as a sedative and in the treatment of hypertension	See reserpine
Sansert (*methysergide maleate*)	Treatment of severe migraine	See ergotamine tartrate

INTERACTIONS

See progestin

Psyllium may decrease absorption of drugs and nutrients due to more rapid passage through the gastrointestinal tract.

See diphenhydramine

See reserpine

history of mental depression, stomach or intestinal ulcers, heart problems, epilepsy, or allergic reactions such as bronchial asthma. Avoid during pregnancy as may produce breathing difficulties in the newborn. Also should not be taken when breastfeeding. Should not discontinue medication unless directed by your physician. Take with food to minimize stomach distress.

Alcohol
Combination enhances depressant effect.
Antidepressants
Reduce effectiveness of reserpine.
Barbiturates
Combination enhances depressant effect, resulting in low blood pressure and slow heart rate.
Digitalis
Combination results in irregular heartbeat.
Diuretics
Combination enhances lowering of blood pressure.

Ephedrine
Reserpine inhibits action of ephedrine and vice versa.
Muscle relaxants
May enhance the psychological side effects of reserpine.
Propranolol
Combination produces excessive sedation.
Stress
Sudden stress such as surgery combined with reserpine therapy may have profound effects on the heart and vascular system, and death may ensue.

See aluminum hydroxide
Tetracycline
Combination should be avoided.

See thyroid

See reserpine

See ergotamine tartrate

DRUG	USES	SIDE EFFECTS
Seconal *(secobarbital)*	Barbiturate used for treatment of insomnia and as a sedative	See phenobarbital
Senokot *(senna concentrate)*	Treatment of constipation	None with recommended doses. May become habit-forming with prolonged use.
Septra *(sulfamethoxazole and trimethoprim)*	Antibiotic. Used in urinary tract infections.	See Sulfonamides
Sominex *(pyrilamine maleate)*	Antihistamine used as a sleep aid	See diphenhydramine
Sudafed *(pseudoephedrine)*	Decongestant	See ephedrine
Sulfonamides *(for example, sulfamethoxazole and sulfisoxazole)*	Antibiotic. Used in treatment of urinary tract infections.	Common but usually mild. Nausea, vomiting, lack of appetite, fever and drowsiness. Also headache, fatigue, diarrhea, thyroid problems, inflammation of the mouth, arthritis, sleeping difficulties, depression, incoordination. Kidney complications resulting in lower back pain and blood disorders may also occur. Late in treatment, allergic reactions may develop, and cross-sensitivity is common between different forms of sulfonamides. Hepatitis (liver disease) has been reported to occur within 3 days of therapy and may be fatal.
Synthroid *(levothyroxine sodium)*	Treatment of thyroid deficiency states producing a general increase in metabolism	See thyroid
Tagamet *(cimetidine)*	Treatment of stomach ulcers	See cimetidine

INTERACTIONS

See phenobarbital

Senokot may decrease absorption of drugs and nutrients due to more rapid passage through the gastrointestinal tract.

See Sulfonamides

See diphenhydramine

See ephedrine

Sulfonamides should not be taken when previous sensitivity has been shown, with jaundice, or during pregnancy and breastfeeding.

NOTE: Sulfonamides vary in their ability to remain in solution, and may crystallize out of solution. To guard against this, drink plenty of fluids. Also solubility increases with pH (becoming more alkaline) so sulfonamides are frequently given with alkalinizing agents to prevent crystals from forming in the urine and causing kidney problems.

Alcohol
Drug reduces breakdown of alcohol, causing intolerance.
Anticoagulants
Drug further increases blood clotting time.
Antidiabetics
May enhance antibiotic activity of sulfonamides. Also combination may produce hypoglycemia.
Aspirin and other pain-killing drugs
Enhance antibiotic activity.
Para-aminobenzoic acid (PABA)
Decreases activity of sulfonamides. Should be

avoided.
Penicillins
Combination may alter penicillin and sulfonamide activity.
Sunlight
Direct exposure should be avoided due to sun sensitivity produced by sulfonamide.
Vitamin C
Since vitamin C is acidic it may increase risk of crystals forming in the urine due to the acidity (see Note under side effects). Also sulfonamides may increase vitamin C excretion.

See thyroid

See cimetidine

DRUG	USES	SIDE EFFECTS
Temaril (*trimeprazine tartrate*)	Treatment of itching and other skin problems	See trimeprazine tartrate
Tenuate (*diethylpropion*)	Weight-reducing aid	See dextroamphetamine sulfate
testosterone Oreton	Treatment of breast cancer and endometriosis	Increase in lean weight, sodium and water retention, suppression of ovarian activity and menstruation. Large doses produce symptoms of masculinity such as hairiness, deepening of the voice, decrease in breast size and endometrial tissue in the uterus,
tetracycline	Antibiotic	Nausea, vomiting, diarrhea and other gastrointestinal disturbances are common with high doses. Overgrowth of resistant organisms such as intestinal bacteria and *Candida albicans* may occur, resulting in mouth infections, pruritis ani, and diarrhea. Allergic reactions may occur, including sun sensitivity. Should not be used with renal disease. Occasionally severe and sometimes fatal liver damage has occurred in
theophylline Elixophyllin	Treatment of asthma. Also used as a diuretic.	Nausea, vomiting, gastrointestinal bleeding, visual disorders, insomnia, headache, anxiety, confusion, rapid

INTERACTIONS

See trimeprazine tartrate

See dextroamphetamine sulfate

acne, increase in libido, and decrease in breast milk. If taken orally may produce inflammation of the mouth. Should be avoided during pregnancy as may cause irregular sexual development of the fetus. Also avoid when breastfeeding.

both pregnant and nonpregnant women treated with tetracycline, especially when given intravenously. Vitamin deficiency may occur especially with prolonged dosage. May be deposited in teeth causing discoloration, and in bones and nails. Should not be taken during pregnancy as can interfere with bone growth of the baby, particularly if taken during the late stages. Should also be avoided when breastfeeding.

Anticoagulants
Drug further increases blood clotting time.
Antidiabetics
Drug may enhance lowering of blood sugar.

Barbiturates
Reduce effectiveness of tetracycline due to increased breakdown.
Corticosteroids (e.g., cortisone)
May lead to development of an infection resistant to tetracycline therapy.
Diuretics
May cause kidney disorders leading to an increase in tetracycline levels. Complications which may be fatal may result, particularly during pregnancy.
Metals
A number of metals combine with tetracycline to form tetracycline-metal complexes which are not readily absorbed from the gastrointestinal tract. This means many antacids, dairy products, dietary sup-

Antihistamines
Reduce activity of testosterone due to increased breakdown.
Barbiturates
Decrease effectiveness of testosterone.

plements and drug products will inhibit tetracyclines. Oral tetracyclines should be taken 1 hour before or 2 hours after these substances. (Metals include aluminum, bismuth, calcium, iron, magnesium.)
Milk
Lowers antibiotic level (see Metals at left).
Penicillins (some types)
Reduce effectiveness of tetracycline.
Sodium bicarbonate
Reduces gastrointestinal absorption of tetracycline, resulting in diminished effectiveness.
Vitamin K
Tetracycline alters the intestinal bacteria which produce vitamin K, reducing its activity.

breathing, irregular heartbeat, irritation of the stomach. Caution with heart disease and during pregnancy.

NOTE: Theophylline, like caffeine, is a central nervous system stimulant which will enhance or inhibit other drugs depending on their action on the central nervous system.
Ephedrine
Toxic reactions have been reported with combination.

DRUG	USES	SIDE EFFECTS
thyroid S–P–T	Treatment of thyroid deficiency states producing a general increase in metabolism	At the beginning of treatment, heart problems, muscle cramps, weight loss and menstrual irregularities may occur. If treatment proceeds too quickly, rapid heart rate, diarrhea, restlessness, insomnia, tremors, irregular heartbeat (particularly in
Tofranil (*imipramine*)	Treatment of depression	See imipramine
Totacillin (*ampicillin*)	Antibiotic. Treatment of urinary tract infections.	See ampicillin
Tranxene (*clorazepate dipotassium*)	Treatment of anxiety	See diazepam
trimeprazine tartrate Temaril	Treatment of itching and other skin problems	Drowsiness, dry mouth, weakness, lowering of body temperature, rapid heart rate, sleeping difficulties, constipation, depression, sun sensitivity and skin rash. Also blood disorders and sensitivity reactions may occur. May cause menstrual irregularities, weight gain and decreased libido. With high doses may cause profound depression of the central nervous system.
Tylenol (*acetaminophen*)	Relief of pain such as headache	See acetaminophen
Valium (*diazepam*)	Tranquilizer	See diazepam

INTERACTIONS

the elderly), headache, flushing, fever, vomiting, excessive loss of weight, muscular weakness and coma may occur. Large doses may be fatal if the condition is complicated with heart disease. Should also be avoided with hypertension.

Anticoagulants
Combination increases blood clotting time.
Antidiabetics
Combination may increase blood sugar levels, increasing antidiabetic requirement.

See imipramine

See ampicillin

See diazepam

Caution with heart disease or any condition which affects blood pressure. Also with breathing difficulties, liver complaints, stomach ulcer, or respiratory impairment.

Should not be used by women of childbearing age. Withdrawal symptoms may occur if the drug is stopped suddenly.

See also diphenhydramine.

Alcohol and other central nervous system depressants
Enhance side effects of trimeprazine, notably drowsiness. Avoid.
Antacids
Reduce activity of trimeprazine due to decreased absorption.
Antidepressants
Enhance side effects of drug, notably drowsiness and depression. Avoid.
Antihistamines
Enhance depressant effects of drug.
Blood pressure drugs
Combination may cause severe low blood pressure. Avoid.
Diuretics
Combination has been shown to cause severe low blood pressure and shock.
Muscle relaxants
Combination may cause breathing difficulties. Caution.

See acetaminophen

See diazepam

DRUG	USES	SIDE EFFECTS
warfarin **Coumadin** **Panwarfin**	Treatment to prevent blood clotting (anticoagulant)	Major risk of hemorrhage from almost any organ in the body. Others include loss of hair, fever, nausea, vomiting, diarrhea, and hypersensitivity reactions. Early signs of overdose are mild bleeding from gums and red blood cells in the urine. Should not be taken during the late stages of pregnancy or when breastfeeding.

INTERACTIONS

Acetaminophen (and other painkilling drugs)
Anticoagulant response may be enhanced by combination. Possible hemorrhage may occur after acetaminophen is withdrawn.

NOTE: Acetaminophen is preferable to aspirin for patients on anticoagulants.

Alcohol
May increase metabolism of anticoagulants and may adversely affect the liver, leading to an increased sensitivity to anticoagulants. Should be avoided.

Antibiotics
Enhance activity due to reduction of vitamin K, important in clotting of blood. Tetracyclines themselves have anticoagulant activity. Risk of hemorrhage.

Antidiabetics
May enhance anticoagulant activity.

Barbiturates (including sedatives)
Serious and fatal hemorrhage has been reported after withdrawal of phenobarbital in patients on oral anticoagulants.

Corticosteroids (e.g., cortisone)
Severe hemorrhage has occurred with combination, possibly due to ulceration of the stomach.

Diuretics
Combination produces reduced effectiveness of both drugs.

Estrogen
Has both a cholesterol-lowering effect (which tends to enhance anticoagulant activity) and a blood-clotting effect (which antagonizes anticoagulants). Caution.

Insulin
Combination enhances lowering of blood sugar.

Radioactive compounds and x-radiation
Enhance anticoagulant effect, leading to hemorrhage.

Vitamin B complex
Enhances activity of anticoagulants.

Vitamin C
Combination results in reduced effectiveness of both drugs when used in large doses. Caution.

Vitamin E
Enhances activity of anticoagulants which may result in hemorrhage with vitamin K deficiency.

Vitamin K
Combination results in reduced effectiveness of both drugs.

Xanthines (coffee, tea, chocolate)
Large amounts reduce anticoagulant activity.

EMPTY NEST BLUES

I can't seem to get a grip on myself.
Everything feels so up in the air.
After my daughter leaves home, I
don't care what happens to me
because my life is just not that
significant.
            —*Comment from
            a 52-year-old woman, 1950.*

The children's leavetaking won't
be painful for me at all. After all
those years of being responsible for
them, I'm at the point where I want
to scream, 'Fall out of the nest already, you guys. It's time!'
            —*Comment from
            a 48-year-old woman, 1980.*

The woman who couldn't get a grip on
herself, dismayed and tormented by her
daughter's impending departure from
home, was said to be in the throes of the
"empty nest" crisis. Indeed, the very
phrase evokes an image of a depressed
and frightened woman clinging to an
outmoded identity as she languishes in
her lonely house.

That woman of 30 years ago presents
sharp contrast to the mother today, eager
to be liberated from childrearing duties
to pursue a new life of her own.

According to David Chiriboga,
Ph.D., a psychology professor, the
"empty nest" most likely is a difficult
period for no more than five percent
of middle-aged couples. "It *can* be
an overwhelming experience," concedes Dr. Chiriboga, who is part of the
Human Development and Aging Program at the University of California in
San Francisco. "Especially," he notes,
"for a woman whose whole identity is
wrapped up in being a mother."

Former studies may have exaggerated the severity and prevalence of
the "crisis," he told us, because they
were rooted in psychiatric reports two
and three decades ago of women hospitalized or receiving therapy for depression. In recent years, however, this
so-called traumatic time has been
reevaluated and reinterpreted by sociologists and psychologists drawing from
community data. Even so, clinical
journals still frequently feature adver-
tisements trumpeting antidepressants
and tranquilizers—especially Valium—
for women suffering from this "empty
nest syndrome."

In his own work, Dr. Chiriboga has
learned that most middle-aged parents
pull through the transition quite
smoothly. Other current studies increasingly support this view. The children's exit isn't necessarily the wrench-
ing parental ordeal it's cracked up to be.

To be sure, it may signal a critical
readjustment and serve as a pointed reminder of advancing old age for some
women. Most studies, though, conducted over the past decade, found that
the youngest child's approaching launch
into the world is generally greeted with
relief, not dismay. For mom and dad,
then, the "empty nest" heralds a second
honeymoon, a renaissance of once-
abandoned dreams.

The possibility for self-growth, maintains Lillian Rubin, Ph.D., a sociologist
and psychologist at the University of
California at Berkeley, has become an
exciting reality for women who told her,
"My only career has been my children."
For most, she says, motherhood had
meant sacrificing their own desires and

subordinating their own needs to the children's. So, says Dr. Rubin, "It's not surprising that when day-to-day care ends and the children leave, relief comes."

Consider the sigh of relief expressed by a 55-year-old mother of two: "It's time for me now. I feel like a cactus finally blooming after 30 years."

Or this 48-year-old mother of three, who wondered where the "brainwashing" about the supposed midlife crisis was coming from: "Everything just falls into a pattern when you're ready."

"I'm ready." That's what Dr. Rubin heard again and again from 160 women she studied, aged 35 to 54, mostly eager to be released at last from childrearing responsibilities. It is true, concedes Dr. Rubin in her book *Women of a Certain Age: The Midlife Search for Self* (Harper & Row, 1979), some women are lonely, depressed, hesitant and mostly frightened as they face an uncertain future. However, she points out, only one mother interviewed suffered classical "empty nest" blues.

Donald Spence, Ph.D., who directs the gerontology program at the University of Rhode Island, agrees that earlier studies overplayed the "empty nest" stage as a terrible upheaval. "It's not nearly as traumatic now," admits the sociologist, whose own reports dating from the 60s characterized that transition as an unhappy time for women.

New Times, Fresh Attitudes

In part, he believes women's new exultant attitude reflects changing times. Not only are women more career-oriented now, he says, but their children are adopting more conventional lifestyles. In the turbulent 60s, he notes, many young people rebelled against their parents' traditional values by dropping out of school and taking drugs.

Of course, because every family's childrearing patterns are different, there are no simple solutions guaranteed to ease this potential crisis period. Current data reveals that women who suffer most from the break are disappointed in their children and have poor relationships with them. These women may feel their mothering role isn't over yet and still need to control the lives of their offspring.

Researchers point out, however, that one of the best preparations for the separation is thinking about it and accepting it as inevitable before it occurs. They suggest several measures that will not only enable you to cope well with the "empty nest" process, but even welcome it with an open mind.

- Develop new hobbies and interests to fill the expanded leisure hours. Now's the time to try your hand at gardening, tennis, weaving, ceramics or whatever grabs you. Exercise such as jogging, swimming and bicycling will help you stay fit and healthy as well as relaxed.
- Donate your skills and time to a worthy cause or organization. Volunteering at schools or with youth groups can fill the void left by your own children's absence.
- If you've always yearned to study Shakespeare or learn furniture refinishing, enroll in university or adult education classes.
- Study a foreign language and then visit the country.
- Try out a parttime job or return to the fulltime career you suspended during your childrearing years.

- Plan to enjoy a second honeymoon by doing more things with your spouse or partner, like taking long walks in the evening, traveling, dining out, or just playing games together.

- Broaden your social circle by joining clubs and making new friends.
- Discuss your fears with a family counselor or other parents who've been through the transition already.

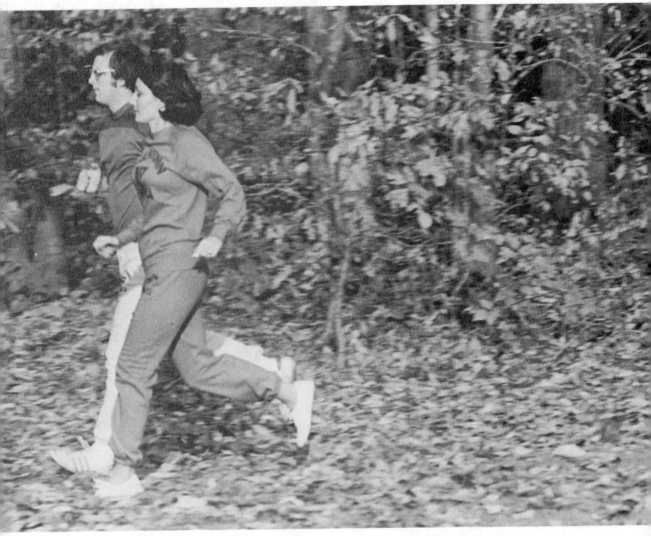

T. L. Gettings

The term "uterine cancer" is a confusing one since both the cervix and the endometrium (the lining or body of the uterus) belong to the uterus. Nevertheless, uterine cancer is used interchangeably with endometrial cancer. And there's no mistaking this disease for the one that strikes the remote portion of the uterus which juts down into the vaginal vault, the cervix.

First of all, cancer of the endometrium strikes older women: 75 percent are postmenopausal women over age 50. Second, it is somewhat less treacherous—usually signaled by symptomatic bleeding early enough to permit effective treatment—and less likely to spread beyond the pelvic reproductive organs. Third, because of its hard-to-isolate location in the uterine lining and the age of women who develop it, uterine cancer practically always results in hysterectomy, even when discovered in its early stages.

The risk factors for endometrial cancer differ as well. Unlike cervical cancer, which is more prevalent in sexually active women—especially those in the lower socioeconomic class—data shows endometrial cancer affects mostly overweight, childless women in the upper socioeconomic group.

Diet may be an underlying culprit with the typical American smorgasbord of fatty meats, salty seasonings and sugary desserts paving the way for many more problems than bargained for. After all, statistics indicate that women who are diabetic, hypertensive or overweight (three problems that can be directly related to poor eating habits) are more likely to develop endometrial cancer. And these are no small risks.

A profile derived from the work of several investigators and compiled by Gary H. Johnson, M.D., of the University of Utah College of Medicine, Salt Lake City, suggests that a woman 30 to 50 pounds overweight is 3 times more likely to develop uterine cancer than another woman of average weight. If she is more than 50 pounds above her ideal weight, she's 10 times more likely to suffer from the disease. (Still waiting to slim down?)

Another theory is that this curious cancer is caused in part by some basic genetic or metabolic disturbance. This is based on evidence that women who were plagued with irregular periods, didn't ovulate regularly, had trouble becoming pregnant, went through a bloody menopause (a "change of life" characterized by heavy and prolonged menstrual bleeding) and didn't reach menopause before age 52 seem more susceptible to its development.

A growing body of evidence suggests that the lining of the uterus in some women may be supersensitive to estrogen. There's no way to predict who those women are. But when they use estrogen, they may be vulnerable to endometrial cancer. Actually, within the last five years, reports of a link between estrogen replacement therapy and endometrial cancer have progressed from vague observations of a possible association to large-scale, carefully controlled studies which suggest a definite cause and effect relationship. For example, a recent study by Hershel Jick, M.D., and associates at the Boston Collaborative Drug Surveillance Program found that for postmenopausal women who did not take estrogen the incidence of endometrial cancer was about 1 in 1,000; for those who did, the incidence was closer to 10 to 30 per 1,000 (*New England Journal of Medicine,* February 1, 1979). See Estrogen Replacement Therapy.

Obviously, it's within your power to avoid many of these risk factors—such as excessive weight gain and estrogen use. And, as with any type of cancer, early detection is the key to effective treatment.

Signs of Trouble

Unfortunately, the trusty Pap smear becomes somewhat undependable when it comes to detecting endometrial cancer. In fact, less than half of the women who have endometrial cancer will discover it through their annual Pap tests. Of those remaining, most will be unaware of any problem until a bloody pool sends them panic-stricken to an M.D. Bleeding between periods is one sign that something may be amiss, as is any bleeding in postmenopausal women who have stopped their menstrual periods altogether. Of course, this bleeding can be indicative of other problems as well, but it's best to get yourself to a gynecologist and let him or her make the diagnosis. If endometrial cancers are detected at the onset of symptomatic bleeding, it is usually early enough to promise effective treatment.

Of course, nabbing a cancerous condition before any symptoms erupt is even better. How? Well, according to many gynecologists, there is one diagnostic test called endometrium aspiration which should be done along with the Pap smear and pelvic exam on menopausal women who fall in the high risk category—that is, those with a his-

tory of infertility, who are overweight, diabetic, have high blood pressure, or are taking any form of estrogen. Or, to be on the safe side, John Mikuta, M.D., gynecologic oncologist at the University of Pennsylvania School of Medicine, recommends this test for *every* woman over the age of 40. After the physician finishes taking the Pap smear samples, he expels the air from a small bulbous syringe, inserts the tip through the cervical canal and into the uterus, where he releases the pressure so that mucus and cellular debris from the uterine walls is sucked into the vacuum. The contents are then emptied out onto a slide for examination. Because the cervical canal is somewhat sensitive to invaders, the passage of the syringe might cause cramps. Since the test takes only a few seconds, the discomfort will subside.

Should the cancer weasel by the Pap smear and aspiration without detection and abnormal bleeding begin, your doctor will probably recommend a diagnostic D and C, or dilation and curettage (a surgical procedure in which the cervix is dilated and either a spoon-shaped instrument known as a curette or a suction device is used to remove the contents of the uterus). This will help to differentiate between bleeding caused by fibroids or other benign condition and cancer (see Fibroid Tumors).

And should the D and C confirm cancer, a hysterectomy is considered your safest and best existing method of treatment. In fact, endometrial cancer is considered one of the few absolute indications for hysterectomy. And since most women with uterine cancer are already past menopause, and since uterine cancer can spread to the ovaries, this is one time when a hysterectomy is almost sure to include removal of the ovaries and fallopian tubes.

Endometriosis (pronounced en-do-me-tree-O-sis) remains an enigma to those in the medical profession. They don't know what causes it, and they're more or less at a loss as to how it's best treated. In fact, in the century or so since this pelvic disease was first diagnosed, the only thing we've managed to learn from them is what it is.

In endometriosis, fragments from the endometrium, or uterine lining, somehow become misplaced during menstruation. Instead of flowing out of the uterus via the vagina, a few leave by way of the fallopian tubes and spill out into the pelvic cavity. There they become embedded and grow on the outer wall of the uterus, along the fallopian tubes, or around practically any other pelvic structure.

Although the condition is not cancerous or life-threatening, it can swaddle the pelvis in a mass of scar tissue, creating a mess of trouble. The most common complaint is pain—increasingly painful periods after perhaps years of relative comfort, a nagging soreness in the lower abdomen which precedes menstruation by two or even three weeks, and an unbearable shot of pain on deep penile penetration during intercourse.

But what many women find even more distressing is their inability to conceive. If the fallopian tubes are tied up with endometrial adhesions, there's no way they can swing over to the ovary and scoop up an egg at ovulation. As a result, approximately 40 percent of women with endometriosis are infertile despite regular periods, normal monthly ovulation and open fallopian tubes.

As a matter of fact, endometriosis affects *only* women who menstruate and ovulate regularly, usually young women between the ages of 25 and 45. And this is one reason why it has become known as the disease of career-conscious women. Apparently, the longer a woman goes without interruption of her normal ovarian function—that is, without getting pregnant—the greater her chances for developing the disease.

For younger married women who might already have symptoms of early endometriosis—and who might have been postponing parenthood—the best solution might be to get pregnant. With the nine-month leave from ovulation and menstruation, areas of endometriosis often shrink and may even disappear. Of course, regression isn't the rule. But for some lucky women the problem leaves with the pregnancy and never returns.

Older women might do well to just sit tight till menopause. The cessation of menstruation and ovulation often brings a spontaneous improvement of the condition.

Options in Treating Endometriosis

For those whose thoughts are too far from childbearing or "change of life" to do them much good, we have several other options. But before you select your mode of treatment, make sure your condition is properly diagnosed.

Because endometriosis affects the pelvic cavity *outside* the uterus, internal exams won't be of much help. Also, endometrial adhesions are not easily distinguishable from normal tissue using bimanual palpation (a diagnostic procedure in which the physician inserts two fingers into the vagina while pushing gently on the lower abdomen with the other hand). The only sure way to make the diagnosis is by laparoscopy—that's one-half of the "Band-Aid sterilization" procedure.

Granted, this is not the easiest diagnostic procedure. Under either local or general anesthesia, the physician will make a small incision just below your navel. Carbon dioxide will be pumped into the abdomen to lift the outer covering of skin and muscle tissue away from the internal organs. Then, using a laparoscope, a kind of slender telescope, the physician can check the pelvic organs for any endometrial adhesions.

Once diagnosed, endometriosis is usually treated one of two ways: medication or surgery. Until recently, the only medication available was hormones. Doses of estrogen or progesterone much higher than those available in the Pill are administered by mouth or, more commonly, through injection to bring on a state of pseudopregnancy by temporarily suspending ovulation and menstruation. It works all right. The adhesions melt away and the pain subsides. The only problem is that long-term use of these synthetic hormones brings on a whole host of adverse side effects, and short-term use offers temporary relief from symptoms but no relief from the progression of the disease.

Recently, a new drug called danazol has come onto the medical market. Unfortunately, danazol is not without potential side effects; namely, it may produce masculinizing reactions such as acne, mild hirsutism (abnormal hair growth), decrease in breast size, slight deepening in the voice, oiliness of the skin or hair. Of course, those don't occur in every woman who tries it. For those women so affected, the distressing problems usually last only as long as the medication is taken but may persist for a few months after treatment stops. And, according to one physician, those effects are "trivial" compared to the potential adverse effects of hormonal agents commonly used for endometriosis. Besides, the benefits may be great.

Although danazol is a newcomer in the treatment of endometriosis, reports of its effectiveness have been very promising. In one small study of women suffering from infertility as a result of endometriosis, half became pregnant after danazol treatment. In another investigation, more than 50 percent of the endometriosis-afflicted women treated with danazol were found to be completely free of any pelvic disease upon laparoscopy exam.

An alternative to danazol treatment is conservative surgery in which a lower abdominal incision is made and the endometrial adhesions removed without removing the uterus. But if fertility is not the main aim of endometriosis therapy, many physicians favor hysterectomy (usually total abdominal hysterectomy plus the removal of diseased fallopian tubes and ovaries)—particularly for older women with severe pain.

ESTROGEN REPLACEMENT THERAPY

Think of a menopausal woman you may know. What image comes into your mind? Well, if you're a drug company advertising estrogen replacement therapy (ERT) to doctors, then you would no doubt want to perpetuate the myth of the menopausal woman as a wrinkled harpy harrowed by trivial everyday occurrences or as a disheveled old woman in a tattered bathrobe obviously unable to cope with getting dressed, let alone doing something useful like ironing her husband's socks.

And that's just what the drug companies have done in their effort to sell doctors on prescribing estrogen replacement therapy. One particular ERT product advertised in a popular medical journal shows a middle-aged woman too pooped to get out of her chair. In her hand are airline tickets for a long-awaited trip. Behind her stands an impatient husband glaring at his watch. The message reads, "Bon voyage? Suddenly she'd rather not go! She's waited 30 years for this trip. Now she just doesn't have the bounce. She has headaches, hot flashes and she feels tired and nervous all the time. And for no reason at all, she cries."

Fact is, there's no proof that estrogen replacement therapy improves vitality or mental outlook. But that doesn't stop the pharmaceutical companies from unabashedly proclaiming the opposite. From them, we hear that estrogen can avert the aging process by preserving our youthful psyche, libido and skin appearance; relieve depression, irritability, nervousness, crying spells, loss of memory and concentration; alleviate joint pains; and even reduce the risk of heart disease and stroke. And in our youth-oriented society, it's easy to understand how the woman over 40 would be willing to swallow those claims along with the estrogen.

No wonder sales of estrogen increased from $15 million in 1962 to $83 million in 1975, the year Premarin (a brand of estrogen) became the fourth or fifth most popular drug in the United States.

In reality, however, estrogen is not the so-called youth pill that it was originally thought to be. Of the 26 alleged menopausal and postmenopausal symptoms, ERT has been shown effective for only hot flashes and, possibly, atrophic vaginitis.

Even the much-touted beneficial effects of estrogen for treatment of osteoporosis are debatable. It's true it stops bone loss but there's no evidence that it reduces the incidence of fractures. And anyway, after withdrawing ERT, the gains in bone density are rapidly lost (*Lancet*, July 7, 1979). This implies that estrogen therapy would have to be long-term to maintain the benefits, and we now know that the cancer risks with extended use are prohibitive. Besides, calcium supplements will do the same thing for you—and without the harmful side effects associated with ERT (see Osteoporosis).

No Fountain of Youth

Nevertheless, with legions of women and women's doctors totally convinced by the blatant ad campaigns, the Food and Drug Administration in September, 1976, finally had to order manufacturers to state: "Estrogens are not indicated for certain conditions, i.e., nervousness, preservation of supple skin, or maintenance of a youthful feeling."

But, no matter, millions of women still take estrogen to help them through menopause. Problem is, some may be getting more than they bargained for. Like trading off hot flashes for endometrial (uterine) cancer.

American women in particular have a higher incidence of uterine cancer after menopause than women in the rest of the world. That is almost certainly due to the misuse of estrogens, says Dr. John W. Studd of the King's College Hospital in London. The United Kingdom, on the other hand, has only one-third the U.S. incidence. Dr. Studd attributes this to the practice of adding progestin (a synthetic form of the natural hormone progesterone) to a low-estrogen regimen for about 7 to 13 days during each cycle, unlike the American preference for continuous or cyclic estrogen therapy in excessive doses without progestin.

But apparently doctors in this country are starting to catch on to the possible benefits of this regimen. Several doctors we spoke to heartily recommend it and suggest that women question their own physicians about the addition of progestin to the cycle if ERT is being prescribed.

Remember, though, that adding progestin does not eliminate the risk of endometrial cancer, although it does appear to reduce it. While initial reports are encouraging, this method hasn't been around long enough for the statistics to tell us for sure if it's really as good as or safe as it seems.

On the other hand, the statistics on using estrogens alone leave no doubt at all about the dangers of hormone therapy. Since 1975 reports have surfaced linking ERT with a greatly increased risk of endometrial cancer. Generally, they found that women who received ERT were 4½ to 8 times more likely to develop endometrial cancer than were women who did not receive the therapy.

What does this mean in practical terms? Ordinarily a 45-year-old woman would have a 1.6 percent chance of developing endometrial cancer. A sevenfold increase in that risk (which is likely for ERT) would up her chances to 11.2 percent or *one in nine!*

And that's just the average. The risk increases drastically with length of time on estrogen. One study, conducted at the University of Washington in Seattle, showed just such a relationship. While there was only a minimal elevation of risk present during the first 2 years, after about 10 to 15 years of use the risk rose 20-fold (*Journal of the American Medical Association*, July 20, 1979).

This same study also confirmed that the risk of cancer was dose-related, so that taking less than 0.625 milligrams per day of estrogen produced a smaller increase in risk than did other dosages.

More recently, another study—this one from the Harvard School of Public Health—confirmed those results and brought out a few new conclusions as well. Researchers found that the association between estrogen and endometrial cancer is about the same whether you take the estrogen every day (continuous) or three weeks out of four (cyclic) and that you are also at an increased risk of invasive cancer—that is, it may spread outside the uterus (*New England Journal of Medicine*, August 28, 1980). This is not to be confused with the English cyclic method which uses estrogen in combination with progestin for a portion of the month.

Of course, if you had a hysterectomy, there's obviously no way ERT can threaten you with endometrial cancer. But that doesn't mean you're free of risk. That's because taking estrogen has also been associated with breast cancer.

In a study done at the University of Southern California School of Medicine in Los Angeles, 138 women under 75 years of age with breast cancer were compared to control subjects. When the total cumulative dose of estrogen was more than 1,500 milligrams, there was a risk of breast cancer 2½ times greater than for the non-estrogen-taking women (*Journal of the American Medical Association*, April 25, 1980).

To get a better idea of what this means, a 1,500-milligram cumulative dose is equivalent to approximately three years of daily use of 1.25 milligrams of estrogen. A 50-year-old woman who receives this dose of ERT would increase her lifetime probability of getting breast cancer by age 75 from 6 percent to 12 percent.

But cancer isn't all that women on ERT have to worry about—as if that isn't enough. Estrogen, after all, is estrogen, whether it comes in the form of a birth control pill or as ERT. So along with endometrial and breast cancer go the additional risks—like clotting problems, heart attacks and liver cancer, to mention just a few (see Oral Contraceptives). Remember, too, that the risks associated with taking estrogen are much greater after age 40. Yet that's just the time when estrogen is recommended for menopausal symptoms.

Anyway, just because menopause is approaching doesn't mean you have to expect the worst. Symptoms vary among women. For some, they may be mildly bothersome, and natural or nutritional remedies may effectively ease the transition. Of course, menopausal complaints are most severe in those who have had their ovaries removed surgically because surgical menopause causes a more abrupt drop in the body's hormone levels than biological menopause does. Still, less than 20 percent of all menopausal women have symptoms severe enough to even consider ERT.

Minimizing the Risks

If you are one who plans to use estrogen, take every precaution you can to minimize the likelihood of serious health complications.

- View ERT only as a *temporary* treatment for specific symptoms such as incapacitating hot flashes. Don't think of estrogen as long-term therapy for depression and least of all as a means of perpetuating youth.
- Take the lowest effective dose for the shortest possible time. Numerous studies have proven that serious health risks such as endometrial cancer increase dramatically when the dosage is over 0.625 milligrams per day and the length of use is greater than two years. For those who've had their ovaries removed surgically, the benefits of estrogen seem greatest when given soon after surgery, while no additional improvement appears to be achieved by prolonging therapy for more than three years. Also question your doctor about including progestin in the regimen since the evidence indicates a reduced risk of endometrial cancer with this method.

- Request a reevaluation of your need for estrogen at least once every six months.
- Supplement your diet with adequate amounts of vitamins B_1, B_2, B_6, C, E, folate and zinc. Be sure to get enough calcium, too, to stave off osteoporosis.
- Know what you're taking. Some estrogen tablets are laced with tranquilizers, testosterone (a male hormone) and even "speed."
- If any vaginal bleeding (even spotting) occurs during ERT, have it checked out immediately by a physician. It could be a sign of endome-

trial cancer. Your doctor will want to do a D and C (dilation and curettage) to be sure of the correct diagnosis.
- Wean yourself from ERT gradually in order to give your body a chance to adjust to the diminished amount of the hormone. Otherwise the flashes are more than likely to return for the same reason you had them in the first place.

Review the sections on Hot Flashes, Menopause, Oral Contraceptives, and Vaginitis: Atrophic for additional pertinent information. And most of all, if you can possibly do without hormone replacement—skip the estrogens.

FATIGUE

Twenty pounds of laundry but you don't have an ounce of energy. Your kids want a maid, your husband a lover, your boss an invariable whiz—no matter what. Yet all you can think about is hitting the sack—if only that would help! Unfortunately what usually happens is that you're so exhausted when your head hits the pillow that the heaviness hangs in there 8, 10, even 12 hours later. Come morning, you can barely direct enough energy into one little finger to hit the snooze alarm for another seven minutes or so of shut-eye.

And so it goes. Tired upon rising. The midafternoon slump. The after-dinner drag. The weekend washout. For anyone concerned about health, happiness, and living life to its fullest, this kind of chronic fatigue can be utterly frustrating. What's worse, a visit to the doctor is sometimes every bit as frustrating as the symptoms that drove you there in the first place.

One woman we spoke with knew this

all too well. "I was so tired all the time, I was sure something was wrong with me. I had no energy whatsoever. I just couldn't push myself to get up in the morning. And most of the time I walked around in such a fog it's a wonder I was able to function at all. Finally, I made an appointment with an internist. He took a blood sample to see if I was anemic. I wasn't. Then he suggested I have a glucose tolerance test—which I did, but nothing showed up. As far as he was concerned, I was in top physical condition. God knows, I didn't feel it! When I persisted with my complaint, he asked me how my personal life was.

" 'Fine,' I told him.

" 'You must be depressed,' he insisted.

"I wasn't and I was very adamant in pointing that out to him. But, he still insisted that depression was at the root of my fatigue and handed me a prescription for Valium."

Outrageous? No, unfortunately—

this woman's story is fairly typical of the treatment many doctors offer for unexplained tiredness. Look at it this way: fatigue is the most common complaint doctors hear from their patients. But, (and this is why so many sufferers feel frustrated) physicians report there's nothing *physically* wrong with 80 percent of them.

The trouble is, doctors are trained to test for and recognize about three primary causes of chronic fatigue. Anemia. Thyroid trouble. Hypoglycemia (low blood sugar). Then, when all else fails (because you've managed to *pass* the tests in spite of your symptoms), physicians frequently succumb to the irresistible temptation of pinning the blame on anxiety or depression or some other elusive emotional problem.

Actually, we shouldn't come down so harshly on a diagnosis of depression. Fatigue *is* a symptom that frequently accompanies such emotional crises as depression and anxiety. But it's wrong for physicians to think of Valium as a valid wake-up pill (see Valium). And wrong, too, to surmise that just because a patient's fatigue does not appear to be grounded in some physical ailment (at least according to the usual barrage of medical tests), then it must—through a process of elimination—be related to some emotional problem.

The truth is, a person's energy level depends on many factors, in which both physical and emotional health play important roles. But there are times when the physical cause of fatigue does not show up on the usual medical tests and yet the person's problem responds to certain treatment. Treatment which, by the way, may involve safe, natural methods or simple changes in lifestyle.

One good example of this is iron deficiency anemia. We won't go into all the details here since that is discussed fully under a separate heading (see Anemia). But briefly, studies have shown that even in the absence of anemia, iron supplementation can boost energy levels in some persons. In other words, just because your blood test is perfectly normal, it doesn't preclude the possibility that you might benefit from taking more iron.

Likewise, a glucose tolerance test reading in the normal range doesn't necessarily mean that low blood sugar can be crossed off your list of possible causes. As you may already know, hypoglycemia is a confusing, controversial issue in the problem of dwindling energy stores. On the one hand, we have the medical establishment warning that hypoglycemia rarely presents a problem. On the other, we have a small but growing number of professionals contending that it is the most common and most often misdiagnosed cause of fatigue. Who's right? Well, according to Jonathan V. Wright, M.D., a practicing physician in Kent, Washington, there's a little bit of truth in both opinions. The confusion, he says, stems in part from the fact that there are actually two types of hypoglycemia.

Basically, the type of hypoglycemia that physicians learn about in their medical textbooks—and the kind that they test for when a patient complains of symptoms of fatigue—is what's called "primary" hypoglycemia. Primary means that the drop in blood sugar is precipitated by some severe dysfunction in the pancreas which causes a surge of insulin to be released. To be sure, this type of hypoglycemia is rare.

But there is another type of hypoglycemia which is not rare: secondary hypoglycemia—so called because the drop in blood sugar is triggered by something other than an actual disease-related dysfunction in the body's insulin-producing system. Overconsumption of sugar and refined foods or dousing your system with coffee or alcohol can do it. So can certain mineral deficiencies, emotional stress, lack of exercise, food allergies—even something so simple as skipping breakfast.

The "Grandmother" Study

In fact, over 20 years ago, in what became known as the "Iowa Breakfast Studies," lots of time, money and effort were invested to prove what most grandmothers could have told us: if you don't eat breakfast, you won't do as well as you could at school or work. Specifically, these studies showed that test subjects who ate one ounce of protein in the morning were better able to perform specific tasks than those who ate no protein or less than one ounce. One of the measurements made was of blood sugar. Those who ate protein had higher blood sugar levels for longer than those who didn't. The blood sugar levels of the latter went sufficiently low that it began to affect their performance at various tasks.

The interesting thing is that neither group had either hypoglycemia or diabetes. All blood sugar readings on glucose tolerance tests were within normal range. But the lower levels brought on by not eating enough protein weren't enough to sustain optimum performance.

Let this be a lesson unto you. If your energy seems especially pitiful in midafternoon, it could be your morning breakfast habit that's to blame. Think protein. And by that, we don't mean to advocate the traditional bacon-and-eggs breakfast that has become the mainstay of the American morning fare. Bacon is not only full of fat, it tends to be treated with cancer-causing nitrates, and eggs are often fried up with lots of grease. Consider more healthful protein options—items you can even eat on the run. How about a hard-boiled egg? Or a piece of cheese, or a cup of yogurt with fruit.

Remember, too, the coffee-and-a-donut routine doesn't solve the breakfast problem any better than no breakfast at all. Sugar in the morning sends your blood sugar soaring—but only temporarily. When it comes back down, it does so with a bang, dragging your energy down to the pits. In fact, one woman told us that she managed to beat the three o'clock slump simply by omitting sugar from her morning coffee.

Basically, the important thing to remember here is that to keep your energy level high, you've got to keep your blood sugar level moderately high but *consistent* throughout the day. To do this, shun high-sugar and refined foods. Concentrate instead on protein like cottage cheese, lean meat, or grain-legume combinations and complex carbohydrate foods such as fresh fruit and vegetables, and whole grains for all your meals. And instead of the usual three gluttonous meals a day that tend to leave you stuffed and then famished later on, try to eat smaller but more frequent meals throughout the day.

For added energy insurance, supplement your diet with the kinds of vitamins and minerals that count most. Tops on that list is, of course, iron, followed closely by the B vitamins folate and B_{12}.

Minerals That Support High Energy

Moving along to some very important minerals, magnesium is one that should also be on your pep-up schedule. Magnesium sparks more chemical reactions in the body than any other mineral. In a severe deficiency, the whole body suffers. You stumble instead of walk, feel depressed, have heart spasms. Doctors are trained to recognize these and over 30 other symptoms of a severe deficiency. But they aren't trained to recognize a *mild* deficiency of magnesium. It has only one noticeable symptom: chronic fatigue.

"A deficiency of magnesium is a common cause of fatigue," says Ray Wunderlich, M.D., of St. Petersburg, Florida.

But that fatigue can easily be cured.

In a study of magnesium and fatigue, 200 men and women who were tired during the day were given the nutrient. In all but two cases, waking tiredness disappeared (*2nd International Symposium on Magnesium*, June, 1976).

Tiredness is hard to define. But, in many cases, it means tired *muscles*—muscles that feel leaden or drained of energy. A lack of magnesium, which helps muscles contract, can cause that tiredness. So can a lack of potassium.

Potassium deficiency is a well-known hazard among long-distance runners and professional athletes. The mineral helps cool muscles, and hours of exertion use it up. If it's not replaced, the result is chronic fatigue. "When you lack potassium," says Gabe Mirkin, M.D., runner of marathons, specialist in sportsmedicine and co-author of *The Sportsmedicine Book*

(Little, Brown, 1978), "you feel tired, weak and irritable."

But a potassium deficiency and the weakness that goes with it aren't limited to athletes. In one study, researchers randomly selected a group of people and measured their potassium intake. Those people with a deficient intake of potassium—60 percent of the men and 40 percent of the women in the study—had a weaker grip than those with a normal intake. And as potassium intake decreased, muscular strength decreased (*Journal of the American Medical Association*, October 6, 1979).

You could probably put up with a few days of weakness. But after a few *months* you feel terrible. "In chronic potassium deficit," wrote a researcher who studied the mineral, "muscular weakness may persist for many months and be interpreted as being due to emotional instability" (*Minnesota Medicine*, June, 1965).

Could a teary, depressed and irritable housewife be nothing more than the victim of a potassium deficiency? Yes. One physician dubbed the problem "The Housewife Syndrome"—but it's not only the housewives who are susceptible! And if potassium offers relief, the combination of potassium and magnesium could really set you free.

A doctor chose 100 of his chronically fatigued patients—84 women and 16 men—and put them on a supplementary regimen of potassium and magnesium. Of the 100, 87 improved.

"The change was startling," wrote Palma Formica, M.D., of Old Bridge, New Jersey. "They had become alert, cheerful, animated and energetic and walked with a lively step. They stated that sleep refreshed them as it had not done for months. Some said they could get along on 6 hours' sleep at night, whereas formerly they had not felt rested on 12 or more. Morning exhaustion had completely subsided."

And their new energy changed their lives.

"Almost all patients have undertaken new activities," he noted. "Six who had not worked outside the home before obtained parttime jobs. Two of the pregnant patients continued to work for a time. Several of the husbands called and expressed appreciation of the physical improvement and consequent increase in emotional well-being of their wives."

Some of those patients had chronic fatigue for over two years. Yet it took only five to six weeks of magnesium and potassium therapy to clear up their problem (*Current Therapeutic Research*, March, 1962).

One more supplement completes our super-energy list: vitamin C.

A study of over 400 people who filled out a questionnaire that asked them to list their vitamin C intake and their "fatigue symptoms" showed that those who took over 400 milligrams of vitamin C a day had less fatigue (*Journal of the American Geriatrics Society*, March, 1976).

Vitamin C may relieve fatigue by cleansing the body of pollutants, such as lead and cadmium.

A doctor in a Swiss village found that his clients who lived close to a busy highway passing through the town had twice as much fatigue (and insomnia, depression and digestive disorders) as those living 50 or more yards from the road. He treated these patients with vitamin C, vitamin B complex and calcium. Over 66 percent got relief from their fatigue.

More Exercise Means More Pep

Of course, when it comes to programming your body for pep, don't underestimate the power of exercise. A good workout at least several times a week will alleviate fatigue in many ways. For one thing, it tones muscles. And well-toned muscles mean less effort every time you use them.

Muscles are made up of fibers which grow larger and stronger the more we exercise them. Actually what's happening is that they're doing themselves a favor, because by becoming larger and stronger they'll be able to function more efficiently. In other words, a little bit of energy will go a much longer way.

The funny thing is, when you're really out of shape, even the least bit of physical exertion seems to drain your energy stores. But don't get discouraged. The more you work at it, the easier it will become. Muscle fibers are very good learners. If you do nothing more than take a walk every day, your muscles will grow as strong as they need to be to walk easily—without getting tired. If you run, they'll become still stronger. If you swim, your shoulders as well as your legs will become stronger.

To perform well, muscles need not only strength, but also fuel, primarily from energy stored in the form of glycogen, and oxygen. Again, that may seem self-defeating—how do you gain more energy by dishing more out? But when you get a lot of exercise, your body will actually build you a better fuel system to go along with your better muscles.

It works like this. When you exercise, you use up glycogen, which is a kind of starch stored in your muscles.

When the glycogen in your muscles runs low, the body calls on the liver to shoot a reserve supply into the bloodstream. But there's a much smoother flow of energy to the muscles when there's plenty of glycogen right on hand. And when you get a lot of exercise, your body can actually *double* the amount of glycogen it stores in the muscles. That's one reason why people who are fit can walk or dance or do other things much longer than people who aren't.

Glycogen isn't the whole story, though. No matter how much you have in your muscles, eventually it gets used up. Luckily, it can be recycled—but only when fresh oxygen is supplied. And when you go on an exercise program, your body will not only give you more ready glycogen, but will also give you a better oxygen-delivery system.

One way that happens is that the capacity of your lungs increases. You get more oxygen out of every breath of air you take. But oxygen doesn't go directly from the lungs to your muscles. It has to be carried there by red blood cells, so once again the body obliges by simply producing more red blood cells. Not only that, but each new blood cell it makes after you go on an exercise program is actually able to carry much more oxygen than a cell in the body of a person whose only exercise is pushing buttons on a TV set. And that means more oxygen to your muscles as well as to those busy brain cells which will help to keep them fresh and free of fog.

As a final advantage, exercise helps keep you trim as well as fit. And there's something to be said for slimness here again. The chronic tiredness heavier persons tend to experience has often been put down to the effort of dragging around all that excess weight. But in the book *Fat and Thin* by Anne Scott Beller, (Farrar, Straus & Giroux, 1977) the suggestion is made that as more and more fat is stored, less and less is burned for energy release. If that is so, says the author, "the only way to relieve the tiredness may be to get up and take a brisk walk, wash a floor, or cut a cord of firewood."

Finally, as we mentioned at the start of this section, freedom from fatigue involves emotional as well as physical factors. And some of the biggest emotional energy robbers are depression, anxiety and boredom. We discuss depression and anxiety under separate headings in this book, but boredom is something we'd like to briefly mention here.

M. Lucille Kinlein, a visiting lecturer at the University of Wisconsin and founder of a new professional practice discipline, the Practice of Kinlein, has some revolutionary concepts about an individual's self-care. And in an interview she told us that attitude is of the utmost importance in maintaining a good state of health and vitality. To illustrate this, she cites the example of a woman who came to her with a low energy level. Her doctor had told her to trim her daily activities. It hadn't helped. So Lucille Kinlein suggested that she expand her activities in areas she enjoyed. The woman ended up doing more than she had ever believed possible and feeling more energetic.

It really works. Boredom and lack of incentive are major causes of fatigue. But by developing a deep interest—indeed a passion—in something, fatigue will often vanish. Try it!

FEMININE HYGIENE

The ad agencies are brainwashing us about our feminine hygiene habits. Just leaf through any women's magazine. Or switch on the TV in between the afternoon "soaps." You'll find the same sweet smiling faces making the same sweet-smelling claims. They have us believing that a daily douche is as fundamental as a morning shower; that a squirt of deodorant between the legs is worth two under the arms; and that a surefire way to find happiness in love is by having your private parts smelling like a lemon tree or herbal bouquet.

Is it true what they say?

"Not at all," was the resounding answer we got from every gynecologist we queried. In fact, not only are these douches and deodorants unnecessary, they also can be harmful to your health.

"Doctors are seeing more irritations of the vaginal area now than they have ever seen before due to the increased use of commercial hygiene products," says Gideon G. Panter, M.D., a prominent New York City gynecologist and a faculty member at New York Hospital–Cornell Medical Center. "Even such seemingly harmless products as colored and perfumed toilet paper, scented powder and soaps, bubble baths, and certain detergents used to launder underwear may contain chemical agents capable of causing allergic reactions and irritation to the skin."

A two-month study at the U.S. Army Hospital, Redstone Arsenal, Alabama, confirms these claims. Of 348 women, those who had used bubble bath, feminine deodorant sprays and douches had a higher incidence of vulvovaginitis (inflammation of the vulva and vagina) than nonusers.

Of the three products examined, the sprays seemed to be the worst offenders. "It's true," says Dr. Panter. "Vaginal sprays can cause infections, itching, burning, irritation, vaginal discharge, rashes and other problems. Personally, I've had to hospitalize too many patients with severe reactions to these sprays to ever advocate their use."

Not so long ago, as you may recall, these sprays were called "feminine *hygiene* deodorant sprays," but the Food and Drug Administration (FDA) quickly put the ax to that when it found that there was nothing medicinal or *hygienic* about them. In fact, the FDA points out, these sprays carry with them considerable risk to the user and should be labeled as follows:

> Caution—for external use only. Spray at least eight inches from skin. Use sparingly and not more than once daily to avoid irritation. Do not use this product with a sanitary napkin. Do not apply to broken, irritated or itching skin. Persistent or unusual odor may indicate the presence of a condition for which a physician should be consulted. If a rash, irritation, unusual vaginal discharge, or discomfort develops, discontinue use immediately and consult physician.

Think about it. The two circumstances when odor-conscious women are most concerned with vaginal odor—during menstruation and intercourse—are two times when the use of a feminine deodorant spray is clearly contraindicated. Also, when a chemical is known to be irritating to the vaginal mucous membranes, it doesn't make sense to intentionally use it near or around the area to be avoided. And besides, Dr. Panter adds, "There's no evidence that vaginal sprays will combat odor any better than plain soap and water—no matter what the television commercials may say."

Chemicalizing the Vagina, an Idea That Stinks

The latest in this cleanliness craze are deodorant sanitary napkins, tampons and suppositories. "The new herbal-scented product was developed to meet the desire of today's young women, ages 18 to 35, for natural clean fragrances in feminine hygiene odor control," reads a promotional mailer for deodorant suppositories. Again, whether you could call such a product "hygienic" is about as questionable as its safety.

Lynn Borgatta, M.D., a physician previously affiliated with Woman's Hospital in New York City, reports a case in which severe itching and swelling of the vulva and vaginal entrance was brought on by the use of deodorant sanitary pads (*Journal of the American Medical Association*, September 15, 1978).

And as if that weren't bad enough, consider the implications of inserting a product containing similar chemicals directly into the vagina.

"Every time you add something to the vagina, you increase your susceptibility to infection," Dr. Panter notes. "The molecules of that substance can invade the vagina's tender mucous membrane." And that goes for douching, too.

Unfortunately, we have been programmed by generations of vigorous douchers. Our mothers douched, our grandmothers douched and, so it seems, did everyone else. Even the *Codex Ebers*, which dates around 1500 B.C., recommends douches of wine, garlic,

fresh dates, cows' bile and asses' milk. Although those ingredients may have been more natural and significantly less caustic than the agents in our present prepackaged douche preparations, douching was no more helpful then than it is today.

"The days of douching are gone," Dr. Panter exclaims. And most gynecologists, including Gerard T. Cicalese, M.D., associate professor of obstetrics and gynecology at New Jersey College of Medicine and Dentistry, agree. Both Dr. Panter and Dr. Cicalese made it clear to us that douching is of no value in promoting feminine hygiene and, in fact, may be the cause of unnecessary distress.

A 59-year-old Chicago woman found this out the hard way. Though past menopause, she suddenly started bleeding again. This bleeding, however, lasted for two months! She consulted her physician, who through a pelvic exam discovered a large tumorlike mass in her pelvis which extended from an ovary to the rectum and colon. Intestinal involvement was so great that a colostomy (an artificial opening made on the abdomen as a substitute for the rectum) had to be performed.

But what was this strange growth? Well, although it resembled a cancerous tumor in many ways, it wasn't malignant. Microscopic examination revealed it to be a cluster of starch granules—the result of prolonged use of a douche powder and water mixture (*Modern Medicine*, January, 1979).

Your Body Cleanses Itself Naturally

What most people fail to realize is that the vagina cleanses itself naturally. Glands located in the cervix secrete a mucous substance that bathes the vaginal walls and washes away trapped debris and germs.

"Merely wiping the lips of the vagina is then sufficient to cleanse the cavity," Dr. Panter explains. "Douching only washes away the natural mucus and upsets the vaginal ecology." This tends to leave the vagina more susceptible to infection.

In addition, douching with one of the new perfumed or "flavored" douches can cause allergic reactions. And too-frequent use of an undiluted or strong douche solution can induce severe irritation and even tissue damage.

But the dangers of douching don't stop there. Hans H. Neumann, M.D., and Alan DeCherney, M.D., of New Haven, Connecticut, point out that 90 percent of the women they attend with inflammation of the uterine tube or pelvic inflammatory disease are vigorous douchers. Only half that many from a healthy group admitted to douching (*New England Journal of Medicine*, September 30, 1976).

The frequency of douching also seems to be a major contributory factor in the development of pelvic inflammatory disease. Of those in the healthy group who douched, only 18 percent were in the habit of douching more than once a week. But 59 percent of those with symptoms of pelvic inflammation douched with similar frequency.

How does douching affect the well-being of the uterus? Drs. Neumann and DeCherney speculate that the gushing water propels germs and bacteria from the vagina into the uterus and even beyond. They also suggest that an anti-bacteria plug in the cervix that normally prevents the upward movement of infection may be eroded by frequent douching.

The Connecticut physicians conclude: "From our own data on gonorrhea and pelvic inflammatory disease, we look with strong suspicion at the douche as contributing to ascending infections by . . . whatever pathogens happen to be in the vagina."

High-pressure douches created by an improperly suspended douche bag may be a major factor in propelling bacteria into the uterus. The bag should never be suspended higher than two feet above the level of the hips. So, if you've been hanging it on your shower curtain rod, you could be pushing for trouble. Douching with equipment that isn't impeccably clean also increases your risk of transmitting infection.

Hygiene during Your Period

Never douche when you have your period. During menstruation the cervix dilates to permit the downward flow of blood and tissue from the uterine lining. At this time the risk of an upward flow of a douche solution into the uterus becomes even more apparent.

In addition to carrying infected material from the vagina into the uterus, physicians caution that douching may also propel uterine tissue back up into the uterine cavity. This could create a condition known as endometriosis, in which tissue from the uterine lining takes root in other places, often producing pain or infertility (see Endometriosis).

Douching with a bulb syringe or one of the new compact disposable douches can be even more dangerous. "Water propelled into the uterus is one thing," Dr. Cicalese told us, "but air injected into the uterus and beyond could prove fatal." And this is particularly dangerous during menstruation and pregnancy when the cervix is dilated. In fact, there have been several maternal deaths reported due to air embolism (the sudden blocking of an artery or vein by air), where the cause was vaginal douching with a bulb syringe.

So how do you stay fresh and clean and free of infection without taking any unnecessary risks? Well, first off, remember that there's nothing offensive about a healthy vagina. The mucous secretions that continually bathe the vagina are completely odor-free, as is your menstrual blood while it is in the vagina. It's only when this discharge or blood hits the air and mingles with perspiration and other bacteria on the skin that unpleasant odors can develop.

To keep your skin clean and free of bacteria, no one has yet challenged the effectiveness of plain old soap and water. By "plain," however, we mean a mild, nondeodorant soap. Or better yet, try a gentle cleanser designed as a soap substitute for supersensitive skin. Then use a soapy finger to gently wash between the vulvar folds. If you want to clean further, Dr. Panter suggests that you put your finger into your vagina during a shower or bath and enable water to enter. You can even put a little soap on your finger to help loosen any dried material. But be sure not to leave any soapy residue.

And contrary to any misinformation you may have gotten in the past, menstruation is not the time to shirk the shower. Bathing is just as important—if not more so—during your period. There's no evidence that it will bring on cramps or interrupt blood flow. If anything, a long, leisurely soak in a warm tub will relieve cramps by relaxing the muscles and promoting the flow of blood.

Keeping your vaginal area fresh throughout the day means keeping it dry and clean. After you've bathed or showered and patted yourself dry, powder your bottom with cornstarch or powdered natural clay (available at many health food stores). Then slip into a pair of cotton panties. Make sure that your clothes are loose enough to permit your vaginal area to breathe. Also, after using the toilet, always wipe yourself from front to back. Then, if necessary, follow up with a moistened paper towel or toilet paper.

Finally, the most important thing to remember is that if, despite your efforts, an unusual odor persists, it may be a sign that something is awry. Certain conditions such as vaginitis produce a foul-smelling discharge.

On the other hand, don't overreact to normal scents. According to Jane M. Rosenzweig, M.D., a San Francisco physician, women may have a set of scent glands, some of which are located in or around the vagina and vulva. Although these glands have for many years been passed off as nonfunctional, Dr. Rosenzweig believes that they are similar to glands in animals which produce sexually arousing aromas. Perhaps, she suggests, in all our efforts to cover up our female scents, we've not been turning on—but have actually been putting off—the opposite sex.

FIBROID TUMORS

With nearly one-quarter of all women over the age of 30 kicking around with fibroids, it's no wonder most abdominal hysterectomies done in this country are performed for this reason. But despite what you may think, it's not true that most fibroids result in hysterectomy. "For the vast majority of women with fibroid tumors, the only treatment is observation," says Stanley J. Birnbaum, M.D., professor of obstetrics and gynecology at Cornell University Medical College.

To understand why, you've got to understand the nature of the tumor. Basically, fibroids are noncancerous (and non-life-threatening) lumps that erupt in the uterine walls. They're made up of the same smooth muscle tissue as the uterus, plus some fibrous connective tissue—hence the name, fibroid. Fibroids grow very slowly. They can be anywhere from the size of a pea to that of a full-term pregnancy. And, when they occur in multiples, they can give a uterus the curious appearance of a lumpy potato.

No one knows exactly why fibroid tumors develop. It's not even known whether heredity is a factor, since they are as common among friends as they are among sisters. One thing is certain, however: their growth depends on a steady diet of the female hormone estrogen. This is why fibroids are known as the disease of menstruating or estrogen-producing women; why they tend to shrink after menopause; and why, according to Dr. Birnbaum, treatment with synthetic estrogen compounds such as the Pill just makes matters worse by ac-

celerating their growth. Don't let anyone tell you otherwise!

In our investigation of fibroid tumors we discovered some good and bad news. The bad news is that if you're destined to develop fibroids, there doesn't seem to be anything you can do to prevent them. But the good news is that fibroids are seldom cause for serious concern. In fact, the majority of women who have these tumors aren't even aware of them. Others find that they can live with the mild pain and minor inconvenience.

Of course, people's pain thresholds vary—as do tumors responsible for pain. But it's important to keep a clear perspective—to know whether it's pain or fear that's really motivating you to extreme treatment.

"Some women who have a fibroid as big as a pea are going to panic," says Dr. Birnbaum. "Nothing you say can reassure them." One woman's story seems to illustrate this:

"For about a year and a half I was having trouble with my period; I never knew when I was going to get it. When I went to the doctor he found fibroid tumors and recommended a hysterectomy. I could have waited but I was so frightened. It was a Thursday when I found out I needed the surgery and I went into the hospital that Sunday and had it done on Monday morning."

Chances are, this woman would have had the hysterectomy even if she had taken the time to mull over her options. For her, the symptoms were troublesome enough to warrant the surgery. But for others who might not be troubled so much by the symptoms as by the fear of what might happen if they *don't* have the surgery, having it could result in serious consequences.

Just How Dangerous Are Fibroids?

Just to set the record straight, a fibroid does occasionally develop into a cancer, but this is very unusual: "Less than one-tenth of one percent undergo degenerative malignant change," according to Dr. Birnbaum. What's more, there is not much chance of this tumor causing other life-threatening trouble, either.

Alan Kaplan, M.D., chief of the division of gynecologic oncology at Baylor College of Medicine, Houston, Texas, explains the worst that can happen: "If a fibroid is large enough and in a particular location it could conceivably interfere with urinary or intestinal function, but in my practice I've found this to be extremely rare," he says. "Probably the most common health problem associated with fibroids is anemia caused by an excessive loss of blood. That can be serious. But, again, it's not acutely life-threatening."

The main problem with fibroids— and the primary reason why women undergo hysterectomy to remove them—is not so much that they can shorten life but that they make life miserable. Depending on their size, shape, location and the number of fibroids present, they can cause abnormal bleeding—that is, heavy or prolonged menstrual periods— and excruciating pain. *Severity of symptoms usually dictates treatment.*

What's important is that abnormal menstrual symptoms should be discussed with a qualified physician so that he can rule out other serious problems.

Diagnosis is literally in the hands of your physician. By inserting two fingers into the vagina and pressing gently on the lower abdomen (just above the pubic bone) with the other hand, a physician is able to feel any unusual bumps or contours on the uterus. The procedure is known as bimanual palpation and like the Pap smear, is a routine part of every gynecological exam. Unfortunately, however, it isn't as accurate as the Pap smear. In a heavy woman, it's nearly impossible to feel internal organs. And even in a thin woman, a larger uterine growth which juts out on the outside walls near an ovary may be indistinguishable from an ovarian tumor which poses a much greater threat. Surgery is often the only way to sort them out. And many doctors feel that, at that point, a hysterectomy might as well be performed.

Fibroids can also be diagnosed during a D and C (dilation and curettage), an office or hospital procedure in which the cervix is gently coaxed open using a dilator, and a spoon-shaped instrument called a curette or a suction device is inserted to peel off the lining of the uterus. In the process, a physician can usually detect any abnormality in the contours which would indicate fibroids while, at the same time, analyzing the uterine lining to rule out cancer.

During a D and C, small, "pedunculated" fibroids (mushroom-shaped fibroids propped atop a connective stem, as opposed to rocklike masses resting directly on or in the uterine lining) may be removed with little trouble.

If the tumor or myoma is larger and somewhat embedded in uterine lining, it may be removed by itself without taking the uterus in a surgical procedure known as a myomectomy. That is usually reserved for women with one or two fibroid growths; obviously, it wouldn't be practical to poke holes in a uterus full of fibroids. Also, since the chance of hemorrhage is even greater for a myomectomy than for a hysterectomy, most physicians would prefer to use this alternative only for women who are troubled enough by their tumor to request treatment but who are young enough to become pregnant.

Otherwise, for the woman plagued with heavy bleeding and pain who is too far from menopause to grit her teeth and hold out for relief, there's always hysterectomy.

FITNESS

Even if you give your car just enough gas, oil and water so that it'll get you where you want to go, chances are it'll end up in the shop soon enough anyway. Most likely your mechanic is very polite to you when you drop off the car—again—but probably he shakes his head after you leave, thinking that with a minimum of maintenance, you could be saving yourself a lot of time and money.

The vehicle that carts you around once you get out of the car—that skeleton fleshed out with muscles and skin—is treated much the same way, unfortunately. The food goes in, glucose provides energy, and the body functions. But even if you pay attention to good nutrition and avoid chemicals in your food and cosmetics, you probably don't spend the time you need to in maintenance, i.e., staying fit through *exercise*. Toning the muscles, getting your total self in shape so that you go through your days feeling energetic and full of vigor—not draggy and just getting by. And though the body holds out a long time (usually longer than the car before it needs repair!), gradually it slows down, the muscles growing loose and flabby from lack of use, and chronic fatigue sets in. Perhaps *you* end up in the shop.

Exercise to Live

In short, to exercise or not to exercise is not even a question. You can't afford *not* to.

If you do not exercise your muscles to keep them fit, they deteriorate. As a result, the weight of the skeleton and of the entire body becomes more and more difficult to support. Energy and endurance are at a real low, making it hard to get through the day. Many people misinterpret this fatigue, thinking that the reason they are tired is that they've "worked too hard," when, in fact, they've worked too little. Exercise, which essentially means working the muscles, *increases* heart output, *increases* lung capacity, and *increases* blood volume. The heart gradually becomes stronger, breathing is deeper and circulation improves, usually resulting in a slower resting pulse rate. That's what being fit is all about. And there is lots of evidence that people who are fit are less likely to have heart disease than people who are inactive.

Being fit can make a big difference in your life—especially in the way you feel about yourself. There are still very few studies that deal with the mental benefits people experience as a direct result of exercise. But it makes perfect sense that if your body feels responsive and strong, you will feel less frustrated in daily life—more able to cope and more in control of your life. The glow of health will shine from within, and people around you will notice the difference.

More and more women are beginning to realize the benefits of exercise, as they join the ranks of joggers, walkers, tennis players and other fitness-minded men and women.

Special Bonus for Women

And for them, there are special advantages to having an exercise program. Gabe Mirkin, M.D., a specialist in sportsmedicine, has noted that women who exercise regularly suffer less from menstrual distresses, such as cramps, bloating and headaches. "Many gynecologists treat menstrual tension with exercise," he wrote in *Jogger* magazine (September, 1978), "and exercise can make you feel less sluggish—a common complaint during menstruation—by increasing the circulation throughout your body."

Also, as we discuss in the section Osteoporosis, the bone weakening that so many women suffer in later years can be prevented to a great degree by exercise.

Women over 45 are particularly prone to fractures caused by weak bones, but authorities suggest that women *from age 25 on* should protect themselves from bone demineralization through calcium supplements *and* exercise.

Another troublesome, seemingly everpresent problem that exercise can control is overweight. In fact, according to a bulletin from the President's Council on Physical Fitness, a lack of physical activity is more often the cause of overweight than is overeating. Several age levels—teenagers, adults, and older persons—have been studied. "In each instance," the report states, "the findings showed that the obese people did not consume any more calories than their normal-weighted age-mates, but that they were very much less active" (*Exercise and Weight Control*, U.S. Government Printing Office, 1976).

Don't be fooled into thinking you can get those extra inches off effortlessly through spot reducing, either. About the only thing it does reduce is your bank account. A recent editorial in the *Journal of the American Medical Association* (July 25, 1980) reported on a study of the effects of mechanical vibrators, commonly used in health spas, on men—some extremely overweight. They found that you would have to sit through 307 15-minute periods of vibration to lose just a pound! The same goes for those ballooned hipsters, rubber bermudas and a device we found that claimed to melt the fat away with the aid of a vacuum cleaner. At best, these products give only temporary relief from overweight through loss of water as sweat.

In any case, fat will be lost only from the areas of greatest concentration and not your chosen trouble spots—no matter how the exercise is done or what the exercise is. And yes, the only way to lose weight is consistent exercise, especially aerobic exercise that uses the large muscle groups and gets the blood going, such as walking, running or rope skipping.

Turn Those Excuses into Turn-Ons

There is a barrage of excuses *not* to exercise—some of which you are probably quite familiar with, and most of which you aren't really fooled by anyway. Deep in your heart, you *know* that rain, sleet and snow don't prevent you from working out the way you need to. But some women have a real, nagging fear that if they tone their muscles, they will begin to develop bulging, masculine profiles.

Breathe easy. This is where hormonal differences between men and women come into play. Testosterone, a hormone, is what seems to be responsible for the extensive muscle growth that men experience from sports, and especially weight training. Women secrete only 5 to 20 micrograms of testosterone daily compared to 30 to 200 micrograms for men, so any muscle gain in women is negligible. It helps to remember what Bonnie Prudden, well-known author and lecturer on physical fitness, observed about the effects of training: "Beneath every beautiful curve lies a beautiful muscle."

Another consideration for some women is that they might be "too old" to exercise. Just another excuse. Exercise, properly done, can make the later years active years. When you have more leisure, there's all the more reason to keep active. Of course, if you're *very* unaccustomed to physical activity, consult first with your physician, but do go ahead and *start moving!* People who exercise regularly have a longer life expectancy, and that is because exercise compensates for bodily decline by increasing heart output, lung capacity and blood volume. Your resistance to degenerative disease is also boosted.

Exercise can rejuvenate your body, but aside from being better able to keep up with your grandmothering, you will enjoy the degree of independence afforded by exercise and *feel* better about yourself. C. Carson Conrad, executive director of the President's Council on Physical Fitness and Sports, puts it this way: "There is a great psychological and financial advantage in having the ability to plan and do things without depending on relatives, friends or hired help. To drive your own car, to succeed with do-it-yourself projects rather than trying to find and pay someone else for the service, and to come and go as you please in terms of physical ability to do so—these are major assets that we believe regular physical exercise can help achieve."

When to Exercise

Some women just can't bear the thought of exercising in the morning. So who says you can't exercise for a half hour as dinner is cooking? Whatever works for you is best, just as long as you don't exercise before bedtime or in the hour after eating a heavy meal.

Earmark *at least* 30 minutes three days a week for a workout. According to Gail Shierman, Ph.D., and Christine Haycock, M.D., coauthors of *Total Woman's Fitness Guide* (World, 1979), "Scientific evidence has shown that if you exercise or participate in an activity, you can do it for a minimum of three days a week and still get effective results. . . . If you can fit only three days a week into your schedule, try to spread it out over the week rather than cramming it all into the weekend."

Ideally, of course, exercise should become a daily routine, but three to four days a week may work out better for you.

The key to keeping up with a fitness

program is in choosing an activity that you really *enjoy*. Nobody says you have to jog or even do a boring series of "exercises" as your one thing to do. Add a little spice to your exercise schedule, and you'll find yourself looking forward to working out your body. Perhaps you're the type who never *liked* gym class and hates organized sports—but you can easily dig around, weed and wield a hoe in the garden for hours without being conscious of the time passing. So, include gardening as one of your weekly activities. Or maybe you enjoy that once-a-month walk that you and your husband take around a nearby lake. Why not make it part of your weekly program? Or if you're a great listener to music, why not put your movements to melody?

When it comes to activity, there is something for everyone. But if you have been inactive for a period of time, if you are over 35 (unless you're a marathoner!) or if you suffer from weakness, an injury, or a condition such as asthma, angina and so forth, consult with your physician before beginning any exercise program. You don't want to tax your system beyond its limits, although proper exercise *by definition* provides a certain amount of healthful stress so that the muscles can grow strong.

Checking your pulse rate is a good indication of how exercise affects you. Each person differs, but in general doctors and physical educators use the following formula to determine what your pulse should be as you exercise: subtract your age from 220, and then multiply by 0.75. If you're 40, your exercise pulse rate should be 135. It is important, however, that you take your pulse *right after* you exercise. Take the count for 10 seconds and then multiply that number by 6 to get your reading. If you wait

much longer, the pulse may slow down too much for an accurate reading.

Four Points to Remember

Keep in mind four things when you set out to get fit:

1. Take it easy at first and allow your body the time and energy it needs to grow strong. "Frequency of exercise—not intensity—is very important," says Charles Wolbers, Ph.D., professor of health and physical education at East Stroudsburg State College in Pennsylvania. "You're not competing against anyone. Your exercise, to be beneficial, must be continuous over a period of time," he says.

2. You are bound to be somewhat sore at first, and it *may* hurt to a certain extent. In fact, *expect* some soreness. You may interpret this as "pain." But it's not the searing, excruciating, I-think-I-tore-a-ligament pain—just a sort of mild aching.

3. After the first few weeks of your exercise program, it will all become easier, and you'll start to feel better—more limber, more energetic and more in tune with yourself. So don't give up! Lots of women quit doing exercise just as they approach the point when they'll benefit most.

4. Vary your exercise routine enough so that your body improves in three distinct areas: flexibility, strength, and endurance, or cardiovascular fitness.

Loosening up Tight Muscles

Stretching your body through its full range of motion will make your joints and muscles elastic and supple. For arthritis sufferers, working toward being flexible may prevent tight joints—all over. Bending, stretching and reaching are natural body movements, movements that should not be avoided at any stage of your life. So moving your appliances and shelves to where they are all within easy reach will only insure more tightness in the joints. But whether or not you have arthritis, being flexible is essential to your well-being and your image of yourself. Mainly, it will keep you looking and feeling younger. The daily stresses of life—mental, emotional and physical—all tend to tighten you up. Stretch to release tension—not only as part of your exercise routine but at your desk, whenever you feel under pressure, or when your body has been in one position for a long time.

Dance and yoga are two activities that have flexibility built in as one of their benefits. Ballet is a very disciplined form of dance, and builds flexibility and leg strength. Modern dance, jazz or belly dancing may suit you better, for there is more room for individual differences, and most modern dance technique is based on natural movements, paying lots of attention to the torso. Yoga is excellent for flexibility, as you are concentrating on stretching and breathing and feeling controlled. While it may not do anything for strength and endurance (you can always run to class!), yoga can make you feel much more in tune with your body and at peace with yourself.

In order to build strength—especially in your upper body where most women tend to be weakest—you must do exercises that offer resistance to a muscle group. Often that means raising and lowering a weight, such as a rock or a book, which you may find difficult at first. Within a very short period of time, however, you will find your exercises

are easier and easier to do—and your whole upper body will look toned and firm *without any significant increase in muscle size!* Many YWCAs now sponsor weight training programs for women, in an atmosphere where women are encouraged not to be embarrassed but to feel good about working out their long-neglected upper bodies.

The Chest Muscles

Of course, there are lots of ways you can build strength without dumbbells or a Universal Gym. To firm up the muscles that support your breasts, the pectoral muscles, try these two:

1. Lie on the floor with your arms straight out from the shoulders, palms up. Slowly bring your arms up, keeping the elbows straight, so that they meet in midair above your chest. Cross them lightly forward and then back and lower again to starting position. Repeat 7 times and work up to 16 times.

Progression: Try doing this exercise holding a lightweight object in each hand, perhaps two hardboiled eggs to start, and progressing to increasingly heavy, yet safe and manageable, weights such as rocks or cans.

2. Find two books of equal weight (not heavy ones!) making sure that you can grasp them easily. Lying flat on the floor with bent knees, hold the books directly above your head (straight up along your ears—arms extended) and slowly raise them toward the ceiling until your arms are extended straight above the chest. Slowly lower the books, returning them to the floor above your head. Raise again slowly 4 times and gradually increase the number of lifts to 16.

Upper Arms

One of the best ways to make your arms and chest strong is to do push-ups. Unfortunately, for most of us, even the thought of a push-up makes us feel tired.

1. Wall push-ups are good to start off with, since regular push-ups are extremely difficult for most women to do. Stand a few feet away from a wall and lean forward, supporting your weight with your arms stretched out directly from the shoulders, palms on the wall (fingers facing up). Your back and elbows are straight. Then bend the elbows and slowly lower your body against the wall as far as you can go, still keeping a straight back. Push out again. Repeat 7 times and build to 16.

2. A modified push-up is also good for building up to a full push-up. Stretch out your body on the floor in the "up" position of a regular push-up, that is, your arms and back are straight, palms beneath shoulders, and fingers pointing ahead. Your weight is supported by your arms and bent toes.

Lower yourself all the way to the floor by bending your elbows, keeping your body straight like a board. Then raise yourself back up to starting position *without worrying* about your stomach and body dragging. Do 2 or 3 of these at first, gradually strengthening your upper body until you can do 16.

Hand and Forearm Muscles

Building up your hand and forearm muscles can be done while sitting at a table.

Place one arm palm-down on the table so that the wrist is off the edge. Hold a rock that weighs about one pound and raise it, keeping your forearm flat on the tabletop, and then lower it. Repeat seven times. Next, try this with your palm up, raising and lowering the rock eight times. This exercise may be repeated eight times with the arm lying on its side, thumb up, and then eight times with the thumb pointing toward the floor.

Progression: Try a heavier weight when you feel a minimum of strain with the one-pounder. If you are a handball enthusiast or enjoy other activities that involve wrist strength, you will want to practice these often.

Aerobic Exercise for the Heart

Endurance, or stamina, depends on the health of your heart, circulation and lungs. And for that, it is vitally important for you to include some type of an *aerobic exercise* in your fitness activities. Aerobic exercise is a term made popular by Kenneth H. Cooper, M.D., of the U.S. Air Force, and it means any strenuous, rhythmic activity that stimulates the heart and lungs. During aerobic exercise you breathe deeply and your heartbeat speeds up, so that you are giving your system a real workout. Table tennis, golf and bowling do not qualify. Walking, running, swimming, cycling and rope skipping *do*.

There are lots of books written on aerobics and individual aerobic exercises, including a book exclusively for women written by Dr. Cooper and his wife Mildred, *Aerobics for Women* (M. Evans, 1972). The most important thing to remember is to start slowly and gradually build up your endurance, so that you don't place undue strain on the heart.

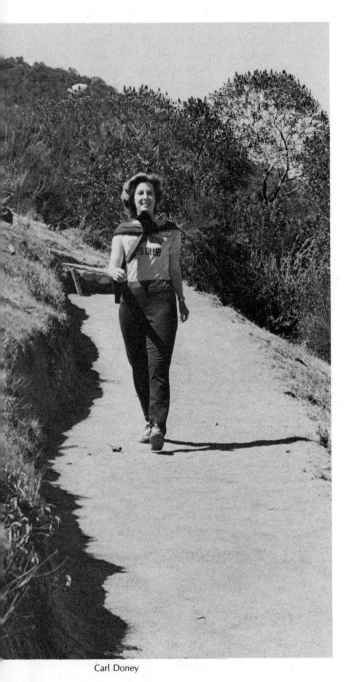

Carl Doney

Get Out and Walk

The key to your physical fitness may be something as simple as walking. A good aerobic exercise, walking seems to especially appeal to women. Charles Kuntzleman, Ph.D., national YMCA fitness consultant, says that in his experience, women take to organized walking programs more than men. (Men, he suspects, feel they have to live up to a "macho image," so they turn to running.) "In terms of health and wellness," Dr. Kuntzleman says, "walking is as good as jogging. Unless you are training for a marathon or some other athletic event, walking is enough. It decreases body fat, increases the strength and endurance of the leg muscles, and relieves stress and anxiety."

The national studies done on fitness in America point out that walking is the single most popular exercise in the country. And well it might be. First of all, there is no special gear required (except a comfortable pair of shoes with good soles). Second, there is no special skill required. In addition, walkers suffer a minimum of injury, and see more of the world right up close.

Research shows us, too, that walking is the type of activity that is good insurance against bone loss due to osteoporosis. And walking protects against heart disease. California endocrinologist Dan Steja, M.D., advises, "To favorably alter cholesterol, to lower sugar, insulin and triglycerides, and to lose weight, walking will do it. I expect it would lower blood pressure as well." To begin a walking program, Dr. Steja says, "I would suggest starting by walking one mile and checking the time it takes. Then I would try to increase both the distance you walk and the time spent walking. I feel people should walk about four to five miles a day, including the walking they do around the house or at work." The physician also suggests that buying a pedometer is a good idea, so you can know how far you actually walk in a day.

Bicycle riding and swimming are two more activities that you should consider for aerobic exercise. Cycling is good for the legs and cardiovascular system, but you must be sure to cycle in combination with stretching and strengthening exercises.

Swimming, by contrast, is an excellent all-around activity. If you use a variety of strokes, good form, and swim in laps, you'll be stretching (flexibility!), working against the force of water (strength!) and giving your heart and lungs a healthy workout (endurance!). So if you already spend time in the water every summer, consider joining a YWCA or other program that has a pool to continue through the year. Through swimming, your breasts probably will look and feel more lifted and firm since you are exercising the pectoral muscles. If you're just getting into the water again, try to swim for 2 straight minutes before resting, and add a minute each session until you can swim 15 to 30 minutes without stopping.

At-Home Aerobics

Running in place and rope skipping are also effective aerobic exercises. Unlike jogging and walking, they can be done at home in one place. Jack Galub writes in *The U.S. Air Force Academy Fitness Program for Women* (Prentice-Hall, 1979) that it is important to wear sneakers or jogging shoes, even if you are running in place on a carpeted floor. Lift your knees also when you run and begin with two minutes at a moderate pace. As with all exercises, build your endurance slowly by increasing either your running time or your speed.

Rope skipping is an activity acceptable and familiar to most women since girlhood. And it is *excellent* for strengthening your cardiovascular system. Keep a steady rhythm (one woman we know regularly skips rope to music on the radio and says that 10 minutes pass by almost before she knows it!), and vary your jumping style from straight up-and-down jumps to "skipping style," where your feet alternate jumping. Depending on your physical condition, begin jumping from 20 to 50 times, keeping count as you go. Increase to 100 jumps and then start counting the minutes until you can jump rope for 8 to 10 minutes. You will find yourself gaining not just endurance but *agility* as well.

Fitness Routine

For an exercise routine that does it all—improves flexibility, strength and endurance while at the same time working on those major muscle groups to burn calories better than anything else—slip into something loose and comfortable like a leotard or sweat suit, switch on the stereo and sail through the following routine.

A 20-Minute Routine That Does It All

Our routine is made up of basic movements that flow into each other in sequence. It takes only about 20 minutes or a side of your favorite record (medium tempo is best). They are marked out in series of eight counts (shown in parentheses) to give you an idea of how fast they should be.

NECK LOOSENERS

1 **2** **3** **4**

Stand comfortably and breathe deeply several times. Drop your head forward and circle to the right (8 counts). Then circle to the left. Repeat.

SHOULDER LOOSENERS

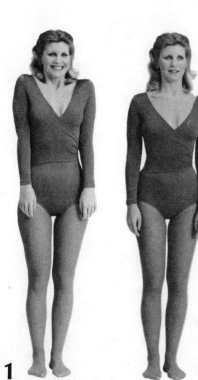

1
Lift your shoulders in a shrugging motion. Hold (4).

2
Slowly release (4) and repeat four times.

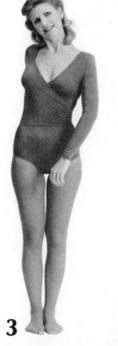

3
Then, keeping your arms loose at your sides, lift your left shoulder up and forward, while lifting your right up and back (2).

4
Reverse in a smooth motion (2), then repeat four times.

Circle your shoulders back (4) and forward (4). Repeat twice.

5
As a variation, walk back four paces while circling your shoulders back.

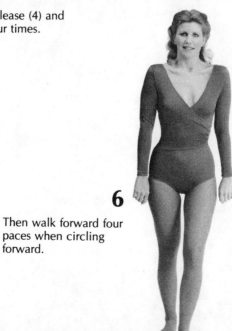

6
Then walk forward four paces when circling forward.

232

BODY ROLL

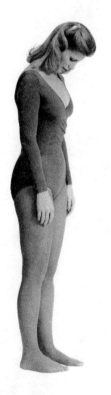

1

Hold your stomach firm,
tuck your chin in,

2

and slowly roll over taking
4 counts to the waist.

3

Then release to the ground
(4).

4

Come up slowly to the
waist (4), then clench your
buttocks, hold in your
stomach and return to standing,

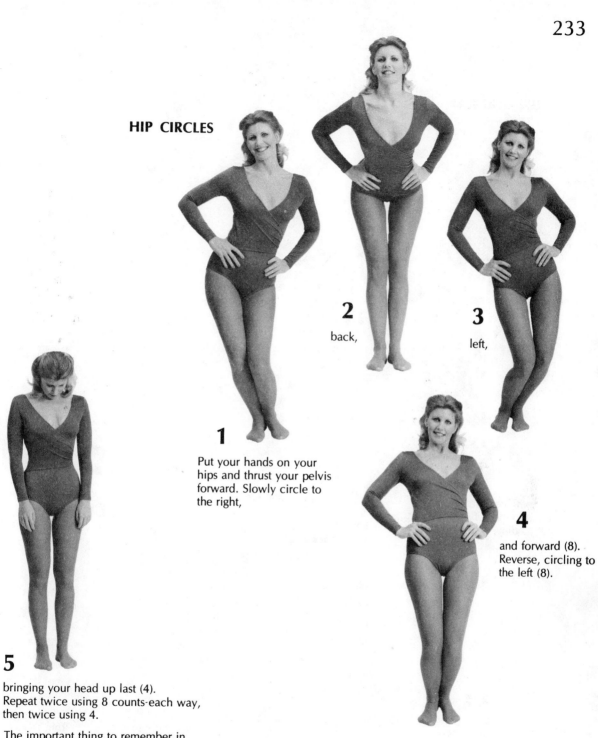

HIP CIRCLES

2 back,

3 left,

1 Put your hands on your hips and thrust your pelvis forward. Slowly circle to the right,

4 and forward (8). Reverse, circling to the left (8).

5 bringing your head up last (4). Repeat twice using 8 counts each way, then twice using 4.

The important thing to remember in this exercise is that the power is in your stomach and your pelvis. Avoid letting go and allowing your stomach to sag.

SIDE STRETCH

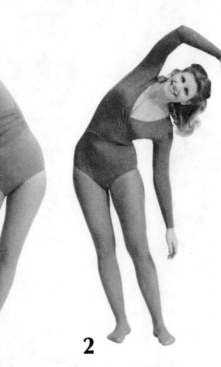

1

Keeping your arms loose, bend to the right (4); return to standing,

2

then bend to the left (4) and hold (4).
Repeat. Bend only enough to feel the stretch.

SIDE LUNGING

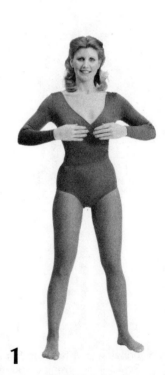

1

Stand with your feet comfortably apart and hold your hands in front of your chest, elbows out to the sides.

The power in this exercise comes from your thighs, so concentrate on contracting the thigh as it comes up from the bend. Also make sure that your feet are far enough apart to feel the stretch when you are lunging.

4

Bend your right knee, open your arms and hold (4).
Return to standing (4). Repeat. Then do twice using 2 counts to bend and 2 counts to straighten.

3

Return to standing, bringing your hands in (4).

2

Bend your left knee, open your arms to the sides, keeping them relaxed, and hold (4).

FORWARD LUNGING

1 Bring your feet into a V-shape, hands held in front of the chest.

2 Slide your right foot forward, open your arms to the front and back, and bend your right knee, turn to the left to look behind you (4).

3 Return to standing by sliding your right foot back to V-position, hands in front of chest (4).

4 Repeat with left leg, then do the sequence four times.

WALL PUSH-UPS

1

Stand facing a wall an arm's length in front of you. Lay your palms on the wall.

2

Slowly bend your elbows and, keeping your heels on the floor, lean forward (4).

3

Push against the wall, straighten your arms and return to standing (4). Repeat four times. Then four times again using 2 counts for each movement.

AEROBICS

Run in place while breathing evenly, and thrust your arms in front of you alternately, opening your hand in the thrust forward and closing it as you pull your arm back. Continue as long as you're comfortable and not out of breath (up to five minutes). (If you'd prefer, try rope skipping instead of running.)

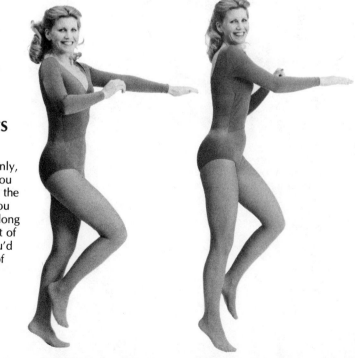

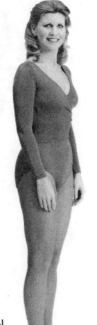

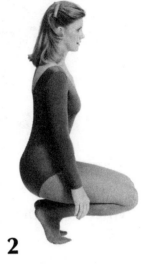

TRANSITION

1

Stand with your feet parallel.

2

Bend your knees and slowly squat, raising your heels off the floor (4).

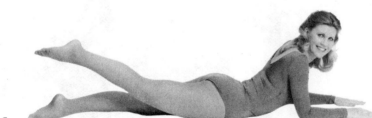

4

and slowly lower your right leg (4). Repeat with each leg. Then repeat two times using 2 counts for each movement.

3

Bring your right leg back, straightening it,

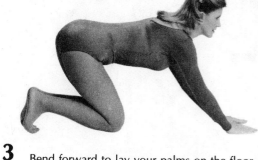

3 Bend forward to lay your palms on the floor,

4 and slide your hands forward, slowly lowering your pelvis to the floor.

LEG POINTERS ON STOMACH

1 Lying on your stomach, legs straight back, raise your torso, leaning on your elbows, hands palms down. Lift your right leg,

2 and, bending your knee slightly, raise your leg up and back over the left leg, touching the floor behind you with your toe; allow your right arm to straighten for balance (4).

TRANSITION

Raise your right leg up and
roll back over to the left.

BODY REACH

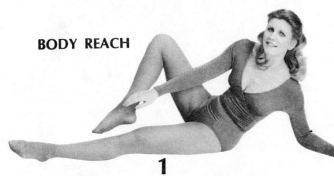

1

Slide the right foot up to
the left knee (8).

2

From this sitting position, bend toward
your left knee, allowing your arms to
hang loosely in front (4). Return to
sitting upright (4).

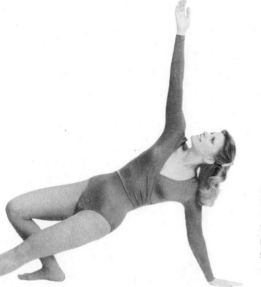

Slowly lower your body, turning your torso to the front. Straighten out your right leg and repeat the sequence, this time sliding your left foot up to your right knee. Repeat once more on each side.

3

Slide your left hand back behind you and lift your body using your right leg and left arm, look upward and reach with your right arm (4).

FOOT CIRCLES

Straighten both legs in front of you. Lift your left leg just off the floor (leaning on your hands behind you if you need to for balance) and point your toes. Circle your foot outward eight times and inward eight times.
Repeat with the right.

SIT-UPS

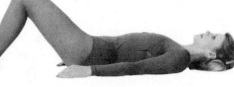

1

Slowly lie down on your back and bend your knees (8).

2

Hold your stomach firm, tuck in your chin and roll up to your knees, using your stomach muscles to pull you up, arms held loosely at your sides (8).

3

Roll down onto your back vertebra by vertebra (8).

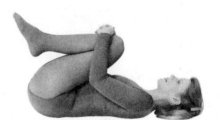

5 Lying on the floor, bring your knees to your chest and hold there with your arms. Relax and breathe evenly for 16 counts.

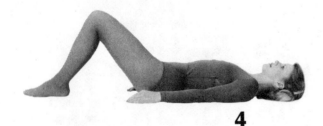

4

Repeat four times using 8 counts for each movement, then four times using 4 counts. The important thing to remember is to use your stomach muscles in this exercise and not to strain your neck.

REST

LEG POINTERS ON BACK

1

Remain on your back, straighten both legs and allow your arms to rest at your sides, hands palms up. Bend your right knee, sliding your foot along your left leg until it rests next to your knee (8).

2

Point your toes, straighten your leg upward,

3

and lower to the side over left leg until touching the floor with your toes (8).

4

Lift your right leg and return to pointing upward and slowly lower to the floor, keeping your leg straight (8). Repeat with each leg four times.

TRANSITION

With your legs straight, slowly sit up and open your legs as far as you can without straining. Point your toes and hold your arms loosely in front of you.

BODY STRETCH

2

and return to upright position (4).

1

Bend toward your right knee, bringing your arms forward (4),

Repeat the movements, this time bending over your left leg. Do the exercise four times over each leg.

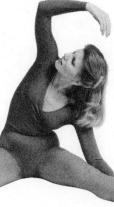

8

Circle your right arm in a counterclockwise direction upward and brush past your right ear.

9

As your arm drops, allow your torso to return to an upright position.

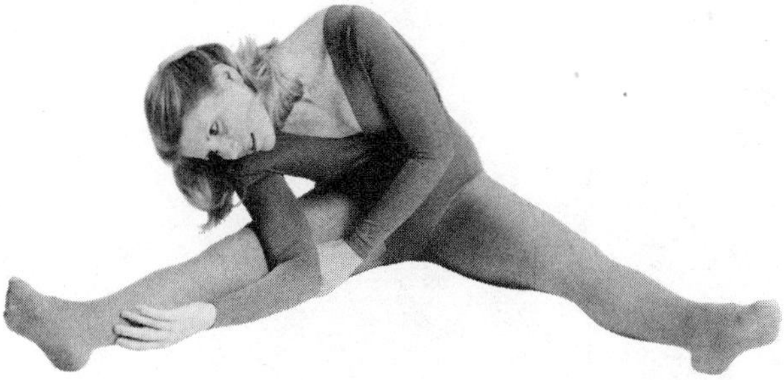

3

Bend toward your right knee again, this time tucking your right hand, palm up, under your right calf so that your torso is held over your right leg.

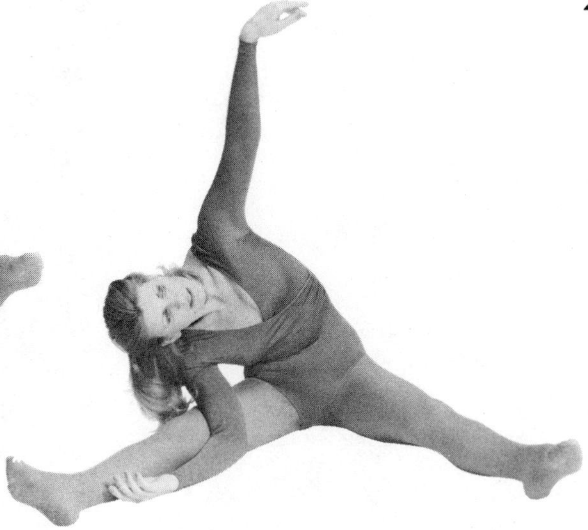

4

Circle your left arm in a counterclockwise direction forward, to the left, upward,

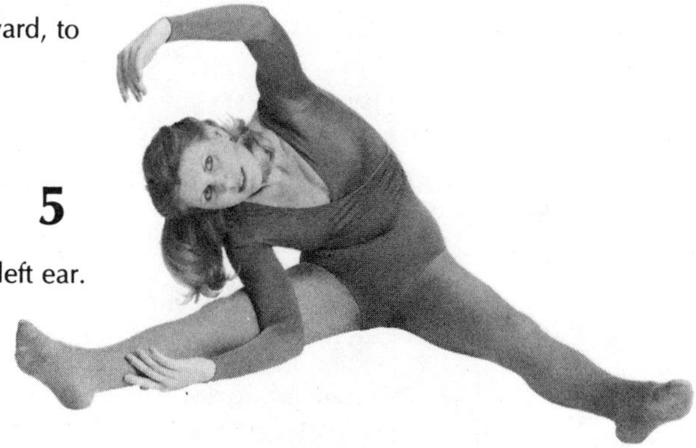

5

and brush over your left ear.

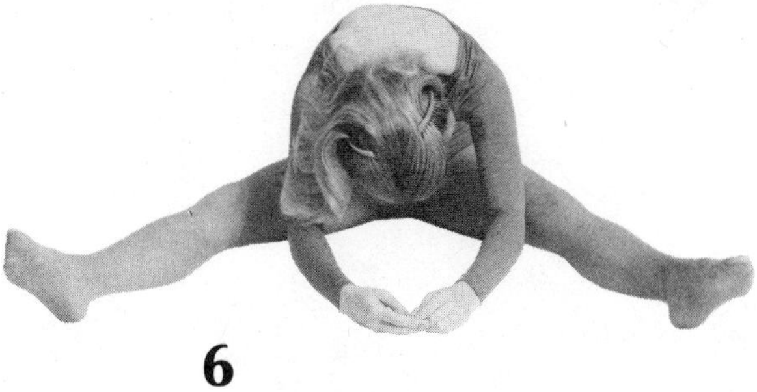

6

Allow your left arm to drop next to your right, and then stretch both your arms forward.

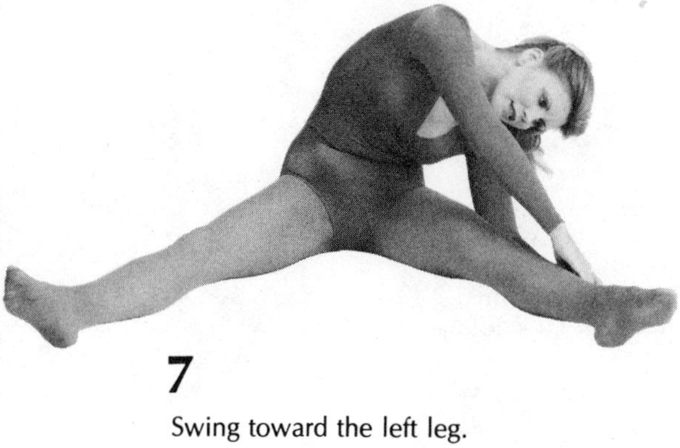

7

Swing toward the left leg.

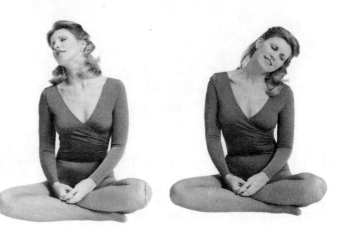

PAUSE

Bring your legs into a cross-legged position, straighten your back and circle your head to the right (8) and to the left (8).

UPPER BODY STRENGTHENERS

1

Hold your hands in front of your chest, lock them together and pull with your left arm to the left, your right resisting the whole way (4). Then pull to the right while your left arm resists (4). Repeat four times to each side.

2

Unlock your hands and press the heels of your hands together.
Repeat the exercise, this time pushing from side to side.

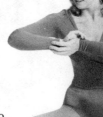

TRANSITION

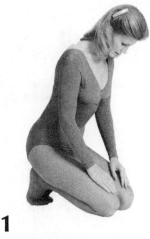

1

Shift to kneeling position,

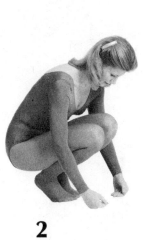

2

then into a squat, resting on the balls of your feet

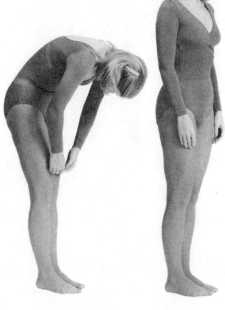

3

Lower your heels, straighten your legs and roll slowly to a standing position, holding your stomach firm (8).

STAR FINISH

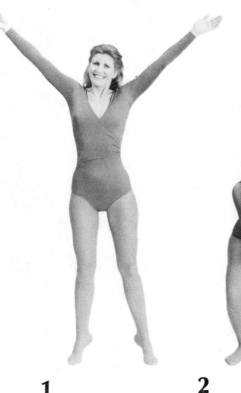

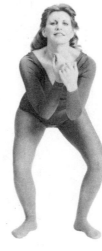

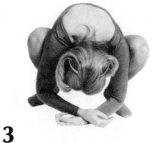

1
Stand with your feet comfortably apart. Reach upward from the balls of your feet, legs and arms stretched out, buttocks clenched, fingers extended, and smile (2).

2
Slowly release like a rag doll—drop your arms, bend your knees,

3
drop your head, allow your buttocks to stick out as you bend over and brush your palms on the floor (6).

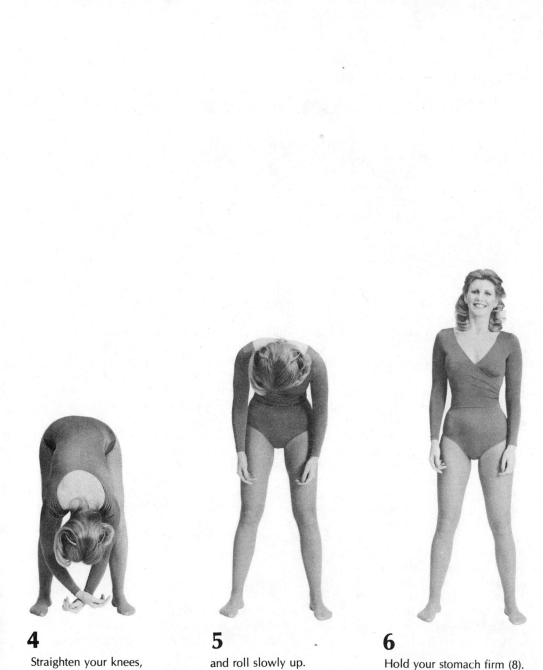

4

Straighten your knees,

5

and roll slowly up.

6

Hold your stomach firm (8).
Repeat.
Shake your body out and lie down on
the floor and relax for several minutes.

GALLBLADDER DISEASE

If it seems to you that more women than men develop gallbladder problems, it could be because they do. Published estimates say that 20 percent of American women compared to only 10 percent of American men between the ages of 55 and 60 have gallstones this very minute. These same figures, based on autopsy reports, claim that one-quarter of the ladies but only one-tenth of the men of any age in this country will develop gallstones some time before they're 60.

Actually, the reason any gallbladder is vulnerable to disease is somewhat of an occupational hazard. Its job is to break down food. Not just any food, but fatty foods only. To do that it receives, stores and concentrates bile produced by the liver, its upstairs neighbor, which it then sprays on our food at an appointed time during digestion. The bile contains an optimum balance among cholesterol and two emulsifiers, bile acids and lecithin, and those emulsifiers hold the fat in the cholesterol in solution until it can be whisked down the intestine's drain.

It's just like Dash in your washer.

Cholesterol is the "greasy dirt" in your kid's dungarees. Bile acids are the detergent in the soap. And lecithin is the water softener that most laundry products contain to neutralize minerals in water which block the action of detergents. If you have the right amount of detergent and the proper measure of water softener, the dirt your child grinds in doesn't stand a chance. If liver bile contains 3 cups bile acid and ¼ cup lecithin to each ¾ cup cholesterol, everything's peachy. But when more cholesterol is added to the bile, or more dirt

to the jeans, things start to go wrong, and the "grimy oil" doesn't come out in the wash. People with gallbladder disease, especially those with gallstones, have so much cholesterol in their systems—and hence their liver bile—that these proportions are knocked out of whack.

But why are women so lucky?

One reason is that we are the chosen childbearers. Three out of four women who suffer from gallstones have been pregnant at least once in their lives. During pregnancy, a woman's body produces more cholesterol, the stuff that gallstones are made of. In addition, a higher estrogen level during pregnancy saps a woman's smooth muscle tone—and, since the gallbladder is a muscular organ, it has a tendency to empty more slowly during pregnancy. That allows cholesterol to stagnate so that stones have a chance to form. Still, the gallstones that form before a child is born are usually small and "silent"; that is, they cause no symptoms. It's just that as the years go by and the woman puts on weight (or fails to lose the weight she gained during pregnancy), they grow in size and become more meddlesome.

The Link with Estrogen

Curiously, however, many doctors have noticed a recent rise in the number of slim, childless women among their gallbladder patients. A survey of 24 Boston area hospitals was conducted to find out why. From that came the interesting discovery that a woman's gallbladder becomes saturated with cholesterol during a normal menstrual cycle and that this saturation reaches dangerous richness when she is taking any kind of estrogen therapy—either an oral contraceptive or hormone replacement supplement during menopause (*New England Journal of Medicine*, January 3, 1974). That saturation, of course, invites the formation of gallstones.

In a parallel study at New York City's Mount Sinai Hospital it was discovered that women who use birth control pills are twice as likely to develop gallstones as those who do not, and that women who receive estrogen for menopausal symptoms are 2½ times more susceptible to them than those who deal with menopause without drugs. The role of estrogen and estrogen therapy in gallbladder disease accounts for the greater number of female victims. It probably also accounts for the relatively recent decrease in the age of victims. Gallstone sufferers have become younger as the Pill has become more popular.

Obviously, then, the avoidance of any unnecessary additions to natural hormone levels—such as the use of oral contraceptives or estrogen therapy during menopause—can be of great help. But if you're being sabotaged by your own natural hormone production, what you need is a way to keep excess cholesterol in solution so it doesn't have a chance to crystallize into annoying little gemstones.

One way to do this, some doctors tell us, is with a neat little drug called chenodeoxycholic acid or chenic acid (for short) or cheno (to its friends). Cheno not only keeps gallstones from forming, it can actually dissolve those that have already taken shape—at least, it did in about half of the people it was tested on at the Mayo Clinic in Rochester, Minnesota. Unfortunately, 20 percent of the people who stopped taking cheno and who were available for reassessment

had stones again (*Journal of the American Medical Association*, March 13, 1978). But the worst part was the unpleasant side effects of the treatment. Like stomach cramps and diarrhea. And the possibility of liver damage, and the worry of fetal damage in women of childbearing age. Further tests at the Mayo Clinic and elsewhere have shown that the liver damage cheno does to laboratory animals is *not* a factor with human subjects. The specter of birth defects, however, has not been exorcised.

At the time of this writing a nationwide study of cheno involving 1,000 persons is underway. It may teach us things that will make the treatment seem more acceptable. But as far as we're concerned, swallowing a powerful mixed blessing every day for the rest of one's life is no solution to any problem. Especially when there's a natural alternative.

According to Dr. K. Holub and associates of the Wilhelmina Hospital in Vienna, Austria, prevention of gallstones may be as close as your nearest grocery and health food stores. Based on their research, corn oil and pyridoxine (vitamin B$_6$) taken together may provide a better and safer solution to cholesterol saturation (*Acta Chirurgica Austriaca*, vol. 8, no. 4, 1976).

In a carefully controlled study, the bile from 22 gallbladder patients was evaluated three days after surgery. Then the same patients were given one tablespoon of corn oil and two 25-milligram tablets of B$_6$ at 7 P.M. and midnight on one day and at 4 A.M. the next day. Bile samples were again taken and analyzed to determine whether there was any change in the cholesterol-dissolving capacity of the bile.

Indeed there was! Of course, the bile's ability to dissolve cholesterol differs greatly from individual to individual. But according to the Austrian research team, *all* patients were better able to keep their cholesterol in solution after treatment with corn oil and B$_6$. In fact, depending on the patient, the bile in the sample taken after the treatment was able to dissolve anywhere from 43 to 86 percent more cholesterol than before the administration of the corn oil-pyridoxine combination.

Like cheno, however, the effectiveness of this treatment may depend on long-term use. But at least there are no ill effects associated with either the corn oil or the vitamin, say the doctors. Besides, they're so easy to take. A tablespoon of corn oil can easily be added to a salad at lunch and again at supper. It may be a little bit more difficult to disguise the corn oil in your morning meal. But you can swallow your tablespoonful and follow it with a chaser of orange juice. Pyridoxine may be purchased in a health food store in 25-milligram tablets. Just take two with each meal. And keep in mind that the oil and B$_6$ should be taken together.

To take prevention one step further, you may want to sprinkle your morning cereal and evening fruit cup with a few tablespoons of bran. (By the way, be sure to drink lots of water with your bran, or let it soak thoroughly in milk before eating.) A study by Eru W. Pomare, M.D., Kenneth W. Heaton, M.D., and two colleagues at the University Department of Medicine, Royal Infirmary in Bristol, England, showed that raw wheat bran may also help to reduce the cholesterol saturation of the bile (*Digestive Diseases*, July, 1976).

During their study, a minimum of 20 grams (a couple of tablespoons) of bran was added to the daily diets of six gallbladder patients.

Within four to six weeks the researchers noted a significant reduction in the cholesterol saturation in the bile of their subjects. Moreover, in two patients the bile became unsaturated. Although the results of this experiment and other similar ones remain inconclusive, they do suggest that lots of fiber in the diet tends to lower cholesterol saturation in the liver bile.

Finally, there is some reason to believe that supplements of vitamin C and lecithin (which is one of the natural "detergents" in liver bile) do help improve the bile's ability to hold cholesterol in solution and hence to get rid of it and gallstones. These experiments—at Mount Sinai Hospital and at the Institute of Nutrition in Bratislava, Czechoslovakia—are extremely tentative, but they do suggest that there are ways of at least limiting the formation of gallstones which do not require the flooding of one's body with strange, powerful and relatively unknown substances.

And remember, even if your gallbladder problem is aggravated by a menacing hormone, a proper diet would soften its blows. In fact, the most important preventive measure anyone can take against gallstones involves the foods she eats—that is, which ones and how much.

A true low-fat, low-animal-protein diet should be adopted. That does not mean giving up the occasional cheeseburger as it did under the traditionally recommended regimen. It means eating a great deal less red meat and going lightly even on chicken and fish. It means learning about vegetable proteins and the theories of complementary protein sources in books like Frances M. Lappé's *Diet for a Small Planet* (Ballantine, 1975).

It means—above all—losing weight

if you should. Study after study has shown that fat people suffer more gallbladder trouble than thin people, because they produce more cholesterol. And because women have a natural predisposition toward excess poundage—again due to the female hormone estrogen—they must be extra careful of their weight. After all, it does no good to cut down on the fats your mouth puts into your liver bile if you don't also cut down on the cholesterol your body itself manufactures.

Even after the removal of a stone-loaded gallbladder and the resulting increase in bile acid production, a tubby patient's level of cholesterol will remain higher than her "detergents" can manage, because her fat-factory continues at full steam. In the famous heart study of 5,000 people in Framingham, Massachusetts, it was learned that folks who weighed at least 20 percent more than the average poundage for their height, frame and sex were *twice* as apt to get gallstones as their normal neighbors. The Pima Indians of Phoenix, Arizona, are nearly all overweight, and they have become famous in gallbladder annals, because almost 70 percent of the tribe develops gallstones. And a survey of deaths due to gallbladder complications in a Los Angeles Veterans Administration hospital revealed that just about half of the dead were 20 or more pounds overweight. A person who weighs 300 pounds will produce *twice* as much cholesterol as a 150-pound person.

What's more, the National Institute of Arthritis, Metabolism, and Digestive Diseases says that this imbalance gets even crazier during the periods of weight fluctuation that chronic dieters undergo. The moral for everybody, according to the Institute, is: Get Thin, Stay Thin, and Avoid Gallstones.

One way to help in this area is to get regular exercise. Vlado Simko, M.D., of the University of Cincinnati Medical Center and a leading researcher in the field of exercise and cholesterol reduction, sent us a fat packet of graphs and charts to document his claims and said:

> Even mild exercise (walking three miles/hour) decreases in human volunteers cholesterol in the red blood cells and increases the output of cholesterol and bile acids in the bile. From several studies in rats we know that if mild exercise is regularly repeated, besides decreasing cholesterol in the red blood cells, it leads to less cholesterol in the bile. (Higher output of cholesterol into the intestine during exercise probably leads to higher losses of cholesterol in the stool.) Decreased cholesterol content of the bile means better solubility of cholesterol in the bile and lesser propensity to form cholesterol gallstones (which are very prevalent in the technological societies).

Think what more than "mild exercise" could do.

We'll even go one step further and suggest that what's good for prevention may be good for treatment, as well.

The only surefire way of coping with gallstones—the ones, of course, with no symptoms or only moderate ones—is to *completely* change those rotten habits. If eating lots of fats, lots of animal protein, and getting too little bulk in one's diet and too little exercise in one's life can cause gallstones, then reversing that trend can help get rid of them, or can, at least, help control them. If being fat causes gallstones, then getting skinny can help get rid of them. And if these ways are naturally your ways, then you stand to avoid gallbladder hassles.

GYNECOLOGISTS AND THEIR ALTERNATIVES

Feminists are currently caught up in a controversy over gynecological care. And it's left many of us in a quandary over the medical men in our own lives. On the one hand, it seems we can't do without them. No matter how well we take care of ourselves there are inevitably times when we'll need someone who specializes in obstetrics and gynecology. But on the other hand, the more we hear of their nonchalance in dishing out drugs and surgery—and the insensitivity of these mostly male physicians to the concerns and problems of women—the more we wonder whether we might do just as well without them.

It's an understandable predicament. Try as we might to trust them, the statistics just do not stack in their favor.

- Hysterectomy is now the number one surgical procedure in this country. And what's even worse, a recent study sponsored by the American Medical Association reveals that hysterectomy and dilation and curettage (D and C), are second among unnecessary surgical procedures, surpassed only by knee surgery.
- Cesarean sections are on the upswing. Estimates maintain that today as many as 25 percent of all delivering mothers in the United States will have c-sections, a surgical procedure once reserved for specific medical problems.
- In spite of (or some may say because of) all our "advances" in obstetrics, the United States still ranks 12th among the developed countries in fetal mortality.
- Minor tranquilizers, such as Valium, are prescribed to women more than twice as frequently as to men.

- Synthetic hormones—in the form of birth control pills, the morning-after pill, or DES (diethylstilbestrol), and estrogen replacement therapy—are still prescribed to millions of women (often with no caution concerning their side effects) despite the overwhelming evidence that they increase the risk of blood clots, stroke, gallbladder disease and cancer.

Of course, all of these pitfalls of modern gynecology and obstetrics are somewhat avoidable—at least to the extent that we can question their necessity and do our best to steer clear of frivolous or overzealous treatment. But something we can't always guard against is attitude. And let's face it, the physician's attitude plays a big part in the way women perceive the whole gynecological experience. Understandably, that experience is often less than positive. In fact, any uneasiness you may feel with your gynecologist and with the gynecological exam is echoed by nearly every other woman.

For example, when 75 students and faculty members at a community college were asked to re-create the feelings they had during their last pelvic exam, 85 percent responded very negatively. Their responses ranged from "nervous, uneasy, apprehensive, anxious, frightened, worried, can't wait for it to be over with, dreading it" and "undignified, awkward, self-conscious, degraded, dehumanized, treated in assembly-line fashion," to "physically uncomfortable, distasteful, horrible, one of my least favorite things, mad, painful." Any of these ring true for you?

Moreover, while 43 percent answered more favorably to the second question concerning attitude toward the physician during the exam, 41 percent again reported negative feelings. Their major complaints involved feelings of being rushed, impersonal, patronizing, condescending, lack of genuine concern (*Obstetrics and Gynecology*, July, 1979).

A Study on Male Attitude

A physician's attitude, the way he treats you, can have a tremendous impact on your health and well-being. Probably more so than you think. And, while we don't want to appear sexist in *our* remarks, after all our research on this subject we can't help but think that men's general attitude toward women is an unavoidable issue here.

For one thing, most physicians are male. It's a fact; 90 percent of all physicians and 91 percent of all ob-gyns are men. And much as we hate to admit it, men in medicine have a tendency to view women a little differently than they would other men.

That was demonstrated quite clearly in a study published in the *Journal of the American Medical Association* (May 18, 1979). Karen J. Armitage, M.D., and associates at the University of California, San Diego, reviewed the medical records of 104 men and women (52 married couples) with such complaints as back pain, headache, dizziness, chest pain and fatigue who had been to one of nine family physicians (all male) for diagnosis and treatment. Interestingly, these physicians—all of whom had distinguished reputations in the community and held important positions in hospitals and in various medical societies—were more careful about pinpointing an underlying cause in the men than

in the women. More specifically, for every single complaint—but especially for symptoms of low back pain and headache—the men received more extensive diagnostic workups than the women. Their conclusions: "Physicians—who in this study were all male—tend to take illness more seriously in men than in women. And, in doing so," they add, "they might be responding to current stereotypes that regard the male as typically stoic and the female as typically hypochrondriacal."

Perhaps also because of this all-pervasive attitude that women are hypochondriacs, and because men will never experience menstrual cramps or labor pains, there seems to be an overwhelming temptation among male physicians to brush off such complaints as mind over matter. In fact, some gynecology texts (obviously written by men) state that "the pain of dysmenorrhea [menstrual cramps] is always secondary to an emotional problem."

Penny Budoff, M.D., clinical associate professor of family medicine at State University Medical Center in Stony Brook, New York, discusses this point in a chapter on health problems of women in *Women In Industry* (University of New York Press, 1977). "Our male-oriented society has never come to grips with menstruation," she says. "Since antiquity, problems and pain related to menstruation have been regarded by many physicians as unimportant, a sign of woman's weakness, either mental or physical. Even today, the most common treatment prescribed is advice to go home, stay in bed, and the pains will go away. It is curious that in this day and age when we are probing outer space, we permit more than half of the population of the world to suffer from menstrual cramps."

Diana Scully, Ph.D., a sociologist who spent hundreds of hours observing ob-gyn specialists in training, noted a similar attitude among males. In her book *Men Who Control Women's Health* (Houghton Mifflin, 1980), she writes, "Residents were encouraged to suspect that many female complaints, including menstrual pain, were psychosomatic, but female residents were less likely than their male counterparts to accept these explanations." To illustrate this, Dr. Scully quotes a female physician as saying, "Well, if you have a patient with severe dysmenorrhea, this patient is really suffering every month. They [the males] will tell her, take some aspirin. They will never know....Dysmenorrhea—they just think the patient is having some cramps. They probably had some diarrhea in their life and they think this is the same. They won't understand that the uterus is contracting and is giving pain to the woman in the same way that cervical dilation is painful in a woman."

Dr. Scully also noted a marked difference in the way male and female residents responded to labor pain. For example, a male physician told her that he imagined the pain of labor to be "less than a kidney stone but more than a sprained ankle." By contrast, a female physician looked at it this way: "When I am at the bedside of a patient feeling her painful contraction, trying to give her some relief, I feel it much more than the men can. I am involved. The man can feel she has a pain; probably give her something. I will suffer with the patient; they won't, never, never."

Well, maybe not *never*. One male resident confided this: "I was taught in medical school how pain is psychological," he said. "Then when I would see a girl in labor and she would be holler-

ing, I would think it is all in her head, it's nothing. When my wife went through it—she isn't the kind of girl that says ouch very much—and when she said ouch, I said this isn't psychological, this is real pain." Nice of him to notice.

It's hard to say how women came to be categorized as wimps. Part of it may stem from the old idea that women are the weaker sex—presumably in mind as well as body. But, more probably, the fact that women seek out medical attention with greater frequency than men adds some fuel to that way of thinking—albeit in a twisted way.

It is true: women's office visits to physicians are 37 percent higher than men's. And although some may argue that women live longer and have to contend with the medical needs of pregnancy and childbirth—which would tend to drive their medical visits far beyond any male's—one study did show that even with all that taken into consideration, women report more serious and chronic illnesses than men.

We have no way to explain that. But the point we do want to make is that women, much more so than men, are in contact with physicians and the health care system. And because of specific needs involving their reproductive organs—namely, menstrual problems, routine Pap smears, prenatal and postnatal care, birth control information, infertility problems and menopausal symptoms—there is a tendency for women today to rely heavily on their gynecologists—often for *all* their health care needs.

Is there anything wrong with that?

Could be. First of all, physicians, ob-gyns included, vary in their experience and expertise of training. You may know one who meets all your health care needs very nicely. But generally speaking, it's not considered a good idea to rely on the ob-gyn for more than specific gynecological problems.

Need a Gynecologist?

"Certain problems should be treated by a gynecologist. Abnormal Pap smears. Fibroid tumors. Cancer. Ovarian cysts," says Alice Rothchild, M.D., herself a practicing ob-gyn and clinical instructor at Harvard Medical School. But, she told us, a gynecologist's training is not appropriate for other problems that may seem related to women but are not related specifically to a woman's anatomy.

Sexual counseling is one area where ob-gyns seem to be undereducated but overconsulted. While it may seem a logical step from the mechanics of birth control and infertility to discussions of sexual difficulties, the truth is that few ob-gyns know enough about the psychological makeup of a woman to offer substantive help in that area. Dr. Scully, who witnessed the training of ob-gyns firsthand at two medical centers, told us that taking your sexual problems to a gynecologist won't get them solved—they are just not equipped to handle those kinds of problems. Besides that, she says, research indicates that many have biased attitudes on female sexuality anyway—so why bring it up in the first place? A paragraph taken from her book sums up the situation:

> During my period of observation, neither institution offered instruction on female sexuality (though Elite [a pseudonym she uses for one of the medical centers] planned to initiate a program the following year). Residents stated that the board qualifying examinations of the American College of Obstetricians and Gynecologists contained only a few super-

ficial questions of sexuality, from which they inferred that the subject was not important. When asked where they acquired their knowledge of human sexuality, answers ranged from *Playboy* magazine to the army. Only a few had read even parts of Masters and Johnson.

Nutrition counseling is another area where your physician may be uninformed. While most schools teach some nutrition in conjunction with other courses, only a quarter of all medical schools include a required nutrition course in their curriculums. Seventy percent do offer elective courses in nutrition, but there is some speculation that with so many required courses to take, many students do not enroll in those electives.

"In nutrition, one of the problems is that it's the more intelligent women who are doing all the reading in nutrition," says Richard Rivlin, M.D., professor of medicine and chief of nutrition at Memorial Sloan-Kettering Cancer Center and the New York Hospital–Cornell Medical Center, in a recent magazine interview. "But the physicians, not being educated in this area, are uncomfortable in answering questions. 'Should I take vitamin E?'—that type of thing. The physician loses credibility, because he cannot really answer these questions, and so the patient is unhappy, or dissatisfied with his answer and then turns elsewhere. I think part of the difficulty lies, really, in the process of medical education" (*New York State Journal of Medicine*, February, 1980).

Even worse than a physician who's ignorant of nutrition is one who's ignorant and hostile to any mention of the topic. In a treatise on women's liberation and the effect it's had on the physician-patient relationship, Alexandra Symonds, M.D., associate clinical professor of psychiatry, New York University School of Medicine, relays the difficulty one of her patients had getting nutritional information from M.D.'s:

> One patient of mine was a woman who had been chronically depressed. She had a long history of skin problems and a long history of medical care. She had always passively followed the instructions of her physician. Recently, as a result of therapy, her depression lifted. For the first time she began to take an interest in her condition and tried to become more informed about the details. She read up on nutrition, read labels of food carefully, patronized health food stores, and tried to get detailed information from her various physicians as to the nature of each medication. She was an intelligent woman who made good use of this knowledge and was able to improve her overall condition as a result of her reading and active participation. However, each time she asked her various physicians for further information, they reacted negatively. One said derogatorily, "Oh, I see that you are one of those health nuts."
> —*New York State Journal of Medicine,*   February, 1980

If you are faced with a similar response, don't be too dismayed. "There's no question about it, nutrition should be stressed more in medical training," Dr. Rivlin told us. "But until we get to that point, women have no choice but to go to a library or specialist who's active in the field to have her nutritional questions answered."

Still the major problem—and possibly a danger—in running to the gynecologist for all that ails you is that it equates the ob-gyn with the general practitioner when there is really nothing *general* about his training. In fact, there are those who would argue that going to a gynecologist for routine check-ups is like going to a general surgeon to check your blood pressure. An absurd analogy? Not when you consider that ob-gyns are actually *surgical* specialists. They are surgeons who specialize in disorders of the female pelvic organs.

Where to Go for Primary Medical Care

If you've read anything at all about avoiding unnecessary surgery, know that rule number one is don't see a surgeon first. Because his forte is surgery, he's more likely to recommend surgical over nonsurgical treatment. And, with so many women seeing gynecologists routinely, is it any wonder that gynecological surgery has one of the worst reputations for unnecessary procedures?

All this has led many women's self-help groups to take the speculum into their own hands. Armed with gynecology texts and self-help manuals, and guided by sympathetic medical personnel, they are learning how to give themselves pelvic exams—and seeing themselves in a whole new light, we may add.

Of course, it isn't for everyone. And if this, the ultimate in medical self-care, makes you just a little bit uptight, relax. There are ways for you to work within the framework of conventional medical care and maintain a healthy advantage.

First of all, we do want to point out that your options here depend in part on where you live and what is available in your community.

For some women, a qualified and caring GP may be the answer. That is especially true in a smaller town where there may be only one or two very busy gynecologists and the family practitioners are frequently called on to do the routine breast exams and Pap smears. On the other hand, it seems some GPs prefer *not* to perform these exams at all—and may not be well qualified to do so. Speaking at a 1979 conference on Women in Medicine at Cornell University Medical College, Lila A. Wallis, M.D., told the audience that in her 28 years of private practice as an internist she heard many complaints from women patients that their family physicians had frequently omitted breast and pelvic exams from their comprehensive physicals. "There is a discrepancy," she says, "in the time and effort which is devoted to women's health problems compared to the time and effort devoted to, say, rheumatic heart disease, for which there are maybe 5,000 to 10,000 new cases each year. Breast and pelvic cancers account for 200,000 new cases each year."

One reason for the inadequacy of some family physicians in conducting breast and pelvic exams may be found in the inadequacy of their training, Dr. Wallis suggests. In spring of 1978, the leaders of the previously mentioned conference at Cornell sent out 98 questionnaires to American medical schools inquiring about their methods and requirements in the teaching of breast and pelvic exams.

Of the 39 schools that responded in any detail, 4 said that they omitted the breast exam altogether in the course on physical diagnosis, and 10 didn't teach the pelvic exam. What's more, Dr. Wallis adds, "in over half of the responding schools the teaching of breast and pelvic exams hasn't changed substantially over the last quarter century despite the fact that women comprise over 51 percent of the population and account for over 60 percent of all patient/physician encounters."

Of course, that's not to say that all family practitioners—or even the majority—are ignorant of women's reproductive organs. Some are well trained and well experienced. But if you don't know for sure "how well," you might be better off looking for someone else.

The Nurse Practitioner and Nurse-Midwife

A good alternative is to go to an ob-gyn nurse practitioner, clinical nurse specialist or nurse-midwife for routine and prenatal care. An ob-gyn nurse practitioner is a registered nurse who has completed a formal and accredited obstetric-gynecologic nurse practitioner's educational program or has work experience with an ob-gyn and passed a certification examination. With a master's degree in nursing, she or he is called a clinical nurse specialist. Both are qualified to do routine breast and pelvic exams including Pap smears, order and interpret routine laboratory tests, treat mild gynecological problems such as vaginal infections, offer birth control information, and provide routine care for all healthy nonpregnant women.

The nurse-midwife is similar in her training and qualifications. She is again a registered nurse who has completed the minimum of a one-year study program followed by a stringent exam for certification. While the emphasis of midwifery training is, of course, on obstetrics, many modern nurse-midwives handle primary gynecological care as well. Sandi Perkins, a nurse-midwife with McTammany Nurse-Midwifery Center, Inc., in Reading, Pennsylvania, describes it this way: "Nurse-midwives are trained to attend to women during their childbearing years—that is from early teens through their fifties—although women still come to us after menopause," she told us. "In our practice we have about half as gynecological patients. The services we provide don't just begin with pregnancy and end with childbirth but continue throughout a woman's life."

And the advantages of both the ob-gyn nurse practitioner and midwife over the ob-gyn and GP for routine gynecological care are many. For one thing, because they see women day in and day out for breast exams and Pap smears, they are usually more experienced in recognizing problems than the GP who does a pelvic perhaps once a week—if that often. Second, because of their basically different orientation—the training of an ob-gyn stresses surgical skills whereas the training of a nurse practitioner or nurse-midwife stresses caring and human relations skills—there is a marked difference in the direction your treatment's likely to take. And also, because the large majority of ob-gyn nurse practitioners and nurse-midwives are women, there's a unique understanding and bond that develops between patient and nurse that's practically impossible to achieve with a male physician.

A woman we spoke with—who happens to be a registered nurse married to a general surgeon—admits that the nurse practitioner can often provide the kind of practical advice that you can't always get from an M.D.

"One time I developed an annoying vaginal infection. The gynecologist I was going to at the time diagnosed it as *Monilia [Candida]* and prescribed My-costatin. It didn't help. In fact, the condition just worsened," she told us. "Then I got to thinking maybe it's not *Monilia*; maybe it's *Trichomonas*. So I mentioned it to him at my next visit.

"'OK,' he said. 'Here's a prescription for Flagyl.' Just like that. He didn't take a culture or anything. Then to top it off, he added as he handed me the prescription. 'Don't take this with alcohol.' 'Why?' I asked. 'Just don't,' he snapped back.

"I gathered from that that he was either too busy to go into detail or too much of a chauvinist to think I'd understand his medical explanation. Or maybe he didn't even know the answer himself. Anyway, I went home and looked up Flagyl in our PDR *[Physicians' Desk Reference]* and found out that the combination of Flagyl and alcohol could cause nausea and vomiting plus some other side effects. Now why couldn't he just tell me that?

"Anyway, the experience so turned me off that I decided to see a nurse practitioner whom I had heard about. She was wonderful. After doing a complete exam, and taking a culture, we sat down and talked. It was sort of a woman-to-woman talk. She told me that she had had the same problem and that one of the most important things to keep in mind is that all these treacherous little organisms thrive in a warm and moist environment and that by keeping yourself cool and dry you can discourage their growth.

"'Do you wear nylon panties?' she asked. 'They're the absolute worst. They trap in the moisture and heat. They don't let you breathe. Always wear cotton underwear. When you're at home, don't wear any at all. And when you step out of the shower and blow dry your hair, use your hairdryer on your bottom as well.'

"Well, it all sounded so simple. But it made a lot of sense. And, do you know, it really works. I haven't had any problem since I started following her advice."

One common argument against nurse-midwives' participation in childbirth has been that they are not experienced enough to recognize problems, so they jeopardize the life of mother and child. Dr. Diana Scully, however, says that research indicates the opposite. "In one controlled study, it was found that nurse-midwives were able to recognize deviations from normal in the obstetrical patient, would ask for medical consultation promptly, and could render safe, effective service themselves to about one-third of a high-risk obstetrics population."

Then, speaking from her own experience, Dr. Scully further elaborates on the competency and compassion of nurse-midwives in everyday gynecological services.

Nurse-midwives gave more thorough examinations. For example, they always included a breast examination as well as instruction, with the use of a rubber model, on self-examination. Nurse-midwives, unlike residents, always explained what they were doing and why, as well as teaching their patients about their bodies. Because the interaction was relaxed and friendly, as opposed to hurried and impersonal, the nurse-midwives' patients usually felt free to ask questions. In contrast, clinic nurses told me that the residents' patients often complained because they were told to "get dressed" before they could ask a question. In short, nurse-midwives informed while residents confused their patients.
—*Men Who Control Women's Health*

Dr. Scully goes on to explain that, at least in her experience, the difference between the way an obstetrician and a nurse-midwife approach childbirth was apparent in the way each defined his or her role. "Midwives have traditionally defined their role in childbirth as assisting women in the natural process of giving birth," she says. "Physicians view childbirth as a medical process."

To get in touch with a nurse-midwife near you, you can write to the National Association of Parents and Professionals for Safe Alternatives in Childbirth (NAPSAC) for a directory of Alternative Birth Services ($5.25 each), or the American College of Nurse-Midwives (see *Appendix* for addresses).

Or contact gynecologists, women's health clinics, or women's self-help groups near you for information. In most areas, ob-gyn nurse practitioners and nurse-midwives work *only* in association with an ob-gyn or clinic such as Planned Parenthood. And actually, because of the limitations of state law and medical insurance companies, it's just as well that they are so affiliated. As illogical as it may sound, insurance companies will cover treatment administered by a nurse-midwife or nurse practitioner if she belongs to a conventional ob-gyn office arrangement. If she's on her own, so are you when it comes to paying the bill.

Unfortunately, however, there just aren't enough nurse practitioners or midwives to go around. But Dr. Scully claims that if more women requested or demanded them, in time there'd be a practitioner or midwife for every ob-gyn—and to everyone's benefit.

In the meantime, many of us have no choice but to seek out an ob-gyn for routine gynecological care. Others, who may be lucky enough to find a nurse-midwife or the like for routine care, may nonetheless require or prefer professional ob-gyn treatment. Remember there's no substitute for the specialized training of an ob-gyn when it comes to assisting problem pregnancies, or treating any kind of abnormal condition that may show up on a Pap smear, as well as problems such as endometriosis, fibroid tumors, or ovarian cysts. That's what they're there for!

Choosing a Gynecologist

Chances are you have already faced the prospect of choosing a new gynecologist, and know what a difficult task it can be. Perhaps you wondered even then: Do I take a stab from the telephone directory? Or rely on my best friend's advice? Can I contact the American Medical Association (AMA) for a more professional referral? Or should I embark on a door-to-door campaign to shop around for a physician whom I can relate to?

Well, it's hard to say what's the best way to zero in on a gynecologist that's right for you. For one thing, there are many variables and what may be of utmost importance to one woman may be a secondary consideration to another. But we can tell you, the *worst* way to go about choosing one is to rely on the Yellow Pages. With a minimum amount of contriving, Joe Schmoe can have his name embellished with an M.D. and listed in the telephone book. Unbelievable but true. Calling the AMA isn't too much better, says Dr. Scully. "They will only give a random list of names. So you might as well have gotten the names from the telephone book."

Asking your general practitioner for a referral may work—so long as you know your referring physician well and thor-

oughly trust his judgment. If you don't know him, you'll have to be on guard that his choice of an ob-gyn for *you* doesn't hinge on *his* friendship or some favor he's returning a fellow physician.

Probably, your most reliable referral sources include women's self-help groups and clinics such as Planned Parenthood which are familiar with physicians in the area and do get feedback from patients who've visited them. If you're near a medical library, you could also check the *A.M.A.'s Directory of Women Physicians in the U.S.* (American Medical Association, 1979) for a female gynecologist in your area.

Another avenue to explore is hospitals. For example, if you happen to know that a certain hospital in your area has a good reputation, call up and ask for the names of the ob-gyns who have privileges there. After all, if the hospital has a good reputation, it's usually because of the doctors who practice there. Teaching hospitals in larger cities are always good bets from this standpoint. In fact, says Dr. Scully, there is some advantage in choosing a physician who is on the staff of a good teaching hospital—not only is he under careful scrutiny day in and day out, but you can be pretty sure he keeps up with the latest medical literature.

Still, it's a good idea to double-check his credentials. The best way to do this is to look him up in the *American Medical Directory* (American Medical Association, 1979), which should be available in your local library, hospital or county medical office. There, you will find out his age (ideally he shouldn't be too old or too young); his medical education, and any medical affiliations. More important, you'll learn if he is board-certified, which means that he has successfully passed a certifying exam conducted by the American Board of Obstetrics and Gynecology.

Of course, it's especially important that you weigh these credentials very carefully. Remember, even if he did attend a top-notch medical school, there's a 50-50 chance that he graduated in the bottom half of his class. Also don't be overly impressed if the initials FACOG follow the M.D. in his title. This only means he is a Fellow of The American College of Obstretricians and Gynecologists, a *voluntary* organization of ob-gyn physicians.

To increase your odds for a satisfactory experience, look to other women. Ask around. You can start with your best friend—but don't stop there. Try to get a good survey and see which names keep cropping up. And while you're asking other women who they go to, find out *why*. What do they like most about him? Least? Have they had any disappointing experiences with him? Is he easy to communicate with? Of course, you should judge these answers very carefully. Remember, your best friend may feel comfortable in the child role to the father image of her gynecologist. You may not.

To evaluate the more technical skills, ask other medical personnel who they go to. Nurses are an excellent source of this kind of information. So are female physicians—and physicians' wives. These women have the background, insight or coaching to recognize good medical skills—and if they feel comfortable with his abilities, chances are you'll be in good hands as well.

One important thing we'd like to mention here: the sex of the physician. As we mentioned earlier, there is a tendency for women to be more receptive to the problems and feelings of other women. But that doesn't mean that you should forsake other qualifications in your search for a female physician. For one thing, there just aren't that many around. Also, not every female gynecologist will meet your specific needs and requirements. And you may overlook a well-qualified and considerate male physician in your quest for the ultimate female.

Don't Be Afraid to Shop Around

Of course, even if you've carefully chosen your gynecologist, the most critical evaluation comes at the actual time of your visit. Until then, there is no way you can absolutely know whether he or she is right for you. In fact, some women narrow their selection down to two or three physicians and then make appointments with all of them in order to make the final selection based on personal interviews. "We see this most often with pregnant women," Dr. Alice Rothchild told us. "They have certain demands. They know what kind of childbirth experience they're looking for. And they want to be sure that the obstetrician will respect and hopefully share her views."

Of course, we've got to warn you, this can be an exhausting and costly procedure. If you're not pregnant or sick and are looking for a gynecologist for routine care, we feel that you'd do just as well screening your physician as best as you can beforehand. Then, if you don't care for his approach, try another for your next appointment. In some cases, you may even be able to call up the doctor's office and ask pertinent questions about the kind of care he offers. That will save both time and money.

Still, some things can't be ascertained without a firsthand visit. For example, a few sources suggest that a reliable guide to a doctor's competency and compassion is the amount of traffic in the waiting room. The best doctor is likely to be busy—but not so busy that you're kept fumbling through old magazines for an hour, then whisked through your appointment in 10 minutes.

Once in his solitary chambers, you'll have the opportunity to judge his merit face to face. Dr. Rothchild gave us some pointers as to what to look for. "There's no way that I can say what's a good and bad patient-physician relationship. Much depends on individual preference," she says. "But I can give you some clues as to what I would look for. Does he explain what he's doing? Does he answer my questions? And most importantly, do I feel satisfied when I leave? From my point of view, every visit to an ob-gyn should be an educational experience.

"Having a healthy relationship with your physician depends on good communication and mutual respect," she told us. "Some women still feel comfortable in a child-parent type of relationship with their M.D. and that's fine, if that's what they want. But from my way of thinking, the best patient-doctor relationships are those in which the patient is considered an intelligent partner in the health care system; one in which the patient is considered an equal to the doctor."

Remember, when it comes right down to it, it's your body, and no one knows it or cares about it the way you do. So don't be afraid to ask questions, to demand a full explanation of your condition or treatment, and to be informed of all potential medication side effects so that you can weigh the consequences and decide for yourself whether or not to take it. "A woman should definitely ask when she has a question—and she shouldn't be afraid to ask constantly," Dr. Rothchild advises. "Be aggressive. It may be a pain in the neck for your doctor, but it's your body and you have the right to know."

And while you're asking questions, try to be specific. For example, if your periods have been unusually heavy lately, don't just ask, "Is everything okay?" Make a list of specific questions in advance.

And while you're preparing your questions, prepare a personal health record to take with you to the exam. This should include the date and length of your last menstrual period, any health or gynecological problems in the past, any medications you might have taken, what type of birth control method you use, plus the family history of gynecological problems. This will help medical history taking.

If you're shy about asking questions or just feel uncomfortable alone during an exam, bring your husband, friend or mother along for support. And if your physician gives you flak about it, get another doctor.

In fact, most of the people we interviewed for this section agreed that if for any reason the gynecologist does not fulfill your needs, feel free to change doctors. They also believe that you should be assertive about why it is that you're unhappy and the reason why you won't be coming back. "Physicians' attitudes have got to change," Dr. Rothchild told us. "And one way we can all help is by pointing out the problems so that they can work at improving their health care."

Some women don't give a dandruff's flake about how their hair looks. For them, a weekly wash is ordeal enough. At the other extreme, we find devotees of a rigorous regimen which subjects their hair to perming, bleaching and plaiting—not to mention such tortuous procedures as teasing and tinting the hair every shade from coal black to powder blue. When these ladies aren't tied to the beautician's chair, you can usually find them wrapped up in rollers or wielding a hot, steamy curling wand. And for what? Ironically, they answer, "for beautiful hair." But the truth is, there's nothing more self-defeating than this type of "pampering."

And no one knows this better than Philip Kingsley. A trained trichologist (a British specialist in scalp and hair science) and author of *The Complete Hair Book* (Grosset & Dunlap, 1979), Kingsley has personally coaxed hundreds of horrendous hair problems—

many of them caused by the kinds of treatment we just mentioned—back to beauty. He's a firm believer that there's nothing more attractive than *healthy* hair and that healthy hair is not only an outgrowth of sensible hair care but of a healthy body.

And it's this commonsense, no-nonsense approach to hair care that has won him quite a following including such celebrities as Candice Bergen, Audrey Hepburn and the British royal family.

We caught up with Philip Kingsley in his New York City salon where this very British gent with a whimsical smile let us in on some of his not-so-secret secrets for healthy hair.

Question: Some old wives' tales about hair care have been around so long we don't even bother to question their validity. Maybe you could help us sort out the good from the bad. For example,

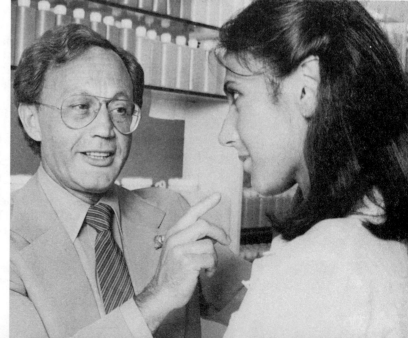

Renowned hair specialist Philip Kingsley does not offer his clients cuts, perms, or colorings. What he does offer is deep conditioning treatments and a wealth of sound scientific advice for healthy hair.

can brushing the hair 100 strokes a day bring back the shine?

Philip Kingsley: Definitely not. Brushing is said to stimulate the scalp and to an extent that's true—but proper massage stimulates the scalp very much better. It's also said that brushing cleanses the hair but shampooing does that so much better. What heavy brushing does do is break the hair and pull it out and scratch the scalp. I'm not saying don't brush at all. But don't use brushing in place of a good saw cut-tooth comb. Rather, brush to smooth the hair as a final step in hair grooming. And don't let the bristles dig into the scalp.

Question: Does hair grow faster when it's cut more frequently?

Philip Kingsley: Nonsense. I think this old wives' tale evolved from observations of men shaving. If a man shaves every day, you'll notice a stubby growth in 12 hours. But if he has a beard, you don't notice the day-to-day growth, so you assume that it's not growing as fast. The truth is, cutting or shaving doesn't make any difference in the rate of growth.

Question: Does frequent cutting have any effect on hair thickness then?

Philip Kingsley: No. It's just an illusion that comes with length. A short hair will feel hard like a short bamboo cane and a long hair—the same hair—will feel thinner and bend like a long bamboo cane.

Another thing—if a man or woman has very long hair it's certain that not all of the hair shafts will be the same length because each hair is at a different stage of growth. What happens is this: a hair grows for a designated period of time. Then the follicle sheds that hair and goes into a resting phase before it begins

to produce another hair. Each day you may lose 40 to 70 hairs as a result of this periodic shedding—which gives you some idea of the many different stages each shaft is at at one time. Of course, a person who gets his hair cut often and keeps it fairly short will have very many more hairs at the same length—and therefore it will appear thicker—than a person with very long hair who may have one-third less hair at the ends than at the scalp.

Question: I've read that another reason longer hair tends to look thinner is that the hair shaft tends to break down as a hair gets older. Is that true?

Philip Kingsley: Oh, no. It's quite the contrary. The longer a hair has been around, the *thicker* the shaft becomes. The reason for this is that exposure to the sun, wind, environmental pollutants and so forth cause the cuticle to swell. To a lesser extent, this is the same kind of damaging chemical reaction that occurs when you bleach your hair. Bleach swells the hair shaft and makes it feel thicker.

What Does Shampooing Really Do to Your Hair?

Question: Some people complain that frequent shampooing makes their hair greasier, while others say excessive washing dries their hair out. Which is true?

Philip Kingsley: Neither. I think hair should be washed every day. After all, you wash your face every day and you take your hair to the same places you take your face.

The reason people think that the more they wash their hair the more oily it becomes is similar to the analogy I made about men shaving. If you wash your hair clean, you immediately notice when it begins to get a little oily. But if you let it get oily, you don't notice it getting *oilier*. The only time shampooing may make your hair oilier is if you've used a very harsh shampoo which absolutely strips the hair and scalp. Then your oil glands may work overtime to undo the damage.

Question: After using one shampoo for several weeks, it often seems like it isn't affecting your hair as it used to. Is it possible that your hair can develop a resistance to certain shampoos?

Philip Kingsley: Just because germs build up a resistance to antibiotics, it doesn't mean that hair builds up a resistance to shampoo. The same shampoo used on the same hair under the same set of circumstances will have the same effect. What happens, though, is that the hair itself changes depending on what you do to it—like perming it, or bleaching it, or tinting it or spraying it—or due to environmental change or job change or nutritional change or physiological change.

I've been doing some research which so far seems to indicate that the menstrual cycle has a profound effect on hair condition. I'm now willing to wager that the time a woman would change her shampoo is immediately before or during the first day or two of her menstrual cycle. The skin secretions and scalp secretions change during that time because of premenstrual tension and also due to hormonal swings. So it stands to reason that the hair changes slightly around the menstrual cycle, too. Usually what happens at this time is the hair gets more oily. If she has a dandruff problem, it gets worse. If she has a tendency toward hair fall, more falls out. It's probably also at this time that she says, "Oh

my goodness, this shampoo isn't working anymore. I'd better switch to another brand." She'll go out, buy another shampoo for a couple of days, say "Ah, yes, this is better." Then she goes back to her normal hormone balance and she thinks again that she's gotten used to this shampoo and goes out to buy another.

Question: So how should she resolve this situation?

Philip Kingsley: Either stick with the same shampoo, or have two shampoos on hand—one to use for three weeks and the other to use for one week.

Can Stress Give You Gray Hair?

Question: Can stress and anxiety give you gray hair?

Philip Kingsley: Well, stress tends to make you gray faster. The interesting thing is, researchers have done experiments in which black rats were put on a diet deficient in B vitamins and their hair turned white. When they were again given B vitamins their hair regained its color. What's so fascinating about all this is that personal stress demands more B vitamins because the body uses more of it up. In fact, the B vitamins have become known as the "nerve vitamins." So, it wouldn't seem unreasonable to conclude from that that stress could have an effect on the graying of hair.

Question: With so many shampoos on the market, how does a person go about choosing one?

Philip Kingsley: One day I went out in New York and bought $400 worth of shampoo, which was about one-fourth of all the shampoos on the pharmacy shelves. Then I took them back to my clinic and blind-tested them: that is, I put them in numbered but unlabeled bottles and gave them to my staff in London and New York. They used them for four months and then wrote down their comments.

The outcome was very interesting indeed insofar as the expensive shampoos came out worst of all. The reason being not only do the expensive shampoos have more expensive scents and more scents (perfume), they also have many more additives, like protein and placenta and all the other rubbish the manufacturers try to put in them. The best shampoos were the middle to lower price range because they don't have as many additives in them.

Also, we discovered that the thicker shampoos weren't any stronger than the thinner ones. Sometimes the *thinner* ones were more concentrated. After all, you can thicken up a shampoo very easily by adding certain things to it.

But perhaps the most fascinating thing of all was that every single shampoo worked better in dilution. And by diluting any shampoo on the market by 50 percent with distilled water you not only use less shampoo, but you'll have better control over it. Some shampoos we tested worked best at 90 percent dilution—that is, one part shampoo to nine parts water.

Having said all that, the basic problem of choosing a shampoo should be resolved through trial and error because what might suit you won't suit me. The thing to do is go out and buy a shampoo, dilute it by 50 percent, try it out for a few weeks, see its effect. If you're not happy with it, go out and buy another. Read the label and the next time buy something with different ingredients. Eventually you'll come across the right shampoo for you.

What About the pH of Your Shampoo?

Question: Does it help to buy a shampoo that's pH-balanced?
Philip Kingsley: It doesn't really make much difference. But a shampoo with a slightly acidic pH would tend to slightly shrink the hair cuticle, which would perhaps give the hair more shine. Perhaps. And acidic shampoo is definitely better for bleached or tinted hair. On the other hand, a shampoo with a slightly alkaline effect tends to slightly swell the hair shaft, which would give the hair a little more body. So, it's six of one, half a dozen of the other.

Question: Does a protein shampoo have any great advantage?
Philip Kingsley: Actually, it has a deleterious effect. We experimented with protein shampoos when they first came out, about seven years ago. Not only did we find that they are useless but in some cases we found that they are more harmful because they brittle-ize the hair. They coat the hair shaft. The ads claim that protein heals split ends. But that's impossible. What they do is momentarily stick the splitting hair shaft together.

They also cause a certain amount of scalp irritation. The trouble is, where you find protein in shampoo you also find preservatives. And it's not only the protein that's detrimental to the hair and scalp but the preservatives which are usually strong antiseptics. So the combination of protein and preservatives is not good.

Question: How do you feel about shampoos with built-in conditioners?
Philip Kingsley: Terrible. You cannot effectively have a combination shampoo

and conditioner. First of all, the ingredients of a shampoo and the ingredients of a conditioner are contrary to each other. One has positive charge and the other has negative charge. They don't have an affinity for each other.

Second, these shampoos tie you down to how much shampoo and how much conditioner you must use. And generally speaking, you'll use less conditioner than shampoo. You're also tied down to conditioning your whole head, scalp included, when in fact you'd hardly ever want to use a conditioner on your scalp. A conditioner belongs on the ends only.

The Best Approach to Dandruff

Question: Do dandruff shampoos work?
Philip Kingsley: I think most dandruff shampoos are rather harsh. And a shampoo that is too harsh can result in an overproduction of oil—which means more dandruff. I'd much rather see a person who has dandruff use a bland shampoo, and then apply a mild antiseptic such as diluted witch hazel or Sea Breeze or a zinc cream to the scalp.

Question: Did you say that an overproduction of oil means *more* dandruff? Isn't dandruff the result of excessive dryness?
Philip Kingsley: Actually, more often than not dandruff is caused by oily scalp. What happens is, people see flakes and they say, "Oh, my goodness, my scalp is dry." But generally these flakes are composed of a lot of oil. The reason dry hair seems to accompany dandruff is that these oily flakes clog the hair follicles and prevent the oil from traveling down the hair shaft. Between the flakes and the dull, dry hair, it looks like what you need is a shampoo for dry hair when

what you really need is a shampoo that will clear up the overly oily condition of the scalp.

Question: Is there a right and wrong way to shampoo the hair?
Philip Kingsley: Oh, absolutely! Many people pour a ghastly amount of shampoo on their heads, rub vigorously till they've worked up a lather (sometimes piling the hair on top of the head and rubbing it about). Then they rinse, repeat the same vigorous lathering procedure and rinse again, very quickly. Finally, they give their hair a rough towel-rub, as if they were polishing brass. Shampooing that way can do enormous damage to your hair.

I always tell my clients to start with a good hair soaking. If you wet your hair well before applying the shampoo, you won't need to use as much soap to work up a lather. Then pour a small amount of diluted shampoo into the palm of your hand—not directly on your head. Rub your hands together and then smooth the shampoo over your hair using the palms of your hands. Gently work up a lather by massaging the head using the fingertips (but not fingernails—that can scratch the scalp) to knead the scalp and then drawing your fingers through your hair to the ends. Don't scrub or rub.

When you rinse, rinse well. I can't overemphasize that point. Shampoo left on the scalp can be very irritating. So after you think you've rinsed your hair completely, rinse again!

If you shampoo your hair every day, as I believe you should, you'll only need one lathering. If you don't, then of course you'll need two.

In any case, after it's completely clean and rinsed, apply a small amount of conditioner or cream rinse—working it gently through your hair with your fingers. Remember, keep it on the hair, not the scalp. Then rinse again. *Completely.*

Now for drying. The worst thing you can do is rub your hair dry with a towel. Just pat it dry and use a very wide-toothed comb to ease out the tangles. This brings to mind another old wives' tale which says that blow drying is bad for the hair. Blowing the hair from wet to damp does absolutely no damage at all. It's going from damp to dry that the potential damage is done. But even that's okay so long as you stop as soon as it's dry. If you keep the dryer on for another 10 extra seconds or so, that's when the trouble comes in. Temperature is another thing. Use the lowest possible warm setting, or even cool. It may take you longer to dry your hair this way—but it's worth it to the health of your hair.

Oily vs. Dry Hair

Question: Can you offer some specific washing instructions for oily hair?

Philip Kingsley: First of all, never use a shampoo formulated for oily hair. They're almost always too harsh. Rather, use a normal mild shampoo. Also, it's a good idea to give extra-special attention to your scalp. You probably won't need a conditioner or cream rinse, but if you do, just apply it to the ends. Then after you're all done with your washing routine, dab a mild astringent to the scalp, using a cotton ball. I recommend a 50 percent dilution of witch hazel and distilled water with just a dash of fresh lemon juice.

Question: What do you recommend for dry hair?

Philip Kingsley: Shampoos formulated for dry hair are generally okay. And always use a conditioner or cream rinse afterwards. You may also want to give yourself a hot oil treatment once a week. Use a light vegetable oil—corn, sunflower, almond or olive, if your hair is very dry—warm it to lukewarm, then apply to your hair using the palm of your hand. Completely coat the hair shaft, and in this case, massage it into the scalp. Then cover your hair with a plastic bag and let it sit—preferably overnight. In the morning wash out the oil completely.

Question: How would you treat hair that may be a different condition at the roots than at the ends?

Philip Kingsley: Some people say they have dry scalp and oily hair. That's an impossibility. But as I said before it is possible to have an oily scalp with dry hair especially when there is a heavy accumulation of dandruff on the scalp. The key here is to keep the scalp immaculately clean using the kind of astringent I suggested for oily hair, and the ends well conditioned with a good conditioner.

Question: Is there a hairstyle that's somehow easier on your hair?

Philip Kingsley: Definitely one that doesn't require a lot of fuss. Hair that needs to be styled, set, hotcombed, teased and otherwise abused is bound to look pretty miserable in spite of your efforts. And sleeping on rollers... that's one of the worst things you can do! They tug on the hair and can eventually damage the hair follicle, causing hair loss. Incidentally, ponytails and "corn row" braids which are now very much in vogue cause similar damage.

I say, the prettiest heads of hair are those that look natural and healthy. What I suggest to my clients is that they determine what type of hair they have, be it naturally straight or curly or whatever, and choose a cut that makes the most of it—something that looks good with a minimum of styling trouble. If your cut falls into place with simple air drying, so much the better.

Your Health and Your Hair

Question: In what ways does your hair reflect your overall health?
Philip Kingsley: In practically every way. If you're not eating properly, or exercising regularly, or if you've been under a great deal of stress, the effects are bound to show up in your hair. I always know when my clients who have a tendency toward dandruff are under especial stress because their dandruff acts up. Changes in your hair condition, or even hair loss, can be a symptom of a much deeper underlying problem like anemia, thyroid or gynecological problem. The kinds of food you eat and medication you take are also reflected in your hair.

Question: You mentioned diet. What is the optimum diet for healthy hair?
Philip Kingsley: The same as the optimum diet for a healthy body. Things like excessive animal fat, excessive salt and excessive sugar are terrible for your health and terrible for your hair. On the other hand, plenty of fruits, plenty of fresh vegetables, plenty of whole grains, plenty of salads, plenty of water (which, incidentally, people don't drink nearly enough of—I recommend that my clients drink eight glasses a day), plus lean fish and poultry are great for your hair and health.

Question: Can you recommend vitamin supplements that are good for your hair?
Philip Kingsley: Oh, yes. I think the B vitamins are extremely important—so I always suggest that my clients take brewer's yeast every day. If they have dry hair I also recommend vitamin E and cod-liver oil tablets. And for a woman who might be suffering from anemia, I tell her to take iron in the form of defatted liver tablets, plus a good iron supplement.

Question: How does exercise benefit the health of the hair?
Philip Kingsley: Exercise is very good because it helps with our circulation. It's also very relaxing.

HAIR LOSS

"The incidence of hair loss in women is increasing at a rate so rapid that it is startling to the doctor as well as the patient," Irwin I. Lubowe, M.D., a New York City dermatologist wrote in 1971 (*Soap, Perfume and Cosmetics,* June, 1971). And there's every reason to believe that the trend continues today. Philip Kingsley, a trained trichologist (a British specialist in scalp and hair science) and author of *The Complete Hair Book* (Grosset & Dunlap, 1979), recently reported that his London and New York hair clinics are treating 25 percent more women for hair loss and thinning than ever before.

Why?

Both cite anxiety and tension as an important—if not *the* most important—influencing factor and suggest that women's advances in the working world may be responsible for their increasing problem with hair recession. "Career women experience more stress," says

Philip Kingsley. "And stress can cause hair and scalp disorders such as dandruff, oiliness, even hair fall." His advice: take it easy!

If you're in a career situation or personal situation that causes a lot of stress, make time for relaxation. A regular exercise routine is a must for relieving tension and also improving circulation. Massage (the whole-body kind) is also a wonderful way to unwind. A good masseuse can knead away knots of tension across your neck and shoulders, which may be impeding proper circulation to the head. Also, says the hair specialist, eat well (low-fat, low-sugar and low-salt foods) and get plenty of sleep (see Hair Care).

Whatever you do, don't panic. Panic over hair loss can create yet more stress, says Philip Kingsley, and contribute to additional hair and scalp problems. Remember, too, everyone loses from 40 to 70 hairs a day. Perhaps your loss is perfectly normal.

Albert Kligman, M.D., Ph.D., professor of dermatology at the University of Pennsylvania Medical School, agrees to a certain extent that stress can cause hair loss, but "not just any old stress," he says. "It's got to be very bad—like going through a divorce, or the trauma of childbirth and new motherhood."

Speaking of motherhood, Dr. Kligman was one of the first to explain exactly why some women tend to lose a lot of hair just after the birth of a child. "Each hair has its own life cycle. It grows for a number of years, then it falls out and the follicle rests for a few months. Somehow or other, pregnancy resets that arrangement. Lots of hair follicles go into a resting phase at one time, usually just after you deliver. What happens is all these hairs fall out at the same time and you think you're going bald.

But you're not. It's just the synchronization of 100,000 hairs."

Of course, not all hair fall is related to pregnancy or stress. Sometimes a hormone imbalance is at fault. And yes, male pattern baldness can affect women, but not nearly to the extent that it does men.

Good Nutrition for Healthy Hair

Low iron is by far a more common cause of hair loss in young women, says Dr. Lubowe. So, eat more liver or take iron tablets and folate, which is also very important to healthy hair (see Anemia).

Another mineral, zinc, may help as well. New evidence suggests that premature loss of hair and perhaps even balding may be linked to a shortage of this mineral. "Animals fed zinc showed a six-to-one difference in hair growth when compared with zinc-deficient animals," Jeng M. Hsu, D.V.M., Ph.D., told us. Dr. Hsu, who is chief of biochemistry research projects at the Veterans Administration Center in Bay Pines, Florida, also found changes in the hair protein structure when zinc was withheld from the animals. But most important, he noted, was the "drastic quantitative reduction of the growth of hair" when zinc was deficient in the diet.

Crash diets can make you lose more than weight. Your hair can go, too. Even when accompanied by vitamin and mineral supplements, a severe diet can trigger severe hair loss. Although generally temporary, it's obviously no way to treat your crowning glory.

As a matter of fact, poor treatment is at the root of many a hair problem.

"Vigorous manipulation of the hair, whether by massaging, shampooing, drying, brushing or combing, tends to break hair mechanically and thus produce characteristic artificial alopecia [baldness]," says Joseph B. Jerome, Ph.D., of the American Medical Association's department of drugs. "The hair roots are still healthy and viable, but there is not much to show for it above the scalp." The key is to be gentle whether shampooing or drying. And avoid scalp massage—neither the scalp nor the hair roots need it.

The way you wear your hair also plays an important role in whether or not you're going to lose it. The ponytail style, tight braiding of the hair, and curling of the hair with rollers, especially the brush rollers, contribute to hair fall-out, warns Dr. Lubowe. Because of the continuous strain and pulling of the hair by these mechanical devices, the shaft is drawn out of the follicle and, in severe cases, the hair loss may be permanent. Usually a change to a more relaxed hairstyle restores the growth of the hair. (Clinical Medicine, March, 1972).

Persistent teasing, bleaching and stripping of the hair may also adversely affect the growth of the hair shaft.

And finally, certain medications can contribute to a hair crisis—most notoriously oral contraceptives (probably for the same reason that pregnancy does, since the synthetic estrogen tends to simulate pregnancy) and certain chemotherapy drugs used to treat cancer.

A. L. Leiby, M.D., a dermatologist in Akron, Ohio, finds that hair loss brought on by the Pill can sometimes be treated effectively with vitamin B_6. The hormones present in oral contraceptives have been associated with a deficiency of this vitamin, which is essential to the health of the hair (Skin and Allergy News, August, 1973).

Similarly, loss of hair is known to occur following the use of methotrexate, an anticancer drug, which has a damaging effect on the metabolism of folate. This B vitamin, so important to the blood, is recommended by Dr. Lubowe as an additional supplement that may favorably affect hair growth.

Also, a simple, natural treatment may stop hair loss in cancer patients undergoing chemotherapy. Peter Boasberg, M.D., a physician from Santa Monica, California, has found that ice applied to the scalp sharply reduces the hair loss in most patients.

According to Dr. Boasberg, "A specially designed ice bonnet, or even a simple ice pack, is placed on the patient's head for 15 minutes before and 30 minutes after an injection of Adriamycin or another anticancer drug. The object is to try to prevent the scalp from receiving an initial rapid, or peak, absorption of the drug.

"Without the ice pack, 90 percent of the patients on Adriamycin lose all their hair. But, if the pack is used, 50 percent can be expected to retain all their hair, and 25 percent can be expected to retain a portion of their hair," he told us. "Occasionally, some patients develop a mild headache, the only discomfort associated with using the ice pack."

The most beneficial aspect of the ice pack treatment is psychological, according to Dr. Boasberg. "Patients feel better when they can face the mirror."

HEADACHES

"Not tonight, dear, I have a headache."

We've all heard that tired old joke about that tired old excuse. What's so maddening is that it's always the woman who's put in the bellyaching (or, more precisely, the headaching) position. And even if you haven't the slightest inclination toward bra-burning feminism, the sexist overtones of that are enough to get you fired up. But before you do, let's just say this: while the joke may be totally unfounded, the idea that women get headaches more than men isn't. In fact, for two of the most infamous types of headaches—migraine and tension—women sufferers outnumber men at least three to one.

Exactly why that is, is difficult to say. But hormones probably have something to do with it. It seems that, for some reason, fluctuations in female hormone levels appear to trigger migraine attacks. For example, many female migraineurs (migraine sufferers) have come to expect the worst just before, during or after their menstrual period or at midcycle during ovulation. Likewise, these often debilitating headaches are rather rare before puberty and after menopause but strike with even greater frequency during the stormy hormonal swings that mark the transitional phase of both.

Pregnancy presents a complex series of hormonal happenings, which also affect migraine—for better or worse. Actually, it's for better *and* worse. What happens is, initially, as hormone levels are changing to meet the demands of the new situation, migraine attacks may increase. However, after the first 12 weeks or so, hormones begin to level off, and during the last uninterrupted six-month stretch some women can expect relative freedom from migraines.

Based on that, one would think that the birth control pill with its even dose of estrogen would ward off headaches. But no, says Robert E. Ryan, Sr., M.D., professor of otolaryngology at St. Louis University School of Medicine and director of the Ryan Headache Center. Migraine headaches as well as headaches related to depression are *more* frequent among oral contraceptive users. In a study he conducted, 40 women were randomly assigned to two test groups. Alternately, each group received oral contraceptives for two months, and nothing for another two months. The women reported *more* headaches during the two months on oral contraceptives (*Headache*, January, 1978).

Again, the reason for that can probably be explained in terms of hormonal fluctuations. According to Dr. Ryan, the women in the above study reported more severe headaches during the last week in each month—when they switched off estrogen. Also, the pills with the higher estrogen content seemed to trigger the worst headache reactions, presumably because coming off them for a week created an even more pronounced hormonal imbalance.

Of course, migraine is such a complicated phenomenon, it's impossible to put all the blame on fluctuating female hormones. It could, as some researchers are now suggesting, involve other substances common to both men and women—namely serotonin—which causes constriction of blood vessels—and prostaglandins—which have the ability to lower blood pressure.

What appears to happen is that, for whatever reason, be it changing levels of estrogen, serotonin, and/or prostaglandins, the blood vessels in the head constrict slightly, then rapidly dilate. Or, they simply dilate without warning. But it is this rapid dilation that creates pressure on the walls of the arteries (which contain sensitive nerves) and causes the pain—often excruciating, disabling pain.

Once an attack like that takes hold, your only hope lies in rest, dark, quiet rooms, cold towels or ice packs on your brow, coffee (the caffeine in which helps to constrict those dilated blood vessels) and probably the most potent pain reliever you can get. In fact, we'd be the last to criticize anyone for taking medication to quickly relieve the agony of this type of intense pain. The only trouble is, many of these potent pain relievers are addictive and some—like propranolol and clonidine—carry terrible risks if you're pregnant. So if your migraines recur frequently—and even if they don't—you're better off doing your bit for prevention. *No* pain, after all, is a far cry better than a deadened one.

Is It a Tension Headache or a Migraine?

But before we get to the hows, it's important and interesting to note that while the term migraine has come to be associated with severe head pain, it isn't always so. In fact, of the estimated 16 million men and women who are predisposed (usually through a family history), some experience only mild pain which is often mistaken for a tension or other type of headache. But there is a clear difference.

According to Seymour Diamond, M.D., adjunct associate professor of neurology at the Chicago Medical School and director of the Diamond Headache Clinic in Chicago, there are specific characteristics of a migraine which set it apart from all other headaches. For one thing, it is always one-sided, creating pain in one or the other half of the head. Second, it does not occur on a daily basis. Third, it is usually accompanied by one or all of the following symptoms: nausea, blurred vision, or supersensitivity to light and noise.

By comparison, the tension headache feels more like a tightened band around the forehead rather than a pounding above one eye. It can recur daily but it never triggers vomiting or visual problems. And while this kind of head throb might be intensified by excessive noise, chances are the sound of a leaky faucet won't drive you as wild as it would if you had a migraine.

The pain mechanism is different for both as well. As we mentioned, migraines occur because of sudden changes in blood vessels and as such are considered vascular headaches. Tension headaches are the result of a contraction of the scalp or neck muscles and are appropriately referred to as muscle-contraction headaches. However, it's not always that easy to separate them since there is often an overlap between muscle and blood vessel contributions to a given headache. Besides that, both are known to be triggered by stress.

Stress is a very elusive type of thing. Most of us relate it to anxiety. But stress can come from lack of sleep, a change in your usual routine such as staying out late then sleeping till noon, or overwork. For a tension headache, then, the reference is to tension in the muscles rather than to nervous tension per se.

FIFTEEN UNSUSPECTED CAUSES OF HEADACHES

1. The Caffeine-Withdrawal Headache is the one coffee drinkers get when they pass up their brew for 18 hours or more. Caffeine constricts blood vessels. So when the daily dose disappears, the blood vessels in the head dilate a bit too far and cause pain.

2. The Premenstrual Headache can accompany cramps and other premenstrual discomfort. Some suggest that it may be a result of water retention within the brain tissues. And if so, relief may be speeded along with vitamin B$_6$ (see Cramps and Other Premenstrual Miseries).

3. The Chinese-Restaurant-Syndrome Headache usually takes the form of pressure or throbbing over the temples and a bandlike sensation around the forehead. The culprit: monosodium glutamate (MSG), a flavor enhancer which is also used in many processed foods such as canned soups.

4. The Hot Dog Headache is also caused by a food additive. This time, it's the sodium nitrate and nitrite processors added to hot dogs and other meats such as ham, bacon, lunchmeats and sausage.

5. The Overexertion Headache occurs with strenuous exercise. What happens is, the smaller blood vessels don't expand fast enough to accommodate the stepped-up blood flow in the larger ones. At the same time, pressure of backed-up blood builds up in the large arteries, painfully stretching the walls.

6. The Salt Headache is caused by—you guessed it—eating too much salt. John B. Brainard, M.D., from St. Paul, Minnesota, tried restricting the salt intake of a group of 12 people who regularly suffered headaches. They were told to avoid all salted snack foods such as pretzels, nuts and potato chips. Only two of the people reported no reduction in their frequency of headaches. And in three people, headaches disappeared entirely (*Minnesota Medicine*, April, 1976).

7. The Hunger Headache might be your problem if pain strikes between meals, just before meals, or when you've skipped a meal entirely. The cause is low blood sugar, or hypoglycemia, which can usually be avoided by making sure you get adequate amounts of protein and complex carbohydrates throughout the day and by eating smaller, more frequent meals.

8. The Noxious Fumes Headache gets you while riding home in bumper-to-bumper rush-hour traffic. Breathing unhealthy concentrations of carbon monoxide, a main ingredient of automobile and truck exhausts, can give you a headache—or kill you if the concentration is high enough and the exposure long enough. Improperly adjusted coal, oil or gas stoves and heaters can also give off carbon monoxide fumes.

9. The Change-of-Habit Headache gets you if, for example, you've gotten to bed in the wee hours of the morn and slept till noon.

10. The Turtle Headache comes after a fitful night's sleep that's left you crouched with your head beneath the covers. Actually, the headache is caused by a buildup of carbon dioxide and a reduction in the oxygen supply. The same thing can happen when you're trapped in a stuffy smoke-filled room or automobile.

11. The Bruxism Headache is one that is caused by a nervous grinding or clenching of teeth in the absence of TMJ syndrome. According to William R. Cinotti, D.D.S., and Arthur Grieder, D.D.S., of the College of Medicine and Dentistry of New Jersey, four out of five bruxists are women. inner conflicts are usually the cause, they say, and the problem can best be resolved if the bruxist learns to relax and reduce stress (*Dental Survey*, February, 1976).

12. The TMJ-Syndrome Headache refers to a headache related to abnormalities of the temporomandibular joints (TMJ, for short), which are often caused by malocclusion, or improper meeting, of the upper and lower teeth. In many people one or both TMJs have been forced out of place, according to Harold Gelb, D.M.D., a New York City dentist who has spent most of his career studying this joint and its effects on muscles, bones, nerves and blood vessels of the face, head, neck and shoulders. Irregularities of the TMJ often result in the "TMJ syndrome," of which headache is a common symptom. Dr. Gelb says that "90 percent of all headaches are muscle-contraction headaches, and a good portion of those are TMJ-related." Other indicators are persistent jaw clenching, a "clicking" jaw and chronic bruxism (grinding or shuffling the teeth). Such dental problems as frequent cheek or lip biting, inexplicable fracturing of teeth and fillings, and worn teeth can also result.

13. The Sunstroke Headache can strike when you spend too much time in the sun unprotected by clothes, a beach hat or common sense. Your body becomes dehydrated and the fluids around the brain and the spinal column become depleted and the blood vessels rub painfully on surrounding tissue. If slowly replacing the lost body fluids by drinking small amounts of warm water over a two- or three-hour period doesn't relieve the headache, your sunstroke may be more serious. Consult a doctor.

14. The Postural Headache is one in which the pain in your head is actually a pain in your neck that radiates upward—a result of poor posture. When your head is thrust forward for prolonged periods of time—for example, if you work at a typewriter all day or sleep with two hefty pillows under your head at night—the muscles at the top of your spine must work extra hard to keep your head erect. This eventually can send waves of pain up the spine and into the head. Also, according to David A. Zohn, M.D., chief of the department of physical medicine and rehabilitation, National Orthopedic and Rehabilitation Hospital in Arlington, Virginia, similar problems can occur from depression which causes a person to slump. "We stand as we feel," he says. Likewise, he cautions, women with large breasts whose bras do not provide adequate support are particularly susceptible to this type of headache, as are persons with ill-fitting bifocals (*Female Patient*, April, 1979).

15. The Ice Cream Headache results from a sudden cooling of the roof of the mouth and the throat, which overstimulates the nerves there and causes pain.

As for migraines and other vascular headaches, which involve a far more intricate chain of reactions, stress is only one of many factors known to set it off. Certain foods are also known to pull the trigger.

For example, when Edda Hanington, M.D., consultant to two London migraine clinics, questioned 500 migraine sufferers on which foods appeared to precipitate their attacks, the foods cited in order of frequency were: chocolate, cheese and dairy products, citrus fruits, alcoholic drinks, fatty fried food, vegetables (especially onions), tea and coffee, meat (especially pork) and seafood.

You may ask, what's left? Well, probably not very much if you did avoid all of those items. But usually, you don't have to. Migraine attacks are very individualized—which means that just because some people get migraines after eating oranges, it doesn't mean you will. What you've got to do is be very careful about the things you do eat and avoid those which you know from experience are likely to bring on an attack.

For a significant number of persons, however, the most treacherous foods are those that have been aged or fermented. That's because these foods tend to contain tyramine, a chemical that appears to work on the vascular system and can trigger migraines in susceptible persons. Cheese is tops in tyramine content—although the amount of tyramine in cheese varies according to the type of bacteria used in the aging process, the length of time that it's aged, and the details of manufacturing. Even the same brand and type of cheese can vary from one batch to another. But generally speaking, Stilton, cheddar and blue cheeses such as Roquefort are the worst in this regard.

Alcoholic beverages can also have devastating effects for the same reason.

And, as with cheese, beware of those that have been aged for considerable lengths of time such as cognac and expensive red wines.

Tyramine is also found in other foods to a lesser degree. These include avocados, raspberries, plums, oranges and bananas.

Another condition that appears to precipitate migraines is low blood sugar, or hypoglycemia. James D. Dexter, M.D., John Roberts, M.D., and John A. Byer, M.D., all of the University of Missouri–Columbia School of Medicine, tested over a three-year period the effect of diet on the frequency and duration of migraine attacks. They found that among 74 people suffering migraines, 56 were hypoglycemic and 6 were diabetic.

All those people were put on a six-meal, low-carbohydrate, high-protein diet with a daily calorie total ranging from 1,000 to 2,500. The diet did not allow refined sugar. All six diabetic persons showed an improvement greater than 75 percent in their migraine symptoms. Three of them were headache-free. Of the subjects who had hypoglycemia and returned for follow-up, 63 percent showed greater than 75 percent improvement (*Headache*, May, 1978).

But perhaps one of the most universal triggers of migraines is something you may never have questioned in this regard—the sun.

Researchers at the University of California at Davis studied 263 patients to see if the sun was a precipitating factor in headaches. They found that the sun triggered migraine attacks in 30 percent of the patients. "Exposure to sun, therefore, is a more frequent precipitating factor in migraine than diet and hormonal changes, which are more often mentioned and discussed in the literature," the researchers concluded.

Although no reliable data could be obtained regarding the duration of sun exposure or the height of temperature, the patients generally needed to be out for more than 30 minutes to an hour and the sun had to be "bright" (*Headache*, January, 1980).

The thing to remember in all of this is that the causes of a migraine tend to be cumulative. In other words, an attack is more likely to strike when more than one factor is present. That explains why a wine and cheese party doesn't trigger an attack on one day but half a cheese sandwich does on another—perhaps when you've been under some stress. Or why it is possible to prevent an attack during headache-prone periods of your menstrual cycle by steering clear of the other triggering factors. That is, be sure to get plenty of sleep, don't overwork, keep your blood sugar level consistent, shun all tyramine-containing foods, and stay out of the sun.

Preventing Headaches with Biofeedback

If all this sounds a little bit too iffy for you, another avenue of headache prevention involves biofeedback. According to Dr. Diamond, biofeedback reduced the frequency of migraines in 70 to 80 percent of the patients he so treated. The most receptive patient, he told us, tends to be a female under 30 years of age who is not hooked on pain medication or saddled with depression.

Biofeedback is a very interesting type of therapy which involves the conscious alteration of seemingly unconscious body functions, with the help of a machine that measures these changes and gives you feedback as to when they are occurring.

In the case of migraines, the biofeedback technique is based on the fact that the majority of sufferers also tend to have cold hands. But when they are taught to consciously warm their hands, they are able to redirect blood flow away from the sensitive blood vessels of the head and avoid the onset of a headache.

Skeptical? Well, admittedly, this technique does sound a little unbelievable at first. But not when you consider that you've probably done this same kind of thing many times before. That's right, you have. Have you ever dreaded or worried about something so much that you broke out into a cold sweat or felt sick to your stomach? You might even have vomited. Whatever it was you were dreading or worrying about hadn't actually happened. But you so convinced yourself that it had that your body reacted as if the act were actually committed. Well, if you can do that, you can convince your hand that it's hot and, in doing so, prevent a migraine from happening.

Usually, it takes anywhere from 4 to 16 training sessions before a person is able to warm her hands at will. But after the initial program you're on your own and the treatment becomes self-help.

According to Steven L. Fahrion, Ph.D., of the Menninger Foundation's Biofeedback and Psychophysiology Center in Topeka, Kansas, the training sessions go something like this: first, the trainer will attach a kind of sensing device to your hand. This sensor is capable of recording small changes in your skin temperature and registering changes on a meter in front of you. A baseline reading is taken. Next you are given instructions on how to go about raising the temperature in your hands. You can begin by saying several times to yourself, "My hands are heavy and warm." This helps to keep the purpose of the exercise in your mind. However, because the part of the brain that controls these processes doesn't understand language, it is important to translate this phrase into an image. "If you can actually imagine what it would feel like if your hands did feel heavy or if they did feel warm, that helps to bring on the changes. Or use a visual image: imagine you are lying out on the beach in the sun or that you're holding your hands over a campfire" (*Mayo Clinic Proceedings*, December, 1977).

Your attitude is most important as you do this. For one thing, if you try too hard—getting yourself all uptight about wanting it to happen—chances are it won't. You have to want to create the change but not worry one way or the other about the results. Also you've got to trust your body to do what you're asking it to do.

The biofeedback part of this therapy is to let you know when your body is reacting to the visualization exercises. In time, with repeated sessions, you will be able to know immediately what it takes to evoke the desired body response. And you may even be able to predict when the temperature change will occur even before the change registers on the metering device.

Then, when you get the feeling that a headache is coming on (some migraine sufferers see flashes of light or suffer momentary loss of vision just before an attack, others get a "funny feeling" that something's going to happen) you can immediately bring to mind those images that are capable of warming your hands and thereby avert the attack.

A variation of this type of biofeedback approach can also be used in cases where migraine and tension headaches occur simultaneously, or where tension headache is the major problem. That is, sensors are attached to the forehead to measure muscle tension and the patient is told to concentrate on relaxing images to ease muscle contractions. However, most people feel that a tension headache is better prevented by attacking the uptight feeling that tends to bring on this type of headache through tension-releasing mind exercises, back and neck massage, and general lifestyle counseling to see if certain sources of stress can be eliminated (for more on relaxation see Anxiety).

Exercise Helps Prevent Headaches

A regular program of physical exercise can also benefit people with both tension and migraine headaches. Obviously, in the case of the tension headache, exercise provides an outlet for pent-up anxiety and frustrations while it works out tight, knotted muscles. In the case of migraines, however, the mechanism isn't that easy to define.

Otto Appenzeller, M.D., Ph.D., of the neurology department and headache clinic at the University of New Mexico School of Medicine in Albuquerque, speculates that endurance training such as running, cycling and swimming may spur the body to produce an important enzyme. That enzyme might prevent blood vessels in the brain from expanding and painfully pressuring nerves.

He's seen several patients find relief by jogging seven to nine miles daily at a speed of seven to nine minutes per mile. "I had 18 patients who suffered from migraines. After reaching this level of activity they are headache-free and medicine-free," he told us.

Dr. Appenzeller, who is a frequent marathon runner himself, believes such a program would be good for just about anyone whose health permits it. You'll lose weight, feel better and, he predicts, "you will be cured of all headaches."

Our town has at least five or six of them. And there are thousands more all across the United States. Health clubs. Figure salons. Trim and fitness centers. Call them what you like. They're popping up all over the place and providing patrons with fun, fitness and food withdrawal counseling for the weight-conscious. Many also offer additional relaxation treats—like sauna, hot tub and massage treatments—which not only help to put all that perspiration into perspective, but also make for a wonderful rejuvenating retreat on a dull, frigid day in December. As a matter of fact, the whole concept of an indoor gymnasium for health-minded adults makes exceptional good sense in the cold and rainy months when motivation toward outdoor court and track activities is hard to come by.

But you don't need a spa or health club to feel good—even then. There's practically nothing that they offer which you couldn't do on your own. Yet, very often, you'd have to go some to experience such a wide variety of fitness modes assembled together under one roof (health clubs are often affiliated with tennis or racketball clubs, swimming pools and indoor tracks). Many women also find the camaraderie of fellow fitness buffs provides the much-needed support and encouragement it takes to slim down or shape up—and stay that way. And if you're the kind of woman who prefers structured group exercise classes to solitary sessions at home—or who has trouble incorporating healthful exercise and relaxation activities into your hectic home life—getting out of the house to one of these fitness centers could be your best bet.

Just remember, what you get out of a health club membership is directly proportional to what you put in. That, and of course, how well the club's offerings meet your needs.

Within recent years health clubs have been hit hard with bad publicity. The main gripe is not so much with their equipment or organization as with their sales techniques. We've heard of women hounded to join after just one sneak preview. What's worse, many health club membership contracts carry more fine print and "catches" than an apartment lease. And they're even harder to break. If you're not careful you could be roped in for two years—which isn't altogether bad, unless, of course, the club goes bankrupt and you're left holding the gym bag with a nonrefundable membership card in it.

Buyer beware, warns Charles T. Kuntzleman, Ph.D., national YMCA fitness consultant, and the editors of *Consumer Guide* in their book *Rating the Exercises* (William Morrow, 1978). "Under no circumstances should you feel badgered, embarrassed, belittled, threatened, detained or mocked. If you feel any excessive amount of pressure, leave or at least ask for more time. If you are told this is a once-in-a-lifetime deal or that the rates go up tomorrow, etc., forget it..." they write. "Read the contract carefully. If you want more time, take it. If you feel you should read it at home or want to discuss it with [someone], do so. If the health club won't permit you to take the contract home, steer clear of that organization. Make sure the contract commits you to no more than two years; one year is preferable. All contracts should provide for a minimum three-day cooling-off period; look for a use of facility clause permitting you to use the club during those three days."

How to Find the Right Health Club

A health club membership is an investment. To protect yourself, shop around and get all the details before committing yourself to one club. We've found that the best place to start is probably at your local YWCA. Believe it or not, some of the Y health clubs are every bit as elaborate—and, in many cases, a good bit more dependable—than the privately owned clubs.

The Y is such a long-standing institution that there's probably a one-in-a-billion chance of it going under. And it's just about the only place you can ease into a fitness program without signing on for a year or two at a time. The other advantage of the Y is that it usually has a wide variety of activities. You can test out the jogging track, the racketball courts, the yoga classes, plus all the exercise equipment, sauna, steam bath and so forth, and decide for yourself where your true interests lie. Then, if you like what they offer at the Y, you can sign on for a yearly membership. Or if the facilities you prefer are too crowded or minimal for your enjoyment, you might want to check out other clubs in your area which may specialize in that activity.

Whatever the case, Robert H. Pike, M.D., a former U.S. Olympic team physician in Fort Collins, Colorado, suggests doing a little groundwork before a visit—to any club. "See if the place is reputable and has good relations with its

clients," he says. "Ask around and see if there have been a lot of dropouts."

When you go to visit a club, "sit down and talk with the manager and interview some of the instructors," says Dr. Pike. "Are they cordial? Do they speak authoritatively and sound like they know what they're talking about? Then tour the facilities and see what they have to offer for the price."

The best time to tour a health club facility is the hour when you would ordinarily use it. If you plan to substitute yoga and a sauna for a sandwich at lunch, check out the facilities at noon-time. If Saturday mornings are your favorite exercise time slot, don't jump into a membership commitment based on a Friday night preview. You may discover every woman in town has the same schedule and that the exercise floor is so crowded you can't turn around without tripping over someone else's mat.

And while you're checking out the facilities, chat with the members to see if they have any complaints or misgivings. A truly satisfied customer is a health club's best sales pitch.

The Problems with Some Health Clubs

Ruth Lindsey, Ph.D., professor of health, physical education and recreation at California State University at Long Beach, conducted a survey of health clubs in 1971 and found that some of them were not very reputable back then. A major concern of hers is the caliber of instructors.

Most of the instructors who worked at them had no background in physical education or physical therapy, she told us. "They were mostly hired for their looks and were given on-the-job training which sometimes lasted only a few weeks." Instructors who were not aware of the different muscle groups sometimes misinformed the club patrons about exercise. "In many cases," says Dr. Lindsey, "the exercise wasn't doing what the employees said it was doing."

She stresses that "anyone who says you can get in shape effortlessly is not telling you the truth. There is no way you can do it without effort." Dr. Lindsey found a number of clubs offering exercise programs that were incapable of bringing about *any* change in weight or fitness.

"There was a lot of passive equipment around," she told us. Passive equipment works on the individual instead of the other way around and includes such items as roller machines and belt vibrators.

A vibrating machine with a belt to place around your backside is "supposed to reduce your hips by shaking them and is based on an erroneous principle called spot reduction," according to Gabe Mirkin, M.D., in *The Sportsmedicine Book* (Little, Brown, 1978). "All it does is shake up your bladder and give you a headache. It doesn't make any difference what part of your body you exercise. The only way to rid yourself of fat is to burn more calories than you take in. Then your fat will disappear from the places it is stored."

The point we're trying to get across here is that just because a gym has all the latest equipment, that doesn't mean it's the best place for you. It could be just the opposite. The health clubs with the most to give are very often those with more mats but fewer contraptions cluttering up the exercise floor.

Of course, there are exercise aids that are completely legitimate—the stationary bicycle or Universal Gym (a series of pulleys and weights), for example. But

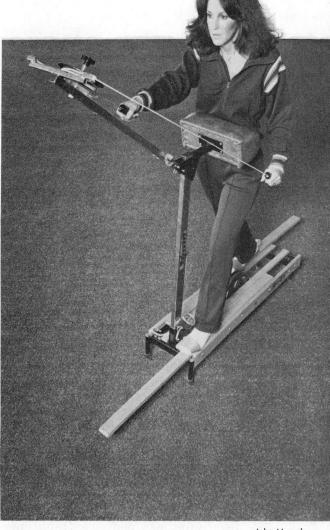

John Hamel

The best type of gym equipment demands physical effort on your part. Take your pick from such equipment as the Universal Gym, stationary bike and the Nordic Trac (above) which simulates cross-country skiing. Beware of "passive" equipment such as roller machines and belt vibrators. Anything that "does the work for you" can't do a good thing for your body.

by far the best way to get in shape is by putting your body through the paces—the right paces. And by that we mean serious exercise workouts which stress flexibility, cardiovascular conditioning, strength and endurance.

Unfortunately, when Dr. Lindsey did observe active exercises in progress at the clubs, "very frequently the exercises were too mild to bring about much of a change. The instructors did not tax the muscles enough," she explains. She also found club members herded through the same exercise program, regardless of their individual needs.

"Some of the classes were doing exercises that were potentially harmful. Double leg raisings can hurt the back and lead to abdominal hernias," she continues. "Doing sit-ups with straight legs is not a good practice for everyone, either."

The authors of the book *Rating the Exercises* recommend finding a club that emphasizes cardiovascular fitness.

"The 'best' [exercise] is cardiovascular exercise, the kind that gets your heart and lungs working harder. It can be any of many activities that are characterized by repeatedly and vigorously moving the major muscles of your body for an extended period of time," they write. "The most important muscle of one's body is the heart, and a good fitness program must recognize this fact. Cardiovascular exercise cannot be neglected."

Dr. Lindsey agrees that a strong heart is a matter of life and death. Forget all those crazy gimmicks. "You should go someplace that offers cardiovascular endurance exercise like jogging, swimming laps and pedaling stationary bicycles.

"You have to work your heart rate up to 80 percent of maximum for 20 to 30 minutes at a time to get any cardiovascu-

lar benefits. An older person would need to work out at 70 percent of maximum, which is roughly 120 beats a minute," she says. Many clubs now offer special aerobic or dancercise classes for this purpose.

Can Women Profit from Weight Training?

If a club keeps good records and measures your thighs, arms, waist, and bust, weight training and body building also can be a valuable part of an exercise program (yes, even for a woman!) says Dr. Pike. The workouts would consist of strengthening and endurance exercises on resistance exercise equipment using ropes and pulleys. And every woman could certainly do with more strength and endurance whether she's struggling to open a jar of beans or running to catch a plane—suitcase in hand.

"I certainly think weight training is essential and a good thing, but don't carry it to extremes," he adds. "It is dangerous to get into a weight training program unless the instructor knows what he's doing. You must start out with low weights and learn how to lift. You can jimmy your back or break an ankle or wrist if you don't do it right."

A weight training program can make you feel and look good, says Dr. Pike. "If your muscles are toned, they will work better and you will function better as a result."

For anyone leading a sedentary life at 35 or anyone over 40 years old, Dr. Pike advises a stress EKG (an electrocardiograph test while on a treadmill) before participating in any strenuous exercise program.

"It's just common sense," he told us. "Probably 90 percent of the health clubs don't require one, but I say let your doctor decide whether an EKG should be done or not. Anyone in my practice above a certain age has the EKG, and that goes as well for people who want to jog and play tennis. It's a valuable preventive tool."

If you have any chronic health problem you should get a physician's approval before using a sauna, steam bath or whirlpool (see also Saunas and Other Hot Baths). When you do use them, go by the rules and don't overdo it.

Also, as a final word before you join, ask if the club belongs to the Association of Physical Fitness Centers. The group is a trade association for full-service health spas and is dedicated to upgrading the industry.

Dr. Lindsey says if you do join a health club, you should not expect any quicker results when it comes to whittling away the pounds and inches. If you lose a pound a week, you're making good progress, she says. "You have to ask yourself, 'What am I going to look like a year from now?' instead of two weeks from now."

HEART DISEASE

Most of us think of heart disease as a man's problem. But today, more and more women are finding that it's suddenly become their problem, too. Speculations on why have largely headed in the same direction. Today's woman is often doing a man's job. She's up against the kind of corporate competition only a man would have known. It only stands to reason that in the process of winning the war for equality, we've lost our natural immunity to heart disease. Or at least, you'd think that has *something* to do with it. But an epidemiologist from the National Heart, Lung, and Blood Institute in Bethesda, Maryland, says guess again.

After eight years of comparing statistics on 465 working women, 466 housewives and 725 men, Suzanne G. Haynes, Ph.D., concludes that the rate of coronary heart disease for working women is not significantly different from that for housewives under 65 years of age.

That's not to say that a hard-driving, achievement-oriented "Type A" personality won't put you at higher risk of heart disease. It will: this kind of self-imposed stress is known to increase blood cholesterol and the blood's clotting tendency as well as raise blood pressure. But it does show that if you are a compulsive person—who can't stand waiting in line or sitting still; who thinks that in order to have something done right you have to do it yourself; or who's fanatical about being on time—it doesn't matter where you are from nine to five weekdays. Your personality, not your job, puts you at risk. Careers don't create competitive personalities. If you're a "Type A," you're just as likely to be demanding and impatient with your children at home as you are with an employee at the office.

So why, then, has heart disease grown so radically among women in recent years?

One reason is that we're living longer than we ever did before. And a woman's risk of heart disease increases as she ages, most notably after menopause. A number of studies confirm this. But one of the most striking reports is a 1978 update of the famous Framingham Study.

That study of residents of Framingham, Massachusetts, began in 1948, when women were enrolled, given a thorough heart examination, and invited to return every two years for new evaluations. By 1978, virtually all of the women in the study had ceased menstruating, and it was possible to look into the connections between heart disease and menopause. The results were striking.

Not one of the 2,873 women in the study had had a heart attack or died of heart disease before menopause. After menopause, heart disease became a common occurrence. For women aged 45 to 54, the incidence of heart disease during or after menopause was *double* the rate before menopause. And the risk was the same whether the menopause occurred naturally or as a result of hysterectomy—and surprisingly, whether the hysterectomy included the removal of the ovaries or not. Also, postmenopausal women on estrogen replacement therapy were twice as likely to develop heart disease (*Annals of Internal Medicine*, August, 1978).

There is a big jump in cholesterol in the blood at menopause, mostly due to a rise in the low-density lipoprotein (LDL) cholesterol, the kind of cholesterol particularly associated with heart disease. Japanese scientists have also found higher levels of triglycerides, another fat implicated in heart disease, in the blood of postmenopausal women (*American Journal of Epidemiology*, April, 1979).

Why Are Young, "Healthy" Women Dying?

But a longer life may be the least of it. Heart problems are now occurring with greater frequency in otherwise healthy *young* women. And this time, the changing trend obviously has nothing to do with the "change of life." Instead, it appears to be a direct result of the growing popularity of cigarette smoking among the under-40-and-female set.

In a study conducted by Hershel Jick, M.D., of the Boston Collaborative Drug Surveillance Program, and associates at the Harvard University School of Public Health, nearly 90 percent of young female heart attack victims were smokers, compared to less than half of a control group of healthy women (*Journal of the American Medical Association*, December 1, 1978).

Another study by Dennis Slone, M.D., of the Drug Epidemiology Unit, Boston University School of Medicine, explores this correlation even further. According to Dr. Slone, the heart attack rate among women smokers is directly proportional to the number of cigarettes they smoke each day. A woman who at day's end is about six cigarettes shy of smoking a full pack is 4½ times more likely to have a heart attack than a woman who never smoked. If, on the other hand, her smoking habit is closer to two packs a day, her risk of heart attack increases by 21 times.

The birth control pill is yet another villain in the conflict between women and heart disease. In Dr. Jick's investigation, 69 percent of the women studied who had heart attacks were on estrogen, compared to only 19 percent of the control group. In addition, Dr. Jick cites a British study by the Royal College of General Practitioners in which 10 of 12 heart attack deaths in women occurred in oral contraceptive users.

A quick glance at the medical literature easily explains why: the Pill, it seems, is capable of creating several problems that are considered serious risk factors for heart disease. First of all, the estrogen in oral contraceptives tends to accelerate the production of certain substances in the blood which cause it to clot more readily. If a clot develops in the heart—or if it first develops in a blood vessel somewhere else but travels to the heart where it lodges and cuts off circulation—a heart attack results. Second, oral contraceptives raise the blood pressure to a certain degree in nearly every woman who uses them. And though the problem isn't severe in all cases, high blood pressure is another significant risk factor in heart disease. Third, according to a study conducted at St. Mary's Hospital in London, cholesterol and triglyceride levels were significantly higher in oral contraceptive users (*Lancet*, May 19, 1979). As you can see, the risks really add up.

Keep Your Risks Down

What's more, women who smoke *and* take the Pill might as well play Russian roulette with their lives. For them, the risk of heart attack can increase by as much as 40 times (*Lancet*, April 7, 1979).

Of course, there are other risk factors involved here. They are hypertension (including a personal history of toxemia in pregnancy), diabetes, angina and a previous heart attack.

Still, the most positive steps you can take to avoid this number one killer of both men and women is to avoid cigarettes and the Pill, especially if you are a young woman.

Also, if you find yourself in constant pursuit of perfection, maybe you need to step back and analyze your priorities. A psychologist who counsels "Type A's" at the University of Montreal says you've got to realize that your compulsion can be nonproductive; you waste energy being angry, impatient, anxious.

Instead, put that "nervous" energy to use doing constructive things—physical things—exercise. Then learn how to delegate authority—even if it's just giving your daughter the responsibility of cleaning her own room—and accept imperfection in everyone, including yourself. Remember, your life may depend on it!

Good nutrition can help you put the odds of developing heart trouble after menopause back in your favor. Lecithin, a substance found in soybeans, eggs and liver, has been effective in lowering triglyceride and LDL cholesterol levels in the blood. Vitamin C has also been used to lower high cholesterol levels. Indeed, Emil Ginter, Ph.D., a noted Czech researcher, believes the recent drop in deaths from heart disease in the United States might be due in part to an increase in the consumption of vitamin C in this country.

And you should probably stick with the vitamin E you're taking for hot flashes (see Hot Flashes) even after you've licked that problem. Vitamin E has been linked in a number of studies to decreased blood coagulation. Vitamin E apparently works by lowering the tendency of platelets, special particles in the blood, to clump together. The clumping together of platelets can lead to a blood clot in arteries feeding the heart or brain, resulting in a heart attack or a stroke.

Magnesium is another nutrient you should be sure you're getting enough of. There is considerable evidence that low levels of magnesium in the heart muscle may contribute to sudden death after a heart attack. Areas of soft drinking water low in magnesium have been found to have higher death rates from heart disease than areas with magnesium-rich hard water.

HEMORRHOIDS

Hemorrhoids wreak havoc with about half of all Americans over 50. And of all these hemorrhoid sufferers, only about half are women. We say "only" because there is a tendency to associate hemorrhoids with women, or at least with pregnant women. But while pregnancy may have a notorious reputation for being a pain in the behind (mind you, we mean that only in the literal sense), it is certainly not the sole contributing factor here. Nor is it necessarily true that a woman who develops hemorrhoids on the delivery table is destined for the operating table in years to come.

But what is a hemorrhoid, anyway?

Well, despite the fact that this one problem is probably kept secretly hidden in more family closets than any other disorder, there's actually nothing mysterious about it. Simply stated, hemorrhoids are varicose veins of the rectal and anal canal. And they seem to be caused by much the same mechanism as those in the legs—that is, by faulty valves in the blood vessels or some other hindrance to proper blood circulation (see Varicose Veins).

In this regard, pregnancy does pose a pretty substantial risk since the swollen uterus restricts blood flow. As a result, much more muscle force than normal is required to recycle blood from the legs and lower torso back to the chest. Coupled with straining during delivery, that can give birth to a very immediate problem or at least leave a young woman with a good headstart toward future trouble.

Primary Cause

The interesting thing about all this, however, is that women of more primitive cultures—who are just as prone to circulatory disorder during pregnancy as we in the "sophisticated" Western world—are bothered by neither varicose veins nor hemorrhoids. The reason, says Denis Burkitt, M.D., a well-known British physician and surgeon, is diet. Hemorrhoids are terribly common among people who eat a highly refined and synthetic diet, and next to nonexistent among folks who favor simpler, more natural fare, explains Dr. Burkitt. His studies have shown that the incidence of hemorrhoids is very high in Western Europe and the United States where white flour and sweets abound, and very low in most African countries, where whole grains and root vegetables are staples. His studies, first reported in the *British Medical Journal* in June, 1972, have even shown that the number of hemorrhoid cases is greater among urban Africans than among their rural neighbors, and that this increase corresponds to the city folks' tendency to adopt the diet of the European colonists who originally built the cities.

The magic ingredient in these "primitive" diets, of course, is fiber. Its presence in food makes for large, soft stools, and they produce less wear and tear—literally—on the anus and rectum. In some ways, then, it doesn't matter what produces hemorrhoids. They usually start out as small problems which are aggravated by things that have nothing to do with their cause. It's the worsening of these aggravating factors and symptoms that we must fight.

Because the large, soft stools of a bulky diet pass easily through the system, they tend not to irritate minor varicose veins in the rectum and anal canal.

African women, as we mentioned, are as susceptible to hemorrhoids during pregnancy as Western women, but the roughage-filled foods they eat keep the swellings small and allow them to be slowly pulled back into place by the natural elasticity of the canal lining. Western women, with their relatively fiberless diet, tend to enlarge their hemorrhoids each time they have bowel movements. The point is that if simple, no-trouble hemorrhoids often become big-trouble hemorrhoids because of hard, small stools, they can be kept down and surgery can be avoided by adopting a stool-softening, high-fiber diet.

The most convenient way to get more fiber into your diet is to make friends with wheat bran. For the best results, get plain, unprocessed, inexpensive bran, not bran cereals. Begin by eating one tablespoon a day mixed into oatmeal, yogurt, soup or even juice. A few days later, raise your intake to two tablespoons a day and see if the results are any better. At some point between one and three tablespoons a day, you should notice the desired effects. Although your stools will be larger, they will be much softer and will pass much more quickly and easily. But remember, in order for bran to do its work, it has to have water to absorb; if you aren't in the habit of drinking much water, add a glass or so a day to your routine.

Other than bran, the kind of fiber you need is also found in whole wheat bread (which contains about four times more total fiber than white bread), whole grain cereals such as oats and corn, as well as potatoes, beans and apples and all other fresh fruits and vegetables.

Natural Remedies for Mild Hemorrhoids

Incidentally, when bleeding becomes a symptom—as it is with early-stage hemorrhoids—doctors often prescribe bulk-type laxatives to soften the stool and chemical suppositories to reduce swelling. A high-fiber diet, however, does better than the foul-tasting laxative, and most suppositories aren't worth what they cost and can be replaced with cold compresses of witch hazel and warm sitz baths. Witch hazel, an astringent, tends to reduce hemorrhoidal swelling as effectively as the more exotic preparations.

Several *Prevention* magazine readers also report relief from hemorrhoids using bioflavonoids and vitamin E. An Illinois woman wrote: "During all three of my pregnancies, I was in such pain with hemorrhoids that I nearly screamed with pain from something so simple as walking. Sitting or lying down became impossible. Then, I sent my husband to the nearest natural foods health center for a bottle of rutin tablets [a bioflavonoid source]. I began taking them immediately (I used three 50-milligram tablets a day). During an extremely restless night I finally must have fallen asleep. When I woke up in the morning the swelling had gone down considerably and by evening, I was able to sit down without wincing. In two days' time the swelling and pain were completely gone!

"Since that time I have been taking three tablets a day and haven't had a twinge of pain. It's been nearly a year and I can't believe it. I firmly believe that this bioflavonoid compound really is a 'miracle' drug for me."

And from a Dearborn, Michigan,

woman we heard: "Although only 22, I have been troubled with hemorrhoids for some time. Nothing relieved the itching and discomfort.

"Since vitamin E has so many uses, I decided to try direct applications (400 international units) three or four times a day. I wasn't really surprised when the itching ceased and the swollen tissue diminished.

"Now whenever I feel the tightness of hemorrhoid distress, I begin the vitamin E applications."

Of course, these natural remedies probably won't do you much good if your problem has already reached the point of severe pain and bleeding. But they're certainly worth a try—even then. Hemorrhoid surgery is tricky business. And should your condition worsen to the point where surgery is a must, we recommend selecting a physician who specializes in the diseases of the rectum and colon and who does a lot of hemorrhoid operations over a general surgeon whose hemorrhoidectomies are few and far between.

HERBS FOR WOMEN

Traditionally, grandmother's bag of home-remedy tricks held a treasury of fragrant herbs. She had peppermint tea to soothe an upset stomach, eucalyptus to clear a stuffy nose, and a terrific camomile concoction to calm a wailing babe better than Brahms' Lullaby.

Today, women are rediscovering the usefulness and versatility of herbs. We're finding, for example, that by cooking creatively with herbs, we can do without, or at least with very little, salt—a rather boring seasoning that puts a tremendous burden on our health. Also, at a time when many of us are rejecting potent drugs for simple ailments and deciding to take responsibility for our health, we are returning more and more to grandma's time-honored herbal recipes. In fact, these age-old herbal remedies can often compete with modern prescriptions for the special health care of a woman's body. No one knows this better than Nan Koehler, a botanist, herbalist, lay midwife and mother of four. Nan and her ob-gyn husband, Donald Solomon, M.D., share a health care practice in Occidental, California. There, her years of training and experience in midwifery and herbalism complement his extensive background in medicine. For the most part the couple finds themselves in complete agreement, preferring natural, nutritional and herbal remedies over drugs and more invasive medical therapies, when at all possible.

We talked with Nan Koehler about the role herbs can play in women's health and have reprinted a portion of the conversation here.

Question: Women have traditionally been the herbalists—the healers with the home remedies. Do you think that there's something about herbs that is more in tune with women's unique sensitivities?

Nan Koehler: Oh, yes, definitely. Women assume responsibility for the health and welfare of the whole family. It starts with food preparation. Traditionally, it is the woman's role to learn to cook. And that's where she first finds out about the usefulness of herbs like basil, rosemary and thyme. But cooking herbs are also medicinal herbs. And one thing soon leads to the other.

Women also have the kind of energy it takes to do gardening—nurturing. I notice this with my children. Even though I offer the same kinds of toys to both my sons and daughters, the girls gravitate toward the toys that show off their nurturing roles—the dolls, the tea-cups. Most of the women I know who are herbalists are also gardeners. It goes together.

Question: In what ways can herbs affect health?

Nan Koehler: Herbs do have medicinal properties. They contain alkaloids and aromatic oils which do have effects on the body.

For example, comfrey leaves and roots contain allantoin, a chemical that stimulates the growth of cells. It has been used since ancient times when it was called "knit-bone" because it helped to heal broken bones and wounds. This has been tested and con- firmed in laboratories.

Herbs are also a good source of minerals. Red raspberry leaf tea is espe- cially high in calcium and magnesium and we recommend it as a daily drink during pregnancy when the body's requirements for these two minerals are greater.

One of the problems of our diet today is that vegetables are often grown in depleted soils, and they don't have the trace minerals that they should. Herbs are concentrated sources for many of the minerals otherwise missing from our diet. That's why I try to include wild greens and fresh herbs in my salads each day—things like dandelion, dock, mulva, miner's lettuce, chickweed. At

first, you may object to the bitterness of some of these plants. But if you take parsley or comfrey leaves, for example, and chop them up very fine and mix them with your leaf lettuce—the ro- maine, or Boston or whatever you're accustomed to—the flavor will be less intense. In time your taste will alter and you'll be able to eat a *whole* salad of wild greens.

Question: Can you recall a specific in- stance where herbs had a dramatic effect on health?

Nan Koehler: When my second son was a year and a half old he got into our bee- hive. He was stung about 25 places on his body. I had read that apple cider vinegar was very good for bee stings— which it is. If you put apple cider vine- gar on the sting as soon as you can, it draws out the poison and there shouldn't be any swelling. So I dabbed the apple cider vinegar over him. It did prevent the swelling but he developed a fever and was very sick nonetheless. I knew if I took him to the doctor, he would give him cortisone and I didn't want him to have that. So before I called our doctor, I looked through my herb books for a home remedy. Over and over I read that basil was good for insect bites. I had basil growing in the garden so I gave him some fresh leaves of basil to eat. Almost immediately his fever went away. The turnaround in his symp- toms was absolutely incredible!

I've since learned that basil is also good to help the liver detoxify poisons. And that's apparently how it helps re- lieve insect bites.

Question: Why is it that some people seem to respond quite readily to the healing properties of herbs while others do not?

Nan Koehler: Oh, there are probably hundreds of reasons. One thing I've noticed is that people who eat a lot of meat protein are less responsive to herbs. It seems that the purer your diet—the less junk food in your diet, the less toxins your body has to deal with—the more dramatically the herbs work on you. I don't know what it is. Maybe it has to do with the kind of person you are—some people may be more psychologically sensitive to herbs.

Another thing I've noticed in helping women birth is that a woman who takes the time to use herbs will almost always have a good outcome with her birth. First of all, it takes a certain amount of care and attention to buy the herbs. Often you have to search far and wide for rare herbs, or you have to harvest them yourself. Then you must figure out what you will do with them and how you'll prepare them. To do all that on a daily basis takes a certain amount of motivation and effort—not like buying a TV dinner. But by doing this every day, the woman reinforces the idea that she's doing everything she can to insure that she will have a healthy baby—a bit of positive thinking.

I've found, too, that women who use herbs also take a lot of care with their diet. It just seems to go hand in hand.

Question: Does the ritual of preparing an herb tea offer some psychological benefit?

Nan Koehler: Oh, yes, it is very soothing, relaxing. In China and Japan they often drink plain hot water. You don't have to have an herb in it. Heating the water, holding the warm cup in your hands and feeling the steam rise up can be tremendously comforting.

Question: How has your knowledge of herbs helped you with your practice of midwifery?

Nan Koehler: I do suggest that the women sip my birthing tea during delivery. It's a wonderfully relaxing and delicious concoction of basil, nutmeg, red raspberry leaf and lavender. The standard birthing tea is a mixture of pennyroyal, cohosh and so forth which causes the uterus to contract. But I've found that once a woman is in active labor, it doesn't matter how hard her uterus is contracting but rather how well she's relaxed that will bring on the birth. The better the woman can relax the quicker the whole process can happen. This tea is sipped between contractions. My husband, who's an obstetrician, kids about the tea. He says it's as effective as Pitocin. It really is a dramatically effective tea.

After birth, I suggest that women drink a lot of comfrey—two to four quarts a day for three to five days. This helps to heal the placenta site so she completely stops bleeding in three to five days instead of dragging on for six weeks. If the woman is instructed to stay in bed and drink the tea she recovers much more quickly.

Classic Herbs for Women

Question: Are there any herbs that you would consider classic herbs for women?

Nan Koehler: Oh, yes. There are many different kinds of plant materials that have in them chemicals that are like our testosterone and estrogen. They're not exactly the same as far as I understand but they are very close and they mimic them enough so that your body reacts as if it were the real thing.

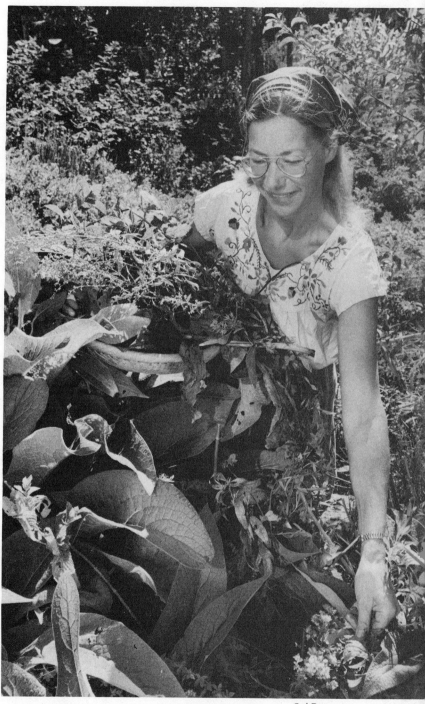

Midwife and herbalist Nan Koehler believes in a type of health care that allows the body the chance to heal itself. Herbs are very much a part of that philosophy, providing gentle assistance for every health need from labor pain to menopausal hot flashes.

Carl Doney

The herbs can affect your pituitary and adrenal glands in such a way that they will regulate the menstrual cycle. We offer a handout in the office that contains an old recipe for a combination of herbs that provide a plant source of hormones plus female regulators, which are herbs used just for women's bodies. The recipe consists of equal parts of sarsaparilla, blessed thistle, licorice root, squaw vine and cramp bark—these are classic herbs for women.

Personally, I think one reason herbs in general are so good is that they are usually high in calcium and magnesium, and a lot of women are lacking in these.

Question: How does this old recipe you mentioned compare to the Lydia Pinkham formula for female complaints? The original formula called for unicorn root, life root, black cohosh, pleurisy root, and fenugreek seed, suspended in alcohol.
Nan Koehler: It's essentially the same. The only difference being that we suggest you drink it in a tea—as opposed to a tincture with alcohol. To me, tea is the more natural way of taking it. The alcohol extract is more potent so you'd take less of it—just a few drops in a glass of water. But many women are dehydrated anyway. And it's good for them to drink a quart or two of tea every day. Very diluted tea. We tell women to sip the tea all day long to keep the level of the herbs up in their body. That should be kept up every day for three whole menstrual cycles.

A lot of women's adrenal glands are overtaxed because of stress and therefore their pituitary isn't functioning properly. The whole endocrine system is such a delicate feedback mechanism that if one gland is out of sync the entire system feels the repercussions. If the pituitary isn't getting the right messages it won't send out the right hormones to the ovaries and your period won't start. That's really a major cause of irregular periods—loss of cyclicity rather than an actual increase or decrease in the amount of hormone.

The best way to deal with this is to give your body a chance to heal itself. Get plenty of rest. And give up meat and other heavy foods for a day or so. We tell women to go on a semifast and drink only the herb tea we just talked about, vegetable broth, and dilute fruit juices.

Question: Are there any types of herbs that may be particularly helpful to a woman at menopause?
Nan Koehler: There definitely are herbs that are used during menopause. They are the same as the herbs used to regulate the cycle. The Lydia Pinkham-type formula will ease the symptoms of menopause. The fenugreek as well as gotu kola, sarsaparilla, licorice root, and wild yam root are natural sources of estrogenlike substances.

Brewing Teas

Question: What's the proper method of preparing herb tea?
Nan Koehler: Use a very small amount of the leaves. Pour boiling water over the leaves either in your cup or preferably in an enamel or ceramic pot with a lid. Always cover the herb tea with a lid because the aromatic oils will evaporate into the air. If you're making an herbal preparation and you can walk into the room and say, "Umm, doesn't that smell nice?" the chemicals are escaping and won't do *you* any good. So always use a lid so that the steam rises and then condenses back into the water.

Also, whenever you make any herbal preparation, be sure that no metal comes in contact with it because the plant alkaloids are very sensitive and are often inactivated by metallic ions. So never use metal pots, metal spoons, or metal tea infusers.

Question: Is there any difference in the preparation of a beverage tea and a medicinal tea?
Nan Koehler: A beverage tea should be a pleasurable experience. So it shouldn't be bitter or dark. It should be just delicately flavored water so that it smells nice and vaguely has the taste of the herb. Most people make the mistake of letting the tea steep way too long. All the tannic acid comes out of the plant cells and it tastes very bitter. That's too much plant material in the tea.

Question: If your intent is to make the most of an herb's healing properties, how would you brew the tea?
Nan Koehler: Generally, it's believed that for healing purposes, you'd want to get as much plant material into the water as is possible. But I think it's more natural to gently coax the body back to good health by preparing a weak beverage brew as just described, and sip it throughout the day. By weak, I mean very weak—½ teaspoon for one to two quarts of water. The idea is that by sipping eight glasses or so of dilute solution you keep a steady concentration of the herbs in your body—which I prefer for healing as opposed to a one-shot, high-potency dose. Again, for best results, you should omit all food from your diet that day and drink *only* the herb tea. If you don't notice an improvement in your condition, then do it again a second day. You should feel better by the third day.

Of course, if you're looking for an instant correctional effect, you can use what's known as a traditional medicinal preparation. To do this, you'd make either a strong infusion or a decoction.

An infusion is made by pouring boiling water over the leaves in a pot and letting it steep until the water turns a deep color. A decoction is made by bringing to a boil the water with the herbs and then simmering it for 5 to 20 minutes or longer. This breaks apart the herb's cell walls to purposely release more chemicals into the water.

Ordinarily you'd make a decoction with roots and bark or berries that are tough. You'd make an infusion with leaves because they are more fragile and break apart easily. Just remember: these are potent herb solutions. Start easy. If you feel sick after drinking a little, discontinue use. It could be that your body's too sensitive for such concentrated doses.

Preparing a Poultice

Question: How would you apply herbs externally to the skin?
Nan Koehler: There are several ways to do that. You can use the herb as is. Just put some crushed fresh herb on the part of the body that's afflicted and wrap it with some type of gauze bandage. Or, you can pulverize the herb with a mortar and pestle and then put it on the area with a wrap. Another way is to put the leaves and a small amount of water in an enameled pot. Bring it to a boil and simmer just long enough to soften the leaves and release the chemicals into the water. Then use the softened leaves with the juice. This is the best way to apply comfrey to your breasts to relieve soreness.

You can also make a lovely massage

oil by simmering the herbs in a vegetable oil such as soy oil or safflower oil. Incidentally, this is a good way to make a garlic oil, which is very healthful for your ears. Crush a clove of garlic in a little bit of vegetable oil—olive oil is the best if you have it. Heat it, not to boiling but just enough so that the garlic cells will open and release the oils into the other oil. Decant that or sieve it off through a piece of cheesecloth into a small container. Just a few drops of this in the ear with an eyedropper will help with ear infections.

Question: Speaking of garlic, certain women's self-help groups suggest inserting a clove of garlic into the vagina to help clear a vaginal infection. Does that sound like a good idea to you?

Nan Koehler: Oh, no. Garlic is a very powerful herb which in concentrated doses can burn mucous membranes. I've talked to women who used garlic suppositories and burned their vaginas. But since garlic does have the wonderful ability to fight infections, I suggest that women crush a clove of garlic in a sitz bath. I think sitz baths are much better than douching. And as long as the garlic is well diluted, there's no chance of harm. This is said to work very well in the treatment of *Trichomonas*.

Question: How can herbs enrich a daily bath?

Nan Koehler: Oh, in so many ways. Here in California, laurel is a common tree. And bay leaves, which come from the laurel tree, are very good for rheumatism and arthritis. The Indians used to put people who had rheumatic attacks into a bay steam bath, and apparently it was a very effective treatment. But I've got to warn you, bay has a very intense aroma much like eucalyptus when you heat or steam it. So you'll only need to use a very small amount.

You can also combine bay with sage. Sage is a muscle relaxant. The bay would be good for sore joints and sinus problems. Camomile and comfrey also make delightful baths.

Take a handful of herbs, toss them into an enameled pot with some water and simmer it for 5 to 10 minutes till it's pretty potent. Decant it or strain it off into the bathtub and dilute it with the bath water. Then hop in and relax. That's really very soothing.

Question: What kind of precautions, if any, should we take with herbs? We've read, for example, that pennyroyal can be harmful—even deadly—when taken internally.

Nan Koehler: All of the herbs I've recommended are perfectly safe when used properly. What happens, though, is that some people think they can make a good thing better by substituting an essential oil for the whole herb. I must caution that while herbs contain essential oils, any concentrated form of these oils can be extremely irritating. When I first became interested in herbs, I decided to try out some essential oils. I put just a few drops of essential oil of cinnamon in my bathtub and my skin got violently red. I didn't realize that these oils can burn you. But they do. Essential oil of peppermint or pennyroyal will do the same thing. And, of course, you can die from taking these oils internally.

AN HERBALIST'S GUIDE TO Herbs for Women

The information in this chart supplied by Nan Koehler should be considered informative, not prescriptive. Always see your doctor when making important decisions concerning your health.

NAN'S NOTE ON PREPARATION:

Herbs can be used individually or together according to taste, she says. Unless otherwise specified, make a very weak brew (1–2 teaspoons in 1–2 quarts water) and sip throughout the day (see text).

Menstruation

To soothe nerves

Clover

Camomile

Valerian root

A general tonic

Mugwort

Do not take in excess.

To promote menstrual flow

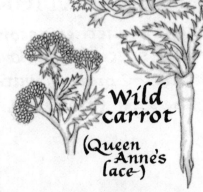

Parsley

Wild carrot
(Queen Anne's lace)

Parsley as a tea helps to relieve cramps. May use directly in vagina. Insert a couple of sprigs with your hand far enough into the vagina so that the stems do not bother you.
Do not use with kidney inflammation.

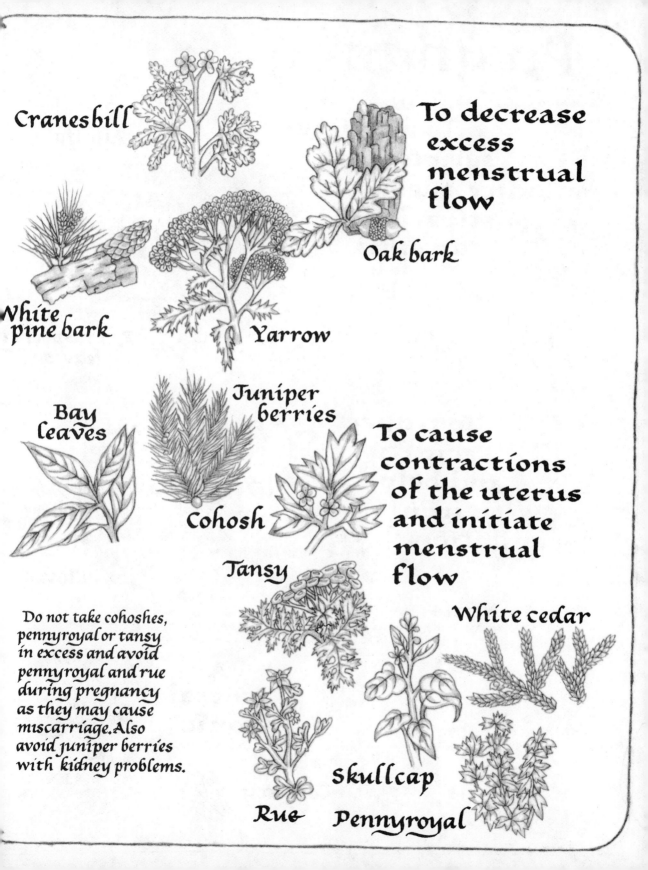

Cranesbill

To decrease excess menstrual flow

Oak bark

White pine bark

Yarrow

Juniper berries

Bay leaves

To cause contractions of the uterus and initiate menstrual flow

Cohosh

White cedar

Tansy

Do not take cohoshes, pennyroyal or tansy in excess and avoid pennyroyal and rue during pregnancy as they may cause miscarriage. Also avoid juniper berries with kidney problems.

Skullcap

Rue

Pennyroyal

Pregnancy

To alleviate symptoms of jaundice, anemia, constipation & toxemia

Alfalfa

Red raspberry leaves

To reduce acidity and help with iron assimilation

Borage

Nettle

Clover

A general tonic

Comfrey

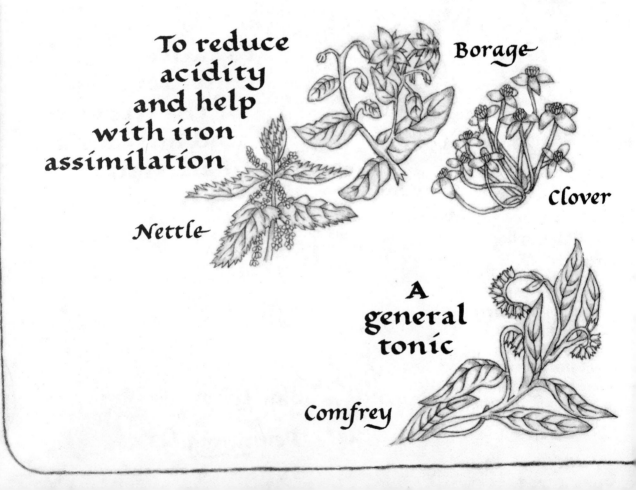

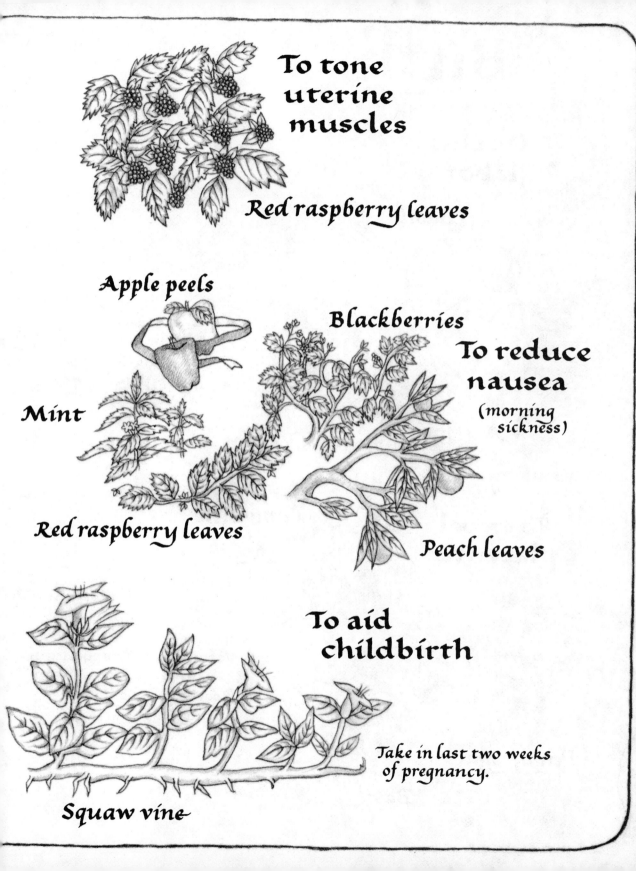

To tone
uterine
muscles

Red raspberry leaves

Apple peels

Blackberries

To reduce
nausea
(morning
sickness)

Mint

Red raspberry leaves

Peach leaves

To aid
childbirth

Take in last two weeks
of pregnancy.

Squaw vine

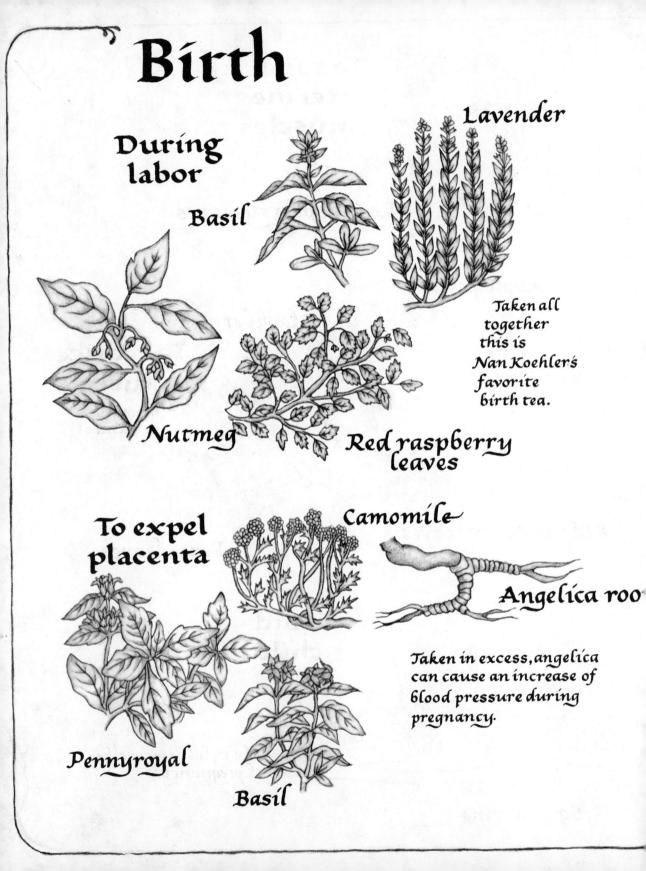

Birth

During labor

Basil

Lavender

Nutmeg

Red raspberry leaves

Taken all together this is Nan Koehler's favorite birth tea.

To expel placenta

Camomile

Angelica root

Taken in excess, angelica can cause an increase of blood pressure during pregnancy.

Pennyroyal

Basil

After birth

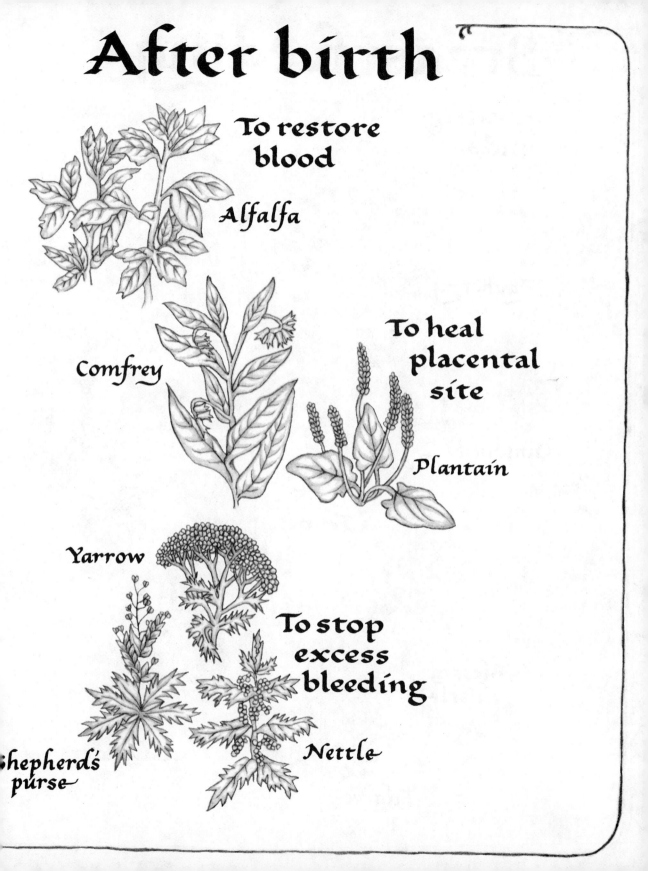

To restore blood

Alfalfa

Comfrey

To heal placental site

Plantain

Yarrow

To stop excess bleeding

Shepherd's purse

Nettle

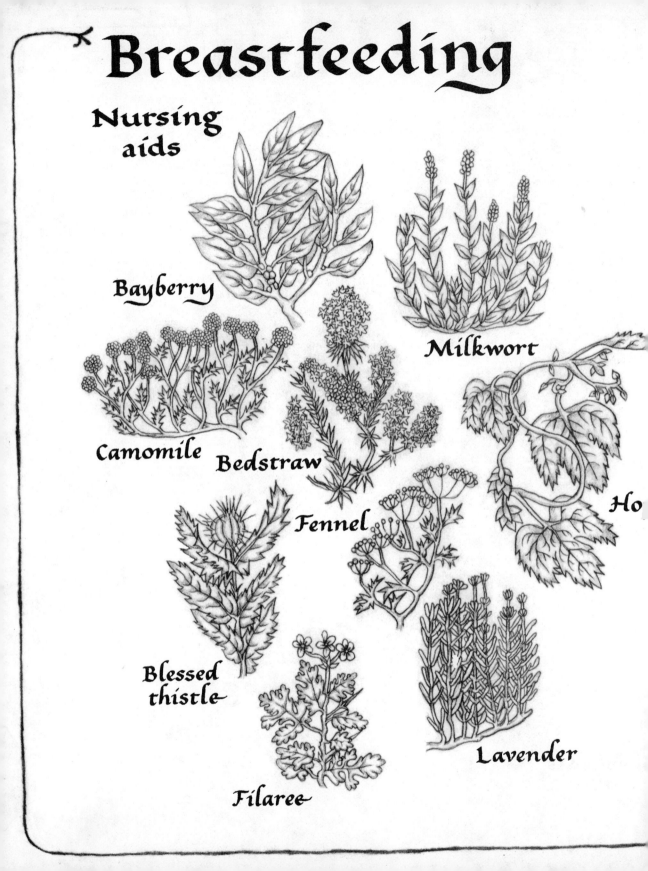

Breastfeeding

Nursing aids

Bayberry

Milkwort

Camomile

Bedstraw

Fennel

Ho

Blessed thistle

Filaree

Lavender

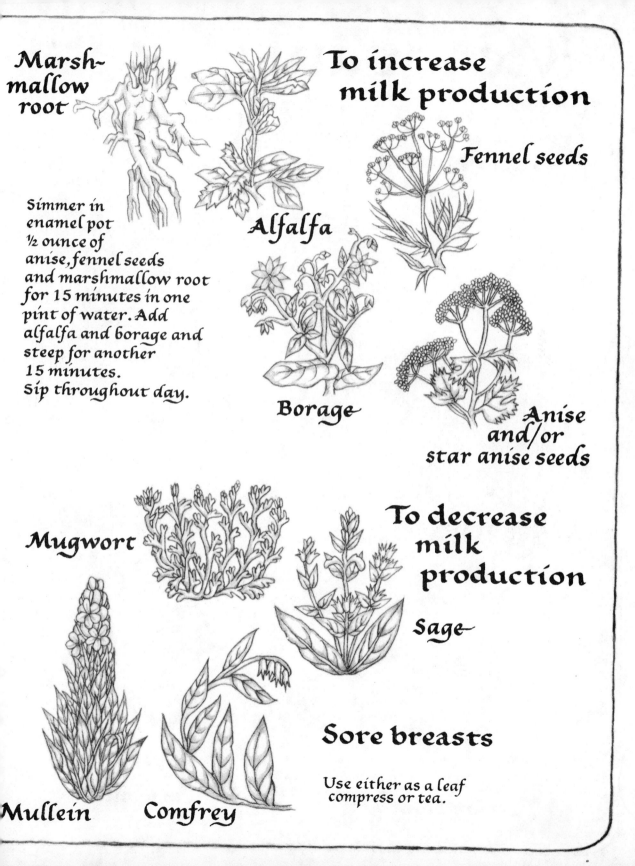

Marsh-
mallow
root

To increase
milk production

Fennel seeds

Simmer in
enamel pot
½ ounce of
anise, fennel seeds
and marshmallow root
for 15 minutes in one
pint of water. Add
alfalfa and borage and
steep for another
15 minutes.
Sip throughout day.

Alfalfa

Borage

Anise
and/or
star anise seeds

Mugwort

To decrease
milk
production

Sage

Sore breasts

Use either as a leaf
compress or tea.

Mullein

Comfrey

Menopause

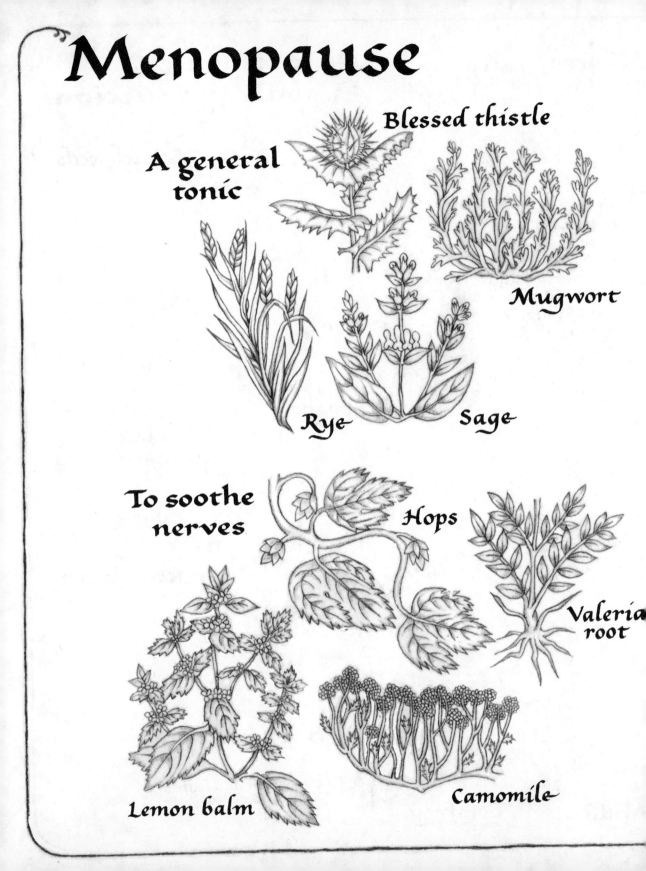

Blessed thistle

A general tonic

Mugwort

Rye

Sage

To soothe nerves

Hops

Valeria root

Lemon balm

Camomile

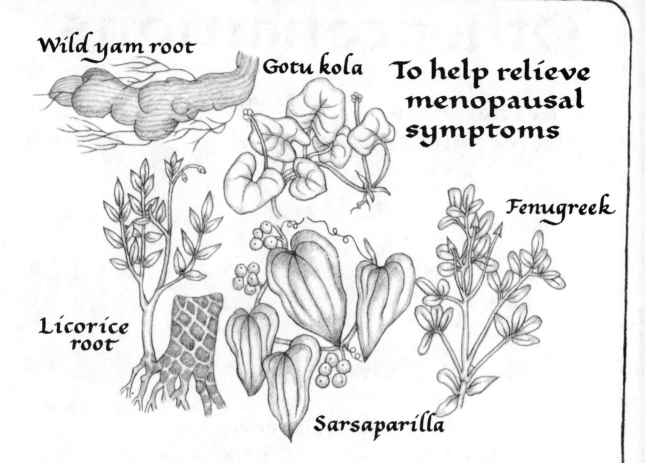

Wild yam root

Gotu kola

To help relieve menopausal symptoms

Fenugreek

Licorice root

Sarsaparilla

For best results, make a tea by mixing 1 herb from each of these groups with an herb high in minerals such as dandelion leaves, alfalfa or borage. Drink the tea daily.

Mugwort and valerian root should not be taken in excess.

Other conditions

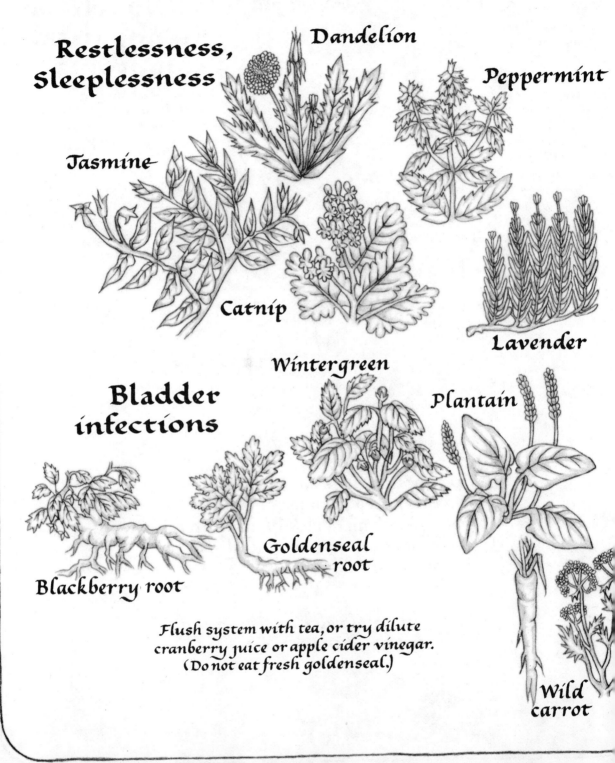

Restlessness, Sleeplessness

Dandelion

Peppermint

Jasmine

Catnip

Lavender

Wintergreen

Bladder infections

Plantain

Goldenseal root

Blackberry root

Flush system with tea, or try dilute cranberry juice or apple cider vinegar. (Do not eat fresh goldenseal.)

Wild carrot

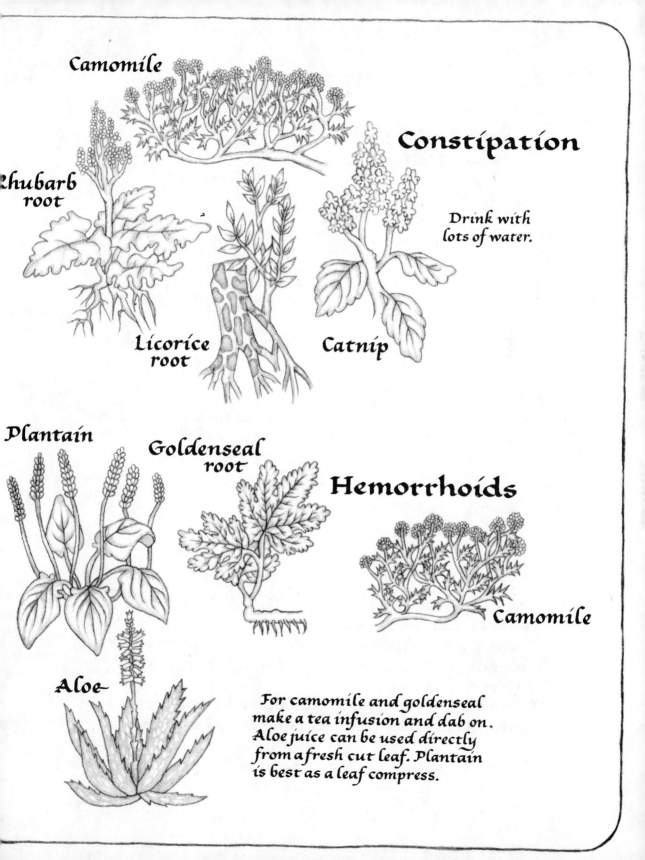

Camomile

Constipation

Rhubarb
root

Drink with
lots of water.

Licorice
root

Catnip

Plantain

Goldenseal
root

Hemorrhoids

Camomile

Aloe

For camomile and goldenseal
make a tea infusion and dab on.
Aloe juice can be used directly
from a fresh cut leaf. Plantain
is best as a leaf compress.

Vaginitis

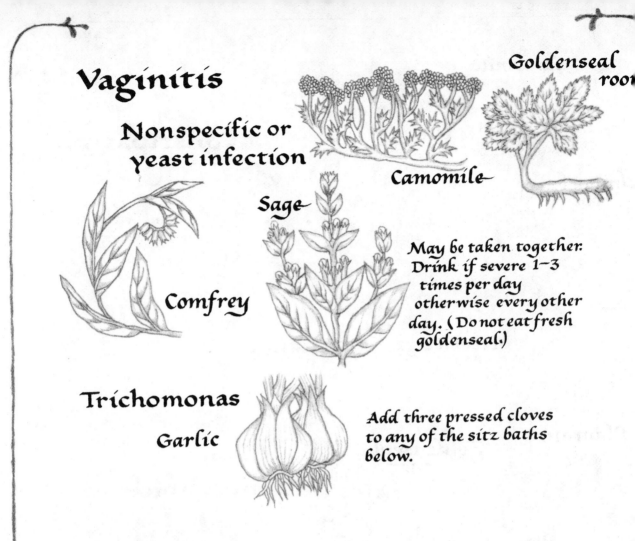

Goldenseal root

Nonspecific or yeast infection

Camomile

Sage

Comfrey

May be taken together. Drink if severe 1–3 times per day otherwise every other day. (Do not eat fresh goldenseal.)

Trichomonas

Garlic

Add three pressed cloves to any of the sitz baths below.

Sitz baths

1. 4½–5 tablespoons Lactobacillus acidophilus in 1 quart warm water, 3–4 times per day.
2. ¼ cup apple cider vinegar or 2 tablespoons baking soda in 1 quart water 3 times per day and taper off over 2 weeks.
3. 2–4 teaspoons liquid chlorophyll in 1 quart warm water 3 times per day and taper off over 2 weeks.

(For specific instructions see also "Vaginitis" p. 310.)

Herpes has been around for a long time. Most of us know it firsthand as the common cold sore. But this peculiar virus comes under many cloaks: everything from cold sores to encephalitis; from shingles to chicken pox. And now, within the last decade or so, still another herpes strain is hitting us below the belt.

Genital herpes (otherwise known as *herpes simplex* virus type 2 or HSV-2) is currently the most common cause of open sores on the female genitalia. According to estimates, 300,000 people in the United States are infected each year. By many accounts, herpes has reached epidemic proportions. And it's no small problem to those unfortunate enough to catch it.

If you're accustomed to wrestling with cold sores, you probably know the pattern. After infection and a couple of days of incubation, the sores erupt. Then, in an agonizing week or two, the painful blisters should regress. That doesn't sound too unbearable except for one thing: relief from the symptoms of herpes is not the same as a cure.

There is no known cure. When the symptoms regress, the virus goes into hiding. For some women it may never rear its ugly head again. But 80 percent of the women who suffer from genital herpes can expect a recurrence in six months. A lesser proportion may be bothered by a lifetime of repeat confrontations. Anything can trigger its reappearance. A menstrual period. Intercourse. Stress. Vaginitis. According to William E. Rawls, M.D., professor of pathology at McMaster University School of Medicine in Ontario, Canada, the pattern varies with the individual.

Most women who suffer from herpes come to recognize what it is that causes flareups. But predicting an episode is little consolation for the pain and discomfort that follow.

Painful red blisters erupt on the vulva (lips of the vagina), the perineum (area of skin between the vagina and rectum) and the buttocks. Inflammation and sores can creep into the vagina and affect the cervix as well. Fever, fatigue, loss of appetite and deep pelvic pain and painful or difficult urination may accompany the infection—especially during the first assault, which is usually the worst.

Aside from creating a temporary hell on earth, herpes poses a small but potentially dangerous risk to unborn children. If the infection occurs during the first 20 weeks of pregnancy, there is a significant risk of aborting. When it occurs after the 32nd week and does not heal by the onset of labor, there is a strong possibility that the infant will develop herpes within a few days of birth—a condition that is almost always fatal to newborns.

Luckily, the chance of this happening is fairly remote. "In my experience in clinical practice, I have seen hundreds of active genital herpes infections in pregnancy, but not a single one has lasted to the actual onset of labor," says New York City gynecologist Gideon G. Panter, M.D., who cites increased body resistance toward the end of pregnancy as a possible explanation. In the extremely rare cases where the herpes is active, with actual pain and blisters during labor, a cesarean section will save the baby from harmful consequences.

Preventing Herpes Infections

Nevertheless, it would be easier to *prevent* herpes in the first place. But that's not as simple as it sounds.

Herpesvirus type 2 is generally transmitted through sexual intercourse. Obviously, then, step number one in prevention is to avoid intimate contact with a partner whose herpes is active, with open oozing sores. Or, at the very least, count on a condom to provide some protection. Just remember: do not touch—any scratch in the skin provides a potential entrance. Dr. Rawls describes an instance where a gynecological resident neglected to don gloves when he examined a herpes patient and picked up the infection through a small scrape on his hand.

To make matters worse, once infected you're liable to find yourself with a headful of misguided information. Even doctors are at a loss as to how to deal with it. As we mentioned earlier, there's no cure for herpes. At best, treatment is aimed at clearing up the symptoms. And at least one popular medical therapy has proven to be more harmful than helpful.

Photodye therapy—which became quite popular a few years ago—involves a two-step procedure: first, the herpes sores are painted with a red dye designed to combine with the *herpesvirus;* then the dyed area is exposed to fluorescent or incandescent light which apparently inactivates the virus.

Unfortunately, several patients treated with phototherapy later developed skin cancer in or near the region of the herpes infection. Still doctors were reluctant to abandon this treatment. "Why frighten a lot of people and deprive patients with recurrent *herpes* *simplex* of a new and hopeful therapy? Why take away something which is so easy to administer and holds such promise of success?" some physicians asked. Why? Because cancer kills; herpes doesn't.

Remember, herpes is self-limiting, which means that even when left untreated it eventually subsides. Moreover, mild symptoms sometimes succumb with little more than warm compresses or a salty bath.

Besides, there are other methods that are proving to be successful (and safe!) in herpes treatment.

The Nutritional Approach to Herpes

At the Shute Institute in London, Ontario, Canada, the world-famous center for vitamin E research, physicians have found that a vitamin E ointment mixed with vitamin C works better than anything else in speeding along the healing process in genital herpes sores. In fact, they have found that application of this mixture can relieve the pain and redness of vulvar herpes sores in 24 hours and completely clear them up in three to four days.

Letters from *Prevention* magazine readers testify to the effectiveness of vitamins E and C in the treatment of genital herpes. "I suffered from *herpes simplex* 2 for two years," a California woman wrote. "I have tried putting vitamin E oil on the pustules and took 2,000 milligrams of vitamin C. To my surprise and delight, it works. Within two days, the herpes was gone."

Another woman tells her story: "I have suffered from *herpes simplex* type 2 for about seven years. Each doctor I've consulted has essentially told me the same thing, there was nothing I could do about it. In January of this year, I started taking vitamins for the first time in my life. After about three months, I noticed that I had not had herpes in all that time. Then I got lax in taking them and got the worst case of herpes I'd had.

"I had some vitamin E in an oil base and decided to put some on the cluster. Within a few hours I saw results and for the next 24 hours I continued to smear the herpes with E. At the end of that time, it had completely cleared up— with not a trace of redness. (For those who don't know, it usually takes any- where from one to three weeks to rid yourself of herpes and even with that, a week later you may have another attack, starting the cycle all over again.)"

A spokesman for the Shute Institute told us that the best form of vitamin E for direct application is an ointment. The vitamin E in capsules is usually too po- tent for this purpose. Instead, look for a salve or ointment containing 30 interna- tional units (I.U.) of vitamin E per gram of base. We found a product which fits that description in a local health food store. It costs about $2 for a 1½-ounce tube.

To that ointment, according to Shute Institute physicians, add some pow- dered, water-soluble vitamin C. Mix as needed in whatever proportion. Or ap- ply vitamin E ointment to the afflicted area, then sprinkle with the vitamin C.

Taking vitamins E and C by mouth may also help to clear up herpes in a hurry. The Shute Institute recommends megadoses of vitamin C (about three grams) and vitamin E (800 I.U.) a day until the symptoms subside. Then, to prevent recurrence, patients at the Shute Institute are advised to take at least two grams of vitamin C and 800 I.U. of vitamin E daily.

Zinc, too, is proving to be an effec- tive weapon against herpes. Zinc has long been recognized for its healing properties, but it was only recently that researchers found out how well it healed genital herpes. It started as a new contraceptive device—a sponge in- serted like a tampon and designed as a sperm barrier. Milos Chvapil, M.D., Ph.D., professor of surgical biology at the University of Arizona, who headed the development of the device, decided to see if adding zinc to the sponges would help to prevent the recurrence of herpes. It worked. Only three of nine women had a reappearance of herpes following treatment with the sponge.

At present the zinc-medicated sponge is still in the experimental stage. But meanwhile, it may not be a bad idea to think about taking an oral supplement of zinc. According to Niels H. Lauersen, M.D., coauthor of *It's Your Body*, (Grosset & Dunlap, 1977), the severity of a herpes infection hinges on the health of your immune system. The first time you're infected with a *herpesvirus*, your body starts producing antibodies to fight it off. These antibodies remain in your system so that the second time you have an attack it will be less severe. Theoretically, at least, when the body develops sufficient antibodies, the re- current episodes of genital herpes should cease. And this is where zinc, as well as vitamins C, E and A, can help. Studies have shown that these nutrients may help to keep your immune mech- anism working at peak performance.

HOT FLASHES

"The first thing to know about hot flashes is that they are harmless," says Rosetta Reitz in her book *Menopause: A Positive Approach* (Chilton, 1977). "They pass quickly and are nothing to be afraid of."

The second thing you should probably know is that they are an extremely common accompaniment to menopause. So common, in fact, that next to menstrual irregularities, hot flashes top the menopausal symptom list for 80 percent of all women.

Rosetta Reitz describes a flash or flush (the two terms are used interchangeably) as "a blush only more so; the redness is deeper and the heat is hotter." It's as if the room suddenly became 20 degrees warmer and you're the only one who's noticed. Your skin turns red; you start to sweat. Sometimes a cold sweat overcomes you. Often you get the urge to run outside and hurl yourself into a bank of snow, but by the time you make up your mind to move, it's passed—gone in less than two minutes.

Actually, it's only been within recent years that research has contributed anything at all to our understanding of menopausal flushing. But what we are now finding out is that there are very real measurable changes which occur in the body at the time of a hot flash. So don't let anyone tell you this menopausal symptom's all in your head!

In a British study, for example, eight menopausal women were carefully monitored for skin temperature, pulse, heart rhythm and so forth, while they were experiencing hot flashes. In every case, the sensation was accompanied by an increased heartbeat (sometimes even palpitations), a dilation of blood vessels of the face and hands, and a rise in skin temperature. Interestingly, the increase in skin temperature, though not very great (it wasn't more than 1°C, though it may rise 3° or 4°), persisted for some time even after the sensation of heat had passed. That finding led the British researchers to conclude that the severity of the hot flash is probably related to the rate of temperature change as well as to the actual temperature increase (*British Medical Journal*, July 8, 1978).

That proves something is indeed happening. But exactly what it is that's causing those changes still remains unclear.

One brand new theory suggests that menopausal flushing is caused by a seesawlike effect between the sloweddown estrogen output of the ovaries and the stepped-up hormone production of the pituitary gland. Normally, in the course of a woman's menstrual years, the hormone production of those two glands is maintained in a delicate balance (see Menstruation).

Of course, this is just a theory and there are some physicians who remain skeptical—but David R. Meldrum, M.D., and Howard L. Judd, M.D., both gynecologists with the University of California School of Medicine, Los Angeles, have studied menopausal women with frequent and severe hot flashes and have found a "significant correlation" between skin temperature increases and the pituitary's release of a hormone.

If it's true what they're saying—and lowered estrogen levels are responsible for kicking off this surge of a pituitary hormone—then it may help to explain how estrogen replacement therapy is able to control those menopausal flushes so effectively.

But progesterone therapy—which carries far fewer health risks than estrogen—may also be effective in preventing hot flashes. A group of physicians at Boston Hospital for Women found that in women who took a certain form of progesterone there was almost a 75 percent decrease in the number of hot flashes (*Journal of the American Medical Association*, September 26, 1980).

Of course, progesterone isn't without side effects either. So unless your symptoms are so severe that you find them absolutely unbearable, you'd be better off avoiding any kind of hormone therapy.

Granted, hot flashes can be very uncomfortable. But they're not painful. And given the swiftness with which they strike and then retreat, they hardly seem worth the risk of hormone therapy—especially with estrogens (see Estrogen Replacement Therapy). Besides the risks, hormones provide only momentary relief from symptoms. You have to continue taking them over a long term to free yourself from these flashes forever.

Natural Ways of Cooling "Flashes"

So what about alternatives?

Well, as we mentioned earlier, the research into this menopausal phenomenon is just getting started. In our opinion, the biggest help in coping with these momentary annoyances is in understanding just how innocuous they are. Hot flashes are really nothing to get all excited about.

Then again, it might be all the excitement that's bringing them on in the first place. In her talks with hundreds of menopausal women, Rosetta Reitz has found that hot flashes seem to occur in many women at moments of high stress. There are no actual studies to back this up, but it is a possible tie-in with some scientific evidence that psychological stress may lower estrogen in postmenopausal women. Perhaps—and this is pure speculation—a stress-related drop in an already dwindling estrogen supply might be just the ticket to tip the hormonal seesaw and set off the series of mechanisms that result in a hot flash. It's a thought, anyway.

Meanwhile, the distinguished group of doctors and gynecologists writing in *My Body, My Health* (John Wiley & Sons, 1979) encourage women to "experiment with practical alterations in [their] daily routine that may help minimize the inconvenience or discomfort of symptoms that [they] do have." In other words, if you—like many of the women Rosetta Reitz interviewed—find that stress brings on a flush, do your best to avoid stressful situations. "Some women also find that an immediate drink of ice water can stop a flush reaction," add the experts in *My Body, My Health*. "A Thermos of ice water on the bedside table may be helpful."

Certain supplements may also be beneficial. Back in the 60s, for example, a published study showed that menopausal flushing could be controlled to a certain extent with bioflavonoids. In a controlled experiment the majority of patients obtained some relief from a combination of bioflavonoids and vitamin C in a preparation known as Peridin-C (*Chicago Medicine*, March 7, 1964).

In addition, more than a few nutrition-oriented physicians report some success in treating their menopausal patients with very high doses of vitamin E—as much as 2,000 to 3,000 international units daily. Jonathan V. Wright, M.D., of Kent, Washington, for one, recommends a combination of vitamin E and kelp, as well as the bioflavonoids rutin and hesperidin. "It's only successful in a minority of cases," he admits, "but for those people, it really works."

Rosetta Reitz has her own nutritional formula to ban the flashes "I have seen flashes disappear completely when the vitamin E is also accompanied by 2,000 to 3,000 milligrams of vitamin C (taken at intervals through the day) and with 1,000 milligrams (also at intervals) of calcium from dolomite or bone meal," she says.

HOUSEHOLD HEALTH HAZARDS

A researcher in Oregon stumbled across statistics showing the risk of dying from cancer is twice as great for housewives as for women who do not work in the home. William E. Morton, M.D., Dr. P.H. (doctor of public health), head of the University of Oregon Health Science Center's division of environmental medicine, told how these figures came to light:

"I was studying the 15-year rate of cancer death in Lane County in Oregon. It's the second largest metropolitan area in the state. I was looking for a specific cancer problem to study—I was actually interested in geographic factors.

"Just for the sake of completeness, though, I included occupation as one of the variables. I looked at housewives because I thought they were a relatively protected group, with a nice low rate of cancer deaths that I could compare with higher rates in industry. But I discovered that for women under 65, the death rate was cut to less than half if they worked outside the home. It was exactly the reverse of what I had expected."

Dr. Morton went back and reviewed his methods, on the chance that he had made some error in his calculations. But the outcome remained the same: for women between the ages of 16 and 64

listed on death certificates as housewives, unemployed, or not in the labor force, the cancer death rate was 102.6 per 100,000. For women listed as employed, the annual death rate was only 51.1 per 100,000. Cancers of the breast, cervix, ovaries, colon and rectum, uterus, liver and gallbladder, brain, lungs, stomach and lymph system were all significantly more common among housewives than among women who worked outside the home.

"Finally, I accepted my findings," Dr. Morton says, "and I began to look into the things that housewives are commonly exposed to in the home. I found that many compounds which require monitoring of the workers' health when used in industry were also commonly present in the home."

Dr. Morton told us that the cancer-causing chemical benzene is an ingredient of window glass cleaners and other common household concoctions. Phenols, which can enhance the cancer-causing effects of other chemicals, are found in many cleansers, "particularly the more potent ones which are used to cut grease," Dr. Morton says. "Any number of lesser substances are suspect, such as aromatic amino compounds. Bleaching agents may be a factor in the overall picture. There are all sorts of possibilities."

No one can say at this point exactly what caused the high rate of cancer among the housewives of Lane County. It may have had nothing to do with household chemicals. But try browsing through the warning labels on the cleansers you keep in your kitchen. It's obvious those chemicals are anything but mother's milk to the human system.

The Problem with Aerosols

Aerosols are among the most hazardous items in our home environment. And they're everywhere you look. Room deodorizers, furniture polish and window cleaners, as well as hair spray, perfume and personal deodorants can all be purchased in convenient spray containers. But convenience doesn't come cheap—and in this case, the price may be your health. In fact, according to a 1974 study by the Consumer Product Safety Commission, "The average severity rating estimated for aerosol-related injuries was higher than the average severity rating for *all other consumer product injuries.*"

The major problem is in the chemicals used to propel these products from the can. As you may recall, there was quite a stir just a few years ago over the fluorocarbon propellants because they are believed to destroy the ozone layer of our atmosphere, our shield against the sun's cancer-causing ultraviolet rays. Banned from using these fluorocarbons, manufacturers then turned to hydrocarbon propellants. But that, unfortunately, has brought the dangers even closer to home.

Hydrocarbons include butane, isobutane and propane—essentially the same highly flammable chemicals you'll find in lighter fluid and gas ranges. As a result, many people have been injured, some seriously, when their aerosols exploded or emitted a torchlike jet of fire. This can occur if the can has been inadvertently punctured or if it's been stored in a hot spot such as a sunny windowsill.

To add insult to injury, some manufacturers are adding methylene chloride, a special solvent, to reduce the pressure and flammability of hydrocarbon aerosols. Methylene chloride, however, caused mutations in laboratory tests on bacteria.

Vincent Simmons, Ph.D., a microbiologist who performed the tests at Stanford Research Institute International in California, is understandably concerned. "I think there's a rush by the manufacturers to sell this product," he says. "I personally, as a scientist, am very concerned about its continued use in aerosols until the long-term experiments with animals presently underway are completed. Knowing the chemistry and other chemicals in that class, my suspicion is that it will turn out to be carcinogenic [cancer-causing]."

Some household hazards don't rely on such indirect methods as cancer to get at their victims. Instead, they simply poison you. Several years ago a housewife in Westchester County, New York, named Jane Darnell, began suffering from nausea, stomach pains, a slight fever, and a general feeling of weakness. Her children began to come down with similiar symptoms. Her eldest teenage son lost 10 pounds, a younger boy developed a hacking cough, and another son suffered from an inexplicable eye infection. One December the entire family came down with an "influenza" that seemed suspiciously like an acute attack of the malady that was plaguing Mrs. Darnell.

As all this was going on, Mrs. Darnell had to contend with problems with her dishwasher. Her husband had repaired the vinyl lining of the washer with a silicone sealant, but it was not effective. Mrs. Darnell's dishes were not coming out as clean as they should have. Twice she had to call repairmen in to work on the machine. The second repairman found the cause of the problem—the sealant was flaking off and slowly accumulating on her dishes in a pattern of specks that nothing seemed to remove.

At this point Mrs. Darnell began suffering from even more bizarre symptoms than she had previously. A painful bump developed on her left leg. Her nose began to bleed and the inside of her lips tore open. One day she rubbed the corner of her eye and blood spurted out.

Arsenic in the Dishwater

Mrs. Darnell decided it might be a good idea to find out exactly what was in that dishwasher sealant. After dozens of calls to the manufacturer of the sealant, she was finally told that it contained a small amount of arsenic to prevent the growth of mildew. Subsequently, in the course of a lawsuit against the manufacturer, testing revealed the sealant contained 17 times the amount of arsenic Mrs. Darnell says she was told was present.

When Mrs. Darnell told her doctor about the arsenic-laced sealant, he concluded she was suffering from chronic arsenic poisoning. He advised her to throw out her dishes and silverware, which she did. Laboratory tests showed that she and her oldest son had high concentrations of arsenic in their systems, and the two had to go through a painful detoxifying treatment, originally developed to treat soldiers who had been the

victims of poison gas. Finally, following the advice of her doctor, Mrs. Darnell reluctantly decided to abort a pregnancy, for fear of what the arsenic might have done to the unborn child. All this to repair the lining of a dishwasher!

Of course, the risks involved in living in an artificial, chemical environment are not confined to the terrors of cancer and arsenic. The price we pay may be a mysterious rash or allergy.

Cleaning up can sometimes be worse for your hands than soiling them in the first place, says Gary S. Nelson, Ph.D., a safety engineer with the Texas Agricultural Extension Service at College Station, Texas.

"Numerous cases of dermatitis are not caused directly by substances used in the workplace, but by materials used to wash up," says Dr. Nelson. "Many times the most available cleaning agent is a dermatitis-producing solvent."

Some of the commonest cleaners around the house and garage—"the prime ones you'd go to," says Dr. Nelson—can be the worst for your skin. Turpentine, gasoline, kerosene and lacquer thinner are the ones that come to mind. Those solvents do their job only too well. Paint and grease aren't the only things they take off.

"You're actually dissolving your hands, that's what you're doing," Dr. Nelson warns.

The skin, he explains, acts as a barrier against injuries and irritants. It's also a two-way water barrier, preventing liquids from seeping into the body and keeping body fluids from leaking out. To do this job, the skin has to be flexible, and it relies on natural fats and oils to stay that way. Strong solvents "defat" the skin and allow it to dry out and crack open. "The solvent will both dry out the skin and then irritate it," says Dr. Nel-

SIMPLE AND SENSIBLE CLEANING SOLUTIONS

Scouring powder: Combine 9 parts whiting (from a hardware store) with 1 part soap granules. This mixture won't scratch surfaces as commercial products do, and it omits the unnecessary chlorine, which could accidentally combine with other chemicals—like ammonia—to produce dangerous chlorine gas.

Brass and copper cleaner: Vinegar and salt paste.

Window cleaner: 4 tablespoons ammonia, 2 tablespoons vinegar, and 1 quart water, followed by hot elbow grease with crumpled old newspapers for a special sparkle.

Drain cleaner: First, try a plunger. Then try ½ cup washing soda followed by 2 cups boiling water. For a stronger treatment, combine a handful of baking soda with ½ cup vinegar. Close the drain and let it sit, then flush with water. (Do this regularly to prevent buildup.)

Washing soda is an alkali much less caustic than lye, but it should be kept locked up. It is dangerous.

Rug cleaner: Get the spill scooped or blotted up fast! Dip a small brush in cold water and work out the spot. For a grease spot, sprinkle a generous amount of dry baking soda or dry cornstarch on the spot. Let it stand for an hour or so, then vacuum. If the grease remains, try the spray cleaner below, and a stiff brush.

Rug shampoo: Mix ¼ cup mild detergent or soap with 1 pint of warm water and 2 tablespoons vinegar. Whip into a stiff foam. First, vacuum the rug thoroughly. Apply the *foam*, and scrub. Let dry, then vacuum again.

Spray cleaner (for surfaces other than varnish, aluminum or asphalt tile): ¼ cup ammonia, ⅛ cup vinegar, 1 tablespoon baking soda, and 1 quart water. Pour into glass or plastic bottle and screw on a handsquirter top.

Spot remover: For fabrics that don't take to bleach, apply ammonia diluted with an equal amount of water. Put paper towels underneath to blot. If the ammonia odor clings, apply a table salt solution. (A last resort for old stains is a dab of vinegar.)

Oven cleaner: Sprinkle spills generously with salt while the oven is still hot. The burned deposit should scrape off with no trouble when the oven cools. For thorough cleaning, set an open shallow dish of full-strength ammonia inside the cold oven. Close the door and let it stand overnight. The ammonia gas from the solution is absorbed by the grease, which ends up like soap. Do not use this method on aluminum. Clean thoroughly.

Deodorizers: Use baking soda here, there and everywhere—down the drain, in diaper pails, refrigerators, cat litter and the kitchen sponge.

son. "Drying out the skin then makes it susceptible to damage by other substances" (see Skin Problems).

Certain fragrance and flavor chemicals, and also certain metal products, commonly bring on allergic skin reactions. Among these are cinnamic aldehyde (cinnamon flavor), hydroxycitronellal (lemon scent) and metal items containing nickel.

F. William Danby, M.D., a practicing dermatologist in Kingston, Ontario, Canada, says that perfume reactions are common among patients who have trouble with their skin. (Fair-skinned people are more sensitive than swarthier types, he says.) But identifying the chemical that caused the reaction can be very difficult. The fragrance in a shampoo, for example, can give some people a rash. But the fragrance itself may be composed of several hundred subingredients, and its exact formula may even be a trade secret. "Even the companies using them [fragrances] don't know what's in them." Dr. Danby says.

Fragrances and other sensitizing chemicals are widely used. Cinnamic aldehyde can be found in soap, toothpaste and ice cream—to name only a few. More than one million pounds of hydroxycitronellal—used to scent bubble bath—are used each year in synthetic perfumes in the United States. Other chemicals that can give people trouble are paraphenylenediamine, an ingredient in hair dye, and formaldehyde, which is found in disinfectants, shampoos, foot sprays, photographic chemicals, high-gloss paper and other items.

It goes to show you, you can't be too careful. But with just a little care, you can reduce your household risks quite a bit. Start by checking out your stockpile of household chemicals and chucking out those that are totally unnecessary. The room deodorizers, for example, and the aerosol dust collectors. Better yet, every aerosol in your house should get the ax. Next try to consolidate cleaning agents. You don't need one for the kitchen sink, another for the bathtub, and so on. See where you can cut back. Then pare down to a few—perhaps bleach, washing soda, and ammonia. You can keep those under lock and key, and use them sparingly. As for all the rest, the o-phenylphenols and isopropanols, we don't need them. Grandmother got on quite well before all these newfangled products came onto the market (see accompanying box, Simple and Sensible Cleaning Solutions, page 319).

Even so, special precautions should be taken. For one thing, never mix two or more potent chemical cleaners together. Chlorine bleach added to ammonia or other acidic products can result in poisonous chlorine gas given off.

Protect your hands from any cleaning solution—even if it's just soap and hot water. Use long-handled brushes and mops instead of hand-held sponges and rags whenever possible. Vinyl rather than rubber gloves are probably better if you are prone to dermatitis. And for home redecorating tasks such as painting and furniture stripping, wear canvas work gloves. As a final note, remove all rings before beginning housework to prevent what is known as "ring-finger dermatitis."

Topping tonsillectomy, hysterectomy has risen to become our nation's number one major operation. And, as if that weren't enough, the figures keep climbing. According to the National Center for Health Statistics, 644,000 were performed in 1978—a 31 percent increase over 10 years ago.

Clearly hysterectomy rates in this country are high—too high, say certain consumer research groups who charge that 15 to 40 percent may be done unnecessarily. What they want to know is:

- Why do American surgeons remove twice as many wombs as British or Welsh physicians?
- Why does our hysterectomy rate continue to soar despite the fact that uterine disease is actually on a downswing?
- Why is it that of all the hysterectomies performed, only about 10 to 20 percent are done to curb cancer or other life-threatening disease?
- And why does the same gynecological complaint result in hysterectomy for one woman, nonsurgical treatment for another, and no treatment at all for still another?

It's enough to make you suspicious, at the very least. But before you become so scalpel-shy as to avoid surgery when it would be in your best interest, there's more to the hysterectomy story than meets the critical consumer eye. For one thing, if money is a motivating factor in recommending hysterectomy—as some consumer advocates have charged— why is it that the operation rate is higher than average in physicians' families?

Confused? So were we. So we contacted several top-notch gynecologists and surgeons to see what they had to say.

"I think you are going to find that there are unnecessary hysterectomies being performed. No question about it," stated John Mikuta, M.D., director of gynecologic oncology at the Hospital of the University of Pennsylvania. "But you have to be careful about what you're calling 'unnecessary.' Sometimes, it's a matter of opinion...."

Stanley J. Birnbaum, M.D., professor of obstetrics and gynecology at Cornell University Medical College, explains, "A prolapsed uterus is a perfectly legitimate indication for performing a hysterectomy. Yet, outside of the body, the uterus appears normal. That doesn't mean that the operation was unnecessary. Sometimes the indication for hysterectomy is not a disease in the uterus; it's a mechanical problem with the uterus. And that's difficult to substantiate with just a pathology report."

At least one stumbling block in determining whether hysterectomy is warranted is the definition of the word "necessary."

Years ago, when hysterectomy was an extremely risk-ridden surgical procedure, it was considered acceptable or "necessary" when the only other alternative was death. In other words, if your life depended on the surgery, you'd have it. And if it didn't, you wouldn't. Simple.

Today, however, since hysterectomy has become a relatively safe surgical procedure (that is, as far as surgery can be called "safe"), it is no longer reserved for life-or-death ordeals. Indeed, the majority of women have them to improve the quality—not the length—of their lives.

That is not altogether wrong. A fibroid tumor may not put a woman's life on the line, but it may cause enough pain to drive her to the brink of despair. Likewise, a prolapsed uterus won't kill you. But if surgery can correct the problem and make life more livable, then why not have it? There are many acceptable reasons for hysterectomy, albeit not exactly lifesaving or "necessary" in the previous sense of the word.

When Is a Hysterectomy Necessary?

The main trouble with this liberalization of hysterectomy indications is that—aside from a few life-threatening conditions including endometrial cancer (cancer of the lining of the uterus), or advanced cervical cancer—there are no absolute criteria for determining when the surgery is warranted. Elective hysterectomies are performed for fallen wombs, fibroid tumors, endometriosis, profuse menstrual bleeding, backaches, headaches and other premenstrual miseries, sterilization and even cancer prevention—again, all possible indications for hysterectomy, but certainly not appropriate to all women, all of the time. Much hinges on the severity of the problem, the degree of discomfort, the age and childbearing status of the woman, the availability of alternative treatment, and the expertise of the physician.

Sometimes the necessity for surgery is easy to evaluate. For example, a 50-year-old woman suffering from backaches and loss of urinary control as a result of a uterus which has fallen to the bottom of her vaginal canal is a prime candidate for a hysterectomy. But a 33-year-old woman who wants another child and whose uterus is only slightly prolapsed isn't. Now, where does that leave the 40-year-old woman with a partial prolapse? Or, the 35-year-old newlywed with a more severe prolapse problem? There are many gray areas.

Unfortunately, if you don't understand the exact state of your condition or the options available in treating it, you could be misled to believe that surgery is the only way out of a gray zone. A New York woman we spoke with discovered this in the nick of time:

"I had been going to a gynecologist for many years, every six months or so. He was a very prominent doctor and a busy man. Every exam, he would ask me if I was losing water and I would say no. This went on for several years. Eventually I did lose a little water—it was just a matter that after urination, when I stood up, a trickle would go down my leg. It was a very minor problem, and if it bothered me at all, I would never have thought in terms of surgery. But since he had been asking so many times, I wondered if possibly it was important and I told the doctor about it. I thought it might have to do with something he was seeing and not telling me about. When I told him about it, he said probably the muscle was a little slack from having two children. He said he could do some plastic work to repair it. He added that when that plastic work was done, he usually would take the uterus, too. Well, that frightened me because I have a very healthy uterus, and I've never had any problems with it whatsoever. I was in my forties. I didn't plan to have any more children, but I saw no reason for having my uterus removed.

"The doctor told me to think about the surgery and he gave me some exercises to do to tighten that muscle. These exercises, by the way, practically eliminated the problem—or else it eliminated itself. I don't know.

"The next time I was in, he asked me if I had been thinking about the surgery. I said I had, and he asked if my husband was in the office. I said yes, and he brought my husband into the office and started showing him diagrams of a prolapsed uterus and said this was what I had. Now I have never had any of the symptoms of a prolapsed uterus and the doctor had never, in all of his examinations, mentioned this possibility to me. He asked us if we thought I would have the surgery and we said that if he really thought it was necessary I probably would. He was a busy and respected man. It certainly never occurred to me that he might want to create surgery.

"So we took it through my union [source of this woman's health insurance] and I decided to get a second opinion. The second doctor told me that my uterus was in excellent condition for a woman my age. He said there was no prolapsed uterus, that in fact my uterus was in a good position.

"Well, that confused me, because here I had this second report conflicting with the recommendation of this doctor I had been going to for years. So I went to a third doctor. He agreed completely with the second doctor and said there was no need for a hysterectomy whatsoever. So, of course, I didn't have it. I never told the first doctor. I just never went back to him."

Fortunately, this woman was spared unneeded surgery. But how many more are less fortunate? Probably more than you'd think. Philip Cole, M.D., professor of epidemiology at Harvard School of Public Health, blames the rise in hysterectomies on what he terms "borderline symptomatology." In other words, the woman's symptoms may just hint of an indication for hysterectomy, and the physician will recommend surgery—often "based on the rationale that if a woman is 35 or 40 years old and has an organ that is disease-prone and of little or no further use, it might as well be removed."

Apparently, too, that is an opinion held by more than a small minority of gynecologists. One woman we interviewed recalls her doctor's words of consolation when she balked at the prospect of surgery.

"Don't look at it *that* way," he admonished her wails over the impending loss. "The uterus is a useless organ anyway—at least once you've had your family. Besides, it's best to get it out now before any *real* trouble starts. Would you rather wait until you got cancer?" he asked, as if the disease were inevitable. "Or risk the possibility of another pregnancy? You're at the age now when you have to start thinking about these things."

Then he said point-blank, with Billy Graham conviction, "In my opinion, every woman should have a hysterectomy by the age of 40."

Another woman we spoke with also objected to her physician's "what do you need it for anyway?" attitude. "He made it sound so insignificant," she said. "You'd think we were discussing the removal of a wart."

Surgical Risks You Should Know About

It doesn't even come close. Hysterectomy is major surgery. And its complication rate is relatively high. For one thing, it presents all the usual hazards of major surgery—infection, hemorrhage, postoperative blood clots and the risks of anesthesia. In addition, because of the uterus's close proximity to other pelvic structures, there's always the possibility of incurring damage or operative trauma to pelvic blood vessels, the rectum, the bladder and the ureters (the tubes connecting the kidneys to the bladder). In fact, one of the more common complications of hysterectomy is the accidental severing of a ureter.

Vaginal hysterectomies, moreover, carry with them the additional risk of creating a somewhat shortened or narrowed vagina, which could make intercourse painful. And if the ovaries are removed, the abrupt drop in estrogen level is likely to cause an immediate "surgical menopause" which is more severe than a natural menopause.

There is even some evidence that the *uterus* itself may influence hormone production. According to D. H. Richards, a physician from Oxford, England, 61 percent of the women under age 45 who had hysterectomies but who had one or both ovaries preserved suffered from hot flashes, urinary symptoms, extreme tiredness, headaches, dizziness and insomnia. Most of these symptoms, he says, can be attributed to a hormone imbalance (*Lancet*, October 26, 1974). A follow-up report from the famous Framingham Study also indicates that hysterectomy patients are at greater risk of coronary heart disease whether or not their ovaries are removed (*Annals of Internal Medicine*, August, 1978).

But by far the most common reaction to hysterectomy is depression. And women who have normal or near-normal uteruses at the time of hysterectomy have more than twice the rate of psychiatric referral. All the more reason to make sure there's good cause to have surgery before you go through with it.

The important thing here is to weigh the odds. Consider the risks and benefits of surgery in terms of your own health and well-being. Understand your condition fully and be aware of alternative treatment should it exist. (For more specifics, see the section of this book that pertains to your individual problem.) Only then can you make an informed decision.

Again, keep in mind that no problem, short of endometrial cancer, is an absolute indication for hysterectomy. And, at least in our opinion, a few indications—including sterilization and cancer prevention—should *not* be handled by hysterectomy.

Yet, one in five hysterectomies is done for sterilization, according to a survey by the U.S. Department of Health, Education and Welfare (HEW; now the Department of Health and Human Services). Imagine. Submitting to major surgery when relatively minor procedures could do the same job.

"It's like cracking a nut with a sledgehammer," says Dr. Birnbaum.

"Subjecting a woman to this relatively dangerous operation for sterilization alone is an outrage," says Sidney Wolfe, M.D., of the Public Citizens Health Research Group in Washington, D.C.

"There's no reason for a woman to submit to major surgery when a relatively simple laparoscopic tubal ligation will do the same job. Better yet, I think that the vasectomy should be given serious consideration by couples desiring sterilization," says Dr. Mikuta.

These assertions are supported by statistics from the Centers for Disease Control in Atlanta, Georgia—which show that reproductive-age hysterectomy patients are over six times more likely to suffer serious surgical complications and five times more likely to die than women who undergo the simpler tubal sterilization.

These opinions sent HEW scurrying to reevaluate their policy and withdraw a popular pamphlet they had distributed entitled "Your Sterilization Operation: Hysterectomy." The new guidelines state that hysterectomy should *not* be performed solely for the purpose of sterilization.

Still, there are physicians who, for whatever reason, are pushing hysterectomies as casually as they dispense Valium. One woman explains:

"When I was 34 years old and had just given birth to my fifth child, my doctor and I discussed the possibility of having my tubes cut and tied. I told him I'd rather wait a few months to be absolutely sure. He said, 'Well, when you come back we might as well do a hysterectomy' (although he assured me that there was absolutely nothing medically wrong). I was so flabbergasted that I left the office and never went back."

There are a couple of exceptions, however, when gynecologists agree that a sterilization hysterectomy is okay or even preferred. That is, when other gynecological problems may require a hysterectomy in the immediate or not-too-distant future. Or when there exists a pelvic condition such as prolapse or fibroids which will probably grow worse.

"We see over and over again, women with minor to moderate gynecological problems who had tubal ligations come back requiring a hysterectomy within the same year," says Alan Kaplan, M.D., of the Baylor College of Medicine in Houston. "This can require two surgical procedures and two anesthetics, thereby doubling the risk."

Just be sure that the "other" reason for the surgery is valid. And beware of the surgeon who might shield the actual reason for the surgery under an umbrella of invented or grossly exaggerated symptoms. According to Jane Hodgson, M.D., professor of surgery at the University of Minnesota School of Medicine, many gynecologists—including those at Catholic hospitals—"cover" sterilization hysterectomies by saying that the reason for the operation is heavy menstrual bleeding, prolapse of the uterus, dysfunctional uterine bleeding or an abnormal (but not cancerous) Pap test. None of these, she states, is justification for subjecting women to the risk of hysterectomy.

One woman we spoke with implied that she may have been so coerced:

"I was thinking of having a tubal ligation but when I brought it up with my gynecologist he changed the subject to hysterectomy. . . . Said I had a slightly prolapsed uterus that would just get worse and I'd eventually need to have a hysterectomy anyway. So why not get it all taken care of at once? The funny thing was, I'd been going to this doctor for several years and he had never before mentioned that I had a prolapsed uterus. Besides that, I wasn't having any discomfort. . . . But he's a well-respected physician in my community and I figured he knew what he was doing so I went through with the operation."

When in Doubt, Get a Second Opinion

An informed health care consumer can immediately spot some flaws in her rationale. For one thing, if she found the prolapse excuse hard to swallow, she shouldn't have bought it so readily. And second, just because her doctor's office sports an impressive sheepskin and a slew of idolizing patients, she shouldn't have assumed him God. *Maybe he was right*. But a second opinion would have certainly cleared up any doubts in her mind. And it may even have freed her from surgery.

Cancer prevention is another poor excuse for hysterectomy. Take a patient who is in the high-risk bracket for cervical cancer. Had her first baby at age 17. Is unmarried and has multiple sex partners. Now let's suppose she shows up at a hospital clinic after having a slightly abnormal (but not cancerous) Pap smear or just walks in off the street and requests a sterilization. There's a good chance that she'll be leaving without her uterus.

They call it "prevention." And, say some physicians, with two strikes against her, this particular lady stands to benefit from the surgery. Number one: her background puts her at high risk of cervical cancer. Number two: if she is sterilized by other means, she probably won't be coming back to the obstetrical service to be screened for cancer.

Removing a perfectly healthy uterus is sometimes justified for persons suffering from cancer phobia (fear of cancer) as well. In fact, it is often the patient who requests the surgery and, says Dr. Mikuta, there may be serious consequences when the physician refuses to comply. Dr. Mikuta tells of a 35-year-old woman who was in good health but who was convinced that because both her mother and sister had died of cervical cancer, it was just a matter of time before she, too, fell victim. She wanted a hysterectomy. But her physician turned her down and told her not to worry, she was fine. About 15 minutes later, the doctor who gave her this advice turned around and saw a body falling past his window. The patient had gone up on the roof and jumped off—all because of her tremendous fear of cancer.

Of course, that is an extreme case. But it does illustrate the fact that indications for hysterectomy are rarely clearcut. Generally speaking, a hysterectomy performed in the absence of disease could hardly be called lifesaving. In this case, it may have been.

Also, physicians maintain that having surgery for sheer prevention is the patient's right. "It's just as valid as having plastic surgery," says Dr. Kaplan. "Of course, I would never push a woman into surgery for this reason. But if a patient says, 'Look, my family history is clouded with case after case of uterine cancer and I'd rather have a hysterectomy now than worry the rest of my life about getting cancer,' she is a valid candidate for hysterectomy. As long as she's completely aware of all the risks involved, then the decision should be hers."

Still, some physicians and consumer research groups would balk. Somehow the idea of thwarting potential but dubious disease at the cost of serious complications, including depression and even death—not to mention hundreds of dollars—just doesn't cut it. Sure, a woman without a uterus is an unlikely target for endometrial cancer. But by the same token, a castrated male is an unlikely candidate for testicular cancer. And you can bet your bottom dollar few men would be willing to put their money and masculinity on the line based on such a flimsy rationale.

If a woman is fearful of cancer, offer her *reassurance*, not surgery, say the consumer advocates. Take the time to explain what cancer is, how it develops, her odds for developing it, risk factors she may be able to avoid, and how regular screening and early treatment can catch it before it kills—often with less mutilation than a hysterectomy. Should this information and education fail to convince her, perhaps she would benefit more from a psychiatrist's couch than a surgeon's table. At least it's worth a try.

Aside from the ethical issue, there's also the problem of justifying the bottom-line benefits. What exactly is to be gained—in terms of life years—by having the surgery before the disease actually occurs? Obviously, those who would have otherwise died from endometrial or cervical cancer stand to gain the most and those who wouldn't have gotten the disease in the first place, the least. But we don't know who's who. So public health authorities and statisticians work with averages. The interpretation of those figures varies with the source.

Those in favor of "preventive" hysterectomy say that women undergoing surgery by the age of 35 have a slightly longer life expectancy than those who do not have the operation. Those against—including Dr. Philip Cole—point out that this increase in life expectancy amounts to an average of only 0.2 years per woman, or roughly 2 to 2½ months. Ironically, this is the time it takes most women to have a hysterectomy and recuperate from the surgery.

Furthermore, in the book *Costs, Risks and Benefits of Surgery* (Oxford University Press, 1977), John P. Bunker, M.D., Benjamin A. Barnes, M.D., and Frederick Mosteller, Ph.D. add an important qualifying remark. According to these men, the increased life expectancy described above relates only to healthy premenopausal women. For the patient who is less healthy or older—for example, a 50-year-old woman with moderately high blood pressure—life expectancy is *shortened* by elective hysterectomy as a result of the tremendous surgical risks.

Discussion shouldn't wind down once the decision to operate has been made. There's much more you should know and there are even a few more decisions you may be involved in.

Will the Ovaries Be Removed, Too?

For starters, find out exactly what your surgeon intends to remove. It may sound silly, but despite the popularity of this procedure, many women are not clear on what a hysterectomy entails. The term hysterectomy refers to the removal of the uterus. Period. Whether your physician chooses to call it a "simple" hysterectomy, a "complete" hysterectomy, a "pan-hysterectomy" or a "total" hysterectomy, technically they all mean the same thing—the removal of the body of the uterus plus its cervix. Two less common procedures include the "subtotal" hysterectomy, which implies the removal of the body of the uterus without the cervix and the "partial" hysterectomy in which only a portion of the body of the uterus is removed. The "radical" hysterectomy, as we mentioned earlier, is a more extensive procedure in which the uterus plus adjacent lymph nodes and possibly part of the vagina goes, usually to stop the spread of cancer.

Whatever the case, you'll notice that none of these terms includes the removal of the ovaries or fallopian tubes. Although about half of all hysterectomies are performed in conjunction with the removal of these adjacent structures, the procedure is referred to separately with a very long fancy term: bilateral salpingo-oophorectomy. Salpingo refers to the fallopian tubes; oophor, to the ovaries; ectomy, to the removal of; bilateral simply means both sides. Therefore, a bilateral salpingo-oophorectomy means removal of both tubes and ovaries.

Unfortunately, even physicians become casual in their terminology and may at times use words like "total hysterectomy" or "complete clean-out" to mean the removal of the uterus plus ovaries. Your best bet is to check with your surgeon and have him or her spell out exactly what you can expect.

If the procedure planned for you includes a bilateral salpingo-oophorectomy, that's definitely something you should know about beforehand. And, depending on the circumstances, it may be one decision in which you'll have a voice.

Every physician we consulted agreed that the patient has the right to decide whether or not she shall retain one or both ovaries. (Most physicians do maintain that retaining one ovary or even a part of an ovary should preserve hormone production.) This, of course, is contingent upon the health of the ovaries and the extent of uterine disease—something which cannot always be determined prior to the surgery. But the variables should be discussed fully and the patient's wishes clearly made known to the surgeon before any consent forms are signed.

Generally speaking, physicians favor the let-be policy for healthy ovaries in any woman under 40 years of age. This woman has not yet reached menopause, so the removal of her ovaries would abruptly cut off her estrogen supply and throw her into a sudden "change of life." And since surgical menopause is notoriously more severe than natural menopause with its gradual tapering off of estrogen, most physicians would just as soon leave the ovaries in if at all possible.

For women over 45 or past menopause, many surgeons believe there's no further need for the ovaries; they've already slowed down their estrogen pro-

duction. And since cancer of the ovary, an extremely virulent and elusive disease, becomes a potential threat in postmenopausal women, physicians often suggest oophorectomy as a preventive measure. In fact, a few go so far as to insist that leaving the ovaries in the postmenopausal patient borders on criminal negligence.

That may be a bit extreme. The mortality rate for ovarian cancer is about 10 per 100,000—less than the number of women who die each year from complications directly attributable to pregnancy and delivery. Also, the ovaries *do* continue to release a trickle of estrogen after menopause—even up to age 60 in some women.

But it is true that the ovaries are susceptible to a whole host of ills. And occasionally, the woman who declines to have them removed at the time of hysterectomy may find herself submitting to a second surgical procedure later to rid herself of a painful or even life-threatening ovarian situation.

On the other hand, the woman who has them removed and then makes up for the lost hormone by taking replacement estrogen may be incurring a whole new set of risks. Of course, as a hysterectomy patient, she won't have to fear the development of endometrial cancer, the major risk related to synthetic estrogen. But other studies have shown that she may have a greater than average chance of developing benign breast cysts and possibly breast cancer (*Journal of the American Medical Association*, October 13, 1978).

Another question to be resolved ahead of time is whether your physician proposes to do the surgery through an abdominal incision or through the vagina. There are advantages and disadvantages to both. For example, those who favor the vaginal hysterectomy point out that postoperative pain, hospitalization, and recuperation time are reduced simply because there is no incision. Also, for some women concerned with scars, this approach has definite psychological benefits. On the other hand, those who prefer to perform abdominal hysterectomies shake their finger at the high rate of infections and possible foreshortening of the vagina incurred during vaginal hysterectomies. They also argue that blatant pelvic disease might be missed by operating blindly from below. To get the full picture of pelvic condition, they say, you've got to go in through the abdomen.

Actually, you probably won't have to wrestle with this decision. It's more than likely that the nature of your problem will dictate the appropriate hysterectomy approach. For example, if you're undergoing surgery for a prolapse problem, the uterus is already on its way out via the vagina; the surgeon has just to complete the job. On the other hand, if the uterus is being removed because of a large fibroid, chances are the physician wouldn't be able to deliver it through the vagina, anyway.

Many times, too, the approach is determined by your physician's area of expertise. Robert Henry Barter, M.D., professor of gynecology at George Washington University in Washington, D.C., and member of the Society of Vaginal Surgeons, believes that although 70 percent of all hysterectomies could be handled successfully through the vagina, most physicians prefer not to do them because they just don't know how. "It's a much more demanding type of surgery," he told us. "You need special equipment, special lighting and so forth. Besides which, you must have special training. There are very few people in this country capable of performing them properly."

Obviously, then, it would do you little good, and possibly some harm, to insist that your physician perform a vaginal hysterectomy when he's skilled in doing abdominal procedures. If you are determined to have a vaginal hysterectomy, you might be better off finding a surgeon who performs them frequently.

Or, if it's just a matter of placating your vanity, talk to your physician about the placement of the incision. According to Dr. Birnbaum, the strongest and least noticeable scar is one that runs horizontally across the pubic hairline. The stress of the muscles pulls the incision closed so it heals very nicely. Also, once your hair has grown back, the scar will be neatly hidden. Who said your two-piece was destined for the Salvation Army?

Fear of a flabby belly following abdominal hysterectomy is also unfounded, says Dr. Birnbaum. Of course, a lot hinges on what you've got to start with. But if you're toned up before surgery, there's no reason why you can't be as firm and flat afterward, because, with rare exception, the muscles are not cut. They're just pulled back, so that the surgeon can get to the organs underneath. That little bit of stretch—nothing compared to pregnancy—can be shaped up with some bent-knee sit-ups and other exercises once the incision is completely healed.

Don't Rush Recovery

It takes a long while to get over the trauma of hysterectomy. You'll feel weak, tired and maybe even a little weepy for several weeks after the surgery. And although physicians insist categorically that recuperation should not take longer than a month or two, sometimes it does. And there's nothing abnormal about it.

One woman we spoke with told us that it took her a year to completely recover from the "wiped-out" feeling. She even felt guilty because her physician acted as if she were dragging out recuperation in order to elicit attention and sympathy. Another woman explained that she had been programmed before the surgery to think that recuperation was going to be a breeze. When the pain, depression and weakness was with her four months later, she sought another physician. The second physician just reiterated the opinion of the first—recuperation from surgery shouldn't take longer than two months. "I know," he said, "I had a hernia operation a couple of years ago."

Unfortunately, some physicians treat hysterectomy as "just another operation." Anyone who's gone through it will tell you that it's just not so. Cutting deep into the abdomen and removing and rearranging internal organs produces deep wounds that take time to heal. In addition, hysterectomy is commonly followed by several distressing symptoms not related to other operations. According to British physician D. H. Richards, 70 percent of his hysterectomy patients had postoperative depression and an almost equal number had hot flashes, urinary symptoms and extensive tiredness. About half suffered headaches, dizziness or insomnia postoperatively (*Lancet*, October 26, 1974).

For that reason, convalescence cannot be rushed. Dr. Mikuta warns his patients to stay away from work for six weeks. And that includes housework. No heavy lifting (more than 5 to 10 pounds). No pushing a vacuum cleaner. Also, hold off with intercourse until your first postoperative check.

Aside from the vast amount of physical mending that's required after this major surgical procedure, there are also psychological wounds to heal. The uterus is a very intimate and personal organ, closely tied up to a woman's image of femininity and self so that feelings of self-doubt, loss of femininity, sexual inadequacy, barrenness and depression frequently follow its removal. And while many women are reluctant to discuss these problems with their physicians, about half suffer some psychological effects within the years following surgery.

"Women need reassurance that the loss of their uterus is not going to alter their functioning as a woman," says Evalyn Gendel, M.D., director of the Human Sexuality Program at the University of California School of Medicine, San Francisco. "It won't make her any less of a woman sexually."

Preparing Yourself Psychologically

Dennis Smith, M.D., a gynecologist and psychiatrist at Case Western Reserve Medical School in Cleveland, goes on to suggest that the psychological trauma of hysterectomy may be prevented or at least lessened with presurgical counseling.

"First of all, a woman has the right to know exactly what she can and cannot expect from the surgery. That way she is emotionally prepared for any consequences," he explains. "For example, women are repeatedly told that the hysterectomy will have *no* effect on their sexual relations. Yet one of the most common problems women report is that the sensation of intercourse is different. They may still enjoy sex and still have orgasm but something has changed. For some women the difference may be the absence of the cervix; perhaps they had gotten some pleasure from cervical contact. For others it may be that the uterus isn't there anymore so they miss the sensation of uterine contractions during orgasm. Actually, it's not too much to deal with—unless, of course, it completely takes her by surprise."

Second, says Dr. Smith, a woman should plunge into her psyche *before* plunging into surgery. It's important that she evaluate her own feelings of femininity and self prior to the surgery. "I can think of a woman right now who has severe pain caused by endometriosis and who would greatly benefit from a hysterectomy," Dr. Smith explains. "She came to me in anticipation of the surgery to discuss a psychological hang-up. Apparently she didn't want any more children but she was having trouble coping with the anticipated loss of her ability to give birth. We discussed

the issue openly. And her eventual decision was to put up with the pain rather than go through with the surgery. I respect that decision. She must come to peace with herself. And this must be done *before* the act is committed.

"Probably the most important consideration is in understanding why the surgery is being performed," Dr. Smith adds. "Pump your physician for information. If you still don't understand, get a second opinion from someone who is willing to sit down and discuss your situation. Don't stop until you can go to yourself and answer without hestitation why the surgery is needed. Women who understand the reason for the loss— even though they may still feel it—are better able to come to terms with any problems that may occur afterwards."

INFERTILITY

It takes two people to make a baby. So if infertility strikes, it's a problem for two people to solve. Contrary to popular belief, it's not always the woman's "fault" when pregnancy fails to occur. In fact, men as often as women have some condition which prevents them from successfully reproducing. Or, in other cases, it's a combination of factors both male and female.

But how do you know if you've even got a problem? Experts say that 80 percent of women (having regular intercourse) will become pregnant within one year, and that increases to 90 percent by two years. So if you have not conceived a baby by that time, chances are something's out of kilter. Of course, if you're over age 30 you probably shouldn't wait around that long before seeking professional help, since the

chances of pregnancy decrease rapidly as you grow older.

Also, if there are any very obvious symptoms such as no menstrual periods or very irregular ones, you should see your clinician right away. (For 10 to 15 percent of couples that's just the case.)

But sometimes the lack of conception isn't due to something so apparent. Fallopian tubes or vas deferens (the sperm-carrying duct) may be blocked (as is the case for 30 to 35 percent of infertile couples), or there may be hostile cervical mucus (20 percent of the cases) or the man may have impaired sperm production or delivery (which happens 40 percent of the time).

To find out what's going on behind the scenes, doctors can turn to a whole battery of diagnostic tests, some simple and some elaborate.

Since it's easier to identify a male-related problem, your doctor will want to start with your partner. That means he will have to submit a specimen of semen for analysis. One look under a microscope and your doctor will know in a flash whether there are enough sperm to make a baby. (It takes at least 20 million sperm per milliliter or 70 million per ejaculation.) He'll also be able to tell if they are champion swimmers (at least 60 percent should be) and whether at least 60 percent are normally shaped.

There are any number of reasons why testes may produce too few or abnormal sperm. Conditions such as mumps, prostatitis (inflammation of the prostate), gonorrhea, hepatitis, hormonal factors—even a testicular injury—can do it. One common cause is varicose veins of the testes (varicocele) which somehow damage sperm. The good news here is that they are easily detected and often correctable with minor surgery.

Sperm Isn't What It Used to Be

A less obvious reason for a low sperm count (but still of great concern because of the implications for future generations) is toxic chemicals in the workplace. It seems that the average number of sperm men are producing has dropped by almost half during the last 30 years according to several studies—from an average of 107 million per milliliter to 62 million per milliliter.

Some researchers point out that during the same 30 years that sperm counts have been declining, our use of toxic substances has steadily increased, with thousands entering the environment each year.

"The so-called eye-opener to the problem of male infertility due to occupational exposure was a pesticide called dibromochloropropane (DBCP)," says Donald Whorton, M.D., a specialist in occupational medicine at the University of California at Berkeley. "It's an emerging field which will require years of research. We do know that the damage caused by DBCP is dose-dependent. And that goes for its reversibility as well. Where the sperm count has been decreased, it takes three months to a year to return to normal. But where the sperm count has been reduced to zero, it may take up to six years to come back—if ever."

Occupational exposure to lead, kepone, microwaves, chloroprene—all have had documented effects on male reproduction.

Even something as seemingly innocuous as excessive heat in the workplace can have adverse effects on male fertility. So can tight underwear, for exactly the same reason—high temperature in the scrotal area.

Heat is deadly to sperm. But that's not all that is. Cimetidine, a drug routinely used in the management of peptic ulcers, will do them in, as will sulphasalazine, a medicine used to treat ulcerative colitis. In fact, coffee, cigarettes, marijuana and alcohol can be sperm enemies, too.

While a controlled study comparing the amount of alcohol consumed to an actual decrease in sperm count has not been done, Jeanne Manson, Ph.D., says the evidence strongly suggests a connection between the two.

Dr. Manson, of the Kettering Laboratory at the University of Cincinnati, also reports that there are studies that do show a connection between *smoking* and sperm. It seems that the percentage of misshapen sperm is directly related to the number of cigarettes smoked daily. And men who smoked longer than 10 years increased their disadvantage (*Work and the Health of Women*, CRC Press, 1979).

Marijuana smokers have abnormal sperm, too—what's left of them. Gabriel G. Nahas, M.D., of Columbia University's College of Physicians and Surgeons, reports that experiments show men who smoked marijuana at least four times a week for six months had a decrease in sperm numbers in proportion to the amount smoked, falling to almost zero in some very heavy users (*Keep Off the Grass*, Pergamon Press, 1979).

Although the effect of caffeine on human sperm has not been studied, its effect on animals has. According to Paul S. Weathersbee, Ph.D., of the University of Washington's Alcoholism and Drug Abuse Institute in Seattle, both rats and roosters showed a complete absence of sperm three weeks after being fed caffeine. That could be of some consequence to the man who normally consumes more than 600 milligrams per day of caffeinated beverages, says Dr. Weathersbee. That's about six to eight cups of coffee a day.

Fertility for the man clearly centers around his ability to produce viable sperm in ample quantities. On the other hand, the woman's reproductive status is, understandably, much harder to assess. After all, the machinery is not only hidden from view but there are more parts that can malfunction.

When It's the Woman's Problem

Still, if the sperm count is normal, the next step is to check out the condition of the woman's fallopian tubes, ovaries, cervical mucus and hormone levels.

Basal body temperature is often the first diagnostic test to find out whether or not you are ovulating (see Natural Birth Control). If your ovaries, pituitary gland or thyroid gland is not up to par in hormone production, then the egg will be released sporadically or not at all.

If the temperature test is inconclusive, then your doctor may decide to do a biopsy of your endometrium (uterine lining). Done in the doctor's office, this test not only measures the hormones progesterone and estrogen, but also can tell whether the endometrium can maintain a fertilized egg. Blood tests will also evaluate the hormone levels, since these substances do circulate throughout the body. A high progesterone level is one way of confirming that ovulation did occur.

But what good does it do to have a readily available egg if the sperm can't get to it? And sometimes the sperm are thwarted in their effort because of hostile cervical mucus. A simple test can be done to determine if yours is setting up barriers to the army of sperm trying to gain entry. The doctor takes a sample of mucus from the cervical canal on the estimated day of ovulation and several hours after sexual intercourse.

As you near ovulation, your mucus should change from thick and sticky to thin and slippery, actually aiding the sperm on their journey. If, upon microscopic examination, however, the doctor sees only dead sperm, then the mucus is not of the friendly variety.

Still, once through the cervical mucus, the sperm need clear sailing through the fallopian tubes. If those are clogged or blocked for some reason, the sperm will never be able to unite with the egg which is traveling up from the opposite direction. Pelvic inflammatory disease (PID) is notorious for causing this condition (see Intrauterine Device [IUD]), as is endometriosis.

Finding out if your tubes are open or closed involves a fairly elaborate procedure. Either the physician can check for the passage of carbon dioxide gas through the tubes (Rubin test) or he or she can use a special x-ray which employs the use of a dye through the tubes (hysterosalpingography). If those methods fail to reveal anything conclusive, then a laparoscopic examination may be necessary (see Sterilization). The laparoscope gives the doctor a bird's-eye view of the condition of the tubes as well as the uterus, ovaries and pelvic cavity. However, this procedure requires a hospital setting and often general anesthesia.

As we said earlier, sometimes the man has a problem, sometimes the woman does, but in about 20 percent of infertile couples, it's a combination of factors.

Of course, any of the above conditions can contribute to that, but there's also the unique condition of sperm antibodies. Sometimes the woman develops antibodies against her partner's sperm, killing them off as if they were invading disease germs. But it's not uncommon for a man to develop antibodies to his own sperm, causing them to clump together and swim abnormally.

Successful Treatments

But whatever the problem turns out to be, there are lots of successful treatments we can tell you about which should bolster your spirits along with your fertility. Some of the methods involve surgery, some drugs, but many are as easy as eating the right foods.

When the problem is obstruction of the tubes, whether fallopian or vas deferens, then surgery, especially microsurgery, can offer a fair chance for success. Cervical mucus consistency can be improved with very small doses of estrogen taken before ovulation. And ovulation itself can be stimulated to occur about 80 percent of the time with the help of two fertility drugs: Clomid (clomiphene citrate) and Pergonal.

Even though the drug claims sound very promising, only about 50 percent of those who ovulate actually conceive and give birth to healthy babies. But you may be able to improve that percentage with vitamin C. This vitamin has been shown to work in some cases where those fertility drugs can't. Masao Igarashi, M.D., a Japanese gynecologist, tried vitamin C, by itself and in combination with the fertility drug clomiphene, in infertile women who had not responded to traditional clomiphene therapy. In two out of five women who habitually failed to ovulate, vitamin C did the trick by itself. Vitamin C and clomiphene combined corrected that problem in five out of five cases, and worked much better than clomiphene alone against several other classes of infertility (*International Journal of Fertility*, vol. 22, no. 3, 1977).

Again the vitamin seems preferable to the drug just in terms of simplicity. Dr. Igarashi describes the case of one sterile woman who did not respond to drug treatment. "In spite of the lack of effect with clomiphene, administration of a daily 400 milligrams of ascorbic acid [vitamin C] succeeded in induction of ovulation and conception. Afterwards, she delivered a normal baby at full term."

In some women infertility is unexplained. But there may be hope for them, too—hope in the form of vitamins B_{12} and B_6.

Speaking recently at a conference on nutrition and reproduction held at the National Institutes of Health in Bethesda, Maryland, Jo Anne Brasal, M.D., noted that some women who cannot conceive—and for whom no medical reason can be found—may be deficient in vitamin B_{12}. Moreover, documented evidence has shown that conception leading to the birth of a normal infant may occur within a few short months of B_{12} therapy.

Others may find new possibilities for pregnancy in high doses of vitamin B_6, according to the findings of two gynecologists, Joel T. Hargrove, M.D., of Columbia, Tennessee, and Guy E. Abraham, M.D., of Rolling Hills, California. Twelve of 14 patients who had been infertile from 18 months to seven years were finally able to conceive after vitamin B_6 therapy. The study participants, ranging in age from 23 to 31, shared one thing in common—premenstrual tension, says Dr. Hargrove. Vitamin B_6 was given daily in doses ranging from 100 to 800 milligrams, depending on the dose needed to relieve each patient's tension symptoms. Of the 13 pregnancies that resulted (one woman conceived twice), 11 occurred within the first 6 months of therapy, one occurred in the 7th and the last occurred in the 11th month of the program.

Although not sure how the vitamin may have helped the patients become pregnant, Dr. Hargrove says there was a significant increase in levels of progesterone (a natural hormone which prepares the lining of the uterus to receive a fertilized egg) in five of seven women studied.

But vitamins and minerals aren't for women only. Men can improve both their sperm numbers and motility (the ability of sperm to move in a forward direction) by downing adequate amounts of vitamins A and C as well as zinc, calcium, magnesium and manganese.

Natural Help for the Male

In one study, male rats were fed a diet low in vitamin A from three weeks to about four months of age. The vitamin A deficiency they developed caused degeneration and loss of sperm cells. The dependence of such cells on vitamin A was supported by the appearance of new sperm within six weeks following vitamin A treatment (*Biology of Reproduction,* November, 1979).

In another study, Earl B. Dawson, Ph.D., of the University of Texas Medical Branch in Galveston, measured the effects of a vitamin C preparation (which also contained calcium, magnesium and manganese) on 20 men with spermagglutination, (a condition associated with antibodies), where sperm stick together in clumps and are unable to swim normally. Seven men were used as controls and received no vitamin C. All 27 men (ages 25 to 38) had been diagnosed as infertile, having decreased motility and relatively low sperm counts, the associated factors which make the clumping problem such bad news.

After 60 days, all 20 men taking the vitamin C preparation (one gram per day) had impregnated their wives, while none of the men in the control group had. And not only had the vitamin C preparation reversed the spermagglutination, but it had also raised sperm *counts* by 54 percent (*Fertility and Sterility,* October, 1979).

"These results," says Dr. Dawson, "suggest the possibility of a cooperative action between the metabolism of vitamin C and the essential metals studied which are vital in sperm physiology."

Spermagglutination has, by some estimates, been implicated as a cause of male infertility in as many as 10 percent of all cases. Which means that over 150,000 men in the U.S. population could have a spermagglutination problem affecting their ability to father children.

"Perhaps," speculates Dr. Dawson, "supplements of vitamin C, calcium, magnesium or manganese can reverse spermagglutination routinely, eliminating the need to use a donor to impregnate the wife [artificial insemination]."

Zinc, too, has been used successfully to improve fertility. Ali A. Abbasi, M.D., an endocrinologist at a Veterans Administration hospital in Allen Park, Michigan, showed that even a mild zinc deficiency caused sperm counts to drop below the point of technical sterility. Supplemental zinc, however, returned sperm counts to normal.

Low semen zinc levels have also been associated with poor sperm motility. But Joel L. Marmar, M.D., a Cherry Hill, New Jersey, urologist, reported boosting the sperm motility index (percent and quality of sperm that move) an average of 33 percent by giving zinc sulfate to men with low semen zinc levels.

The object of supplementing your diet with these nutrients is to improve as many fertility factors as possible—that is, the ones you have some control over.

But along with nutritional supplementation there are other ways both you and your partner can make the most of what you've got. Here are a few quick tips:

- Keep your weight close to normal. Extremes of either kind (whether too fat or painfully thin) may affect the monthly release of an egg from the ovary.
- Keep a record of your menstrual cycles to help you figure out your fertile days. (See Natural Birth Control for information on how to chart your cycle.)
- Have sexual intercourse every 24 to 48 hours during your fertile period. More frequent intercourse will actually decrease your chances because sperm become depleted and need time to regenerate.
- Remain on your back with a pillow under your hips and knees drawn up for 15 to 30 minutes after intercourse.
- Don't douche.
- Men can improve sperm production with exercise and proper diet, by cutting back on alcohol, cigarettes and coffee, and possibly by wearing loose-fitting underwear.
- And both of you should try to relax, since physical and emotional stress can interfere with fertility. Of course you're anxious to have a baby, but you can still have fun while you're trying!

INTRAUTERINE DEVICE (IUD)

"I was pretty sure I didn't want any more children but at 22 I didn't want anything permanently done, like sterilization, and I didn't want to take any chances with the Pill. So my doctor fitted me with an IUD—the coil. Everything was fine—until the seventh year of use. Then the problems started. First there were heavier periods, then spotting between. There was pain, too, which started at about the same time, not a stabbing pain but a steady, constant ache. It even hurt during intercourse, which was something I'd never experienced before.

"My doctor had me come to his office to remove the IUD, but he said he had trouble finding it. He didn't say why or what had happened to it. Anyway, he managed to eventually remove it but it wasn't easy. He then gave me antibiotics to clear up the infection. That's what he said was the cause of all the pain and bleeding. But after three months on medication the pain was still there and my white blood cell count was very high, too, which—I was told—was a sure sign of serious infection.

"At this point I was hospitalized and three other ob-gyn specialists were called in for consultation. Each one examined me. They talked plenty to each other but told me nothing. I guess they weren't even sure themselves what was going on because they said they had to operate to 'take a look.' When I woke up, I found that they took more than a look—they took out my uterus, fallopian tubes and my ovaries. That left me sterile and in menopause. I was only 29, for God's sake!

"Later, I asked the doctor who operated if he thought the infection was due to the coil. He looked straight at me and nodded, 'What do *you* think? Of course.'"

The Heartache You Don't Hear About

That's one woman's story. But, unfortunately, hers is not an isolated case. And the reason we're making a big deal of this is because most doctors don't. You practically never hear about all the heartache that the IUD has caused. What's so ironic, though, is that many women—like the woman who told us her story above—choose the IUD over the Pill because they think it's safe. It isn't.

Infection, also known as pelvic inflammatory disease (PID), hospitalizes about 50,000 IUD users each year. And there are another 200,000 whose infections are mild enough to be treated at home with drugs. But mild or severe, the end results can be disastrous. PID can involve just the uterus or it can spread to the tubes, ovaries and other pelvic structures. When that happens antibiotics may not be effective. That's because the body sometimes fights the infection by laying down scar tissue that is impermeable to drugs. This scar tissue (or adhesions) can also clog the tubes and ultimately cause sterility.

The symptoms as well as the infection can be anywhere from mild to severe, too. The woman quoted earlier actually suffered only mild symptoms. For some women the experience is even worse. Excruciating pain. High fever. Chills. A foul yellow discharge. And vaginal bleeding. On the other hand, it's possible to have no symptoms at all—but that doesn't mean you're out of danger.

With no symptoms, a woman may go on using the IUD until she's ready to have children, only to find out that her fallopian tubes are hopelessly blocked and her chances for motherhood have been destroyed.

True, not all infections lead to permanent damage. Most don't. But if you're a young woman, aged 16 to 19, your risk of infection and possible infertility is 10 times higher than for older women, aged 30 to 49 (*British Medical Journal*, July 12, 1980). And women who've never had children are at greater risk than those who have, no matter what their age.

Infertility is a hard enough pill to swallow when you desire children, but to be thrown into premature menopause is another matter altogether. And that's what can happen if the infection goes so far that drugs are no longer effective and a hysterectomy complete with the removal of the ovaries and fallopian tubes is required.

PID is about the worst possible complication of the IUD but it's certainly not the only one. And others can crop up the minute the IUD is inserted.

The IUD is believed to do its job by altering the lining of the uterus so that a fertilized egg cannot become implanted. It does this by causing a local inflammatory response inside the uterus, much like the local reaction you'd get if you had a splinter in your finger. Except a splinter is a minor inconvenience and your finger heals in a hurry with no lasting damage. No so with the IUD.

Be on the Lookout for These Symptoms

Increased pain and heavy bleeding are the complaints most often heard. In fact, anywhere from 3 to 35 percent of IUD users have it removed for just those reasons. It's not uncommon for the period to last two to four days longer than usual while loss of blood doubles or even triples over pre-IUD amounts. Anyone losing that much blood each month should take an iron supplement to prevent anemia (about five times the Recommended Dietary Allowance).

Increased menstrual cramps or pain from the IUD is common and may be severe at times. But pain can be a symptom of infection, too, so it's important to be able to distinguish one from the other. Cramping is usually intermittent, with real pain coming and going every few hours. But if you have pain that is continuous and lasts longer than

24 hours, an infection may be the cause and it should be reported at once to your doctor.

Some women, especially those who've never had children, cannot tolerate the IUD and the body expels it spontaneously. It may be because they have a small or abnormally shaped uterine cavity or just the fact that the IUD used was too small. At any rate, about 20 percent of those who expel their IUD are totally unaware of its disappearance, because they haven't routinely checked for the strings.

Of course, a missing string doesn't necessarily mean you've expelled the IUD. Sometimes the strings are drawn up through the cervix and into the uterus. Then you have no way of knowing if your IUD is where it should be. Your clinician will try to retrieve the strings by using a special narrow clamp. But if he is not successful, he will have to remove the IUD completely by grasping it with a contraption called alligator forceps.

Your strings may also disappear if your IUD has become embedded in the uterine wall or perforated the uterus completely. Usually that is due to faulty insertion techniques, but occasionally an IUD will gradually migrate on its own and settle in the abdominal cavity *outside* the uterus. In the process, it may entangle a loop of intestine, causing adhesions or dangerous inflammation. With those kinds of complications you'll have pain as the clue. But again there may be no symptoms at all, especially with the newer all-plastic models. Lost IUDs must be removed surgically. Unfortunately, some women don't discover the problem until pregnancy develops.

Although partial or complete expulsion of the IUD accounts for about one-third of the pregnancies, slipups can still occur if the IUD is perfectly in place. And while less than five percent of IUD users become pregnant, the consequences can be grave. The likelihood of miscarriage, for example, is very high—about 50 percent, compared to about 15 percent for other pregnancies. Worse yet, miscarriage often occurs late in pregnancy—after six months—making it even more dangerous with a higher risk of hemorrhage and serious infection. One study revealed that as many as 95 percent of those who miscarry with the IUD show signs of infection (*Journal of Reproductive Medicine,* March, 1978).

What's more, the combination of pregnancy and infection is potentially fatal for an IUD user. Removing the device as soon as a pregnancy is discovered helps decrease the chances of serious infection. And knowing the symptoms to look for can help, too.

The usual signs of infection (abdominal pain, vaginal bleeding) don't always apply when pregnancy is involved. For that reason, don't ignore fever, nausea, headache and muscle aches (usually symptoms of the flu), for they may be the warnings that tip you off. And early diagnosis and treatment can make a significant difference in the outcome.

The likelihood of an ectopic, or tubal, pregnancy can be as much as nine times greater if you have an IUD than if you use any other method of birth control. It's believed that tubal pregnancies are more common in IUD users because of the greater incidence of tubal infections and the resulting scar tissue buildup. If the fallopian tube is blocked, the fertilized egg becomes trapped, implanting itself there instead of in the uterus where it belongs. Unless it's removed surgically, the growing em-

bryo can eventually rupture the narrow tube, causing massive internal bleeding or even death.

Symptoms of pregnancy along with lower abdominal pain and some dark vaginal bleeding should alert you enough to seek medical attention before the possible ectopic pregnancy reaches the bursting point.

Who—If Anyone—Should Use an IUD?

In spite of all the possible complications and risks involved with the IUD, the medical community still views it as a safe and effective method of family planning.

Safer for some than for others, it seems. Planned Parenthood says the "ideal" candidate for an IUD is a woman who is 25 years old, has had one baby, has one sexual partner, has never had venereal disease (VD), and has never had any pelvic infection. And even if you can find someone who fits that description, the statistics tell us she's probably not without risk either.

Still, some women may choose to take their chances in return for a birth control method that practically guarantees effectiveness. Theoretically, the IUD is between 95 and 99 percent effective. And for some women it's so convenient they call it a get-it-and-forget-it method. Except for checking the presence of the strings each month and a yearly visit to your gynecologist, there's nothing else to do.

There are about five popular models on the market right now. The Lippes Loop and Saf-T-Coil are plastic, and the Copper 7 and Copper T are partly wrapped in copper. One type, the Progestasert, releases the hormone progesterone which supposedly reduces heavy bleeding. But no one knows yet what the long-term effects of progesterone might be on the cervix or uterus. IUDs come in various sizes to accommodate different-size wombs. It's important for your doctor to fit you with just the right size. Too small and you may expel it without even realizing it, leaving yourself unprotected. Too large and it may become embedded in the wall of the uterus, or worse, it may perforate it.

Before an IUD is inserted your doctor should do an internal exam and Pap smear. A Pap smear tells him or her whether or not you are free of any infection in the pelvic region. That will lessen the chances of introducing bacteria (which could possibly initiate PID) into the uterus at the time of insertion.

It's best to have the IUD inserted *during* your menstrual period. At that time your cervix is softer and more open and you can also be sure that you're not pregnant. Many women find the procedure quite painful. When nerves are stimulated in the cervical area it can lead to nausea and fainting. For that reason oxygen is usually kept nearby. After it's inserted your doctor should show you how to check for the strings which hang out of the cervix about an inch. That's how you know it's where it should be.

Protection from pregnancy starts immediately upon insertion but additional protection is still recommended during the first month since expulsion rates are highest during that time. Always be on the lookout for complications which could turn up down the road. And see a doctor immediately if something—anything—doesn't seem right.

LICHEN PLANUS

What's a curious skin condition like lichen planus doing in a book on women and natural healing? Well, for reasons yet unknown, lichen planus is twice as common in women as in men. And, according to a couple of fairly recent studies, these unremitting skin eruptions (which were colorfully described by the dermatologist we consulted as "puzzling, persistent, purple, polygonal plaque") do appear to respond to nutritional therapy.

In an Australian study, blood tests were taken on 58 persons (44 of them women) with lichen planus sores in their mouths. Interestingly enough, 41 of the 58 patients were either severely or marginally deficient in various vitamins—most commonly in vitamins B_1 (thiamine), B_6 and C.

According to Mark Jolly, D.D.Sc., professor of oral medicine and oral surgery at the University of Sydney, and Silvia Nobile, Ph.D., director of the vitamin laboratories of Roche Products in Sydney, subsequent vitamin therapy did not completely eradicate the problem. However, 20 of the 41 deficient patients showed "good improvement" and 9 "some improvement" following the supplementation. And 27 of those were able to maintain that improvement during long periods of vitamin therapy—which is as good a track record as conventional treatment with cortisone can claim.

But what makes this study particularly noteworthy is the fact that many physicians believe lichen planus is related to stress. Personality studies of persons suffering from this condition—similar to those studies that linked the "Type A" personality with heart disease—suggest that lichen planus victims are pleasant people who tend to internalize their emotions.

If this is the case, and if stress is the culprit responsible for the disorder, then the B vitamins with C (the so-called stress supplements) may just be the key to prevention in the first place. Particularly for women, who tend to bear the burden of depression and anxiety twice as frequently as men.

In addition to that, vitamin A appears to hold some promise for lichen planus victims. In another study—this time in New Delhi, India—140 patients suffering from this skin condition were given vitamin A in dosages of 100,000 international units a day for 15 days. That was followed by another 15 days of rest with no treatment.

While the dropout rate for this study was very high, those who did continue with the treatment showed significant improvement. For example, after 4 to 6 courses of treatment, 6 out of 19 experienced good to excellent results, and after 10 or more courses, 9 out of 12 patients were practically freed from this incessant problem.

We should mention here, however, that vitamin A can be toxic in large doses. And since this treatment does involve large "therapeutic" dosages, you should proceed cautiously and only under a doctor's supervision.

LIFESTYLE COUNSELING

Chances are we'd all like to nudge our daily routine here and there to make room for more healthful habits and activities. Maybe you've already tried. Perhaps you take a good long walk at lunch. Or swim before you sup. Maybe you've revamped your refrigerator repertoire in favor of fresh, wholesome foods. Or tried to gradually reduce the red meat in your diet. Each one of these efforts is a step in the right direction. But if you really want to make strides toward optimum health, you probably should be doing all that plus more.

"No time," you say.

"What's left?" you ask.

You'd be surprised how many wonderful little health bonuses you can sandwich in in a day. And what a difference each day can make in the way you look and feel.

"The trick is to step back and look for missing links—weaknesses in your lifestyle that could be weakening your health," says Dyveke (pronounced DER-vi-ka) Spino, Ph.D., a dynamic and multitalented lady whose experiences as world-class jogging coach, tennis pro, concert pianist, and psychology professor have given her much insight into the wide variety of lifestyle changes that can put your mind and body in perfect harmony and keep you on the winning side of health. Today, Dyveke directs a training institute in Santa Barbara, California, which sponsors seminars and trainings based on her book, *New Age Training for Fitness and Health* (Grove Press, 1979). She and her staff spend a good deal of time helping men and women imprint their lives with important health habits. Her model of lifestyle counseling has recently been developed into a series of films.

We sat in on a typical counseling session between Dyveke and a female client.

We have reprinted their conversation here as an example of the kinds of changes you may want to make in your own life.

Dyveke Spino: First of all, I'd like to give you a little overview of what we'll be doing today and then we'll go free flow. What I do is look at the full spectrum of your life—your day's schedule, your thoughts, your ideas, your activities. I'd also like to find out who you are; what you want; what your wildest dreams are; what sports you like; what physical things you've done in the past; what hang-ups you have about your body. I'll be looking for the missing links. What we're aiming for is endurance, strength, flexibility, and inner peace or freedom from stress. And, of course, nutrition. Why don't we start out with what your current life is. Tell me a little about yourself.

Client: I'm an assistant manager in a bank. I'm married; no children. My husband and I like to play tennis and bicycle but we've had less and less time for that since we've gotten involved in renovating an old house. Not only that, I grew up in a family of workaholics, so that I feel guilty when I do anything but work.

Dyveke Spino: How old are you and how long have you been married?

Client: I'm 27 and have been married for three years.

Dyveke Spino: Okay. First of all, let's take a look at your work environment. Is there a lot of noise?

Client: Right now, my office opens onto a main thoroughfare. It gets quite a bit of traffic. But that doesn't bother me too much. What I do object to is the fact that I'll soon be moving to another branch where the offices are painted with very bright colors. The windows are high above eye level so that it's impossible to see anything out of them save the sky. They are also tinted and fixed so they cannot be opened.

Dyveke Spino: That doesn't sound good. Health is very much determined by your environment and when you're in an environment that, first of all, you have negative attitudes toward; second, that is painted with bright colors; and third, that has no windows to speak of, that means you have a lack of inspiration.

To counteract the bright colors and lack of windows, hang a mural on one wall—pick a pastoral scene, or something that soothes you. And then fill your office with lots of plants. Potted plants not only give off negative ions but lots of oxygen—two things you may be short of in a small enclosed space.

Do you sit all day?

Client: Yes, most of the day. I do get up and down to greet customers or walk over to the teller's window for one thing or another. But that's just a couple of steps away.

Dyveke Spino: Oh, my goodness. Do you take any breaks during the day?

Client: I do, yes. I can't sit in one place for more than an hour or two. I get up and walk.

Dyveke Spino: That's exactly what you should be doing. Listen to your body—it will tell you that it needs to be moved and stretched. Do you feel under a lot of pressure or do you feel that you have time management under control?

Client: I feel a certain amount of pressure.

Dyveke Spino: So it's a high-pressure job.

Client: It's not a particularly high-pressure job; I believe it has to do with pressure I put on myself. I'm somewhat of a perfectionist and I push myself.

The Overachiever Syndrome

Dyveke Spino: It sounds to me that there's a syndrome here. You've got a touch of the "Type A." High-driving. Perfectionist. A bit of the overachiever. You don't take too much time to play. That's really part of our puritan ethic. You're groomed to feel that way after college. We have to learn to take that step back, and learn to be a little more gentle with ourselves. I bet you're very good at what you do.

Do you like your work?

Client: Oh, yes, very much.

Dyveke Spino: That's very important. If we're not happy with our job—something that, let's face it, takes up a good part of our life—it's bound to show up in our health. Of course, there's a certain amount of stress in any job. But if you like what you're doing, there are ways to deal with that stress. Let's see if your daily routine provides outlets.

Tell me about your morning.

Client: I'm not a morning person. Getting up is a drag. I hit the snooze alarm five times before I roll out of bed.

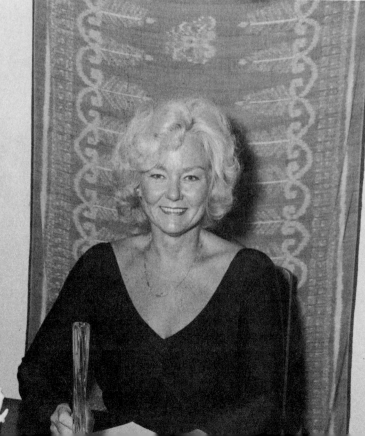

Fred Smith Assocs.

To keep on the winning side of health you've got to put your mind and body in perfect harmony, says Dyveke Spino, a psychologist and fitness expert. To do that, she suggests simple changes in lifestyle.

Dyveke Spino: Have you ever had your thyroid checked?

Client: Yes, I did. I went to see an internist once because I was so tired. He checked my thyroid, did a blood workup to see if I was anemic—the whole works. He couldn't find anything wrong with me. So he gave me a prescription for Valium and sent me on my way.

Dyveke Spino: He gave you Valium? Oh, that is horrible! We've opened up a Pandora's box because fatigue and depression and just feeling blah is the biggest complaint we get from people who come in here. Also all kinds of skin disorders, hair falling out, things like that.

You see, you're not a depressed person. You like your job. You have a good marriage. So you should feel a tremendous bounce in the morning. Excitement to get up. When you get the heaviness there are various reasons for it. Let's see what they might be. What time do you get up in the morning?

Client: Eight o'clock.

Dyveke Spino: That late? And what time do you go to bed at night?

Client: Oh, about midnight. After the news.

Dyveke Spino: You only get eight hours of sleep.

Client: Isn't that enough?

Dyveke Spino: Well, it depends. Everyone's different, you know. But what really bothers me is the time you go to bed. It's very important that you get sleep before midnight because the hours before 12 are the most restful.

You've already got that style of staying up late and then sleeping till 8. If we could switch that and get you to bed by 11 P.M. and up by 7 A.M., that would be much more of a natural rhythm. Maybe

you could get into the habit of watching the news earlier—say at 6 P.M. That would free you up later so you could get to sleep earlier. Besides, those blood-and-guts news accounts are not exactly conducive to restful sleep.

If you get, say, 20 to 30 percent more energy by doing two or three little things, if it's inspiring and fun, then you'll do it. If you don't get the feedback then you won't do it. So let's try that.

Another thing—the atmosphere in your bedroom. Since you live in the East, I assume that your house is heated in the winter. Right?

Client: Yes.

Designing Your Bedroom for True Rest

Dyveke Spino: The oxygen is probably burning out of your air. You should leave a little window open at night. Also, the closed-in, artificial atmosphere of a heated room is very low in negative ions. You know that beautiful feeling you get in San Francisco. It makes you feel exhilarated, alive. Well, that's because San Francisco is a very high negative ion city due to all the crosswinds and water around it. Negative ions are found near high mountains, around pine trees and oceans. What you must do is try to re-create this negative ion density in your bedroom at night so that you wake up exhilarated. The open window will help. So will potted plants which give off negative ions. Natural fabrics like cotton and wool also emit negative ions as opposed to synthetic fibers. So wear a cotton nightgown. And try to have cotton sheets and wool rugs if you can. You'll wake up more refreshed in the morning.

What do you do after you get up?

Client: I go to the bathroom. Let my dog out. Feed my cat.

Dyveke Spino: It's good that you go outside with the dog in the morning—you get fresh air. Doesn't that help wake you up?

Client: Well, I don't actually go out with him. I just open the door and let him romp in the backyard.

Dyveke Spino: Well, in that case, what you should do, at the very least, is take six to eight really good deep breaths at the door.

Being a Californian I never knew what it was like to grow up with any heat. When I was in Illinois, it was unbelievable. I'd wake up in the morning with this heavy head. I just couldn't get started. I just sort of dragged around. So I'd go over to the door and take a few deep breaths. That surge of oxygen to my brain would really get me going.

We're also going to think about getting your circulation going in the morning. What you need is a simple exercise that's non-weight-bearing, that's fun and interesting. See that thing behind you? It's a mini-trampoline. I have a feeling that what would be wonderful would be to have one at the bank (maybe in the lunchroom or women's lounge) which several people could use, and one at home. In the morning when you first get up you should be getting your circulation going, get the lymphatic system going. Just switch on a little music and hop on that trampoline for about five minutes. It will probably change your day. Just sort of dance and play on it.

Now, we've got the lymphatic system working. We're getting oxygen to the brain. You're starting the day with some fun and play that sort of balances out this puritan ethic guilt feeling of taking time for yourself. Also it will give you that additional cardiovascular workout that you need. Incidentally, it would also be a good idea to hop on this little

trampoline when you get home at night. Get a little bit of a workout. Maybe while you're watching the six o'clock news.

Client: Is five minutes enough to get that response?

Dyveke Spino: Oh, yes, one, two, three minutes is a lot on a trampoline. If you put music on, it's a lot of fun. It's playful. I think these trampolines are better than exercise bikes for a lot of people because the springing is non-weight-bearing. Unlike jogging on a hard surface, it doesn't put any strain on the ankles, knees or lower back. And, you see, tension and pressure register in the skeletal muscle system. You've got the beginning of rigidity along your back. And you're just a young woman, but 20 more years of that...this will help to reverse it.

Starting the Day Right

Dyveke Spino: Do you eat breakfast?

Client: Yes. I usually make myself a blender drink with a half cup of yogurt, a small banana, two tablespoons brewer's yeast, two tablespoons wheat germ, and some skim milk.

Dyveke Spino: And that's your breakfast? How marvelous. Do you take any supplements?

Client: When I think of it, but not consistently.

Dyveke Spino: For the stress, of course, you should be taking extra B vitamins and C. I recently worked with a vitamin C expert who worked with Linus Pauling. It's truly a remarkable vitamin. So get used to taking this vitamin C powder all the time. You just suddenly feel much brighter.

I'd sure like to see you take some

ascorbic acid (vitamin C)—at least two to three grams (½ teaspoon) a day. Put it in your breakfast drink. Your skin is a little bit dry, too, so why don't you put some lecithin (a teaspoon) in the drink, too. You won't even taste it. It's good for your skin. And it will keep your arteries clean as a whistle. We're looking at how to balance your body energy systems.

How do you use your lunch break?
Client: Well, I do belong to a health club so I go there at noon for about 20 minutes of exercise. It's not an elaborate setup. They conduct exercise classes and have some equipment, a Jacuzzi and sauna.

Dyveke Spino: What kind of exercises do you do?
Client: Oh, the usual thing. Five minutes on a stationary bicycle. Sit-ups on a slantboard. Toe-raises. Leg-lifts. I've been trying to concentrate on my legs lately. That's my weakest point.

Dyveke Spino: What about flexibility work? Do you do any yoga? Do you push any weights to strengthen?
Client: No.

Dyveke Spino: Yes, well, those are two of your missing links. See, you already have a misalignment in your body. Your head tilts forward. It's from your profession, sitting at a desk all day.

We'll give you a quick and light routine of yoga, The Seven Series (which works your spine in seven directions) to aid your flexibility. The first week, do it twice a week. The second week, take it to three times a week and hold it there for three weeks. Then the fifth week take it to four times a week. Anything after that is gravy. If you find you're doing it five, six, seven times a week, that's total gravy.

But I do think it's wonderful that you take a midday break like that. You'd definitely want to keep up that routine.

Do you go with some of the other women at work?
Client: One other woman.

Dyveke Spino: Great. Particularly with women it's important to have a training buddy. I think what you need to do is have a few more. Then you're bound to keep each other's motivation up.

Do you have a slump of energy in the afternoon?
Client: Yes, usually around 3 P.M. I get sleepy and have trouble concentrating.

Dyveke Spino: That's when the trampoline at work would do you good. The really beautiful thing about the trampoline is, you don't have to change your clothes, or redo your makeup. You don't work up a sweat.

Do you ever eat sweets at that time?
Client: Sometimes I'll have an apple or a banana.

THE SEVEN SERIES

Dyveke Spino's 10-minute yoga routine for a quick whole-body stretch.

1

2

3

Dyveke Spino: That's good. That's what we'd want you to do. Sometimes this slump is caused by low blood sugar or it might be due to a depletion of potassium. Since bananas are high in natural sweeteners and potassium, they make an excellent afternoon snack.

Now tell me about what you do in the evenings.

Client: Usually the minute I'm in the door I start cooking—even before I have a chance to change. While I have the rice on the stove or the chicken in the oven I make my quick change. Then it's back into the kitchen. We eat and then clean up. Then, if we're not out running around—going shopping or whatever—I usually plop into bed with a slew of magazines to read. The trouble is, by nine o'clock, I'm usually bushed.

Dyveke Spino: By nine o'clock? Oh, that's too bad. What kind of food do you prepare for dinner?

Client: Well, I try to make quick meals without compromising nutrition. Many nights I whip something up in my wok—chicken with stir-fried vegetables, pepper steak. Sometimes it's spaghetti with artichoke pasta and my own tomato sauce (which I canned in the summer). We've been trying to cut down on red meat, and since I don't like fish, we eat a lot of turkey and chicken. Once in a while I'll have an omelet and my husband will make himself some fish. I try to make a totally vegetarian meal at least once a week. In the wintertime, I often make a big pot of soup on the weekend which we have during the week. My husband's favorite meal is a bowl of soup and a large salad—usually with tuna fish and Swiss cheese. He's not hard to please.

Dyveke Spino: It sounds to me like you're getting pretty good nutrition. I'm glad to see that you're trying to cut back on the beef and pork. First of all, they're terribly high in saturated fats. And secondly, they're so shot full of hormones and antibiotics, they're just not good for you.

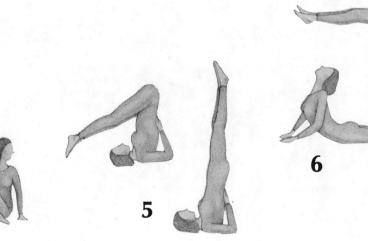

HOW TO MAKE ROOM FOR FUN

The old saying that a woman's work is never done was never truer than today. With families and jobs to juggle, old obligations and new priorities to iron out, plus all those miscellaneous things that demand perpetual care, women are busier than ever. The catch-22 of all this is that as these outside demands leave us less and less time for ourselves, we actually need more and more. But how do you cram fun into an already crowded schedule? Believe it or not, every schedule's got some spare time built in. Here's how to find it:

1. Get yourself a nice big tablet and write down each thing you do in a day and how long it takes you to do it. Include everything. How much time do you spend reading the morning paper? Readying yourself for work? Sipping coffee? Running errands? Preparing dinner? Sleeping?

2. Now, let's look at what you've got. Keep an eye open for dawdlings, time gaps, and unnecessary or redundant activities that take up more time than they're worth. For example, do you linger over a pot of coffee and the morning gazette for an hour and a half? Is your hour's lunch spent amidst friendly chatter and cigarette smoke chowing down a full-course meal, wine included? Do you collapse in front of the TV for an hour or two (maybe three) every evening? All of us have some moments like those—perhaps you even think of them as "time to myself," "time to relax," or even "fun." Stop kidding yourself: they're none of the above. The truth is, there's nothing more fun, energizing, and relaxing (that is, able to release tension and stress) than movement, exercise and its feel-good reverberations.

3. Now let's think of ways to rearrange our activities to free up some time. Some suggestions:

- If you spend two to three hours a night glued to the tube, peel yourself away early and go to bed. Then get an hour or two headstart in the morning—free time before breakfast to do the kinds of things that count.

- If your workday is interrupted by a leisurely lounge at a restaurant at lunch, brown-bag a light meal instead—one to eat at your desk—and spend your lunch hour enjoying yourself. Take a leisurely walk, join a health club, or, as Dyveke Spino recommends, keep a mini-trampoline close at hand and use it during this newfound time.

- If you consistently spend an hour or more preparing supper, get out of the kitchen. Many—and we must add, some of the most healthful—meals can be prepared in 30 minutes or less, and if time is at a premium, you shouldn't have to devote any more time than that at it. Stir-frying, which seals in foods' nutrients, takes about 10 minutes. The most time-consuming part about it is the preparation—cutting the foods into bite-size pieces. But even so, the whole operation should take no longer than a half hour. A pressure cooker can help boil down the usual 45 minutes for brown rice to about 20. Likewise, broiling, which is a very healthful way to prepare chicken and fish, takes all of 20 to 25 minutes. And just think of the time that frees up. Instead of flying home from work and into the kitchen, you can stop for a swim or jog around a park on the way home—and still have dinner on the table at approximately the same time.

- If you spend a good part of the day—every day—running errands, consolidate your efforts. Get into the habit of keeping lists. Grocery lists. Drycleaning lists. Appointment lists. Keep them in a visible spot like the refrigerator door or kitchen bulletin board. Then, on shopping day, or a day that you have a prearranged appointment, check what other errands you can take care of at the same time. Perhaps your dentist's office is just around the corner from a shoe repair place where you've got to go to get your boots reheeled. Or maybe it's a block away from your child's school and you can fill a 2 P.M. time slot and pick little Tommy up after school. It's a case of simple organization.

4. Overcome those guilt feelings. I don't know what it is about women, but we always seem to feel guilty about something. Not being home when the kids arrive from school. Not having dinner on the table for hubby when he steps through the front door. Not checking in with mom on a regular basis. Not being a hundred places at once just so we're available whenever and wherever we're needed.

Let's face it, we can't do it. No one can. And the funny thing is, when you get right down to it, nobody expects you to! In fact, all those people will manage very well without your constant attention. Oh, the initial transition will be touchy—after all, you've conditioned them to depend on you. But think of it this way: are you really giving your family as much as you could if you feel tired, worn out and unhappy? If you're not the best you could be in health and appearance? If you're not in touch with your own feelings, let alone those of everyone else? Ask yourself if it's possible, that by taking time to exercise, to become fit, to become more slender, you might actually be improving your relationship with your family. We think you might be surprised by the answer. Also, you can try these suggestions:

- To counteract strong guilt feelings, you need even stronger feel-good feelings. So choose an activity that you really enjoy—one that really makes you feel good and good about yourself. No one says you have to jog, if you don't like to. Maybe tennis is more to your taste. If you're not sure what kind of physical activity beckons you, choose a place instead. Do you enjoy the open spaces and fresh air of a park? Or the lovely formality and soft fragrances of a city rose garden? Then go to one of these spots and just walk or bicycle or, if the spirit moves you, jog.

- To ease the feeling that you've abandoned your family, take them along. There's sure to be at least one activity that you all can enjoy. Like swimming, folk dancing, tennis, hiking, ice skating or volleyball. Perhaps, satisfy their five o'clock hunger pangs with some cheese or raw veggies, then head off for some predinner excitement. Or make it a Saturday morning event.

What do you do then from 9:00 to 11:30 P.M.?

Client: Read or do work from the office or whatever—usually I'm in bed with the TV on.

Television and Your Energy

Dyveke Spino: You spend 2½ hours a night watching television?

Client: I don't really watch it. It's on for background more than anything else.

Dyveke Spino: That could also contribute to your fatigue. Because you have noise during the day, right? So you really don't have any quiet time. Why don't you start out the first week with one night a week without the TV? See if you feel any different. Also all that mind chatter—blood and guts and noise—goes into your head. There's so much of this mind chatter that we can't get down into our true feelings.

What do you talk with your husband about in the evenings?

Client: We share our day's experiences at work. We talk about our house. Future plans. Trips. Different things.

Dyveke Spino: Do you share any time during the week inspiring one another?

Client: How do you mean?

Dyveke Spino: Maybe reading great thoughts or going to a study group that's really uplifting.

Client: We took a transcendental meditation course once.

Dyveke Spino: Oh, wonderful. Did you keep it up?

Client: For awhile. Then it got harder to get out of bed in the morning. We'd skip that part. Then we'd decide that since we were missing the morning session, the evening wasn't doing us much good, so we'd skip that, too. We gradually drifted away from it. But I do wish we'd start up again. I really felt that it helped to unclutter my mind.

Dyveke Spino: Then you really should do it. Try it once a week to begin with. You shouldn't feel that missing a session a day defeats the whole benefit. You benefit every time you do it. Do you and your husband participate in any physical fitness activity on a regular basis?

Client: No, not usually.

Enjoying Life Together

Dyveke Spino: One night a week you and your husband should get out and play tennis or folk dance—something that is hilariously fun. Keep those interests alive. Chances are you'll develop a whole new set of friends—people who will support your athletic pursuits.

This is the time to lay the bridges for sports that you're going to keep up for the rest of your life. I played tennis the other day with a man who's 68 and he beat me.

Anyway, join the tennis club and you'll find that you and your husband will gradually get away from that evening rut in front of the TV.

It's extremely important to get one or two little things started that you truly play at—you have that sense of a joyous child again. . . . We don't ever really want to lose that.

You've heard them called liver spots and age spots—never sun spots. But that might well be a more appropriate name for those annoying brown splotches.

"At one time, they were thought to be due to liver disease. But they're not. They have nothing to do with age either, except that they tend to occur in older people." says Albert Kligman, M.D., Ph.D., professor of dermatology at the University of Pennsylvania Medical School. "They are areas of skin where the pigment cells are overproducing pigment. And they're entirely due to sunlight. Entirely. It's a foiled attempt to make a tan. You will never find an age spot in the armpit or under a bra."

Dr. Kligman also points out that these "sun spots" are a little different from the brown patches that occur during pregnancy—that "mask of pregnancy," as we know it, or "melasma" or "chloasma" as it is known in the dens of dermatology. Again it's a case of overproduction of pigment. But because they occur in pregnancy and in women who take oral contraceptives, there appears to be a hormone link. We say "appears to be." Dr. Kligman admits that the exact cause of chloasma just isn't known. And while it is known that the sun is *not* the cause, sunlight does activate it, he says. So again, if you don't go out in the sun, chances are you won't be plagued by either type of undesirable skin pigmentation.

But what about "sun spots" you've already got? Well, it's possible that they will fade in time, provided you lead a shady life. Some women also claim that lemon juice dabbed onto the spots daily will eventually lighten them somewhat.

Whatever you do, however, don't waste your money on a skin bleach.

The active ingredient in most over-the-counter skin bleaches today has been changed from ammoniated mercury (which is known to cause mercury poisoning) to hydroquinone, a chemical also used in photographic developers. When applied to the skin, hydroquinone suppresses specific enzyme activity within pigment-producing cells so they are unable to make pigment. The trouble is, says Dr. Kligman, who's spent years studying these bleaches, the low concentration of this chemical that is permitted in over-the-counter bleaches like Porcelana just isn't enough to produce the desired effect. In order to get results you have to use higher concentrations for prolonged periods of time.

According to a medical panel's 1978 report before the Food and Drug Administration (FDA), "prolonged use of high concentrations of hydroquinone with exposure to the sun may produce disfiguring effects." In one study, for example, researchers examined the effects of hydroquinone-containing bleaches on the highly pigmented skin of black women. Interestingly enough, the researchers found that the facial skin overcame the bleaching effect and in some cases grew *darker* than normal—particularly in areas that were exposed to the sun and where the cream had been rubbed in well. Thereafter, "novel" changes occurred in the skin—whatever that means.

For that reason, some skin bleaches now include sunscreens in their formula. But again, evidence brought out at the FDA hearings suggests that will not help. A major problem is that the wavelengths that produce tanning and pigment darkening extend into the visible spectrum. To block these waves, you'd have to use a broad-spectrum sunscreen or opaque sunscreen like zinc oxide.

So given the choice, it seems a good deal more practical to keep to the shade—rather than apply these skin bleaches *and* stay out of the sun.

LOVE

"Love is the total acceptance of another person," says Gerald Jampolsky, M.D., founder of the Center for Attitudinal Healing in Tiburon, California.

"Love is a relationship without shoulds or shouldn'ts. When we are in love, we accept," says Ari Kiev, M.D.

"In an ideal loving relationship we feel safe and accepted no matter what we do, we feel safe to be ourselves. When someone loves us freely, they should have no expectations or demands," says David Viscott, M.D.

Love, these psychiatrists say, is acceptance. And the opposite of acceptance is expectation. Not simply, "I love you," but "I'll love you if . . ." And many of us complete that sentence with: "I'll love you if you love me back."

"We all have a tendency to want to make deals with other people rather than to give without demands," says Harmon Bro, Ph.D., psychotherapist and former professor at Syracuse University in New York.

"It is this manipulative type of loving that blocks the full expression of love in our life," he told us.

"Loving with expectations is love that is conditional love," Dr. Viscott, a California psychiatrist and author of *How to Live with Another Person* (Priam, 1979), told us. "If you need the other person's love to feel good about yourself, you look up to him out of desperation. And you give love out of fear,

constantly worried that he might stop loving you. This isn't love, it's dependency with little joy or happiness in it."

Dr. Kiev, a psychiatrist from New York City and author of *Active Loving* (Crowell, 1979), explained how the marvelous spontaneity of love turns into the drudgery of a relationship full of expectations and demands.

"When we first begin to love someone, everything is new and sparkling. Our tendency is to try to hold on to that sparkle, to structure it, because we're afraid of losing it. But the minute we try to hold on, we destroy the relationship.

"We tend to hide our normal actions because we want to impress the other person to maintain that sparkle or magic feeling. We become afraid of showing our true feelings, or being open and vulnerable, because we think the person will stop loving us if we have imperfections. And since we don't allow the other person to see our imperfections, we usually don't allow them to show us theirs. We put shoulds and shouldn'ts on them that are impossible to meet.

"When we strive for this certainty, we shut off love. A relationship, which to be fulfilling must be sharing, giving and accepting, becomes full of pressures and expectations caused by the fear of losing it. That fear may destroy the relationship."

But it doesn't have to.

"The only way fear—or any other

negative emotion—can destroy a relationship is if we don't let the other person know what we're feeling," says Peter Hansen, a therapist consultant from St. Paul, Minnesota, who has conducted over 500 workshops on love and relationships.

"It's very important to verbalize feelings," agrees Dr. Kiev. "You may think you'll get a negative response, but you probably won't. Everyone really wants to be honest, and it feels so good to just open up and share with someone what you're feeling. They'll appreciate your openness, because it allows them to be open, too, and to share vulnerabilities.

"However, don't say, 'You hurt me,' or 'You made me angry.' Just talk about yourself: 'I feel hurt when you act that way,' or 'I feel angry when you do that.'

"When you express your feelings in this way, you don't attack or accuse or berate the other person, you just communicate. I find that even a bad sexual situation will usually clear up if the communication in a relationship improves."

"What destroys a relationship is dishonesty and a lack of open communication," adds Dr. Viscott. "Dishonesty is one of the two things that block love. The other is not loving yourself.

"You can't receive love from another person unless you love yourself. If you don't love yourself, and a person says, 'I love you,' you think, 'I don't deserve it.' You resist the love because you can't think of yourself as worthy, because you can't value their positive estimation of yourself."

"Only if we love ourselves can we give love to others," says Carol Lentz, director of the Cornucopia Institute in St. Mary, Kentucky, where she teaches a self-improvement program called "The Living Love Way to Happiness."

"When you don't love yourself, you want the other person to love you," she told us. "This demand destroys your ability to accept the other person unconditionally, to love them."

Why You Must Love Yourself

"All the negative emotions—anger, fear, grief—stem from lack of self-love," says Peter Hansen. "When you love yourself, you feel complete and zestful. To see the zestful person in yourself and in others is the essence of loving.

"Love," he continues, "is simply the most creative use of our own energy, and there are many ways to channel that energy. Eating natural foods, getting aerobic exercise, spending time in unmolested nature, praying, meditating—but most importantly, giving someone 100 percent of your attention when you relate to them—are all effective ways to increase loving.

"There are many creative disciplines to enrich our ability to love," agrees Dr. Bro. "Meditation or equivalent methods of quieting the mind such as listening to music or spending time with nature can free us of our hang-ups and mobilize our creative energy to pay full attention to others and love.

"Another discipline is to recognize when you are coming from a bad place, when you are rejecting others, manipulating others, or feeling sorry for yourself. Notice your voice, your choice of words, your manner, and if they're negative or destructive, change them.

"Also, when someone relates to us in an aggressive or defensive or shy way, try to realize the hurt and fear and need for love behind that behavior. We should see someone else's bad behavior as an opportunity to give love, not as a personal affront.

"Yet even with these disciplines, we should realize that love is essentially playful. It is spontaneous, fully present, unguarded and able to be surprised. It is not a heavyhanded kind of virtue, but a flexible and natural process."

And becoming more loving—more natural—has another benefit: better health.

"People who have never developed the capacity for loving find their lovelessness reflected in their body," says Dr. Bro. "That emotional guardedness and defensiveness can express itself physically as muscular tension, shallow breathing, lack of normal sexual function and an uninflected voice."

"When people hold in their feelings," says Peter Hansen, "they begin to feel hopeless and powerless, they give up. That giving up is expressed in the body as sickness. Cancer, for instance, shows up mostly in personality types who have held back anger all their lives.

"But people who are loving—who completely accept themselves and others—are usually full of energy and joy. Love and health go hand in hand."

MARIJUANA

Gone are the days when the term "pot" meant just one thing: a kettle to cook in. "Grass" referred to a short-cropped ground cover, nothing more. And whisper of "the weed" was simply small talk of a death-defying dandelion that staked permanent roots in an otherwise perfect lawn.

Today, the first and foremost thing that comes to mind when we hear terms like pot, grass, and the weed is—you guessed it!—marijuana. And, shocking as it is, it probably won't surprise you to learn that nearly 60 percent of our 18- to 21-year-olds and perhaps 80 percent of the students on some of our college campuses have at least sampled a joint (that's not some sleazy dive, but rather the term for a rolled marijuana cigarette).

Almost one in five of those who try marijuana become regular users. But what's so frightening is that most are convinced it's a harmless habit—or, at least, that it's a lot less risky than smoking Lucky Strikes or swigging Scotch and sodas. Admittedly, there just wasn't enough conclusive research to suggest otherwise. That is, until recently. Today, we've got more than enough evidence to implicate marijuana in cellular damage (possibly leading to cancer, reduced immunity from disease, and genetic defects), infertility, deterioration in mental functioning, and irreversible brain and lung damage.

Those who smoke pot have long contended that marijuana is less injurious to the lungs than tobacco. But according to the most recent series of experiments, rats exposed to marijuana in doses equivalent to a man or woman smoking one to six joints a day for one year, suffered severe tissue damage and inflammation of the lungs. Animals exposed to tobacco smoke for the same length of time did not incur the same type of damage. Another study found that marijuana is as likely to produce lung cancer in humans and more likely to cause alterations in DNA and chromosomes of the lung cells than plain old cigarettes.

There's more bad news for those who think of marijuana as somewhat of a modern-day aphrodisiac. Popular theories insist that pot removes inhibitions and enhances sexual sensitivity. But the latest spate of scientific studies shows that moderate doses may provoke the desire but take away the performance—and, worse, that even small doses can seriously impair reproductive functions.

Wylie C. Hembree, M.D., and Gabriel G. Nahas, M.D., Ph.D., of Columbia University's College of Physicians and Surgeons, have found, for example, that heavy pot users have a lower sperm count as well as a tendency toward malformed and sluggish sperm cells. In a study, 11 young, healthy male volunteers agreed to smoke between 5 and 12 joints a day. The researchers report that after just one month, there was a significantly increased number of abnormal sperm cells among these young men.

Marijuana and a Woman's Hormones

But the most dangerous aspect of smoking marijuana is its effects on young women, Dr. Nahas told us. Just as pot reduces the hormones responsible for sperm formation, it interferes with the brain hormones that regulate the delicate orchestration of functions connected with the menstrual cycle.

Joan Bauman, Ph.D., a research associate at the Masters and Johnson Institute in St. Louis, compared the menstrual cycles of 26 women who smoked marijuana at least four times a week with the cycles of 17 nonsmoking women of the same age. Interestingly enough, the average menstrual cycle of the marijuana smokers was two days shorter than the average cycle of the nonsmokers. In addition, 40 percent of the smokers' cycles—as opposed to only 15 percent of the nonsmokers'—were marked by either a failure to ovulate (release an egg) or a faster onset of menstruation following ovulation.

One obvious implication of this is infertility. According to Dr. Bauman, even if ovulation does occur, the fertilized egg may not have ample time to implant itself in the womb before the lining is shed. And apparently, from what Dr. Nahas tells us, it may not take much pot to evoke such a response.

"It only takes one joint to produce a temporary disruption in the brain hormones which can last for six to eight hours," he says. "So women who smoke as few as three joints a week can have a disruption of their menstrual cycle."

That doesn't mean that pot will replace the Pill as the latest oral contraceptive. Carol Grace Smith, Ph.D., a pharmacologist at the Uniformed Services Medical School in Bethesda, Maryland, points out that THC, the major mind-altering chemical in marijuana, not only affects the hormones that govern ovulation and menstruation, but may have a direct and damaging effect on ovarian function. "We're extremely concerned about the effects of the drug on the developing reproductive systems of female teenagers," she explains. "This phase of development is particularly vulnerable to disruption by drugs." Also, Dr. Nahas adds, when you consider that a pair of ovaries releases a mere 400 eggs in a lifetime compared to the 300 million sperm produced per ejaculation in a man, it's easy to see why women are more vulnerable to toxic substances like marijuana which have such a profound effect on reproductive functions.

Surprise: It Accumulates in Your System

The trouble is, THC makes a beeline from the lungs to the brain, sex organs and fatty tissues. And there it sits. Evidence supplied by Dr. Nahas suggests that it takes about a month to completely rid the body of the THC in just one joint. THC only loses its punch gradually, so that if you smoked one joint a day for one month, you would still have 10 times the original dose in your body by month's end. And there is reason to believe that, for women, THC could be even higher. THC tends to accumulate in fatty tissues and women have a higher percentage of body fat than men, Dr. Nahas explains. The more fat, the more marijuana is stored.

And the more THC in a young woman's fat stores, the greater the potential for harm should she become pregnant. "Smoking marijuana is like playing genetic roulette for a woman," Dr. Nahas exclaims. There is evidence that THC passes across the placenta to a developing fetus. And, at least in rhesus monkeys (which have a reproductive system very similar to that of a human being), a daily dose of THC can be harmful if not fatal to the developing fetus.

At the California Primate Research Center at the University of California at Davis, Ethel N. Sassenrath, Ph.D., found that 40 percent of the offspring of female monkeys given the equivalent of one to three joints a day died before, during or shortly after birth. Monkeys not exposed to marijuana lost just 11 percent of their babies. In addition, while all of the THC-exposed fetuses looked perfectly normal, autopsies showed that each had at least one poorly developed internal organ. In several cases, these problems were associated with abnormalities in the placenta. None of the offspring of nondrugged mothers suffered any such problem.

And what about the babies that survived despite their marijuana-doped mothers? They all appeared normal, Dr. Sassenrath says, although the males did have a lower birth weight than the offspring of nondrugged mothers and most of them had subtle behavioral problems.

Marijuana-smoking mothers who breastfeed may likewise bestow grave consequences on their young. Several studies have shown that THC is excreted in mother's milk. And although there are no human studies on this, suckling rats treated with marijuana for six days after birth suffered permanent hormonal and behavioral changes.

Thoughts of motherhood aside, Dr. Nahas warns all women of the hazards of mixing marijuana with other drugs. Marijuana is a drug and for obvious reasons, then, it can interact with alcohol or medication. The combination of birth control pills and marijuana, for example, may result in midcycle spotting and other menstrual irregularities, Dr. Nahas told us.

On the other hand, Dr. Nahas has information on at least 25 other drugs which have a more potent effect on the body when mixed with marijuana. "THC inhibits the synthesis of a very important enzyme which is involved in the body's detoxification process," Dr. Nahas explains. "Take barbiturates, for example. Barbiturates usually stimulate this particular enzyme production, which in turn increases the elimination of the barbiturates from the body. THC inhibits this process so you will get an exaggeration of the effects of the barbiturates. This occurs with other drugs as well, such as antihistamines. When an antihistamine is taken together with marijuana, your mouth will get drier, you will feel sleepier, and your mental abilities will be even further impaired. The same holds true for the interaction between alcohol and pot. Marijuana plus alcohol will make you drunker than alcohol alone."

I don't remember exactly how Dr. Singermann put it, because, as soon as I got the gist of what he was saying, my head seemed to fill with air and my eyes got hot.

"... definitely something there ... a mass ... good chance of malignancy ... different kinds of mastectomy, as you probably know ... some women say they want a separate procedure ... studies show ... in my own experience ... but, of course, it's up to you."

He stopped. I realized I was supposed to talk now. It sounded as if I was expected to say whether I wanted just to have my breast cut off, or whether I wanted my breast cut off and some other things too.

I turned to Dr. Singermann. I heard myself speak. "Are you saying that you think I have cancer?" (That word had not been used. I soon learned that cancer is a word doctors almost never use.) "I mean, I know you can't know for sure, but what are the odds—what percentage—what is the likelihood. . . ?"

Dr. Singermann smiled and leaned on his desk. "Everyone wants numbers. It's very hard to say, maybe 70–30, 60–40, I don't know."

I heard myself speak again. "Are you saying, do you mean it's 60 or 70 percent *likely*, you mean, it's *likely?*"

It was making him uncomfortable. "Look, percentages are just percentages. People want numbers, you give them numbers, but . . . unreliable . . . you don't really know until . . . but . . ." Then he stood up. Then I stood up. Then I fell down.

I didn't faint, exactly, because I didn't altogether lose consciousness. Nor did I fall far, or get hurt. There was a small sofa in the room, and I remember being placed on it. "I'll be all right," I said. But the line must have convinced no one because as soon as I said it I began to cry, the bad, loud, gasping kind. I wanted to hold something, so I held my face. I held it hard with both hands, as if it were someone else's.

—*First, You Cry*
(J. B. Lippincott, 1976)

In her aptly titled book, NBC news correspondent Betty Rollin relates the hard-hitting reality of losing her breast to cancer—a trauma that more and more women are coming to experience. Each year about 108,000 women are diagnosed to have breast cancer. And about 90 percent have their breast removed in a procedure called mastectomy. For any woman, it's got to be an emotion-packed ordeal like none other—and one that releases more deep-seated concerns and worries in a day than most of us are likely to experience in a lifetime.

Fear of dying. Sadness over the loss—a death—of a part of you. Shock over the suddenness and magnitude of the verdict. Envy for anyone with two healthy breasts. Anger because it had to happen to you. Isolation because you don't know anyone else who's gone through it. Anxiety and apprehension over the looming unknown.

Your head fills with a million questions: Will the cancer be caught in time? What will I look like without a breast? How will my husband (or lover) react? How will I be able to cope with this obvious deformity that strikes such a blow to my femininity?

How? First, as Betty Rollin knows,

you cry. Then you pull yourself together and arm yourself with as much information and knowledge as you'll need to get yourself through with the best possible outcome.

Take Time to Consider Your Choices

Fortunately, today, women are given (and if not given, they *take*) the time to think about their options, to make plans and to take part in those very important decisions. In the past, it wasn't uncommon for a woman to enter a hospital for a simple breast biopsy and leave without a breast—the practice being that at biopsy, a pathologist would examine a tissue sample under a microscope and decide on the spot whether or not it was cancer. If he felt that it was, the breast was removed immediately, and the woman first learned of the decision in the recovery room hours later.

Today many physicians are adopting the two-step procedure (that is, the biopsy done at one time and the breast removed at a later date, if necessary). And if yours hasn't you can request— yes, insist—upon it. There are many advantages to the two-step procedure, which we discuss under Breast Lumps: Benign or Malignant? But briefly, you're better assured an accurate diagnosis, you have the opportunity to discuss options in treatment with your physician, and you can prepare yourself for whatever that treatment is. That is extremely important.

According to the 1979 Final Report of the American College of Surgeons Commission on Cancer, 85 percent of all breast cancers are predictable, while 15 percent vary markedly in their growth patterns. For example, of 23,777 tumors they studied, 14 different types of cancer were found—some slow-growing, some fast, some fast-spreading, others that didn't spread at all (see accompanying box, Breast Cancer Classification System). Ideally, then, treatment should be tailored to the tumor as well as to the extent of the disease.

The type and extent of the cancer are both things that should be carefully evaluated between biopsy and further surgery. For advanced cancer, it involves complete tissue analysis, blood workups, skeletal x-rays, and a very crucial test called an estrogen receptor assay. A biopsy and estrogen receptor assay are sufficient for minimal cancers (those that are small or noninvasive). The assay tests a piece of the cancerous tissue to see how it responds to hormonal drug therapy, which is nontoxic. That information could be invaluable if the cancer has spread or if it recurs.

Unfortunately, though, according to Mortimer B. Lipsett, M.D., director of the National Institutes of Health's Clinical Center, only half of all American women who are diagnosed to have breast cancer this year will have the benefit of this test. More and more hospitals perform this test automatically. But if the hospital where you'll undergo the biopsy isn't equipped to do an estrogen receptor assay, make arrangements with your surgeon to have a sample of your tumor frozen promptly and sent to a laboratory that is.

The idea behind all these preliminary tests is not to determine whether you might need more extensive surgery. What they do is help to zero in on the *minimum* treatment needed to insure maximum chance for recovery. And in many cases they avoid the need for unnecessarily radical surgical procedures.

For example, if the tumor is very small and localized, that is, if it hasn't

BREAST CANCER CLASSIFICATION SYSTEM

Cancer is classed according to stage and type. The stage indicates how far it has spread, and the type denotes how aggressively it behaves or is likely to behave.

Stage is determined by size of the tumor, involvement of the lymph nodes, and metastases. Briefly, this system places the cancer at one of four stages of development:

stage I The malignant growth is confined to the breast. There are no signs that it has spread to the armpit or beyond.

stage II The primary (largest and first discovered) tumor is only at stage I, but there are suspicious lumps in the armpit.

stage III The primary tumor has invaded the skin, chest wall and chest muscles. Lumps can be felt in the armpit, and unpalpable masses may also be present. (That cannot be determined without further surgery. Manual palpation is very unreliable here.)

stage IV The cancer has spread beyond the breast and armpit region, usually to bone marrow, liver or lungs.

SOURCE: Adapted from *Current Medical Diagnosis and Treatment 1978*, by Marcus A. Krupp et al. (Los Altos, CA: Lange Medical Publications, 1978) p. 421.

How aggressively the tumor itself grows may also be used to determine treatment. Based on examination of biopsied cells, cancer can be classified according to its likelihood of spreading to distant organs (metastasizing) and its potential for destroying healthy tissue surrounding it (invasiveness):

type I Rarely metastasizes, not invasive. The cells multiply within but not beyond a local tumor or tumors, which makes them easy to remove surgically.

type II Rarely metastasizes, always invasive. The cells may spread to ducts and other breast tissues, requiring breast removal or radiation.

type III Moderately metastasizes, always invasive. Most of those cancers originate in the ducts themselves and are called invasive ductal carcinoma; the others originate in glands and are called adenocarcinoma. Both are very likely to spread to lymph nodes and possibly the bloodstream, making local control unlikely.

type IV Highly metastasizes, always invasive. Those cells spread directly from the original tumor into the bloodstream. Immediate and sustained drug therapy has made them less lethal than previously.

spread throughout the breast or to neighboring lymph nodes (which act as a transmission center to other areas of the body), then there's no longer any reason to do the more disfiguring radical mastectomy, or Halsted mastectomy, which involves removal of the breast, the lymph nodes under the arm and the chest muscle underneath. By the same token, if the cancer is so far along that it has invaded the lymph system and spread, or metastasized, to other organs of the body, no amount of breast surgery is going to remedy the situation.

What Kind of Surgery?

Actually, that's another thing that's changed in recent years. There was a time in the not-so-distant past when the radical mastectomy described above was the automatic treatment for any and all types of breast cancer—the reason being, the bigger the operation, the more likely the cure. Today, thank goodness, physicians recognize that long-term survival for women who undergo a "modified" radical mastectomy for early breast cancer (stage I and some stage II tumors) is as good as if they had had the standard radical—approximately 80 to 85 percent.

The modified radical mastectomy may sound at first like a contradiction of terms—which is why doctors prefer the term "total" mastectomy with axillary dissection. What it means is that, like the radical, the breast and axillary lymph nodes are removed and biopsied. But here the procedure is modified to the extent that the chest muscles remain intact. The advantages of modified radical over standard radical are not only cosmetic, but functional. Retaining the major muscle avoids a concave hollow below the collarbone which would im-

pair movement in the shoulder and very likely cause swelling in the arm.

The supersleuth of the breast surgery puzzle is Bernard Fisher, M.D., who pilots the National Cancer Institute-sponsored National Surgical Adjuvant Breast Project, an extensive study of the cure rates for all types of surgery and combination therapies. According to Dr. Fisher, "standard radical mastectomies are hard to justify anymore. All our data show no difference in survival for standard versus 'total' mastectomy with axillary dissection."

That conclusion is widely supported. A careful study by Gerald N. Robinson, M.D., and others in the departments of surgery, pathology and epidemiology at the Mayo Clinic showed no significant difference in survival of patients with identical cancers treated by either standard radical or the more modified procedure (*Mayo Clinic Proceedings*, July, 1976).

Responding to those studies, on June 5, 1979, the National Institutes of Health brought together a panel of practicing physicians, biomedical research scientists, consumers and other interested people to reexamine issues concerned with the treatment of early breast cancer. Not surprisingly, the group's recommendation was that the modified radical mastectomy should replace the radical mastectomy as the choice for early breast cancer (classified as stage I) and even for some breast cancers that have spread to underarm lymph nodes (classified as stage II).

For more advanced stage III and stage IV cancers, surgery usually isn't the answer. Rather, physicians prefer to weaken the disease and counteract its physical effect through radiation, hormonal or drug therapy (chemotherapy).

But back to the early cancers—a

small but adventuresome number of physicians would like to pare down the standard surgical procedure for these localized cancers even further. But we must warn you that at the time of this writing, anything less than the "total" mastectomy with axillary dissection is considered experimental and remains unproven in terms of long-tern survival rates. However, today researchers are reevaluating more simple surgical procedures that carry fewer disfiguring effects.

For example, in the past a simple mastectomy (in which the breast is removed but not the lymph nodes) or a lumpectomy (also referred to as a "partial mastectomy" in which only the lump is removed) were combined with radiation therapy to treat stage I cancer. Advocates of this very limited surgery claimed that results equal radical mastectomy—as long as the tumor is caught in time. And therein lay the hitch. The reason these procedures were not embraced by the majority of cancer specialists is that they ignored the lymph nodes. But now, physicians who are experimenting with this technique are removing the lymph nodes as well, biopsying them, and prescribing further treatment if necessary, such as chemotherapy, based on biopsy results.

More Options for Treatment

Samuel Hellman, M.D., of the Joint Center for Radiation Therapy, Boston, suggests a system that combines surgery, radiation therapy and chemotherapy drugs which may just be the answer. "A possible therapeutic approach for early breast cancer would be local removal of the tumor with sampling of the axillary lymph nodes, followed by radiation of the breast, and finally chemotherapy if the axillary nodes show cancer," he explains. "This treatment plan may improve the survival of breast cancer patients and optimize both function and cosmetic appearance."

Another encouraging note—Dr. Hellman, along with Jay R. Harris, M.D., and Martin B. Levene, M.D., reports that the department of radiation therapy at Harvard Medical School has had excellent results in the treatment of early breast cancer with radiation therapy *alone*. Between June, 1968, and December, 1976, 129 women with stage I or stage II breast cancer were referred to the department because they either refused a mastectomy or some medical condition precluded surgery. Six of the patients had cancer in both breasts, bringing the total number of breasts treated to 135. All were biopsied. Radiation therapy was begun and by treatment's end, each involved breast had received about 5,000 rads of radiation (a mammogram delivers one rad—radiation absorbed dose—at most). In 32 patients an additional radioactive implant was embedded at the tumor site.

As of their report in the December, 1978, issue of the *Seminars in Oncology*, only five percent of the breasts showed recurrence and all of those recurrences have been in the breast alone with no lymph node involvement. What's more, the breast cancer control rate is equivalent to that seen with radical mastectomy—as are the 5-year survival rates (91 percent for stage I; 66 percent for stage II). Still, radiation therapy is not without disadvantages, including the destruction of healthy tissue and scarring. Researchers also caution that it's too soon to tell whether this approach will weather as well over the 10-year haul. We'll just have to wait and see.

Meanwhile, if you have a suspicious lump, your best bet is to have the biopsy done as soon as possible, and if the results come back positive for cancer, find yourself a good, well-qualified breast cancer specialist right away. Remember, it needn't be the one who performed the biopsy, though there's no reason it shouldn't if you're satisfied with his attitudes and technique.

Finding the right doctor or surgeon for any problem is always a challenge. But in the case of breast cancer, probably more so. The trouble is, there are few "breast cancer specialists" per se but many doctors who treat breast cancer. There are general surgeons (who also do appendectomies and gallbladder surgery), thoracic surgeons (who specialize in all types of chest surgery—male or female), and oncologists. An oncologist is a cancer specialist, but believe it or not, even that specialty is becoming more specialized. The surgical oncologist specializes in surgical treatments, the radiation oncologist in radiation therapy, and the medical oncologist in chemotherapy. It's confusing, to say the least.

If you discover a lump, your best bet is probably to go first to your primary care physician. He or she can then refer you to one of these specialists if necessary. If you are at a loss and don't know where to begin, call the National Surgical Adjuvant Breast Project Hotline (see *Appendix*). They can explain the available treatments, answer your questions and refer you to a specialist in your area.

Of course, in view of widely varying opinions and discrepancies in the treatment of breast cancer, don't be afraid to get a second opinion.

Rose Kushner, a mastectomy patient and author of *Why Me? What Every Woman Should Know About Breast Cancer to Save Her Life* (New American Library, 1977), knows the benefits of shopping around for a surgeon all too well. Back in 1974 when she suspected she had breast cancer she called 19 surgeons before she found one who was willing to do a two-part biopsy procedure, something that is well accepted today. Later she underwent a "total" mastectomy with axillary dissection at a time when the Halsted radical was all the rage.

Because she realized the difficulty women have in getting the kind of information and guidance they need to make sound judgments concerning breast cancer, Rose Kushner started the Breast Cancer Advisory Center. One woman had been told that she needed a mastectomy right away. Instead she called the Breast Care Advisory Center, where it was suggested that she get a second opinion at Roswell Park Memorial Institute in Buffalo, New York, which was near her home. She did. And to the woman's relief, the pathologist at Roswell Park reexamined her biopsy slides and told her that she did not have cancer. Her lump was a "sclerosing adenosis," which any pathologist could mistake for a cancerous lump but which actually is not malignant.

Once you are absolutely convinced of the nature of your problem, the available options, and the qualifications of your physician, sit down with him or her to discuss the details of treatment fully.

Quality of life after mastectomy is just as important as length of life. Don't hesitate to ask your surgeon any questions about the operation itself, healing time or side effects. He should explain in detail what is to be removed during the operation and why. How much tissue is going to be removed, particularly in the underarm and chest area, influences healing time and arm motion at the shoulder.

The possibility of future reconstruction of the breast may also influence the direction of the surgeon's incision. With the increasing acceptance (and affordability) of breast reconstruction after mastectomy, horizontal incisions are favored. That results in a scar that falls into the skin's natural tension lines, improves the cosmetic effect of reconstruction, and doesn't interfere with the blood supply to the reconstructed breast. (A discussion of breast reconstruction surgery appears later in this section.)

After the breast is removed, the edges of the cut area will be pulled together snugly over the ribs and sewn up. If you have small breasts, it may be necessary to graft some skin from your thigh over the cut area, because there might not be enough of a flap left to sew the wound closed. If the underarm nodes must be removed, tubes will be left in place to drain lymph fluids from the surgical wound for about four days after the operation.

The mortality rate for breast removal surgery itself is relatively low, compared to other surgical procedures—the risks involved are related to the anesthesia.

Although your physician can give you a fair estimate of your chances for a cancer-free life after treatment, he cannot honestly give absolute guarantees. Most patients know that and don't expect any promises. Knowing how long your physical rehabilitation will take and what you can do to speed your recovery is important to your psychological adjustment right from the start.

The Full Recovery: Body and Soul

The road to recovery begins as soon as you wake up from the anesthetic. Taking into consideration how much tension pulls at the incision, how tightly the skin pulls across your chest, and any tubes that may remain in place to drain the wound, your physician will recommend certain exercises to prevent stiffness in the shoulder and arm. You will be instructed by a nurse or physical therapist and perhaps your physician, who will be sure you are exercising correctly.

The easiest exercise is simply brushing your hair, which you will be encouraged to do right from day one. Other exercises include walking your fingers up a wall like a spider, crumpling paper into wads, squeezing a rubber ball, lowering window shades and rotating the shoulder in enlarging circles. Later, when the stitches have been removed, you will be given more vigorous exercises, which will carry over into your daily household activities after you return home.

Dozens of questions will enter your mind. Your physician should answer all of your medical questions to your satisfaction but will probably request that a volunteer from the Reach to Recovery Program visit you in the hospital about the fourth to sixth day after surgery. She will answer your questions about clothing and offer psychological assurance. Also, the shock of realizing what has happened requires that you talk to someone who knows what you are going through.

Reach to Recovery is a service program of the American Cancer Society (ACS) made up of healthy postmastectomy women who have successfully adjusted to their surgery. Just talking with a former patient who is obviously well and energetic is a morale booster that cannot be replaced by even the most understanding neighbor or relative. In fact, according to a survey in the San Francisco area, mastectomy patients rated these talks with other postmastectomy women of utmost importance—especially before the surgery. In any case, after the surgery she will probably offer you a temporary, lightweight, washable prosthesis to slip into your bra. You can walk out looking the same as you did when you entered the hospital, and in a few weeks shop for a more permanent artificial breast. The Reach to Recovery volunteer will also give you an informative booklet prepared by ACS which gives exact details on how to alter your clothing, shop for a prosthesis, exercise at home and so forth. There is no charge for her service.

How long you stay in the hospital depends on your surgeon, but the average is about 7 days. You may remain hospitalized for up to 14 days if you have had skin grafts, because of extra fluids that must be drained from the wound. There is also about a 10 percent chance of infection, which may delay discharge.

Before you go home, you will be advised to take special precautions with your affected arm. Without the lymph glands to fight infection, it will be more prone to infection and burns, including sunburn. Injections, blood tests and blood pressure tests should be done on the good arm. Edgardo Alday, M.D., associate professor of surgery at Jefferson Medical College in Philadelphia, gives his patients plenty of sage advice. "Avoid the smallest kinds of injuries to the affected arm and shoulder. Wear kitchen mitts when cooking to avoid burns, and long sleeves and gloves when gardening. (Don't get pricked by thorny roses.) Don't brush against people wearing corsages. Avoid jostling in crowds or on subways, and take care that people don't greet you with hearty slaps on the affected arm."

The most common but delayed complication after mastectomy is swelling in the arm (lymphedema). Because surgery has interfered with the lymph system, fluids can stagnate in the limb rather than recirculate to the trunk. Varying degrees of swelling show up in about one-third of postmastectomy patients, often not for a few months or even a year or more after the operation. A low-salt diet, arm elevation, an elastic sleeve prescribed by your doctor, and avoiding overweight usually help. Diuretics are sometimes prescribed. Very rarely, uncontrolled swelling requires surgical drainage of the arm.

You'll probably tire easily during your first few days at home. The change from being waited on to facing piles of laundry and empty cupboards can be discouraging, breast or no breast. Don't expect too much from yourself at first. Eventually you'll be washing windows, typing office reports, playing tennis—almost anything. One woman told us that the only thing she couldn't do was knead bread dough and that actually, the more she used the arm, the less it bothered her.

Your own recuperation will depend on your type of surgery and individual stamina. Ask your doctor when you can return to work or whether you should limit your activities in any way. He or she will probably tell you to do as much as you can, without straining yourself.

Improving Your Chances of Long-Term Recovery

Beyond postsurgical recuperation, you may be wondering what, if anything, you can do to insure a complete *long-term* recovery. At this point, however, the only *definite* edge you can give yourself in the race against cancer is early detection. But there are some preliminary studies which suggest that in addition to early detection, women who are not overweight, do not smoke, and do not suppress their feelings over the trauma are more likely to celebrate their 10-year anniversary of breast cancer completely free of this dreaded disease.

Dr. Norman F. Boyd, of the Princess Margaret Hospital, Toronto, Canada, and the Ontario Cancer Institute, examined the various risk factors in the development of breast cancer including age, family history of the disease, menopausal status and so on in 750 women with breast cancer to determine whether these same factors had any relationship to 5- and 10-year recovery rates. Interestingly, he explains, "body weight was the only risk factor found to be associated with significant differences in survival."

Another study, by William L. Donegan, M.D., professor of surgery at the Medical College of Wisconsin, in Milwaukee, showed a similar trend. A graph plotting postmastectomy patients' weights against any future disease flare-up shows the relationship clearly: as the weights of the women in his study decreased so, too, did their rate of cancer recurrence.

Drs. Boyd and Donegan both point out, however, that they have no evidence that weight loss after mastectomy has any effect on long-term survival, although they admit the suggestion that it would is certainly there.

Likewise, there may be some benefit in kicking the smoking habit. Writing in the *New England Journal of Medicine* (June 26, 1980), Harry W. Daniell, M.D., voices his long-held suspicion that breast cancer patients who smoke do not seem to fare as well as those who don't. He further suggests that the link may be in the relationship between cigarettes and estrogen. After all, premature menopause, osteoporosis and infertility—all problems aggravated by an estrogen deficiency—are accelerated by cigarette smoking.

To test his theory, Dr. Daniell examined the biopsy reports and estrogen receptor assays of 78 smoking and non-smoking women with breast cancer. Although this was a small group of women and therefore the results must be considered carefully, they were nonetheless very interesting. In the estrogen receptor assays, he found 61 percent of the smokers had "negative" readings, compared to only 32 percent of the nonsmokers—an indicator that their types of cancer were more likely to recur and less likely to respond to hormone therapy. Likewise he found that lymph node involvement was more common among smokers than nonsmokers.

Mental attitude also appears to enter into long-term survival of breast cancer patients. According to a study by a group of researchers at Johns Hopkins University in Baltimore, Maryland, women who were better able to "externalize and communicate their negative attitudes"—who expressed their feelings of anxiety, alienation, depression and anger—appeared to live longer than those who acted as if they had the whole situation under control—who on the outside appeared to be coping beautifully with the situation but who in reality were suppressing and denying psychological stress (*Journal of the American Medical Association,* October, 1979).

That's not to say don't cope. Just allow yourself time to feel the emotional pain and express it. It makes acceptance later so much easier.

Dealing with the physical effects of breast loss is a small task compared to the psychological readjustment. Many emotions can come into play. In spite of her surgeon's reassurances, the question foremost in a woman's mind may be, "Did he get out all the cancer?" Worry over cure of a potentially fatal disease is compounded by anger and resentment that the whole nightmare has cropped up in her life. Anxiety over survival of her marriage (or future relationships if she is single, divorced or widowed) is likely to develop. Concern for her femininity develops partly because society has often stereotyped the desirable woman as one who displays a perfect set of large breasts. Even if her bosom isn't the *Playboy* ideal, if one breast is removed she may wonder how her husband or companion can ever really love her again in the same way. She may fear that he will pity or be ashamed of her.

The man who shares his life with a woman who has lost a breast to cancer has his own fears and feelings. He must be medically assured that the surgical operation itself will not affect her sexual desire or responsiveness, but that how he and the woman *cope* with the loss can. Even just being held and caressed may be important. That calls for open communication between the doctor or counselor and the woman's husband and also between man and woman. A man may be afraid he is going to hurt her during lovemaking. A simple change in

position to avoid leaning on the operated side may relieve discomfort.

You may want to make love again as soon as you are physically up to it, but your husband may assume that after the operation you don't feel like having sex, and he may avoid normal advances so as not to appear demanding. If he doesn't come up to the bedroom until after you've changed into your nightgown, he may simply be afraid that you'll be embarrassed to undress in front of him anymore. That can easily be misinterpreted by you as rejection. And if you slip into the bathroom to get dressed in the morning because you think he'll be horrified at the sight of your scar, the two of you will never adjust.

Talk about your feelings and assumptions. And remember, he married a person, not an artist's model, and he's mainly glad you're still around to cherish all the more, not less.

One postmastectomy woman, a Reach to Recovery volunteer who counsels other women, describes the readjustments very matter-of-factly:

"It's like an appendectomy scar. At first the scar is red and ugly, and you flinch when you look at it. Once you have overcome that, you don't worry about it as much. If you were relaxed about undressing in front of your husband before, it's not as much of an adjustment to face. I mean, if you've never undressed in front of him before, you shouldn't start now. Although I naturally wish I looked better, I'm not self-conscious about it, although I must admit I don't walk around the house nude.

"Some couples find it difficult to start making love again after surgery. Just the pressure on your chest may hurt. Or the fear of being hurt itself makes it difficult to begin. I think my advice to most women is that she must let her husband know that she's not different, because he's a little apprehensive. He doesn't want to hurt her. She must be receptive and let him know she wants to try.

"I must say that it was difficult and a little awkward for my husband and me at first, but we talked about it and resolved the problems."

Most men, in fact, are not horrified or repelled when their wife or lover loses a breast. Mildred Hope Witkin, Ph.D., associate director of the human sexuality program at New York Hospital–Cornell Medical Center, emphasizes that those couples who deal with the problem immediately—from the day a woman leaves the hospital—lessen the chance of psychological trauma taking root. "It is crucial that the man display his love in very close, physical ways. It doesn't even have to be full intercourse. Otherwise, the woman will continue to feel ugly and undesirable."

Concerning the unattached woman who will worry about facing the intimate side of a future relationship with one breast, Dr. Witkin says, "Nine out of 10 men do not back away when confronted by a lover who has lost a breast. Most single patients later marry or become involved in successful relationships."

Feelings of family and friends have to be dealt with, too. Having been threatened by what they see as a near-tragedy may make them apprehensive. They will try to show concern without pity. You, in turn, may find yourself feeling jealous of women with two healthy breasts. If you have a teenaged daughter, you may dread being confronted by her about her chances of facing the same loss. Younger children will have a lot of unanswered questions which must be answered directly in order to assuage unrealistic, imagined fears. Your actions more than your words will reassure them that you are just as nurturing and maternal as you were with two breasts.

Some women choose to look at it this way: their personality, intelligence, job, family or social life did not all hinge on their breasts before, so there's no reason to feel that loss of one is going to destroy their whole world.

You may go through a month or two of depression or withdrawal, fantasize that your husband is going to leave you, feel that friends are clamming up, or worry that cancer will recur. Those reactions are not excessively morbid. They need to be aired. But try not to prolong your emotional reaction.

You may be reluctant to tell your doctor that you sometimes feel sensations of itching, tingling or even pain in the "phantom breast" after mastectomy. Occasional or daily feelings that the breast is still there may begin just a few days or even a year after surgery, causing apprehension. Although it is disconcerting, you are not crazy. The "phantom limb" feeling is shared by people who have lost limbs. Don't hesitate to discuss such sensations with your doctor.

What You Must Do for Yourself

It is important that you continue to practice monthly self-examination on the remaining breast. Psychologically, that may be difficult, due to anxiety over finding a lump and once again setting off a chain of events leading to removal of your second breast. When you return to your physician for your first postoperative check of the incision, ask him to discuss that with you. Although there is a slightly increased risk of cancer turning up in a remaining breast, in most women it does not, and you are simply playing it safe by checking the breast routinely. For three years after mastectomy, your doctor will probably ask you to return for an office checkup every two to four months. A mammogram will be taken yearly, not only to be certain there is nothing going on in the second breast but also to check for recurrence of the first cancer if you have had a partial. Again, these checkups are sources of reassurance to the patient who has been treated for early cancer.

Examination is then done every 6 months until five years after surgery, and every 6 to 12 months after that.

Choosing a Breast Prosthesis

When you go home, don't immediately clear your closets of all your pretty nighties and evening dresses. Having your breast removed doesn't mean you are doomed to flannel nightgowns and shapeless smocks for the rest of your life. Most women want to face the world—and their mirror—looking their best, and breast prostheses that slip into your bra have now been perfected to the point where you can fool even your best friend. Prices and quality vary from homemade or very inexpensive dacron "falsies" or padded bras to lifelike individually fitted prostheses designed by a postmastectomy woman who, ironically, had previously designed the bosomy Barbie doll, so she knew what she was doing!

Those breast forms are made of sturdy, waterproof polyurethane, filled with liquid silicone. Some "teardrop" styles only replace the missing breast removed by simple mastectomy. Another model is molded to fill up the chest hollow and swoop under the arm, replacing everything cut out by more radical mastectomies. All come in "rights" and "lefts," just like shoes, as well as your cup size. The artificial breast equals your own breast in contour and weight and is soft and yielding to the touch.

Obviously, the latter is the form that most nearly looks—and feels—like a real live breast. It is often impossible to tell the difference, even wearing just a bra in front of the fitting room mirror. And this type is very unlikely to embarrass you by sinking or riding up.

You may have to visit more than one store until you find a satisfactory prosthesis. Good prostheses are available in specialty shops, some surgical supply houses and the intimate apparel departments of larger department stores. You should be assisted by a trained saleswoman in finding a properly fitting bra, because your whole chest may have changed after surgery and, possibly, weight loss. You will then be fitted for a prosthesis just as you would be for any other special fitting problem such as wide hips, broad shoulders or a short waist, rather than for a deformity. The salespeople will also show you how to make slight alterations on your bras and swimsuits so you can wear the new breast under almost anything.

Some insurance plans pay for prostheses and some do not. Check with your carrier. Medicaid will reimburse you, but the amount varies from region to region. In any case, have the salesperson write "surgical prosthesis," plus your size, on the sales slip so you may apply for reimbursement. The cost of breast forms as well as fees for fitting or altering bras is a tax-deductible medical expense.

When shopping for a prosthesis, it is a good idea to wear a close-fitting dress, sweater or clingy blouse that will give you a good view of how your bosom will look in clothing. You may wish to ask your sister or best friend to accompany you to the store.

In spite of these new, better-fitting prostheses, some women still feel that what they'd like more than anything is another real breast. And with today's advances in plastic surgery, some women are finding that breast reconstruction is no problem. Or at least, it's well worth the trouble because it gives them back the self-confidence and freedom they lost with the mastectomy.

Actually, if you have any intention of considering breast reconstruction, it's best to bring it up with your surgeon *prior* to the mastectomy. This may affect certain decisions he'll make early on, which could make the reconstruction easier.

If you haven't already discussed breast reconstruction surgery with your physician, one of your postoperative checkups might be a good time to bring it up. Don't be disappointed if your surgeon or physician glosses over the possibility of rebuilding the breast. His word is not final. Traditionally, surgeons have felt that you should thank God for being alive, and just forget about your silly breasts.

Reconstruction is widely available and can be done after almost any type of mastectomy. It is even possible after the chest muscles have been removed by a standard radical mastectomy, or after the skin has been damaged by radiation therapy. Reconstruction is more likely to be considered when the chance of recurrence is minute (that is, early stage I cancer). Detection of new cancer may be more difficult once the implant is in place. Safety of reconstruction from the standpoint of masking cancer recurrence is under dispute and not heavily documented, so surgeons are still cautious when selecting patients for the procedure.

Many leading surgeons, however, share the view expressed by Curtis M. Phillips, M.D., chairman of the department of surgery at Baptist Memorial Hospital in Jacksonville, Florida, regarding reconstructed breasts for women: "If we can provide a prosthesis for them, without any undue risk, why shouldn't we at least give them this option?" (*Female Patient*, October, 1976).

Considering Breast Reconstruction

A woman has only one life to live, and she very much prefers to live it with two breasts, in spite of cancer. Knowing that reconstruction is a possible option makes a woman less afraid of going to her doctor for early diagnosis of suspicious signs. Even if a woman must face breast removal, the prospect of reconstruction softens the emotional shock that follows mastectomy. How many women, if they lost their two front teeth in an accident, would hesitate to get new "teeth" from a dentist?

Breast reconstruction is based on the surgical techniques first used for breast enlargement and is always done by a plastic surgeon. (Don't get the technique confused with silicone injections. That's a whole different—and unadvisable—ball game.) The results of reconstructive surgery are not absolutely perfect, but are very good. Don't expect guarantees. No surgeon, plastic or otherwise, can give them. But compared to a flat or concave chest, a reconstructed breast is just dandy. You may even come through it with a new nipple.

Breast reconstruction is not usually done much sooner than three to six months after the mastectomy to allow time for the surgical incision to heal, the skin to soften and stretch and to check for recurrence of cancer. It can even be done several years after mastectomy. There is also the possibility that by the time your body is ready for reconstruction, you may be so satisfied with an aesthetically pleasing prosthesis that you may no longer feel reconstruction of the breast, and the pain that goes with it, is necessary.

Because reconstruction is an elective procedure, you have plenty of time to choose your plastic surgeon. Write to the American Society of Plastic and Reconstructive Surgeons, Inc., 29 East Madison Avenue, Suite 800, Chicago, Illinois 60602. They will provide names of qualified plastic surgeons in your area. You can also check the *Directory of Medical Specialists* in your local public library, which lists plastic surgeons certified by the American Board of Plastic Surgery. Ask your prospective plastic surgeon if he does a lot of breast reconstruction work. Complications are minimized when the procedure is performed by a surgeon who is experienced at reconstruction.

You will visit the surgeon at his office for a consultation sometime before the operation. He will examine you, evaluate your particular case and answer your questions at that time. He will also consult the surgeon who performed your mastectomy about your eligibility for the operation.

Reconstruction can be done in one operation if you have enough soft tissue left in the breast area, but is usually done in at least two separate operations, sometimes more if you have had skin grafts or radiation therapy. The technique is being refined to eventually telescope the whole job into one procedure for some patients.

The first stage is always major surgery under general anesthesia. To form the breast mound, the skin on the chest is raised to create a generous, padded skin flap, and a soft, pliable sack of silicone gel is inserted into that pocket. The opening is sewn closed and often left unbandaged for close observation. Antibiotics are routinely given to resist in-

fection, followed by painkillers for several days. Activity will be limited during the initial week or two after surgery.

Two months or more later, the second stage of surgery is done either under general anesthesia in the hospital or under local anesthesia in the office operating room. The surgeon will enlarge the breast, reposition the implant, if necessary, and possibly add a nipple and areola. Those can sometimes be fashioned from the labia (pigmented skin folds just outside the vagina) or grafted from your remaining real nipple and areola. If your nipple was saved at the time of mastectomy—that is, removed from the breast and attached to the inside of the thigh—it can be reapplied to the new breast at this time.

The size, shape, position and appearance of a refashioned nipple may fall short of expectations. Restored nipples lack the sensitivity of an intact or real nipple. But many women are completely satisfied with contour restoration and are not concerned if the nipple is not restored.

You won't look like the Venus de Milo, but the implanted breast will be rather firm and natural-looking. Use of an implant limits its size, so your remaining breast may require surgical remodeling to balance it with the reconstructed breast. If your own breast is large, it will be pared down to match the new one; if it is small, it will be augmented with an implant similar to the one fitted under the new breast; and if it is saggy, it will be firmed up. The goal is a new, symmetrical you.

While most women are very pleased with the results of reconstructive surgery, you should go into it knowing the minuses as well as the pluses. There are a few possible complications. The skin flap between the implant and your body is thin and its blood supply not perfectly efficient, so swelling, discoloration, infection and occasional skin breakdown may occur. Fluid may collect under the flap and persist for weeks. The implant itself can harden or shift. Robert M. Goldwyn, M.D., a Boston surgeon who does a lot of breast reconstruction, feels that complications are fewer when the operation is done in two stages.

Fees for cosmetic surgery—which reconstruction is often considered to be—are high and depend on the extent of the surgery required. Costs may vary slightly from community to community and surgeon to surgeon. The surgeon's fee will be added to hospital costs, operating room charges, anesthesiologist fees and so forth. Costs related to breast reconstruction are not reimbursed by Medicare at this time, but the procedure is currently under review. Your private carrier may reimburse you. Most Blue Cross–Blue Shield plans now cover reconstruction under Major Medical, and the trend is likely to continue. Contact your own carrier to see where you stand.

MASTITIS

If you are breastfeeding and develop pain and swelling in your breast, as well as a painful lump, you probably have a blocked milk duct. But when a blocked duct is also accompanied by redness, fever and a general sick feeling—tired, rundown, aching—you've got a breast infection, otherwise known as mastitis. Don't panic. Mastitis is quite common, and when caught early—particularly before a fever develops—it will usually respond with simple home remedies. Best of all, you might be relieved to know that your breastfeeding schedule won't have to be interrupted.

Actually, there are many causes of mastitis, not the least of which is the tension and stress of adjusting to a new baby. The infection may also be brought on by a tight bra that has somehow plugged a milk duct and stopped milk flow, or by a cracked nipple which is an open invitation to infection.

But whatever you do, don't stop nursing. Women mistakenly believe that their infection will be transferred to the baby and, on top of that, that continued breastfeeding will just make their problem worse. In fact, the opposite holds true. Mastitis will in no way affect the health of your breastfed child. And, while it may be painful to breastfeed, the breast will hurt less afterward because it will be emptied of milk. Any gynecologist will tell you, keeping the breast empty is step one to recovery.

Step two is to take a nice hot bath or shower and let your breast bask in the heat as often as possible. Or relax with a heating pad on your breast. Remember, too, a breast infection is like a throat infection or a cold: in order to feel better faster you'll have to rest and take it easy for a few days. Don't push yourself.

Finally, it's important that you continue wearing your bra—even while you're sleeping. Just make sure it fits properly and isn't pinching you or rubbing deep into your shoulders.

Sore, cracked nipples should be lubricated with a mild ointment such as water-based lanolin or A and D Ointment. Some women have also suggested that the oil from a vitamin E capsule has helped to heal cracked nipples when nothing else worked.

If, in spite of all these measures, your condition hasn't improved in 24 hours or if your fever is greater than 101°F, call your doctor. He or she will probably prescribe antibiotics for a few days. Drugs are passed on to your child in your breast milk in small quantities. But, according to Jennifer Niebyl, M.D., associate professor of gynecology and obstetrics at the Johns Hopkins University School of Medicine in Baltimore, Maryland, the benefits of continued breastfeeding outweigh the risks of taking antibiotics. Only tetracycline can cause teeth discoloration in newborns, she says; penicillin and erythromycin are safer.

MENOPAUSE

Menopause, like menstrual onset, is so wrapped up in rumor and misconception that many women are convinced "the curse" will catch them coming and going. Women who know better, however, know that just isn't so. For them this "change of life" represents a natural transitional period which gives rise to another phase in female maturity—and one that affords a new kind of freedom. The end of menstruation, then, doesn't mark the end of the world but rather the beginning of an exciting and challenging new lifestyle.

Of course, getting there involves a hormonal change of some magnitude. And that's not likely to go by unnoticed. Nor would we want to mislead you by saying it's easy. But the transition can be less traumatic when you know what to expect and why.

The term menopause refers to the actual cessation of all menstrual periods. For some women this may occur abruptly. But for most, menopause is easier to articulate than anticipate. The reason is, it doesn't usually happen overnight. Rather, it is preceded by a gradual slowdown of ovarian function which can span 4 to 6—sometimes 10—years. During this time, estrogen production may taper off gradually, causing the amount and duration of the menstrual flow to decrease accordingly.

More commonly, however, the shifting to a new hormonal equilibrium is jerky and uneven so that periods become increasingly erratic. There may be a heavy flow one month, the next month scant, several months with no period at all, then another flow or two before the period stops altogether. The trouble is, you'll never know *exactly* when you have reached menopause—that is, when menstruation has ceased for good. And the only way to be certain that it has happened is when you've been free of periods for one full year.

For most women, menopause comes between their 45th and 53rd year, although some women continue to menstruate into their sixties. This age is predetermined to a large extent by genetics. So, if your mother stopped menstruating by age 48, there's a better-than-average chance that you, too, will reach menopause in your late forties or thereabouts. However, there are several outside factors that may shift that date somewhat, in either direction.

A couple of years ago, for example, a Belgian study involving almost 4,000 women disclosed that women who weighed more than 132 pounds tended to go through menopause at a much later age than women who weighed less than that (*Maturitas*, September, 1978).

In yet another extensive investigation—this one based on the case histories of more than 3,500 women in seven countries—three Boston researchers made the startling discovery that cigarette smoking may actually foreshorten a woman's menstrual years and bring on menopause at a much earlier age than if she doesn't smoke. The study further suggests that the more cigarettes a woman smokes per day, the earlier her menopause is likely to occur (*Lancet*, June 25, 1977).

At this point, there doesn't appear to be any benefit in extending or shortening your normal span of childbearing years. If anything, the reverse may be true. For example, Barry Sherman, M.D., Robert Wallace, M.D., and Alan Treloar, Ph.D., of the University of Iowa Medical School, found that heavy women—who tend to have a later menopause than thin women—have a higher than average risk of breast cancer. The link, they say, is in their fat stores which supply them with a greater edge in the estrogen department. The more estrogen you've got as you near the menopausal years, the longer you may be able to stave off menopause but the greater your chances of developing breast cancer.

On the other hand, smoking your way down a shorter road to menopause is likewise liable to have you stumbling across some unforeseen health ruts along the way. According to Hershel Jick, M.D., of the Boston University School of Medicine, now that it appears smoking throws more women prematurely into menopause, perhaps it's time to reevaluate our thinking on the actual role menopause plays in the development of heart disease. Since smoking is also associated with a higher risk of heart disease, perhaps smoking—and not menopause per se—is responsible for statistics that note a higher incidence of heart disease in postmenopausal women, he says.

About the only conclusions we can draw from all of this is that menopause involves a perfectly natural physiological transition which takes place according to a built-in biological clock. Anything we can do to keep from interfering with this delicate schedule is probably to our benefit. Of course, at the present time it's impossible to know every factor that should be avoided because of its potential impact on menopause. But we can guess that not smoking and watching our weight combined with sensible fitness and dietary habits are a start.

The important thing to remember here is that menopause is not something to be dreaded like a disease. It is normal for every woman. And while it does signal the end of menstruation, it does not—as is mistakenly believed—involve the abrupt shutdown of estrogen production. Granted, estrogen production will slow down considerably. But your ovaries will continue to produce estrogen for 10 or 15, possibly even 20 years after you pass the menopause mark. The only exception to that is, of course, in the case of surgical menopause, when the ovaries have been physically removed. Then the estrogen reduction is sudden and dramatic, and the symptoms that much worse.

But what about the rest of us, you may ask. Isn't it true that with menopause come symptoms of hot flashes, vaginal dryness, weight gain, wrinkles, thinning hair or baldness, unwanted facial hair, and depression, anxiety, even madness?

Hot Flashes: the Only True Menopausal Symptom

Actually, no. The only symptom above that appears to be a direct result of the body's immediate slowed estrogen production is hot flashes. In one study of tribal South Africa, for instance, Wulf H. Utian, M.D., of Case Western Reserve Medical School in Cleveland, found that in a culture where menopause is embraced as a welcomed passage in life, and postmenopausal women are respected for their experience and wisdom, women rarely complain of menopausal symptoms. "In our culture," says Dr. Utian, "several things often occur simultaneously in a woman's life at about the time of her menopause: her children leave home, she may lose one or both parents, her husband may be faced with work and social pressures, or he may become sick or so successful he has no time for his wife. If she just sits back and acquires a negative self-image, she may develop symptoms which are falsely blamed on menopause."

An explanation of physiological changes at the time of menopause will help you understand why some symptoms are directly related to the menopause while some are not. At some time when a woman is in her midyears, her ovaries get a message from the brain to slow down their estrogen production. The pituitary gland—which also produces hormones at a rate that complements the ovaries' production—misconstrues this ovarian slowdown as a problem. In an attempt to set things straight, the pituitary sends a surge of hormone (the follicle-stimulating hormone, or FSH) to the ovaries in hopes of jarring them back on schedule. It

doesn't work, so the pituitary sends another shot, and another, and another, until you wind up with a hormonal imbalance that involves more than just estrogen, the one you hear most about.

Since the hypothalamus, the master gland in the brain, is intimately involved with the pituitary, any imbalance there has some impact on the hypothalamus. The hypothalamus, not surprisingly, is involved in such body functions as sleep, heat regulation and energy levels, not to mention the vast network of nerves. This is why the symptoms that can be directly correlated to the hormone swings of menopause are hot flashes, tingling sensations, insomnia, heart palpitations, fatigue and occasional migrainelike headaches.

Otherwise, none of the remaining symptoms are the direct result of estrogen cutback. Instead, most follow your individual aging progress; the speed and degree to which they affect you depend on genetics and countless other environmental factors. The only exception to this—that is, the only symptoms mentioned above that have no real connection with either aging or menopause—are the emotional ones: depression, anxiety and madness.

For example, a special form of depression called involutional melancholia—because it is thought to involve a "degenerative" biological change, meaning menopause—is a myth, according to a Yale University psychiatric researcher. After an intensive review of published data and a study at Yale involving 422 women suffering from depression, Myrna M. Weissman, Ph.D., concludes that women between ages 45 and 55 have *no* increase in symptoms or susceptibility to depression (*Journal of the American Medical Association*, August 24–31, 1979).

"Despite popular belief, clinical writings and the official nomenclature, several independent studies fail to show an increase in depression among women in the menopausal years," says Dr. Weissman. "Moreover, depressions occurring in menopausal women do not appear to exhibit a distinct pattern."

So, contrary to popular belief, the menopausal drop in hormones has no effect on depression. It seems that this common phenomenon is spurred not so much by diminishing hormones as by a woman's diminishing self-esteem. Early writings, after all, which talked of menopause as a time of emotional and physical turmoil, gave menopausal women much to be depressed about. The loss of femininity, the irrevocable sterility. But today, brighter, more sensible attitudes are changing all that.

A Boston survey of 484 women from 25 to more than 60 years of age showed that while the younger women had negative feelings associated with menopause, the menopausal women had positive or neutral associations. In general, the younger women were more fearful of the unknown and felt more negative about their own distant menopause. Those women who were between 25 and 40 expressed the more traditional beliefs concerning menopausal symptoms. The women who were experiencing menopause or were postmenopausal, however, felt neutral or positive about their experience. When asked specifically about the loss of childbearing capacity, 90 percent either didn't care one way or the other or were pleased to have passed that part of their life (*Our Bodies, Ourselves*, Simon & Schuster, 1976).

A survey conducted by the National Center for Health Statistics between 1971 and 1975 supports those findings.

Women over 40 (the age at which menopause becomes a pressing reality for most) were less likely to report a nervous breakdown or the feeling that one was coming on than were women who were at that age when they were interviewed 10 years earlier.

Even more interesting was the finding that today menopausal and postmenopausal women are enjoying a more positive mental outlook than women in their twenties and thirties. While 10 years ago these younger women were the ones who carried on as if nothing fazed them, today more nervous breakdowns were reported in women under 45. So look who's happy now!

Sexually, too, menopausal women are more well adjusted today than ever before. Previously, women might well have been influenced by preachings that sexual desire or libido is lost with the monthly menstrual periods, and that as women pass that menopause mark they become less physically attractive. For example, in 1904, a noted sexologist wrote in *Sexology* (Philadelphia Puritan):

> . . . in well-regulated lives the sexual passions become less and less imperious, diminishing gradually, until an average of 45 in the woman and 55 in the man, they are but rarely awakened and seldom solicited. . . . Nothing can exceed the calm of parents descending the downhill of life. . .for whom the present, freed from the torments of excitement, has only the sweet rewards of contentment and repose.
> —*Postgraduate Medicine*, May, 1979

He also commented that "after the 'change of life' sexual congress, while permissible, should be infrequent" for the sake of both wife and husband. The consequences of indulgence, he added, were sudden death by rupture of large blood vessels for the man and cancer of the womb for women.

Thank goodness we've come to our senses. Today the last thing a woman needs is a scare tactic like that. She knows where her libido is. In the Boston survey mentioned earlier, about half of the menopausal and postmenopausal women reported no change in sexual desire, while the rest were equally divided in reporting an increase or decrease in libido. When asked if they felt differently about themselves, sexually, two-thirds said no.

In Shere Hite's famous nationwide study of female sexuality, *The Hite Report* (Macmillan, 1976), the same kind of positive sexual feelings among older women emerged. For example, to the author's questions, "How does age affect sex? Does desire for sex increase or decrease, or neither, with age? Enjoyment of sex?" she received the following sample responses:

"I am enjoying sex more in my forties than I did in my thirties; I enjoyed it more in my thirties than in my twenties. There's a liberating combination of experience, self-knowledge, and confidence, and an absence of pregnancy fears."

"I think that men are conned into believing that it decreases in age for them. I don't think it decreases drastically for anyone, *especially* for women. My best sexual experiences are coming out of maturity and self-confidence."

"Menopause makes everything better, easier, and less dependent on time . . . I went through it fairly easily."

"I am 66 and sexual desire has not diminished. The enjoyment is as great as ever. I think it might diminish if you couldn't have sex. But enjoying it has nothing to do with age."

Granted, there were some women who responded negatively to the same question—women who did not have satisfying sex lives. But the point is, if you have an active sex life prior to menopause, there's no reason why going through the "change of life" should change all that. In fact, there is some evidence that libido should—at least theoretically—increase at menopause, because of the nature of hormonal changes. (Just remember, if you do engage in intercourse, continue to use some method of birth control until a year after your last period.)

Of course, to make menopause a positive experience both psychologically and physically, you can't underestimate the effect of an extra good diet. That's not to say that this is the only time you need to eat right—there are obvious advantages to eating a wholesome, sensible diet throughout every phase of life. But there are special needs and requirements during these menopausal and postmenopausal years that must be met.

For one thing, as we grow older, our bodies require fewer calories for maintenance. Consequently, if you follow your natural appetite, you should be eating less than you did in your twenties. The only trouble is, while our calorie needs decrease, our nutrient needs stay the same or even increase. That means that choosing your foods wisely, including those that are low in calories but high in nutrition, is even more important now. Also, because calorie needs are lower, beware of high-fat and high-sugar foods which can put weight on you faster than ever before.

You've got to remember that there

are a few physical pitfalls of menopause—namely, osteoporosis and heart disease. So your diet should counteract these, and it can if you plan it right. In other words, if you avoid high-fat, high-cholesterol foods and concentrate instead on whole foods—whole grains, fresh fruits and vegetables, and low-fat but high-calcium items such as buttermilk, low-fat yogurt, cottage cheese and skim milk.

For added assurance, supplements are a must during menopause. Specifically, a good B complex supplement and vitamin C to help you cope with stress and prevent depression and anxiety; calcium and vitamin D to strengthen bones and prevent osteoporosis; and vitamin E for hot flashes and more. We say "more" because in a 1974 survey conducted by *Prevention* magazine, over 2,000 women who responded volunteered that vitamin E relieved all their menopausal problems either partly or entirely. The most frequent comments were: more energy and a better sense of well-being; relief of leg cramps; and relief of hot flashes and other problems of menopause. We asked Jonathan V. Wright, M.D., a nutrition-oriented physician from Kent, Washington, and author of *Dr. Wright's Book of Nutritional Therapy* (Rodale Press, 1979) if there was anything else he could add to the list.

"Some women are very successful with very high doses of vitamin E throughout the menopause—2,000 to 3,000 [international] units daily. They say that either it knocked out their symptoms completely—physical symptoms—or at least they became tolerable, and not really as bad as they used to be," he told us. "I found that sometimes a combination of vitamins and kelp helps. In some women kelp seems to do something to reduce or relieve menopause

symptoms. And a third way—bioflavonoids, rutin, hesperidin. So they get bioflavonoids in 500- or 1,000-milligram tablets and take several of those a day. I usually ask people to play with those three things and see if they can use one or a combination of them that's going to knock down the symptoms or at least relieve them enough so that they are tolerable.

"If they are taking estrogen then the thing to do is to take nutritional safeguards against bad effects, mainly to use the whole B complex to detoxify that estrogen in the body, and, as Dr. Carlton Fredericks [a well-known nutritionist] has been pointing out for the last several years, including a source of iodine also, and again you come down to kelp to protect against some of the effects of estrogen."

We'd also like to point out that exercise is just as important during the menopausal and postmenopausal years as it is at any other phase of your life. That's not to say that you need to turn in your favorite rocking chair for a pair of running shoes—though that's not a bad idea. Of course, you've got to consider what kind of shape you're in to begin with. If you've been physically active all your life, there's no reason to stop now. If you haven't, this is as good a time as any to start. It's really never too late—so don't use that one as an excuse. In fact, one of the best exercises for you may be walking. Don't scoff at that. Walking at a fairly brisk pace every day and gradually increasing the distance you walk is probably the safest and most effective way to get in shape. And it's something practically everyone can do. Yoga is another good way to gently limber up and is, by the way, an excellent way to relieve arthritis pain.

In any case, the benefits of exercise at this point in your life are many. It keeps your joints and muscles limbered up and strong. It gives spring to your step and color to your cheeks so you'll look as young as you feel. It helps to build bones and thus prevents osteoporosis. It banishes fatigue and depression. It gives you the edge on heart disease. What more could you ask for?

For more information on related subjects see Fitness, Heart Disease, Hot Flashes, Osteoporosis, Vaginitis: Atrophic, and Wrinkles.

Robert Griffith

Yoga and walking are two excellent but less strenuous ways to get started back on the road to fitness for women who've been somewhat inactive over the years.

MENSTRUAL PROBLEMS

An occasional abnormal period isn't unusual. Almost all of us, at some point in our lives, will experience some kind of problem. A menstrual period may be shorter or longer than normal. Bleeding may be scant or exceptionally heavy at times. Spotting may occur at midcycle. Timing may be off; perhaps your usually punctual period will be a couple of weeks late or several days early—maybe you'll miss a month altogether.

If your schedule goes askew once in a great while, it's probably nothing to worry about. The condition will quickly return to normal. But when the problem persists for three or more months, it's time to ask, Why?

Sometimes these symptoms signal a more serious underlying problem. Profuse and prolonged menstrual bleeding, for example, can be a sign of fibroid tumors, endometrial hyperplasia (an overgrowth of the uterine lining), or even endometrial cancer. Similarly, midcycle spotting may occasionally be just an accompaniment to "mittelschmerz" (pain midway between the menstrual periods) at ovulation—or it could be a warning of some potentially serious cervical condition. And since the menstrual cycle is such a complicated process, pinpointing the problem is often a job for a qualified gynecologist. So for any persistent menstrual complaint, see your physician. If he or she can rule out serious trouble, perhaps the cause is related to your lifestyle— and some simple, natural healing methods can get you back on track.

Actually, there are even certain times when an abnormal period is considered perfectly normal—that is, in the very beginning and toward the end of a woman's menstruating years. During adolescence and again at menopause, ovulation frequently misses its cue. And without ovulation, all kinds of menstrual problems can erupt. Heavy bleeding. Light bleeding. Unpredictable periods. You name it.

What happens is, a woman's hormones need some time to adjust to the various stages of her life. Early on, a girl's circulating estrogen level is gradually rising to a new high. And later on, when a woman reaches her middle years, her estrogen levels begin to taper off a bit. But without just the right amount of this and other very important hormones, ovulation will not take place. And without ovulation, there is no release of progesterone—the hormone responsible for regulating the menstrual cycle.

Otherwise, an occasional miss or fluctuation throughout the reproductive years can be caused by any of a number of factors. For one thing, the menstrual cycle depends on hormonal harmony and since the master gland which regulates our hormones lies in the brain, any kind of mind factor—from anxiety over a new job to the stress of vacation-

ing with two toddlers—can knock a menstrual cycle out of whack. Likewise the effect of various drugs, such as tranquilizers, on the brain can disrupt menstruation in some women.

In addition to emotional health, regular menstrual cycles hinge on good physical condition—the kind that comes with a sensible exercise program and a natural, wholesome diet. How do these factors enter in? You'd be surprised! For one thing, we know that crash dieting is the quickest way to put a dent into a perfectly smooth-running menstrual cycle. And second, women whose poor dietary and exercise regimens leave them either overweight or underweight experience menstrual problems more frequently than do women of normal weight.

Failure to Begin Menstruating (Primary Amenorrhea)

If a girl reaches the age of 16 without menstruating, there is some reason to suspect trouble. But not always—it's not unheard of for periods to begin at age 18. Still, the usual procedure at this stage of the game is to see a doctor. He or she can usually tell whether the gal's just a late bloomer or if her hormones are out of order. One thing he may not consider, however, is her athletic inclination.

According to Allan J. Ryan, M.D., of Minneapolis, one factor which appears to have a profound influence on menstrual onset and "may well be the most common cause of delayed menarche in young women in this country today" is athletic training (*Postgraduate Medicine*, March, 1980). Apparently, adolescent girls who engage in intensive training programs such as running, gymnastics or ballet do not begin menstruating at the usual time. In fact, many fail to menstruate until they stop training. When they do stop, the majority start to menstruate within a few months and continue to menstruate normally without any problems.

Why this is, no one can say for sure. But the most plausible reason has to do with body fat. Like it or not, fat is closely allied with estrogen. And, according to several researchers, including R. E. Frisch, Ph.D., a woman's body build must contain a particular percentage of fat (at least 17 percent) somewhere in order for estrogen production to signal the initial menstrual cycle to begin on cue (*Science*, September 13, 1974).

What this means is that adolescent girls with vigorous athletic pursuits may trim the fat so closely that their hormones go on a temporary hiatus. But it's not only cheerleading practice that's to blame—those quick meals at McDonald's and generally poor eating habits can do a girl in just as surely. During adolescence there is a significant growth spurt. It takes a good healthy appetite to fill out the width to match that sudden soar in height. Likewise, the lean and hungry look of anorexic girls (that is, girls who purposely diet to the point of starvation) may be at the root of their failure to menstruate (see Anorexia Nervosa).

When Menstrual Periods Stop (Secondary Amenorrhea)

It may sound silly, but the most common reasons for suspended menstruation are pregnancy and menopause. Obviously. If you have positively ruled out both of those, consider your lifestyle. Just as a strenuous training program or stringent diet can delay menstrual onset, so can they discontinue a long-functioning menstrual cycle.

For example, biologist Karen A. Carl-berg, of the University of New Mexico, reports that female athletes miss their menstrual periods more frequently than women who have no vigorous athletic pursuits. More specifically, in her study, 12 percent of the athletes as compared to 2 percent of the nonathletes suffered from amenorrhea for between three months and four years. Data compiled by C. Harmon Brown, M.D., director of Olympic development for women's track and field in this country and head of student health services at California State University, Hayward, reveals a similar correlation between athletics and amenorrhea. "About 30 percent [of the long-distance women runners at the Olympic training camp in Squaw Valley, California] had no periods at all during training, while they had fairly regular periods before," he explains.

Dieting, too, can cause a similar disruption. For example, of a group of 170 nonmenstruating women seen at St. Mary's Hospital in London, 39 stopped getting their periods as a direct result of dieting. And while it's true that many of those women suffered from anorexia nervosa, 15 did not. They simply embarked on an ambitious weight-reducing scheme that left their bodies starving for the hormones necessary to bring on their monthly periods. Another study confirms that women suffering from dietary amenorrhea have an impairment in function of the luteinizing hormone (LH) which triggers ovulation (*British Medical Journal*, February 11, 1978).

There is much speculation as to the cause of all this. Some say the mere stress and strain of a severe exercise or dietary regimen is enough to shake the system. Others suggest that in the process of overexercising or undereating, a woman may lose much of her body fat. And, if her fatty stores dip below a certain critical point of perhaps 22 percent (in the average woman, fat accounts for 26 to 28 percent of total body weight), neither ovulation nor menstruation will occur.

Whatever the case, most physicians feel that the condition should not affect future fertility so long as the woman regains those feminine curves of underlying fatty tissue. But putting on pounds can be as difficult to some women as taking them off is to others (see also Weight Control). And it can take from six months to a year before the menstrual cycle will get back on track.

Post-Pill Amenorrhea

You can imagine the disappointment when a woman decides on motherhood but can't muster up even one menstrual period to carry it off. Well, unfortunately, that happens to more than a few women who take birth control pills. For some reason, coming off oral contraceptives can bring menstruation to a screeching halt. And ironically, some of the most susceptible women are those with a history of irregular cycles— which was why many of them got on the Pill in the first place.

In their book, *Women and the Crisis in Sex Hormones* (Rawson Associates, 1977), Barbara Seaman and Gideon Seaman, M.D., cite countless reports of post-Pill amenorrhea and infertility, some of which involved permanent problems. For the majority of women, however, they claim that the outlook is brighter. While most doctors attempt to remedy the situation by prescribing yet more hormones, "most cases of post-Pill infertility and amenorrhea correct themselves spontaneously within a few months to two years," they explain. "With the proper nutritional stimulus, many such cases can right themselves much more quickly than that."

For "proper nutritional stimulus" the Seamans recommend a high-protein diet supplemented with B_6, zinc, folate, C, E, and selenium. "On this regimen, ovulation and menstruation usually return within three to four months," they claim, "unless the amenorrheic woman is underweight as well." In cases where slimness interferes with the solution, the Seamans suggest a higher-calorie diet including wheat germ oil and other forms of vitamin E. "E—especially in the form of wheat germ oil—was demonstrated—long before the era of the Pill—to induce menstruation in women who are malnourished or extremely stressed," they say.

Irregular Bleeding Intervals

Intrauterine devices (IUDs), birth control pills, and ectopic pregnancies (pregnancies that occur in the fallopian tubes) can all present you with irregular periods. Usually, however, bad timing is more closely related to stress or poor dietary habits. And to a certain extent, all of the information that relates to amenorrhea can be taken into account here as well.

More specifically, however, to regulate a sporadic menstrual cycle you may also want to boost your intake of B vitamins with brewer's yeast or B complex supplements. The B vitamins have long been recommended for problem periods (see also Cramps and Other Premenstrual Miseries). And although there is no scientific evidence that they help in menstrual regulation, we have heard of several cases in which they did. One woman writes of her experience with B's:

"Since age 13 (I am now 28) my monthly period has been quite irregular. Occasionally I'd go four to six months with no monthly flow. After consulting various doctors over the years, I concluded that this was the way my system was and accepted it.... Last spring I began taking a B complex supplement... and after five months of perfectly on-time periods, I began wondering about it. My roommate has had the same experience, but she experimented by not taking any B vitamins. Her period became irregular again. No doubt, we'll both stick with the B supplements."

Profuse or Prolonged Menstrual Bleeding (Menorrhagia)

An excessive loss of menstrual blood—either due to an extraordinarily heavy flow or an extended menstrual period—can be a sign of serious uterine distress. It is also frequently encountered in association with the use of intrauterine devices. In fact, an article in the *British Medical Journal* states that "IUDs may increase the incidence of menorrhagia at least fivefold in otherwise healthy women." And, "intermenstrual spotting occurs in about one-third of women" (February, 1976).

But every once in a while, a physician comes across a case of menorrhagia that defies diagnosis. There's no evidence of fibroids. Pap smears are normal. Even a D and C (dilation and curettage) fails to uncover any concealed malady. Basically, the uterus is in A-1 condition but the woman, obviously, is not.

She might be going through 14 tampons a day. Or waiting out a menstrual period that lasts for weeks or even months. Her blood count is understandably low, as is her stamina: she complains that she doesn't have the energy to go to work or take care of her kids.

Unfortunately, what causes this problem is not always easy to assess.

When it isn't related to disease (which should be determined by a Pap smear and, if necessary, a D and C), the condition is simply labeled "dysfunctional bleeding," meaning that it's a result of some functional problem in the reproductive organs. As we mentioned earlier, sometimes—and particularly in women nearing menopause—the problem is in the ovaries' failure to produce eggs, or ovulate.

Typically, medical treatment includes a D and C (dilation of the cervix and curettage of the uterus) to clean out the excess blood buildup and temporarily stop the bleeding as well as to rule out any malignancy, and hormone therapy—usually a progesterone pill or an estrogen-progesterone compound—to signal the periodic shedding.

That combination treatment is often successful in controlling the bleeding, particularly in women who are biding their time till menopause, when dysfunctional bleeding should subside. Yet, hormones are not without their side effects, including the increased risk of endometrial and possibly even breast cancer.

Vitamin A and Heavy Bleeding

For those who'd rather not take the chance, a study published in the *South African Medical Journal* which suggests that moderately high doses of vitamin A can reduce heavy menstrual bleeding offers another, natural alternative. (February 12, 1977).

Although the effect of a vitamin A deficiency on the reproductive systems of women has never been clearly documented, it's known that vitamin A levels in women fluctuate in a cyclic pattern during the menstrual cycle. That—in addition to animal studies that showed a laboratory-induced vitamin A deficiency decreased hormone production and suspended the menstrual cycle—suggests a strong correlation between vitamin A levels and female hormones.

With that information at hand, Drs. D. M. Lithgow and W. M. Politzer of Johannesburg, South Africa, tested the vitamin A levels in 71 women suffering from menorrhagia and found, on the average, only 67 international units (I.U.) of the vitamin per 100 milliliters of blood. By comparison, a group of healthy controls with normal menstrual periods had about 166 I.U. per 100 milliliters—almost 2½ times the amount measured in the first group.

To make sure this wasn't a coincidence, the researchers then decided to treat 52 women with symptoms of dysfunctional bleeding with 60,000 I.U. of vitamin A a day for 35 days. Close to 93 percent of the women treated were either cured or helped by the vitamin A.

One woman we spoke with reported similar success:

"I had been having heavy bleeding during my periods for at least a year. I've never been able to do much on the first day, but this kept me down five days a month. I was hemorrhaging. I had to change every 10 or 15 minutes, and I couldn't do a thing. I went for 1½ years to doctors: first, my family doctor, a gynecologist and a hematologist. The hematologist suggested a hysterectomy. So I went to see the gynecologist again and he was hesitant about operating. He said he hated to do it since internally I appeared to be perfectly normal. However, he wanted to prescribe the Pill. Some choice, hysterectomy or the Pill! About a week later I read about vitamin A for heavy bleeding, so I started taking 10,000 units [I.U.] of the vitamin twice a day. I was due for a period in 2½ weeks. When it came, there was no hemorrhaging. There was a

heavy flow, but I could carry on normal activities. After that my periods were normal. That was several months ago and I haven't been to a doctor since."

(Vitamin A is one vitamin you can take too much of, but 25,000 I.U. a day will not cause adults any problems. Nearly all cases of toxicity involve taking hundreds of thousands of units every day for months or years.)

Heavy menstrual bleeding has also been shown to ease up with bioflavonoids. That, according to a group of doctors at a French hospital who reported that these nutrients gave the women "good to excellent results." Bioflavonoids, usually extracted for supplements from the inner peel and white pulpy portion of citrus fruits, are widely recognized in Europe for their ability to strengthen blood vessels, particularly the walls of the capillaries. In treating menorrhagia patients with bioflavonoids, the French doctors observed "progressive improvement, with the most marked improvement achieved by the third menstrual cycle" (*Family Practice News*, March 15, 1974).

One woman felt strongly enough about the benefits of bioflavonoids to write us:

"For more than ten years I have been suffering from menstrual disorders. My menstrual cycle was shorter than average—25 days—and the flow was much heavier than normal. This caused extra iron loss and tied me close to home during those times. A nuisance to say the least. My doctor suggested a hysterectomy, and warned that such heavy blood loss over the years would be very hard on my body (I am 29 years old).

"Then I read of a European study in which bioflavonoids helped some women with menstrual disorders. So I started taking one gram of citrus bioflavonoids a day. The first month I noticed no change. The second month my cycle increased in length, and the flow decreased considerably. My cycle is now 34 days and I am free to move around any day of the month. I plan on staying on the bioflavonoids indefinitely as my body apparently had a need for more than the average intake."

In addition, no matter what the cause or treatment, heavy menstrual bleeding should be counteracted with a stepped-up intake of iron to prevent anemia. Liver and other meats, green leafy vegetables, apricots and blackstrap molasses are all excellent sources of iron. Dairy products are not (remember that, if you're on a self-imposed cottage cheese-and-yogurt diet). For more on this and the kinds of iron supplements that matter most, see Anemia.

MENSTRUATION

Most women simply think of menstruation as their monthly period. Period. But there's a whole lot more to the menstrual cycle than that. In fact, this bloody inconvenience we so disparagingly chalk off as "the curse" is quite a wondrous occurrence and just one of many intricate and interrelated processes which make up the most complex bodily function known to man—and woman, of course.

The whole business begins in the brain. Along about the time a girl graduates from anklets to knee-highs (at about seven or eight), a tiny but powerful control center in her brain begins bombarding her ovaries with a very special hormone called FSH (which stands for follicle-stimulating hormone). Its mission: to stimulate growth of the infinitesimal sacs, called follicles, which surround each egg. Not every sac is singled out, however. With 40,000 to 400,000 or so immature eggs to choose from, this is a very selective process. But as more and more are selected and stimulated to grow, specific cells within each follicle begin to crank out that more familiar female hormone, estrogen—you know, the one responsible for redistributing baby fat into feminine body contours.

In fact, a young girl's budding breasts are the very first sign that follicles have begun to ripen and release that strictly feminine hormone. More subtle internal changes soon follow. For example, before the onset of the first menstrual period, the uterus blossoms to a new adult size and the lining of the uterus plumps up to soft and sumptuous proportions. All this on account of estrogen.

We are told that the average girl will probably notice changes in her breasts by age 10 and begin menstruating by age 12. But let's face it, few of us are average. And the truth of the matter is, anywhere from 9 to 16 (or occasionally even 17 or 18) can be perfectly normal for you. The age of onset is predetermined, at least in part, by heredity. If your mother began menstruating at age 14, chances are you will, too. And even if you reach your 15th birthday without losing a bloody drop, don't panic. Individual variations are such that no two women—not even mother and daughter—are exactly alike.

In any case, that periodic bleeding, as we know it, is just as remarkable as the initial preparation for it. And, again, estrogen continues to play a crucial role.

As long as the level of estrogen

reaching the uterine lining is maintained above a certain level, the tissue lining continues to grow and thicken indefinitely. It's when the estrogen level takes a slight dip that the lining begins to slough off and bleeding occurs. What causes this cutback in estrogen production?

Well, once again we go back to the brain for the answer. Because the brain is the source not only of FSH, which stimulates follicles to maturity, but also of another hormone called LH (luteinizing hormone), which pricks one follicle open each month to release an egg.

Just before ovulation, the ovary looks perfectly smooth except for one tiny blister on the surface. This quarter-inch bulge is a follicle which has ripened and migrated to the surface of the ovary where it awaits its final cue from the brain centers. When word comes, in the form of LH, the follicle bursts open and the egg catapults into an abdominal void where it is scooped up by the funnel-like hands of the fallopian tubes. Ovulation has occurred.

Interestingly enough, the shredded remnant of the egg's last nest not only continues producing estrogen after ovulation, but the ruptured follicle now pours out another important hormone, progesterone. By stimulating the growth of specialized cells which produce nutrients to sustain a developing fetus, progesterone further readies the uterine lining to accept an implanted egg.

When the egg doesn't happen to meet up with a sperm and become fertilized, word spreads fast. Somehow the remaining follicle back in the ovary gets wind of it, and, probably realizing that there's no longer any need for a luxuriant uterine lining to bed the egg, it simply shrivels up. As it does, the production of estrogen and progesterone slowly shuts down. Without these hormones, the uterine lining begins to fall apart, pouring its blood and guts into the vaginal canal. The menstrual period has begun. At the same time, the brain centers are alerted by the lower hormone levels that the project was aborted before it was begun. In response, follicle-stimulating hormones are released and the cycle starts over again.

Menstrual bleeding usually lasts anywhere from three to seven days, with the heaviest flow occurring early on. For example, in one study it was found that 91 percent of total blood loss occurs by day three in a five-day period. By period's end, total blood loss averages about 1/2 cup.

Menstrual blood consists of red blood cells, tissues from the uterine lining, cervical mucus, cervical and vaginal cells, bacteria and enzymes. That's it. And contrary to the old wives' tale that drinking cold beverages or taking a cold shower will bring on clot formation—menstrual blood does not clot. It can't. It doesn't contain fibrinogen, the blood-clotting substance in red blood cells. What you perceive as a clot is just a blob of mucus around which some red blood cells have clustered. Nothing serious.

Understanding Your Unique Cycle

Actually, while all menstrual cycles function essentially the same way, there are variations in all women, so that your menstrual cycle is as unique to you as your fingerprints. It's part and parcel of your identity. And there are certain things you should know as part of your personal health record.

For example, at the very least you should know the length of your menstrual cycle—that is, the interval between periods. The most common menstrual cycle runs 28 days—much like the cycle of the moon. But that doesn't mean that if the onset of your next menstrual period doesn't fall on the mystical 28th day, your body rhythms are out of sync. In an extensive study of some 20,655 cycles in 2,316 women, researchers found that cycle lengths varied from 24 to 32 days. In fact, less than one-sixth of the cycles coincided with the lunar 28.

To see where you fall in all of this, take a calendar and for the next few months (at least three) note the first day of every period. Then count up the days between periods. The first day of bleeding—even if it's just a drop or two—is considered day one of your menstrual cycle. So include that day but not day one of the following cycle. In other words, if your period begins March 1 and your next period begins March 30, your cycle length is 29—not 30—days. The reason it's a good idea to repeat this countdown three or four times is that cycles can fluctuate somewhat—they can swing off schedule for any of a number of reasons including stress, travel or illness. But if you come up with the same cycle number two or three months in a row, you can consider it your lucky number.

If you'd like to take this body awareness one step further, you can calculate when ovulation occurs. Generally, ovulation takes place 14 days (give or take a couple of days) before your next period. For example, a woman with a consistent 28-day cycle may ovulate anytime from the 12th to 16th day. But again, all women are different so that rough estimate can vary even more.

To determine more precisely when your ovary releases an egg each month, you'll have to keep fastidious records of your basal body temperature and changes in cervical mucus—at least for three months or so until a pattern emerges. We discuss the full details and how-tos of this under Natural Birth Control. But briefly, this is what you're looking for: just before ovulation there is a slight but significant drop in basal body temperature followed by a sharp rise the following day. That is due to the hormone progesterone, which is released after the follicle bursts and the egg is released. Likewise, cervical mucus becomes increasingly transparent and elastic (just like raw egg white) before ovulation. Then after ovulation and the production of progesterone, the mucus reverts to its scant, sticky and cloudy "infertile" stage.

Interestingly, some women don't need to rely on an elaborate charting system for this. Each month, as the egg springs forth from its follicle, they feel a characteristic pain in the lower abdomen called "mittelschmerz" (middle pain). Some women describe it as a quick, sharp pain, others as a dull, monotonous pain much like menstrual cramps. But whatever the case, it does appear to be a very real phenomenon. Until recently, however, we could only speculate as to the cause.

Utilizing the new diagnostic method, ultrasound, a group of radiologists at Massachusetts General Hospital finally have evidence that mittelschmerz is clearly fact, not fantasy. Sixteen healthy women who did not use oral contraceptives or IUDs (intrauterine devices) were tested with the ultrasound scanner within 48 hours of ovulation. Eight of those examinations showed small amounts of fluid in the pelvic cavity—possibly blood spilled from the ovary as the follicle broke through. And since four of those eight women did experience sharp lower abdominal pain at

HOW HORMONES CONTROL YOUR MENSTRUAL CYCLE

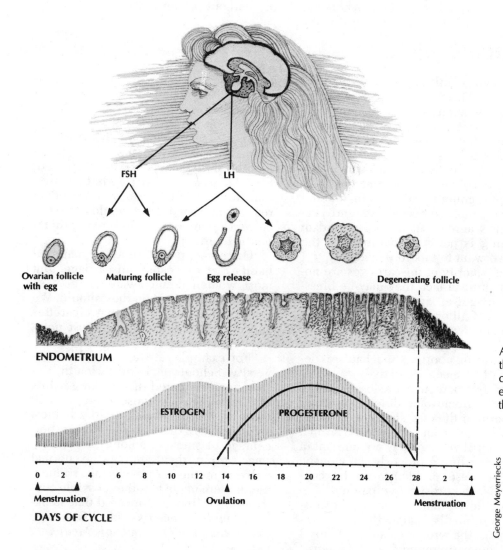

FSH

LH

Ovarian follicle with egg Maturing follicle Egg release Degenerating follicle

ENDOMETRIUM

ESTROGEN PROGESTERONE

A control center in the brain begins the complex chain of events that make up the menstrual cycle.

0 2 4 6 8 10 12 14 16 18 20 22 24 26 28 2 4

▲   ▲   ▲   ▲   ▲

Menstruation Ovulation Menstruation

DAYS OF CYCLE

George Meyerriecks

midcycle, researchers suggest that this little bit of blood could cause internal irritation and pain in sensitive women (*Journal of the American Medical Association,* June 22, 1979).

It's also possible to spot at ovulation—though this is fairly unusual and it would be wise to have any midcycle bleeding checked out with a physician.

As a matter of fact, any kind of unusual menstrual occurrences, especially changes from your norm, which persist through two or three cycles should be discussed with a qualified physician. And that, after all, is one reason why getting so intimate with your menstrual cycle is important. When you get to know what "normal" is for you, it's a cinch to spot abnormalities—even slight ones which could lead to big trouble without proper treatment.

MISCARRIAGE

More than a million women miscarry each year. That's 10 to 15 percent of all pregnant women—a fairly common occurrence. In this case, however, having company doesn't ease the misery. The loss of a baby—even if it's less than three months in the making—often stirs up all sorts of feelings of grief and guilt. We're not going to say too much about the grief; most gynecologists and psychologists agree that a brief period of mourning is perfectly natural. It's the guilt we want to talk to you about.

The majority of miscarriages are nobody's fault. In fact, they may be blessings in disguise, says Lucienne Lanson, M.D., a California gynecologist and author of *From Woman to Woman* (Alfred A. Knopf, 1975). It's nature's own built-in abortive mechanism designed to reject defective embryos. Twenty-five percent of the losses are the result of chromosome defects in either the sperm or the egg, she says. In other cases, the sperm and egg may be normal but the fertilized egg may not implant in the uterine lining properly. Obviously, none of these problems can be controlled by the prospective parents.

Trouble is, many women who miscarry continually blame themselves—and for all the wrong reasons. "If only I hadn't gone swimming" or "I knew I shouldn't have overdone the day's activities" are common self-accusations. But if you're used to swimming or cycling, or whatever, those activities aren't going to harm you or your baby—even in the first 12 weeks of the pregnancy when miscarriages are more apt to occur. If the egg is healthy and firmly attached to the womb, there's no chance that you'll be able to shake it loose.

Also, the superstition that insists that to avoid miscarriage you'll have to avoid intercourse during the first three months of pregnancy is also unfounded. Says Dr. Lanson, "It stands to reason that if an early pregnancy could be so readily disturbed there wouldn't be the current lineup of women seeking therapeutic abortions."

Of course, there are a few maternal habits that can cause miscarriage. But most women aren't aware of them so they don't worry when they should. We think you should know that cigarettes and alcohol are among the most notorious abortive agents.

For example, at the Columbia University School of Public Health, researchers compared the smoking habits of 574 women who miscarried and 320 women who delivered healthy babies. Interestingly, there was a higher percentage of smokers among the miscarriage group than among the normal delivery mothers. And even after adjustments were made for other possible contributing factors, it appeared that smoking *doubled* the risk of miscarriage (*New England Journal of Medicine*, October 13, 1977).

Furthermore, you don't have to be an alcoholic to lose a baby to alcohol. According to a recent study, even moderate drinking once or twice daily may cause miscarriages. Analyzing data from 32,019 women early in their pregnancies, researchers at the National Institute of Child Health and Human Development in California discovered that women who drank alcohol daily had a higher spontaneous abortion (miscarriage) rate than nondrinkers— regardless of smoking habits, age, previous childbirth or abortion. Those who took over three drinks daily were 3 1/2 times more likely to have a miscarriage during the second trimester (15 to 27 weeks) of their pregnancy than non-

drinkers. Women who drank once or twice daily still faced almost twice the risk of abstainers. No problem was found for women who drank less than once a day (*Lancet*, July 26, 1980).

So if you want to do best by your baby, avoid the spirits as well as the cigarettes. If then, in spite of your precautions, you miscarry, at least be reassured that it was through no fault of your own. It was probably meant to be.

MORNING SICKNESS

I've got to stop this throwing up all the time. My obstetrician says I might have to go in the hospital on I.V.'s if it gets much worse. I don't want to do that, but I can hardly keep anything down and that's not good for the baby either.

Sound familiar? For about half of all expectant mothers, morning sickness is one of those not-so-pleasant symptoms of pregnancy that can really obscure the anticipated joy of motherhood. Most cases are not as severe as the woman's above—sometimes it's just a slight nausea that completely dissipates after the 14th week. Other times, however, it can become so persistent it's downright sickening. And incidentally, it doesn't strike only in the morning. Morning sickness can last straight through into the evening, becoming particularly severe at mealtimes.

It's hard to believe that there's anything positive to say about such a nauseating problem. But here's something that may give you some consolation. While no one knows for sure what causes nausea and vomiting during pregnancy, it is known that women who do go through that ordeal are more likely to have a normal delivery and baby.

An interesting study at the University of Washington and Albany Medical

College may shed light on our understanding of this. Researchers found that women who smoke and/or drink during pregnancy are actually *less* likely to suffer nausea. It's possible then, some scientists suggest, that the reason women who are nauseated have better pregnancy outcomes is that they are less likely to be smokers or drinkers, since both habits have decidedly ill effects on the developing baby (*Acta Obstetricia Et Gynecologica Scandinavica*, vol. 58, no. 1, 1979).

What they may not have considered is that women who are nauseated usually can't stand to drink or smoke. Which leads us to speculate: could it be that nausea is a kind of extreme preventive measure taken by nature to discourage us from exposing our unborn children to toxic substances during the critical early months of their development? An interesting thought, anyway.

The trouble is, while morning sickness may be nature's way of protecting our offspring from potentially harmful substances like alcohol, cigarettes and even coffee, it can become so troublesome that it drives us to drugs, which likewise hold hazardous consequences. Medications like Bendectin and Bonine are frequently prescribed to ease nausea in pregnancy even though both have been shown to cause fetal abnormalities in laboratory animals, and, in the case of Bonine, in humans as well.

Thank goodness there are some natural alternatives that appear to work just as well. Vitamin B_6, for one, is prescribed by many nutrition-oriented physicians for their patients with morning sickness—in doses ranging from 10 milligrams a day to 200 milligrams three times a day, if necessary.

Best of all, there's no evidence that B_6 poses any health hazard to pregnant women or their developing babies. At worst, very high doses of B_6 during pregnancy can create slight problems after the birth—problems that can be easily avoided. "Six hundred milligrams of pyridoxine [B_6] daily has been found to shut off nursing, so that amount has to be cut back after childbirth," says Jonathan V. Wright, M.D., a practicing physician in Kent, Washington. "Secondly, if the baby is exposed to high amounts of B_6 before it's born and then very little immediately after birth—for example, in a commercial formula—it could possibly have withdrawal seizures. However, both these theoretical hazards are easily avoided by nursing the baby while continuing to take 20 to 30 milligrams of B_6 a day."

Two other nutrients that appear to take the queasiness out of pregnancy are vitamins K and C. Actually, this isn't new. Richard L. Merkel, M.D., first reported the benefits of these vitamins in the treatment of morning sickness in the August, 1952, issue of the *American Journal of Obstetrics and Gynecology*. Benefits which, by the way, were experienced by 64 out of 70 women he so treated.

Dr. Merkel's recommendations are for very small doses of the vitamins (5 milligrams of K and 25 milligrams of C a day) which on the average are taken for only 30 days. He does point out, however, that neither vitamin C nor vitamin K worked by itself. They had to be taken together.

Dr. Wright, who has prescribed Dr. Merkel's regimen to several patients who did not respond to B_6 therapy, agrees that it can be very effective and stresses the importance of choosing the right form of vitamin K, which will probably have to be purchased through prescription.

"Vitamins K_1 and K_2 are the naturally occurring forms. Pharmaceutical textbooks say that vitamin K_1 appears to be nontoxic," Dr. Wright says. "Vitamin K_3, a synthetic form, is theoretically toxic in very large doses. K_3 is actually the type used in Dr. Merkel's report, but I'd still rather stick with K_1."

Just how safe is vitamin K in the low doses recommended for morning sickness?

"Safer than any drug that's prescribed for it," Dr. Wright asserts. "Remember, we're talking about small doses of K. And vitamin K is the same vitamin given to all infants just after they're born to prevent hemorrhagic disease of the newborn, which is nothing more than bleeding from vitamin K deficiency. Since I discovered Dr. Merkel's article about vitamin K stopping nausea and vomiting in pregnancy, I've been wondering if there isn't a connection. Why else should so many babies require vitamin K, if their mothers get enough?"

Doctors often suggest these additional tips to ease nausea in pregnancy:

- Drink plenty of fluids to avoid dehydration.
- Eat small, frequent meals interspersed with high-protein snacks.
- Limit sweets, animal fats, heavy and fried foods, and spiced dishes.

Taking the plunge without a parachute? The mere thought sends shivers up your spine. And for some, natural birth control doesn't sound any better. But with careful observation of an intricate set of body signs, it can be as safe a method of preventing pregnancy as many others—and quite a bit safer from a health standpoint than some!

We're not talking about the rhythm method, although that is a "natural" method of birth control and one that is commonly used. The trouble is, it doesn't have a very good track record. And no wonder! All it amounts to is calculated guesswork.

The rhythm method is based on the general concept that ovulation occurs 14 days (give or take a few) before your next period. By keeping track of your periods for 6 to 12 months, and averaging out ovulation based on that 14-day standard, you're supposed to get some idea of when you ovulate. But "some idea" isn't always good enough.

It doesn't take into account that all women are different; for you, the 14-day standard may be way off base. Nor does it consider that ovulation can fluctuate from one month to the next because hormones are affected by what affects you. Stress, illness, travel—even more exercise than usual—can change the pattern of your cycle. Depending on when these circumstances occur, you may ovulate earlier or later than usual. And with the rhythm method, there's no way to predict these fluctuations. That's not to say you won't know—just that if you do, it's too late to do anything about it. Get the picture?

Fortunately, there is another method of natural birth control that is more scientific and precise in its calculations. It involves a careful observation of subtle changes in your body—more specifically, changes that occur in basal body temperature and cervical mucus.

Your monthly menstrual cycle, which is determined by a delicate balancing of hormones, culminates in an ovary's release of an egg. When this happens, the welcome mat goes out for the sperm. In preparation for its arrival, vaginal temperature (basal body temperature) rises, presumably creating a more inviting atmosphere, and the cervix steps up its production of mucus so the sperm will be able to slip and slide up the birth canal to its destination. If conditions and timing are just right, the rendezvous of sperm and egg will take place.

But this is where you can do your meddling. Once you learn to recognize when conditions are just right for fertilization, you can make sure the timing is off by abstaining from sexual intercourse at ovulation and for a few days before and after. But first you've got to keep track of those changes.

Charting Your Fertility

The best way to organize your observations is in the form of a chart. Take a piece of graph or plain paper and number from 1 to 35 across the top. These numbers represent the days of your cycle. Just above these numbers leave a space to fill in the day of the week and date—beginning the first day of your menstrual period.

On the left-hand margin of the paper, starting at the bottom, list the degrees Fahrenheit of temperature beginning

BASAL TEMPERATURE AND MUCUS CHART

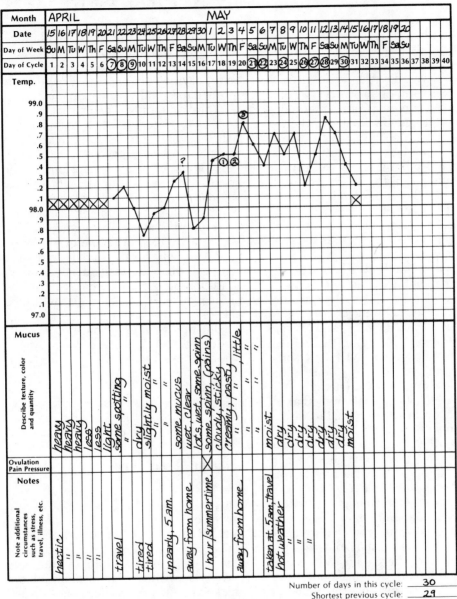

Month	APRIL															MAY																								
Date	15	16	17	18	19	20	21	22	23	24	25	26	27	28	29	30	1	2	3	4	5	6	7	8	9	10	11	12	13	14	15	16	17	18	19	20				
Day of Week	Su	M	Tu	W	Th	F	Sa	Su	M	Tu	W	Th	F	Sa	Su	M	Tu	W	Th	F	Sa	Su	M	Tu	W	Th	F	Sa	Su	M	Tu	W	Th	F	Sa	Su				
Day of Cycle	1	2	3	4	5	6	7	8	9	10	11	12	13	14	15	16	17	18	19	20	21	22	23	24	25	26	27	28	29	30	31	32	33	34	35	36	37	38	39	40

Number of days in this cycle: __30__

Shortest previous cycle: __29__

This is a sample chart of a woman who has 30-day cycles. Here ovulation probably occurred on day 16 since the temperature rose 0.6°F higher after that day and remained high for three consecutive days. Also the mucus changed from the *Spinnbarkeit* form to the creamy, scant form indicating that ovulation had occurred.

with 97.0° and ending with 99.0° or thereabouts. Underneath leave a space for recording mucus changes and a line for marking your estimate for the time of ovulation. Leave a line or two at the bottom for adding any comments on the circumstances of each day, such as "emotional," "depressed," "illness" or "travel." Then put away the chart in a safe spot till your period begins.

On the first day of your period, mark the date just above cycle day number one on the chart. There's no need to record your temperature during your period though you might like to indicate the amount of flow in the space left for mucus observations. Just cross these days off the chart with an X. Immediately after your period, start recording mucus and temperature changes.

Checking your cervical mucus may sound like a rather icky method of assessing the situation. But you've probably already noticed changes in mucous discharge when you've wiped yourself with bathroom tissue. Some days, nothing. Other days, it appears white and pasty, or clear and watery. You may not have even given it a second thought.

All along your cervix there are about 100 tiny glands which respond to hormonal instructions and produce varying amounts of mucus each day. Just before your period begins, when estrogen levels plummet, the mucus is scant, sticky and white or cream colored. After your period, there may be a few days when you are completely dry. Then, as the estrogen levels gradually increase in preparation for ovulation, the quantity of mucus gradually increases. It also becomes clearer and thinner the closer you are to ovulation. At the estrogen peak, just before ovulation, you'll notice a profuse discharge of perfectly clear mucus which is uniquely elastic. Taken between two fingers, it will stretch to a slick, shimmering strand. At this time, the most fertile time of the month, mucous secretions soar up to 10 times what they were just after menstruation to serve as a slippery guide for sperm.

Then, after ovulation, the production of progesterone, which is responsible for a rise in basal body temperature, also inhibits the mucus-producing cells of the cervix. Once again the mucus becomes scant, sticky and cloudy.

To see the pattern of these changes firsthand, check your mucus each morning, beginning the day after your period ends. Consider its color (clear or milky white), consistency (thick and pasty, thin and watery, glossy and stretchable), and quantity (scant or heavy). Make note of these changes at the bottom of the chart (see sample).

Intercourse can also change the appearance and amount of mucous secretions. So, to keep the chart as complete as possible, circle the dates of sexual intercourse.

Checking Your Basal Temperature

Another method to be used in combination with observing your cervical mucus is recording your basal body temperature.

Your normal body temperature is 98.6°, but as you sleep your metabolism goes into a state of semihibernation and your temperature dips somewhat. How low depends in part on where you are in your menstrual cycle. In order to record these changes, it's important that you take your temperature first thing on awakening—before your morning pilgrimage to the john, before a glass of o.j. and before so much as one toe inches its way toward the bedroom floor.

To facilitate this, shake down your thermometer the night before and place it next to your bed. You may want to

INTERPRETING CHANGES IN CERVICAL MUCUS

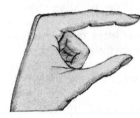

Dry: infertile.

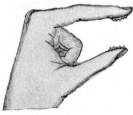

Thick and Pasty: in the beginning and end of cycle. Probably infertile.

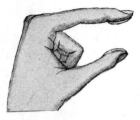

Thin and Watery: approaching ovulation. Fertile.

purchase a special basal thermometer, which more accurately registers fractions of degrees and is easier to read in the wee hours of the morn. Then, when your alarm sounds, roll over, put the thermometer in place (temperatures taken vaginally or rectally, inserting at least halfway, are usually more accurate, but you can take it orally as well), hit the snooze alarm, and relax for five or six minutes more. At the alarm's next buzz, take out the thermometer, throw open the shutters (or simply turn on the light) and record your temperature on the chart.

As you join the dots on your graph you should be able to determine when you ovulate. For the first few days after your period, and barring any unusual circumstances such as illness or travel, your temperature will probably be pretty stable—usually not fluctuating more than 0.2°. Then, at the time of ovulation, your temperature will drop to a point *lower* than any of those recorded on the previous few days. The following morning, your temperature will jump 0.4° to 1.0° *higher* and remain elevated until about two or three days before your next period, when it will drop to the preovulation level.

Failure to register this change in basal temperature probably indicates that you haven't ovulated. Don't worry if

it happens once—it's perfectly normal to miss a month occasionally. On the other hand, if your temperature doesn't return to the preovulation level just before your period is due, it could be a sign that you're pregnant.

Once you get into the habit of doing this each day, it will become as automatic as your morning stretch-and-yawn routine.

Now you can determine when you've ovulated using all the indications available on the chart. But you must also allow for those days before and after ovulation when conception is still a possibility.

The *length* of fertile time is at best only an estimate. Sperm can remain viable one to three days after launching, maybe even longer. If the egg is released during this period, there's a good chance it'll meet up with the ever-ready sperm. Unfortunately it's difficult to estimate beforehand when ovulation will take place. Generally if there's any cervical mucus present, you should avoid making love, which means allowing for at least five days before your usual day of ovulation.

It's much easier to determine when ovulation has occurred. The egg lives for 12 to 48 hours after its release from the ovary. Ovulation causes a rise in temperature of about 0.6°, which may occur in a

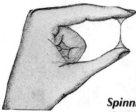

Spinnbarkeit (the ability to be stretched into a clear, shimmering strand): just at ovulation. The most fertile time of the month.

George Meyerriecks

day or over a period of several days. You must record *three* consecutive temperatures that are at least 0.4° higher than the average of the four days previous to the rise (see sample chart). It is fairly safe to make love after this point, providing your cervical mucus also indicates that ovulation has occurred. Again, to be even safer, don't have intercourse if there is any mucus present.

How Risky Is "Going Natural"?

Unfortunately, there is always an outside chance of what is called spontaneous ovulation, the release of a second egg which may occur at times other than midcycle. And there may be no observable sign to indicate that this has taken place.

However, if you follow your chart closely and avoid taking risks, this method can be as safe as any other. Remember, it takes a few months before you really know your body enough to read your fertility signs accurately and prevent conception. If you've never used this method before, it's fairly safe to combine it with the diaphragm, foam or condom during probable fertility times, till you become more familiar and comfortable with it. We must caution you, however, that gynecologists frown on this for the reason that spermicides interfere with the interpretation of the cervical mucus readings. For long-term use, they say, mixing the natural methods with others could present more of a liability than added insurance.

So, once you get on to it, you're on your own...literally. There are no pills or gadgets to back you up. This is one birth control method in which success or failure is measured in terms of human effort. And, considering the ever-present possibility of error, we feel that this natural method is most appropriate in a situation that would be supportive should a pregnancy occur.

Ideally, too, this method should be cooperative—involving both people. So encourage your partner to be aware of your fertility cycle. The more he knows, the more responsibility the two of you will share. Unfortunately, some men can be resistant to learning about the mysteries of a woman's body. And, face it, you're the one who has to say, "No, not tonight, darling" or live with the uncertainty that follows taking a risk. So, despite what the manuals on this method state, the responsibility ultimately falls with you. Let the decision whether to "go natural" or not be yours.

Editor's Note: This section should be taken as informative and not prescriptive. There are always exceptions and variations in natural birth control which must be taken into account to be reasonably safe. We suggest obtaining a book on the subject that covers a wider range of possibilities than we could cover here. One we find particularly helpful is *A Cooperative Method of Natural Birth Control* by Margaret Nofziger (Summertown, Tenn.: The Book Publishing Company, 1976). The publishers also provide a kit including a basal body thermometer and charts along with the book on request.

ORAL CONTRACEPTIVES

Most oral contraceptives (OCs) are a combination of estrogen and progestin, two powerful synthetic hormones similar to our own natural ones. But when they're added to the ones we've already got, they create such an unnatural hormone imbalance that something so natural as "sperm meets egg" is out of the question. There are several ways that happens. First, they inhibit the release of FSH (follicle-stimulating hormones) and LH (luteinizing hormones), the pituitary hormones that stimulate your ovaries to release an egg (see Menstruation). As long as you take the Pill, ovulation is suppressed. Second, the progestin in the Pill produces such a thick cervical mucus that it would take a pretty super sperm to get through. And as a final safeguard, the Pill alters the uterine lining in such a way that even if ovulation did manage to occur and the egg was fertilized, implantation would be unsuccessful.

Sounds like it's virtually impossible to get pregnant if you take a pill every day. And that's just about true. Theoretical effectiveness is 99.5 percent, and for human beings who have been known to goof up, practical effectiveness is still about 96 percent.

Take a pill, forget pregnancy. If only it were that simple.

Twenty years ago, when the Pill was first prescribed in this country, it seemed like the answer to everyone's dream. An easier, neater or more convenient method had never been discovered and what's more, it worked.

But the same 20-year span also produced scads of research studies which, from the beginning, cast doubt on the safety of the method. At first the reports were ignored or downplayed. But the voices of dissension became louder and more persistent, until the disturbing results about the Pill finally reached the women taking them. Even so, an estimated six million women each year still expose their bodies to these potent chemicals which leave no tissue or organ untouched.

Health risks run the gamut from minor inconveniences to fatal mishaps. Length of use, dosage and potency of estrogen, age of user, whether smoking is part of the picture—all contribute to the severity of the risks. And stopping the Pill does not necessarily reverse or even decrease the damage already done.

What the Pill Does to Your Blood

Blood-clotting disorders head the list of dangerous side effects. And here the evidence is staggering. The estrogen in the Pill is responsible for an increase in certain substances in the blood which cause it to clot more easily. That's okay when you're bleeding from a cut finger, for example, but blood flowing in your arteries and veins is supposed to stay fluid. If it doesn't, all sorts of problems can result. If a blood clot breaks off from the wall of a vein, it will travel through the circulation until it gets stuck in another blood vessel too small to let it pass. Big clots plug up big veins. But even a little clot can cut off circulation to a vital organ, causing damage or even death. A blood clot in the heart causes a heart attack; one in the brain is called a stroke. At any rate, death from these diseases occurs about 5 times more frequently in Pill users than in nonusers and 10 times more frequently if you have been taking the Pill for five years or longer.

If you happen to be a smoker, too, you're really taking chances with your life. Smoking 25 cigarettes or more a day increases the risk of a heart attack by 20 to 40 times over that for women who don't smoke or take the Pill (*Lancet*, April 7, 1979).

High blood pressure is also associated with heart disease. So the 600,000 women who develop this condition from the Pill have reason to be concerned. Although high blood pressure usually occurs within the first six months of use, you're still not out of danger after that time. Oral contraceptives raise the blood pressure to some degree in almost all women who use them even if they don't develop severe hypertension. What this means over the long haul nobody knows for sure, but even a small rise may prove to be potentially dangerous.

If heart disease and stroke don't scare you off, then how about cancer?

Oral contraceptives have been strongly associated with liver tumors, both benign and cancerous. Known as hepatic cell adenoma, the incidence of this once extremely rare cancerous tumor has shown a rapid increase since the inception of the Pill. The risk of developing this potentially fatal disease increases drastically with length of use, so that a woman using the Pill for eight years or longer faces a 500-fold increase in her chances of developing liver cancer over someone who has used the Pill for a year or less.

Of added interest is the fact that liver involvement can be detected as early as six months after Pill use begins. Doctors at Vanderbilt University School of Medicine in Nashville discovered that liver size increased by 17 percent in women using OCs and this enlargement may be associated with hepatic adenoma (*Ob. Gyn. News*, December 1, 1978).

But the liver isn't the only organ that can be hit by cancer. Another study done in California found that malignant melanoma, a very serious type of skin cancer, was twice as likely to occur among Pill users as among those who had never used the Pill (*British Journal of Cancer*, vol. 36, 1977).

And if that's not enough, there is also some disquieting evidence that links estrogen with increased rates of breast, cervical and vaginal cancers. Along these lines, women with noncancerous breast disease show an increased risk of developing cancerous breasts if they start taking the Pill.

Also, several other studies have disclosed an increased rate of cervical dysplasia (abnormal growth of cells on the surface of the cervix), a condition which has been known to precede the actual onset of cervical cancer in some women. And, once again, the risk of this increases with the length of time on the Pill.

It's also interesting to note that users of one particular type of OC (a sequential preparation called Oracon) showed a sevenfold increase in endometrial cancer, and it has since been removed from the market.

Of course, not all risks of oral contraceptives are that lethal. And although they won't kill you, they sure can mess up your body's chemistry.

Diabetes, Heart Trouble and Other Side Effects

Most notable are the effects on carbohydrate (sugar) metabolism. Women who take the Pill for a year or longer show altered glucose tolerance levels similar to those of diabetics, even though there may be no symptoms of the disease at the time. Doctors refer to this as chemical diabetes, a condition that can lead to the type of diabetes that may develop in middle age. While 60 to 70 percent of Pill users show a mild deterioration of glucose tolerance, 13 percent (about three-quarters of a million women) actually develop chemical diabetes.

Lipid, or fat, metabolism is closely linked to carbohydrates so it comes as no surprise to learn that oral contraceptive users face significant changes in blood fats as well.

Cholesterol and triglyceride levels were significantly higher in OC users than in nonusers, according to a study done at St. Mary's Hospital in London. Abnormal cholesterol levels occurred three times more frequently in the high-estrogen Pill users than in the controls and twice as frequently as in the lower estrogen users. High-dose and medium-dose estrogen use also significantly raised triglyceride levels (*Lancet*, May 19, 1979). The implications of this altered fat metabolism are frightening when you consider that cholesterol and triglyceride increases have been connected to high blood pressure, blood clotting and the associated risks of heart attack and stroke.

But cholesterol is also involved with the formation of gallstones which may form within the bile when it is overly saturated with the substance. And women on the Pill have been shown to have an increased concentration of cholesterol in their bile. Maybe that's why gallstones—those requiring surgery— are 2½ times more common in women on oral contraceptives than in non-Pill users.

Some side effects get you in the gut, but others are literally in your head. Migraine headaches for one; dizziness (vertigo) for another; and eye disturbances for a third.

One recent study done at the St. Louis University School of Medicine tested 40 women for migraine headache before and after oral contraceptive use. Headaches were worse when taking the Pill in 28 of the 40 women in the experiment. The researchers also noted that the incidence of headache rose to 60 percent when pills containing higher dosages of estrogen were used, and that oral contraceptives may actually initiate headaches in women who had never had them before (*Headache*, January, 1978).

As for dizziness, an ear, nose and throat specialist in Liverpool, England, noted an increasing number of young women suffering from vertigo, a condition that usually occurs in older age groups. The common thread in all these women (who were in their twenties and thirties) was that most of them were taking oral contraceptives and could attribute the onset of symptoms to the time when Pill use began.

While vertigo and headaches will usually subside after discontinuing oral contraceptive use, some of the eye complications may not. Most serious is a blood clot in the retinal vein or inflammation of the optic nerve, both of which can cause blindness. Double vision, blurred vision or loss of part of the field of vision have also been known to occur. Less dramatic (but still worth mentioning), Pill-related fluid retention may change the contour of the cornea, so that contact lenses which used to fit comfortably no longer do. In fact, some Pill users can't tolerate lenses at all.

Still other women have trouble tolerating life itself. Mild to severe depression is much more common among OC users than many realize. Depressive personality changes occur in about a third of all Pill users while 3 out of 50 actually become suicidal. Because the symptoms may build slowly from cycle

WHAT SIDE EFFECTS TELL YOU ABOUT YOUR ORAL CONTRACEPTIVE

TOO MUCH ESTROGEN	TOO LITTLE ESTROGEN	TOO MUCH PROGESTIN	TOO LITTLE PROGESTIN
Nausea, bloating, dizziness	Early and/or midcycle breakthrough bleeding	Increased appetite	Late breakthrough bleeding
Cervical discharge, polyps	Increased spotting	Persistent weight gain	No menstrual period or heavy menstrual flow
Brown patches on face and body	Decreased menstrual flow	Tiredness, fatigue	
High blood pressure		Decreased menstrual flow	
Migraine headache		Acne, oily scalp	
Breast fullness or tenderness		Hair loss	
Fluid retention		Depression	
Uterine cramps		Excessive facial and body hair	
Contact lenses don't fit		Vaginitis (*Candida*)	
		Decrease in breast size	

NOTES: Chart compiled by Stephen H. Paul, Ph.D., chairman of the department of pharmaceutical economics and health care delivery of Temple University in Philadelphia, Pa.
The side effects listed may occur when the amount of estrogen or progestin is too much or too little in relation to your own normal hormone balance.

to cycle, often it's observant friends or relatives who notice the destructive changes more than the Pill user herself.

Pill Users and Vitamins

The fact that mood changes build slowly suggests that there may be a metabolic reason for it. And that's just what researchers have found. Many cases of Pill-induced depression are the result of vitamin B_6 (pyridoxine) depletion. That's because the estrogen in the Pill prevents the body from absorbing B_6.

Armed with that knowledge, several researchers (independent of each other) tested women on OCs suffering depressive symptoms. In one study 50 milligrams per day of vitamin B_6 was given to 58 women. Considerable improvement or complete recovery occurred in 76 percent. And those women noticed the benefits of B_6 within one day of administration (*Lancet*, April 18, 1970).

More recently, a study showed significantly elevated mood in 56 percent of women receiving B_6 for Pill depression. But in this study, the results were achieved with only 30 milligrams per day (*International Journal for Vitamin and Nutrition Research*, vol. 49, no. 1, 1979).

But vitamin B_6 isn't the only nutrient affected by the Pill. Riboflavin (B_2), folate, vitamin B_{12}, thiamine (B_1), zinc, and vitamins C and E have all been shown to be depleted in OC users.

This apparent vitamin deficiency may also help explain why women on the Pill seem to be more prone to viral and bacterial infections. But researchers have also found that certain blood proteins (called gamma globulins) which help protect us against infections and diseases are significantly lower in OC users than in nonusers. Furthermore, as the dose of estrogen is increased, the concentration of gamma globulins is decreased.

Bladder and kidney infections are commonplace, but even diseases such as laryngitis, bronchitis, influenza and pleurisy are not uncommon. A loss of immunity to chicken pox is creating a separate stir, probably because that virus is a member of the herpes family. And herpes has had a lot of bad press recently due to its possible connection to cancer of the cervix.

The implications of OCs to your own health are one thing, but what about the possible effects on any children you may plan to have? Studies have shown that women taking the Pill before conception or accidentally during early pregnancy were at a five times greater risk of giving birth to deformed babies. Common sense says to wait about six months after your last Pill before even trying to conceive—that is, assuming you can even become pregnant.

After coming off the Pill, some women have trouble getting their menstrual periods back on schedule. Post-Pill amenorrhea (a condition in which menstrual periods stop completely) usually corrects itself in time, but it can take anywhere from a few months to two years. Nevertheless, fertility in post–Pill users lags behind that in never-users from 3 to 42 months, according to recent information. And for some unfortunate women, fertility never returns.

If all these side effects aren't enough to turn you off, here are a few more to think about: inflamed gums, decreased sex drive, elevated white blood cell count, stunted growth in young teens, hair loss, nausea, vomiting and water retention.

No wonder 45 to 75 percent of Pill users discontinue using them before one year is up! We can't imagine anyone who is aware of the risks even trying them in the first place.

Nevertheless, for some women the assurance of *not* getting pregnant is worth every other risk the Pill carries. If after considering all alternatives, you still feel that the Pill is the best birth control method for you, try at least to minimize the health risks.

Here Are the Troublemakers

All of the potentially fatal and most of the serious side effects are due to the estrogen component of the Pill—which would lead you to believe that it's best to take a Pill with the lowest estrogen possible. And for the most part that's true. But just because you use a Pill with a low estrogen *dose* doesn't necessarily mean you are taking one with the least risk. That's because there are two types of estrogen used. One, ethinyl estradiol, is about two times as potent as the other type, mestranol. For example, Demulen (which contains ethinyl estradiol) is twice as potent as Norinyl 1/50 (which contains mestranol), even though both contain 50 micrograms of the estrogen component.

The progestin (a synthetic form of the natural hormone progesterone) portion of the Pill has five common pseudonyms. You may see them written as ethynodiol diacetate, norethindrone, norethindrone acetate, norethynodrel and norgestrel. The last mentioned is anywhere from 1 to 30 times more potent than the others. Since the progestin component is mainly responsible for annoying side effects such as acne, oily

ORAL CONTRACEPTIVES ACCORDING TO ESTROGEN–PROGESTIN BALANCE

ESTROGEN-DOMINANT	INTERMEDIATE	PROGESTIN-DOMINANT
Enovid-E	Ortho-Novum 1/80	Zorane 1.5/30
Enovid 5 mg.	Norinyl 1+80	Loestrin 1.5/30
Ovulen	Ortho-Novum 1/50	Zorane 1/20
Ortho-Novum 2 mg.	Norinyl 1+50	Loestrin 1/20
Norinyl 2 mg.	Ovcon-50	Lo/Ovral
	Norlestrin 1/50	Ortho-Novum 10 mg.
	Zorane 1/50	Norlestrin 2.5/50
	Demulen	
	Brevicon	
	Modicon	
	Ovcon-35	

NOTES: Chart compiled by Steven H. Paul, Ph.D., chairman of the department of pharmaceutical economics and health care delivery of Temple University in Philadelphia, Pa.
Brand names are listed as they appear on the product. Numbers included in the name refer to hormone content. Check with your physician or pharmacist for information regarding specific levels of estrogen and progestin in your brand.

skin, increased facial hair, smaller breasts, increased appetite and weight gain, as opposed to serious health risks, choosing a low-progestin pill is not nearly so critical as choosing a low-estrogen one.

That's the reason most doctors start their patients with a low-estrogen pill. And that's exactly as it should be. But before we leave you, there is one more consideration: that is, compatibility. Specifically, the oral contraceptive you use should suit your individual body chemistry. All women are different and, consequently, produce different amounts of their own estrogen and progesterone normally, says Stephen H. Paul, Ph.D., chairman of the department of pharmaceutical economics and health care delivery at Temple University in Philadelphia. Ideally, the particular pill you take should lock into your own natural balance.

If it doesn't, you'll know soon enough by the side effects you experience. If they don't go away in a month or so, it may be necessary to change the product or the strength of the OC initially prescribed. Many of the more common side effects are brought on by an incompatibility between the potency or dominance of either the estrogen or progestin in the Pill as they relate to your normal hormone balance. We listed the most typical reactions you may experience on the accompanying chart.

By openly discussing all your symptoms with your doctor, he or she will then know how to modify the chemicals in the Pill so that your side effects are lessened or even eliminated. Hopefully the one your body can tolerate most comfortably will also happen to be one of low estrogen content.

Some women may want to try the relatively new all-progestin birth control pill, known as the minipill. True, the proven side effects are mainly nuisance ones, but the effectiveness is less than the combination Pill (reports range from 87 to 98 percent), and there is also the troublesome side effect of intermittent breakthrough bleeding. Since detailed studies on safety have yet to be completed, it's hard to say now what lies ahead for this method. But the Food and Drug Administration has decided that for the present it's best to presume that the real health risks are the same as for the combination Pill.

Since the Pill depletes your stores of many essential vitamins, it's also important to supplement your diet with adequate amounts of vitamins B_1, B_2, B_6, B_{12}, C, E, folate and zinc. Just to give you an idea of the importance of this: one specialist at the University of Alabama School of Medicine found that young OC users with mild to moderate cervical dysplasia had significant improvement in this condition after taking 10 milligrams of folate orally for three months (*Journal of the American Medical Association*, August 15, 1980).

Some clinicians further recommend that users take a vacation—that is, a vacation from the Pill. Opinions vary on length of Pill-free time. Some say to quit permanently after five consecutive years of use, while others recommend that women go off the Pill about two cycles per year so that possible suppression of the natural hormone cycle can be detected early.

And finally, if you are seriously considering the Pill, please think twice—and then again—if any of the following pertain to you:

- Cigarette smoking.
- A tendency to develop blood clots (or a history of this condition). That includes phlebitis as well as remote problems such as impending surgery, leg casts or serious leg injuries (these are prone to deep vein thrombosis) as well as the obvious ones like strokes and heart attacks.
- A personal or family history of coronary artery disease, high blood pressure and high cholesterol levels.
- A personal or family history of cancer or the existence of a "precancerous" condition. That goes for hepatic adenoma or impaired liver function along with cancer of the breast or reproductive system, fibrocystic breast disease, even a precancerous Pap smear, or past exposure to diethylstilbestrol (DES)—whether your mother took DES when she was pregnant with you or whether you have taken it yourself.
- Pregnancy, or termination of a pregnancy within the last 10 to 14 days, or breastfeeding.
- Age over 35 or under 18.
- A personal history of severe headaches (both vascular and migraine), diabetes or a strong family history of diabetes, gallbladder disease, varicose veins, depression, epilepsy, recurrent urinary tract infections or kidney disease, asthma, acute mononucleosis, or sickle cell disease.

In osteoporosis, once-strong bones that could take whatever life dished out become as fragile as china. Porous as a spider's web and as easily broken, they snap at the slightest bump—stepping off a curb, brushing into a table—and often at no bump at all.

Every year *six million* people with osteoporosis—five million of them postmenopausal women—suffer these bone fractures, often spinal fractures that crush the delicate vertebrae, stealing inches from their height and, in the case of women, saddling them with a "dowager's hump."

But the bone injury that adds an even worse insult than shrinking is a hip fracture. One out of every six people who have a hip fracture because of osteoporosis dies within three months, literally wasting away in a hospital bed.

Bone loss, while found predominantly in older women, is not restricted to them. A survey of "healthy, normal" people, consisting of 3,000 women and 1,000 men from the ages of 10 to 95, showed that bone density in women reaches its peak between the ages of 35 and 45, and declines *rapidly* afterward. Women as young as 25 were found to have bone density levels from 10 to 25 percent below average (*Family Physician,* October, 1978).

Yet postmenopausal women are still singled out as the most likely victims of this disease—with 90 percent of all postmenopausal women losing "a significant amount of bone tissue" (*Geriatrics,* September, 1977).

At menopause the production of the female hormone estrogen slows down. And while estrogen controls the menstrual cycle, it also acts to hold calcium in the bones. With less estrogen, calcium trickles out of the bones in a steady, year-after-year flow until, shrunken and weak, they collapse.

Some doctors have tried to solve this problem by giving women estrogen. But there's just one problem: cancer—cancer of the ovaries, cancer of the uterus, breast cancer. (For more on this, see Estrogen Replacement Therapy.)

Keeping Strong Bones without Hormones

Thank goodness, that's not our only option. Strong bones can be maintained through the menopausal years with an increase in the dietary supply of calcium—the thing that bones are made of.

In fact, in a recent study comparing estrogen and calcium treatments, calcium proved to be no small competition. Sixty-one postmenopausal women were divided into three groups. One group received no treatment, another group 800 milligrams of calcium, and the third estrogen. The size of their bones was measured when the study began, and again two years later (*British Medical Journal,* September 24, 1977).

"The untreated group continued to lose bone during the two years," write the researchers, while "the estrogen group lost none." Those in the calcium-treated group lost some bone mass, but far less than the untreated group. And without cancer as a side effect!

What's more, another study shows that it's possible to enjoy even better bone response to calcium. For while the women in the study comparing estrogen and calcium took 800 milligrams of calcium and still lost some bone, a study by Herta Spencer, M.D., and two colleagues at the Veterans Administration Hospital in Hines, Illinois, showed that an intake of 1,200 milligrams of calcium puts a halt to calcium's loss from the bones (*NIH Record*, May 7, 1974.)

And a two-year study published in *Annals of Internal Medicine* (December, 1977) showed that 22 postmenopausal women who took 1,400 milligrams of calcium a day had *no* measurable bone loss.

It works like this: a person's bones and teeth contain 99 percent of the body's calcium. But calcium is a must not only for strong bones but for the health of every cell in your body. If these cells cannot get enough calcium through the food you eat, your body will literally eat itself, sucking calcium from the bones and leaving them shrunken and weak. In fact, most middle-aged people are "calcium cannibals."

A U.S. Department of Agriculture Survey of 5,500 women over 45 showed that their average intake of calcium was 450 milligrams per day—not even half of what they should have been getting to prevent osteoporosis!

Bones are not static organs. In all of us, they are constantly being formed and broken down. At menopause the rate at which women's bones lose substance increases dramatically. At the same time, scientists at the Creighton University School of Medicine in Nebraska have shown, a dramatic shift in the body's calcium balance takes place. The body loses more calcium than it takes in, partly because less calcium is absorbed in the intestines, and partly because more calcium is excreted in the urine.

"Both changes are quite small," Robert Heaney, M.D., and his associates report, "but are nevertheless sufficient to explain both the balance shift and the rate of bone loss known to be occurring in postmenopausal women. The relation between calcium balance and calcium intake observed in these women is such as to suggest that the change in balance performance can be offset by an increase in the dietary calcium intake" (*Journal of Laboratory and Clinical Medicine*, December, 1978).

Dr. Heaney reports that even in the women he examined who were still menstruating, the calcium requirements were about 25 percent higher than the government's Recommended Dietary Allowance (RDA) of 800 milligrams. The women who had gone through menopause needed from 50 percent to 100 percent more calcium than the RDA.

Obviously, then, the younger you are when you begin supplementing your diet with calcium, the better you'll be able to stave off bone problems in later years. But no matter when you start, you're bound to benefit—even if some damage is already done.

It's Never Too Late to Turn Back the Clock

Anthony Albanese, Ph.D., Edward Lorenze, Jr., M.D., and Evelyn Wein at the Burke Rehabilitation Center in White Plains, New York, conducted studies to determine the relationship of calcium and bone loss in elderly women. They wanted to find out if bone loss in the elderly could be slowed down or even reversed by calcium supplements. In their experiment, 67 women from 37 to 73 years old were divided into two groups. One group was given 750 milligrams of calcium and 375 international units of vitamin D daily as supplements to their regular diet. The second group was given placebo, or "dummy," pills. After three years, the first group's bone density *increased* an average of 12.5 percent. The placebo group's bone density had *decreased* an average of 6 percent.

That could be good news to older women who may already be experiencing bone loss and are thinking it's too late to do anything about it. Studies indicate that it's never too late to benefit from calcium. Even people who stop taking the supplements and later begin again get results. Eight of the 67 people studied decided to stop taking their calcium supplements. When they later reentered the program, tests showed their bone density had deteriorated after they stopped taking calcium. Their bone density improved after they began taking supplements again (*Family Physician*, October, 1978).

Of course, we should point out that osteoporosis is of sufficient complexity that no two women respond the same to supplements. In some of the women in the above study, for example, only a mild increase in density resulted after more than three years. In others, density increased remarkably. One 62-year-old woman, who started out with bones more porous than six other women aged 36 to 54, ended up, three years later, with bones denser than those of the youngest of the six.

In general, the women's bones did not respond with calcification until six to nine months of day-in, day-out supplement taking had elapsed. "In some of those women, bone loss has been going on for 20 years. You can't expect to put it back so fast," Dr. Albanese told us.

The older you are, the longer you have to wait for better bones. At a Rye, New York, nursing home, women whose average age was 84 took a year and a half to respond to supplements. But when they did, their bones grew denser by 11 percent, while a nonsupplemented con-

trol group experienced an 8 percent decrease in bone mass during the same time period, Dr. Albanese said.

Bone density is actually the last thing to fall into place on Dr. Albanese's program. "Their leg cramps go in about a month or two, and their lower back pain disappears in about six months," he said.

A major argument Dr. Albanese makes for calcium supplementation is the scarcity of calcium in people's daily diets. Milk, as everyone knows, is a good source of calcium. But it's not *the* answer—because to get your 1,200 milligrams of calcium from milk, you'd have to drink at least three glasses a day along with your regular diet. These three glasses are packed with calories and fat. So you have to ask yourself two questions. One: can you afford the extra fat—in the milk and on your waistline? And two: even if you drink skim milk, are you going to drink three glasses of milk every day, day after day?

If the answer is no, don't take a chance. Perhaps you should opt for food supplements, either calcium itself, or calcium-rich bone meal or dolomite. Bone meal also contains phosphorus, and dolomite contains a good proportion of magnesium, which are both as essential as calcium for healthy bones.

Of course, stepping up your daily intake of calcium is only half the battle—you've got to absorb the mineral if you want to win the war against osteoporosis. Studies show that your ability to absorb dietary calcium goes downhill steadily with age. By the time you're getting on in years, the amount you absorb and are able to deposit as bone is less than the amount you're continually losing.

And this is when vitamin D can help. "Probably the most important factor affecting calcium metabolism is a sufficient supply of vitamin D," says an article in the *American Journal of Clinical Nutrition* (June, 1974).

Without vitamin D, you could drink milk until the cows come home and still not get enough calcium. Vitamin D helps the body absorb calcium, getting it out of the digestive tract and into bones.

While moderate sunning at the seashore is an excellent way to build up vitamin D in young people and middle-aged adults, older women may have to rely on supplements year-round for their vitamin D. In a study of 62 geriatric patients, ranging in age from 65 to 95, sunlight appeared to have no effect on vitamin D levels in their blood. The levels *did* increase, however, after the patients were given vitamin D supplements. The study concludes that older people may benefit more from taking vitamin D supplements than from depending too much on sunshine (*Gerontology*, vol. 24, no. 2, 1978). Apparently, as we grow older, our bodies may not be able to manufacture vitamin D from sunlight as well as in our youth.

Exercise Also Strengthens Bones

Exercise is another great way to build bone. Bone is like muscle. It will grow stronger as greater demands are placed upon it. Research indicates that no matter how old we are, exercise can increase mineralization of bone.

In a study at Oregon State University, for example, each of 90 participants ranging in age from 20 to 25 was classified according to the amount he or she normally exercised. High-, moderate- and low-activity groups were defined. The high-activity group was measured and found to have denser bones than both the moderate and the low groups. The researchers also found that calcium intake significantly influenced the bone density of participants. They concluded that an increased calcium intake, combined with adequate exercise, results in stronger bones.

Vigorous physical activity for young girls during their growing years also was recommended as a safeguard against early onset of osteoporosis. The exercise, they concluded, would help to build maximum bone strength and bone density in the young women.

Exercise was recommended not only as a safeguard against osteoporosis but also as a treatment for it. Scientifically prescribed exercises for osteoporosis were recommended to be used in conjunction with calcium and vitamin D supplementation (*Nutrition Reports International*, June, 1978).

People at any age seem to benefit from exercise, so saying it's "too late" won't work as an excuse here either. A group of 18 menopausal women was divided in half to see if exercise could modify their bone loss. One group did warm-up, conditioning and circulatory exercises for one hour three times a week. The other 9 women did not exercise. After one year, calcium in the body had *increased* in the exercise group. Body calcium *decreased* in every woman who did not exercise. The researchers learned that aging and frail bones did *not* have to be accepted as a package deal. Even women after menopause could continue to build their bones instead of losing them if they exercised regularly (*Annals of Internal Medicine*, September, 1978).

Of all the routine medical tests, the Pap test (or Pap smear) is probably the least objectionable and most widely accepted. Developed in the 1920s by George Papanicolaou, M.D., it's fast, simple, painless, and, unlike other diagnostic procedures, it involves no physical risk to the patient. Best of all, it's capable of detecting precancerous conditions of the cervix long before a full-fledged cancer develops.

Doesn't sound like there's a thing wrong with it. And there probably isn't—not theoretically, anyway. But within recent years, there has been some flap over the Pap. The controversy centers on how frequently a woman needs to have the test in order to detect cervical cancer early enough to insure 100 percent cure.

Before anybody even thought to question this most sacred of all cancer screening methods, women accepted the Pap test as an indispensable part of their yearly pelvic exam. Today, however, the same organization that publicized the importance of yearly screening—the American Cancer Society (ACS)—has just amended its recommendations: for most women having a negative Pap test two years in a row, a test every three years thereafter is sufficient. That's not to say that the rest of the medical community immediately adopted the same guidelines. The American College of Obstetricians and Gynecologists (ACOG), for one, officially repudiated them, pledging continued support for the annual Pap test. And the National Institutes of Health (NIH), which brought together a committee of 14 specialists to settle the discrepancy, emerged with a solution that only added to the confusion. With com-

mittee members split 50–50 on the issue, the NIH finally reached a settlement that straddled both viewpoints. Their recommendation: that smears should be taken at intervals ranging from one year (as urged by the ACOG) to every three years (as proposed by the ACS) or periods in between.

Obviously, it's no easy issue to sort out. But understanding exactly why it's an issue at all helps in our overall understanding of the Pap smear. First, some background information.

The Pap smear shouldn't be unfamiliar to you. A recent Gallup poll tells us that nearly 80 percent of American women over the age of 20 have had at least one in their lives. Yet, there is a certain mystique associated with a procedure which takes place under the cover of a white sheet.

What Happens in a Pap Smear

Actually, what occurs in those few minutes takes longer to explain than it does to experience. First, the physician inserts an instrument called a speculum into the vagina. Once in place, the two shoehornlike prongs are spread apart to permit a clear view of the cervix. Then, with the blunt tip of a depression stick or a cotton swab, the doctor will take two or three sample scrapings: one from the outer cuff of the cervix, one from the area just inside the cervical canal, and possibly one from the vaginal wall.

Aside from some discomfort caused by the pressure of the speculum, you shouldn't feel any pain. For one thing, the cervix has no nerve endings. And second, since the cervix is shedding cells all the time, only this loosened cellular debris is scraped away to be smeared onto slides for microscopic analysis. Indeed, some women remark that the most painful part of the procedure is waiting to hear the results.

And, says Robert Bowser, Ph.D., program director for gynecologic cancer of the National Cancer Institute, even that's uncalled for. The vast majority of Pap smears are normal. Even if a woman is called back for a follow-up test, it doesn't mean she should panic. She could be asked to return for any of a dozen reasons. Maybe the slide wasn't prepared properly. Or she might have a vaginal infection. Or maybe it's some slight abnormality labeled "precancerous" which might disappear on its own.

Unfortunately and understandably, though, there's more than one woman confused by Pap test terminology. After all, what health-minded person can comprehend that a "negative" test result could bring anything but bad news? But it's actually good news. Negative to the physician means negative for disease. It means that the cells of your cervix are normal; there's no sign of cancer.

"Positive," on the other hand, implies the presence of cancer. But again, don't panic. Some physicians use the term "positive" to describe any Class III to Class V abnormality—which, as you can see from our chart on Pap smear classifications, covers a lot of ground. Furthermore, any precancerous condition and even early cervical cancer is very treatable and curable. In fact, thinking in terms of cancer or surgery at this point is jumping the gun. No competent doctor would base a diagnosis solely on the findings of a single Pap smear. Besides, physicians tell us, if you've been having Pap tests regularly, chances are *extremely remote that the first hint of trouble is going to signal a serious invasive cancer.*

How Often? Well, It Depends

That brings us back to our original dilemma. How regularly should you have a Pap test to insure early detection?

Well, according to the July/August, 1980, guidelines of the American Cancer Society, all healthy women age 20 and over, and those under 20 who are sexually active, should have a Pap test for two consecutive years. If those tests are both negative—and if the woman is not considered at high risk of cervical cancer because of an early age of sexual intercourse, multiple sexual partners, or a history of genital herpes—then she should continue to have Pap smears taken at least every three years.

Exceptions to the rule, according to the ACS, include women who are at high risk of cervical cancer and therefore should be screened more frequently, and those who are relatively inactive sexually and may consequently prefer longer intervals between the tests.

Also, although the original Pap test procedure has been modified to include screening for endometrial (uterine) cancer, it is much more accurate in screening for cervical cancer. The ACS nevertheless suggests that at menopause, the time at which a woman becomes more susceptible to cancers in the lining of the uterus, every woman should have a complete pelvic exam, including a Pap test. If she is at high risk of endometrial cancer because of a history of infertility, excessive weight, abnormal uterine bleeding or estrogen replacement therapy, she should probably have a Pap test every year thereafter.

There are several sound arguments in favor of the ACS's more lenient guidelines for cervical cancer screening. First of all, cervical cancer is neither

PAP SMEAR CLASSIFICATIONS

CURRENT GUIDELINES*

Classification	What It Means
Class I	Negative = Normal
Class II	Inconclusive = Abnormal changes in cell formation, which could be anything from a *Trichomonas* infection to an early precancerous problem
Class III	Suspicious = Abnormal cellular changes which are insufficient for a definitive diagnosis
Class IV	Highly Suspicious = Markedly abnormal cellular changes which, however, cannot be definitely called positive
Class V	Positive for cancer

NEW GUIDELINES PROPOSED BY THE NATIONAL CANCER INSTITUTE

Unsatisfactory Cellular Specimen	Slide quality too poor to obtain an accurate reading
Normal Cellular Pattern	Normal
Benign Cellular Changes	Any abnormal changes caused by infection or injury, none of which are precancerous
Dysplasia	Mild, Moderate or Severe = Abnormal cellular changes thought to be precancerous; rated according to the proportion of abnormal to normal cells present on the slide sample as well as degree of change in size and shape of abnormal cells
Carcinoma in situ	A localized cancer condition
Invasive Carcinoma	A cancer that has invaded the underlying tissues of the cervix

* This is an example of the type of classification system used in some Pap smear screening laboratories. There are slight variations, however, from one hospital to the next.

a major cause of death among American women nor is the cervix a leading cancer site for women. What's more, women who are at risk of developing the disease are easily identifiable (see Cervical Cancer). As a result, there is an un- derstandable skepticism over the importance of a major screening effort to detect a relatively minor medical threat—especially, adds New York University health researcher Anne-Marie Foltz, since the women who are most conscientious about having their annual exams (that is, educated middle-class women) are precisely the ones who are at low risk of developing the disease anyway.

Second, evidence points to the fact that cervical cancer tends to develop very slowly and is preceded by several precancerous stages that are easily detected and treatable years before a full-fledged cancer rears its ugly head. The length of this latent period varies from one study to the next but even the most conservative estimate places the early warning phase at eight years. Other studies have shown that it may take 30 years before cervical cancer becomes a threat to life. "If detection and treatment any time in these stages deliver virtually perfect cure rates," the ACS declares, "it is extremely hard to justify an annual examination. If anything, the interval could be longer than three years."

The Trouble with Too Many Pap Smears

Third, there is some concern that, in repeating the test every year, a certain percentage of women may be subjected to unnecessary treatment. That may occur because a smear is misread or because a "precancerous" condition may never progress to a true cancer or, in certain cases, may actually regress without treatment.

As an example, a recently published study disclosed that of a group of 53 women with "positive" Pap smears who refused follow-up diagnosis or treatment, 19 returned two or more years later with "negative" Pap results (*Lancet*, August 26, 1978). Either the original test reports were mistaken or the "cancers" had completely disappeared.

Although the proportion of precan-cerous conditions that regress is unknown, a 1956 study showed that those that did regress did so within a year of diagnosis. Not knowing the length of time those conditions existed before diagnosis, it is difficult to translate that finding into practical advice on frequency of testing. But, says the ACS report, "one thing seems certain: less frequent examinations (e.g., every three years) will reduce any risk [of unnecessary treatment] by at least one-third."

Admittedly, the American Cancer Society presents some pretty convincing arguments on behalf of the three-year Pap test (after two consecutive negative tests). But the other side—those that still favor the annual exam—has sound justification for its views and should be heard out before you make your own decision.

One very important point made by advocates of an annual exam actually coincides with something mentioned by the ACS—that is, that Pap smears are only as accurate as the person reading the slide. While human error accounts for a certain percentage of negative (harmless) smears being misinterpreted as positive (cancer), which could result in some unnecessary treatment, an error in the other direction (that is, a truly cancerous test misread as harmless) can have much more serious consequences.

Actually, sorting out the good slides from the bad ones is not as easy as distinguishing between black and white. There's "positive" and there's "negative" and then there's the "suspicious" group.

"It's like how do you recognize your grandmother.... Well, she has gray hair, a long nose and wears glasses," explains John Seybolt, M.D., chief of the cytology laboratory at the New York Hospital–Cornell Medical Center. "Now you look at someone and say 'Well, she has gray hair only.' That's not enough to call her your grandmother. You need more criteria. The same holds true for classifying Pap smears. A slide may have two or three criteria for a 'positive' classification but if it doesn't have enough of them, it doesn't qualify."

The trouble is, it sometimes takes a very trained eye to detect the difference. And most pathology labs, because of the huge volume of slides they must examine each day, leave Pap smear readings up to laboratory technicians with limited training. Depending on state requirements, a cytopathologist (a physician who specializes in interpreting cell samples) may be required to review a certain percentage of those slides. But obviously, there is the possibility that a cancerous slide may be misread by a lab technician and never reviewed by a cytopathologist.

Errors can occur before the slide even reaches the laboratory. "How the Pap smears are done, reported, and handled is crucial," says Anthony DiDomenico, M.D., a New York City obstetrician and gynecologist. "In a San Diego study, for example, they reevaluated why 76 cases of cervical cancer found in a year hadn't been detected sooner. They learned that physicians had erred in 40 of these cases.

"Errors were also made by laboratory personnel," Dr. DiDomenico adds. "They had destroyed some smears so there could be no follow-up; some positive smears were erroneously reported as negative" (*Female Patient*, March, 1979).

With that in mind, many physicians continue to support the yearly Pap test, emphasizing that it betters your chances of catching the cancer in time—if only by reducing the margin of human error. They have other reasons for the yearly exam, but none so strong as that one.

Of course, choosing your gynecologist carefully and knowing the reputation of the lab that reads your slides is your best assurance that your Pap test results will be accurate. Sometimes, however, even that's not enough.

Obviously, then, it's impossible for us to recommend an optimum frequency of Pap smears. Discuss it with a physician or medical personnel whom you trust. Perhaps every other year is a good compromise. Or, if you opt for the yearly exam, follow abnormal cervical lesions for a year before subjecting yourself to treatment—especially conization and hysterectomy, which carry considerable risks. Remember, too, no treatment should be undertaken on the basis of a Pap smear alone (see Cervical Cancer).

POSTPARTUM SHAPE-UP

You've had your baby. But don't be too upset that you're still in maternity clothes, unable to squeeze into the "skinny" clothes that made up your wardrobe before you became pregnant. Obviously, your body has been through a major redesigning. You put on more weight than the birth took off and your muscles did a lot of stretching to accommodate.

We know your initial urge will be to slim down as fast as possible. It's understandable. You've spent nine months feeling out of shape, and now you're anxious to get your old body back. But be patient. You'll get there—but not just yet. Remember that your body is in the process of healing itself and, if you're breastfeeding, it's got to work at building up its milk supply, too.

"It is important that you not go on a crash diet to lose weight because you need all the essential basic foods and vitamins to build yourself up," says Gideon G. Panter, M.D., a prominent gynecologist in New York City and coauthor of *Now That You've Had Your Baby* (David McKay, 1976). "The way to lose weight now is by gradually cutting down high-carbohydrate and high-caloric foods, but still eating the foods that you need for energy and body building."

It's particularly important that you insure yourself a high protein intake. To avoid shortchanging yourself, continue taking in the same amounts you did during pregnancy—at least 75 to 100 grams of protein.

For most women gentle postpartum exercises (similar to those done during pregnancy) can begin within one to two weeks of delivery—no sooner, especially if you plan to breastfeed.

"A woman gets very discouraged when she doesn't have enough milk to feed her baby," says Sandi Perkins of the McTammany Nurse-Midwifery Center in Reading, Pennsylvania. "When this happens, we ask about her activities throughout the day. Often she's just not resting enough. We suggest resting one to two weeks before starting an exercise program so that a good milk supply can be established. Then she can build up her strength gradually with very mild exercises over the next month."

As a general rule, always consult your physician first before changing your diet or beginning an exercise program. (Of course, cesarean mothers should follow special exercises supplied by cesarean section groups or their doctors.) And don't expect miracles to happen overnight.

Your belly is apt to be closer to the size it was when you were five months pregnant, but now you don't have that taut look. To get that abdomen in shape again, you must work on strengthening the muscles—carefully, gently and gradually. But before you begin, it is important to check your stomach to see if the abdominal muscles have separated. Four sets of muscles—the recti mus-

Exercise for Separated Recti Muscles

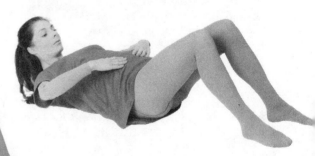

Lying on your back with knees bent, put your hands on each side of the abdomen.

Take in a deep breath, and as you exhale, lift your head up,

cles—surround your abdomen much as a corset would, and there is a seam between the right and left halves which is formed of thick connective tissue. This line extends down the middle of your abdomen, and it may have darkened during your pregnancy. In some women this strip of tissue actually stretches so far that the recti muscles separate like a zipper opening under stress. This can show up during the latter part of your pregnancy, or more commonly, in the postpartum period.

Physical therapist Helene Yocum, who is vice chairman for the section on obstetrics/gynecology of the American Physical Therapy Association, says, "If the separation is large or allowed to continue untreated, you will have permanent weakening of your abdominal wall," which leads to lower back problems and other discomforts. To check for separated recti muscles, she suggests this method: lie on your back with your knees bent and tighten your belly muscles, pushing down into the floor with the small of the back as your pelvis tilts forward. Curl your head forward and

place your fingers on the line right around your navel. If you can fit more than two fingers in the space between the bands of muscle, then you should do the following special exercise from *The Pregnancy-After-30 Workbook* (Rodale Press, 1978) for 10 repetitions at least five times a day.

Follow your body signals when you exercise and ease up if you need to. If an exercise strains the pelvic floor, discontinue it temporarily and work instead on contracting the pelvic floor with Kegel exercises (see Pregnancy and Fitness). Kegels should be continued throughout the postpartum period (and long afterward) as they help tighten up the vaginal area as well as the supports that keep the uterus in place.

Don't jump into anything very vigorous at first. There are certain movements that may do more harm than good. We suggest beginning with the exercise routine outlined in the section Pregnancy and Fitness. Gently work up to doing the routine several times before attempting more strenuous exercise.

and later your shoulders, at the same time gently pushing the underlying muscles together toward the midline.

Lie back slowly. If you are faithful with doing the exercise, the gap should return to the normal half inch within a week or so.

PREGNANCY AND FITNESS

All of us have heard tales of women who work in the fields right up to the moment of giving birth...and then go back out to the fields an hour after the baby is born. Today, such behavior would be unthinkable. Doctors would be horrified, the neighbors would talk, and your husband would turn you over to the authorities.

Somewhere along the line, everything changed for pregnant women. Not a little bit, either. More like 180 degrees. Their "condition"—that of bearing a fetus for nine months—took on the aura of a debilitating state, with doctors and specialists in charge. The hospital, an institution associated with sickness and crippling disorders, became The Place to have a baby. Everything the mother-to-be did as a *normal* part of her everyday life became open to public scrutiny and concern—even her slightest movements. Unconsciously or consciously, attitudes developed toward pregnant women which come across in all sorts of subtle and not-so-subtle ways. You may notice that your partner becomes particularly protective, opening doors for you and urging you to "take it easy" while he plays step-and-fetch-it. Your friends, too, may suddenly start to mother you—some to the point that you feel totally invalided.

Now, there's nothing wrong with a little pampering when you're expecting. After all, being pregnant and giving birth *are* "biggies" in the realm of life events. But there's a point at which all that babying may be more harmful than helpful. Inactivity is as detrimental as overexertion during pregnancy.

Get the picture? Exercise says it all. The word is out: pregnancy is *not* the time to lock yourself up in a castle. Physical educators and gynecologists alike are now agreeing that pregnant women should make every attempt to stay fit. Diana Simkin, a Lamaze instructor and director of exercise at the Elisabeth Bing Center for Parents in New York City, told us, "There is a mythical history of pregnancy as a delicate condition. Women in their third month who are not yet showing will come in and say they're afraid to sleep on their stomachs for fear of squashing the baby." She added, "We need to get away from all the fears surrounding pregnancy."

Studies of female athletes who married and had children show that they had a greater number of complication-free pregnancies and easier deliveries. In one study of outstanding female athletes in Germany, duration of labor for them was significantly shorter than for the control group of women, and, in fact, the third phase of birth lasted only half as long. What's more, some of the women attained their best performances after giving birth to the first child. Female athletes in a Hungarian study also had shorter than average labor and the necessity for cesarean section was nearly 50 percent less than in the nonathlete control group. They also had fewer complications in pregnancy, especially toxemia (*Physical Fitness Research Digest*, July, 1978).

When you think about it, it makes a lot of sense. By improving your flexibility, building muscular strength and strengthening your cardiovascular system, you are preparing your body to handle all aspects of pregnancy— the increase in weight, strain on the back and abdominal muscles, the need for getting maximum oxygen to your blood vessels and, of course, labor and delivery with all the exertion those entail.

Making sure you get regular exercise can lessen your chances of tearing muscles during delivery, and this makes for faster postpartum recovery. Says Christine Haycock, M.D., assistant professor of surgery at New Jersey Medical School and fellow of the American College of Sports Medicine, "Muscle-strengthening exercises can help you give a good squeeze when the time comes. And exercise helps you to relax, which is very important in delivery."

What Kind of Exercise Is Safe?

What kinds of exercise can I do? you may ask. Is there something I shouldn't do? "As far as that goes, a pregnant woman can do anything she pleases—*except* contact sports," says Dr. Haycock. "I've known women who jogged five miles a day up to the day of delivery. Tennis, horseback riding, anything. As long as it's a normal pregnancy," she stresses, "with no bleeding or spotting or other symptoms of complications."

Of course, those women were all accustomed to strenuous exercise prior to their pregnancies. "Don't begin an activity such as jogging when you get pregnant. Walking—or 'wogging' [fast walking]—yes. Jogging, no. The increase in total body volume during pregnancy is about 10 percent, and that takes an adjustment."

Lonnie Holtzman Morris, C.N.M. (certified nurse-midwife), director of The Childbirth Center in Englewood, New Jersey, advises prospective mothers to "continue whatever they've been doing for exercise—even tennis

and skiing." She also recommends the YWCA special fitness classes for pregnant women and tells mothers-to-be to get out and walk every day. "The uterus is a muscle," she says, "and when it's flabby, it won't work as well. Generally, at the center, we find that labor progresses more normally when the mother is in good physical shape."

The Childbearing Center in New York City, which is sponsored by the Maternity Center Association, follows basically the same guidelines regarding exercise. Gene Cranch, C.N.M., Dr. P.H. (doctor of public health), assistant director at the Maternity Center Association, told us that most of the women who come to the Childbearing Center to have their babies are already involved in exercise—yoga, running, and so on. If they have not exercised, they are advised to follow the exercising guidelines in Elizabeth Noble's *Essential Exercises for the Childbearing Year* (Houghton Mifflin, 1976). Otherwise, they are told to continue doing what they have been doing for exercise—walking, biking, jogging, tennis, dance—as long as their body says it's okay (that is, no spotting, no pulling of the muscles, reasonable weight gain). "One woman at the center was doing quite a lot of exercise, which was normal for her. But she wasn't gaining weight like she should," Dr. Cranch told us, "but when her body told her to cut down on the exercise she began to gain her proper weight.

"Swimming," Dr. Cranch adds, "is really one of the best activities during pregnancy—the mothers say they feel fantastic in the water. At about 38 weeks or so, the woman's body says 'Slow down,' and the nesting instinct takes over."

Diana Simkin prefers an exercise program that blends modern dance and yoga, rather than calisthenics, which she describes in her book, *The Complete Pregnancy Exercise Program* (New American Library, 1980). "I like people to feel the connection between breathing and moving—using breathing as an aid to facilitate movement, "she told us. "And a dance approach to exercise helps you build up strength, stamina and flexibility in a graceful way. You learn to move efficiently—relax what you don't need and work what you do."

Elizabeth Noble, a registered physical therapist who specializes in obstetrics and gynecology, and author of the book recommended so highly by Dr. Cranch, cautions that you should avoid exercises that strain the lower back or overstretch already strained abdominal muscles. Do *not*, for instance, do straight-leg sit-ups or double leg raises. (Bent-knee sit-ups are okay.) The bicycle exercise, where you boost your hips into the air and pump your legs above your head, is also a no-no, as are exercises that have you lying on your back with legs resting perpendicular against a wall, since this hinders circulation.

Exercising the muscles that control the pelvic floor is also essential if you want to avoid prolapsed uterus, urinary incontinence (the release of urine when you laugh, cough or sneeze), and a host of other related problems. While you may never have thought of yourself as having muscular control "down there," the picture is this: the pelvic floor is made up of sheets of muscle suspended beneath the uterus from the pubic bone up in front to the tailbone in back. They support the uterus, bladder and bowel. To find that group of muscles, the next time you are urinating, try to slow down or stop the flow of urine. Your ability to control the flow is an indication of how strong your muscles are.

For toning these muscles, Kegel exercises—designed by a University of California, Los Angeles, surgeon, Arnold Kegel—are your best bet. Think of your pelvic floor as a slow elevator, and your normal state as the first floor. Slowly tighten the muscles, imagining that the elevator is moving up to the second floor. Then tighten a little more and move to the third floor. Count to five before tightening even further, moving up to the fourth floor. At that point, you

Spare-Moment Exercises That Help

Some things you *can* do in your everyday movements to prepare you for childbirth include:

Sitting tailor-fashion whenever you can,

and squatting when you go to lift objects or small children (instead of bending at the waist).

relax *just slightly,* making stops at the third floor, second floor and the first floor. Then go down to the basement, which means your muscles actually bulge outward a little. (This stage correlates with the bearing down during second-stage contractions in the birthing process.) Do 5 Kegels at least 10 times a day for a total of 50 times. That may sound like a lot. But luckily, it's the kind of exercise you can do anytime, anywhere—at your desk, washing dishes, talking on the telephone—and no one (except you) will ever know. Having control over your pelvic floor muscles will insure good tone and support for the pelvic organs and will help you to relax as you give birth.

As for your own total exercise program, it should be as individual as you are, for each woman has her own threshold of discomfort during pregnancy. Whatever you do—whether you keep up your square dancing and badminton or take up special exercises at home—you should let your doctor know what you're up to.

At any rate, the first trimester of pregnancy tends to be the time when

your work capacity (in terms of exercise) is lowest. On the other hand, according to an article in the *Female Patient* (February, 1979), "the ability to do work then increases to nonpregnant levels during the second trimester coincident with improvement in blood volume and hemoglobin." Diana Simkin noticed while teaching her exercise classes that "in the first trimester, a lot of women just don't feel their best, so they may not feel up to exercising. The important thing to remember is that this feeling is only temporary. It will pass—and when it does that's the time to start your exercise program. Even if you get a late start, you're bound to benefit."

Pregnancy Exercise Routine

After consulting with many experts in pregnancy and exercise, we combined the best advice of all of them to design the following routine for you—one that offers relaxation while strengthening and toning muscles you need to make labor and delivery more comfortable. And help you regain your strength after childbirth.

The movements are adapted from modern dance, yoga, Tai Chi, belly dancing (which has its origins in childbirth movements), and some of the specific exercises recommended to pregnant women by the experts we interviewed. Best of all, they can be done by almost anyone. (A woman who has a pregnancy with complications should seek special exercises from her physician.) If you are an active person, you are likely to be more flexible and toned than a woman who did not exercise regularly before becoming pregnant. But, done every day, this rhythmics program will serve to keep you in tune with your body, give you confidence and prepare you for the exciting day when you give birth to your child.

Also, rotate your ankles when you're sitting down or elevate your feet on a pillow. That will reduce cramping in the lower legs.

418

Step-by-Step Health for Two

For a slow, steady pace, try following this routine with music, such as a piano concerto.

Begin by standing with your feet comfortably (but not too far) apart. Breathe deeply, in and out, several times. Then continue in the following sequence.

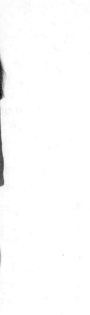

PELVIC TILTING

Remain standing comfortably.

1

2

Draw your hands up along your sides and as you go, flatten the small of your back and tighten your abdominal muscles, tucking under with your pelvis. (Do not squeeze the buttock muscles, as this will strain your back.) Breathe normally!

HOLDING THE WORLD

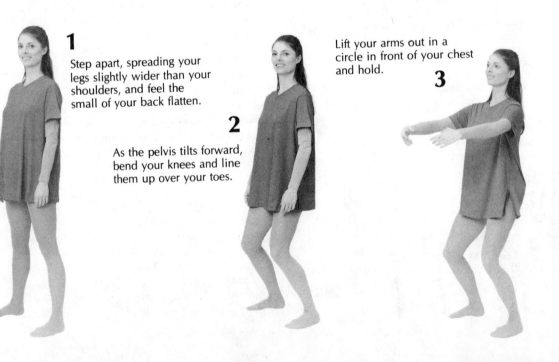

1

Step apart, spreading your legs slightly wider than your shoulders, and feel the small of your back flatten.

2

As the pelvis tilts forward, bend your knees and line them up over your toes.

Lift your arms out in a circle in front of your chest and hold.

3

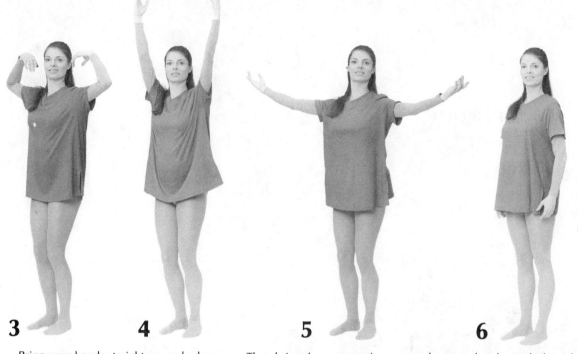

3 Bring your hands straight up and when they brush the tops of your shoulders, extend them up into the air over your head.

4

5 Then bring them out and down (without bending your elbows),

6 and as your hands touch the sides of your thighs, release your abdomen, forcing out the tension, and begin again.

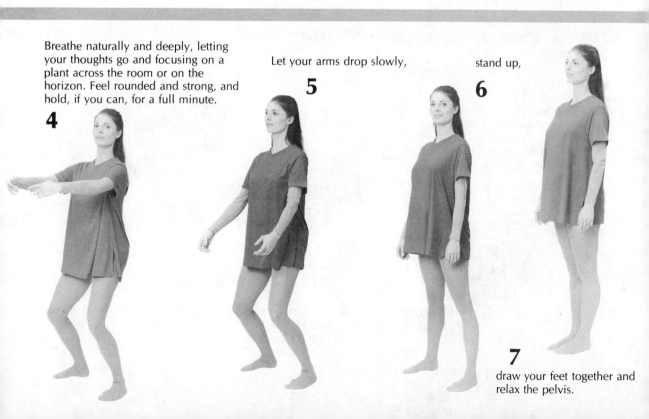

4 Breathe naturally and deeply, letting your thoughts go and focusing on a plant across the room or on the horizon. Feel rounded and strong, and hold, if you can, for a full minute.

5 Let your arms drop slowly,

6 stand up,

7 draw your feet together and relax the pelvis.

CALF STRETCH

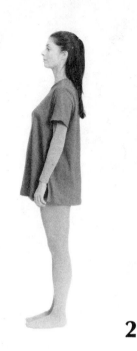

1 Stand facing a wall about three paces away.

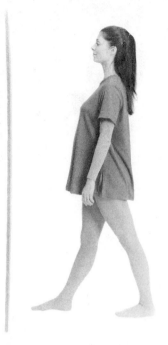

2 Step forward with your right foot,

BODY ARCH

Move to all fours, and hold your back in a tabletop position so that the small of your back is flattened, not hollowed. (Do *not* let go and allow the weight of your belly to sag and pull your back into a curve.)

1

2 Contract the stomach muscles and buttocks, pushing up and rounding with the lower back.

Hold this for a few seconds,

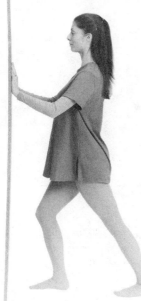

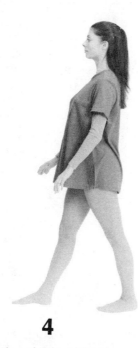

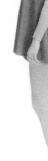

3

then bend your right knee slowly, keeping your left leg straight, heel on the floor. Use the wall to steady yourself,

4

then slowly straighten your right leg.

5

Step back, then forward with your left leg and repeat, keeping your weight evenly distributed between your legs.

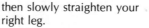

FETAL SIT

Squat with your spine held straight and the pelvis tilted back, using doorknob handles or a heavy piece of furniture if you need to. As the small of your back relaxes, your calves get a good stretch, especially if you keep your heels on the floor. Let your elbows rest on your knees if you are not holding onto a support, and just rest in this position for a minute, while the force of gravity is on *your* side. (This exercise is not necessary during postpartum.)

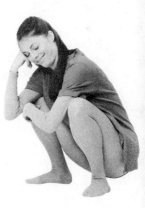

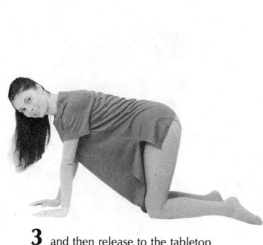

3 and then release to the tabletop position. Repeat.

LEG STRETCH

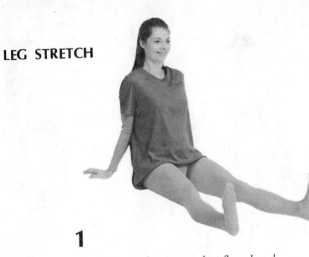

1

Sit with your legs apart, feet flexed and hands supporting from behind.

2

Point your toes and circle back to flexed position and point again. Repeat eight times with each foot.

FOOT WHEELS

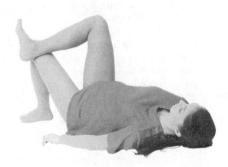

1

From the lying-down position, knees bent, place your right ankle on the left knee so that your foot has full range of motion. Rotate your foot in large, slow clockwise circles (about eight times) and then reverse the circles.

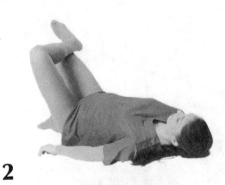

2

Repeat on the other side, propping the left ankle on the right knee. Exercising your feet will increase circulation and relieve cramping.

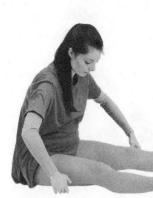

3

Slowly bend forward as far
as is comfortable,

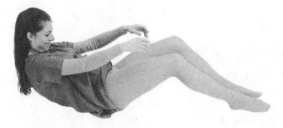

4

then pull your legs together, bend your
knees,

5

and let your body down to the floor,
vertebra by vertebra as if you were
laying down a string of pearls.

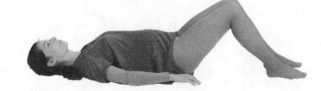

6

Take a minute to rest.

424

CURVE-UPS

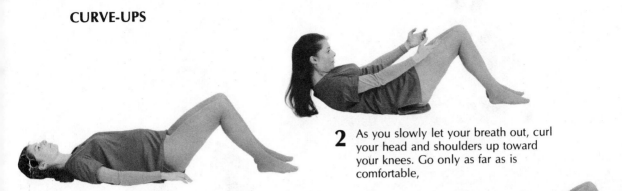

1 From this relaxed, lying position, allow your hands to rest at your sides. Take a long, deep breath.

2 As you slowly let your breath out, curl your head and shoulders up toward your knees. Go only as far as is comfortable,

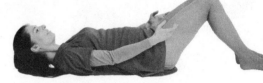

3 and then slowly unfold your back to the floor, vertebra by vertebra, and breathe naturally.

DIAGONAL CURVE-UPS

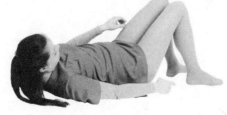

1 Next, try rolling up diagonally to the right side,

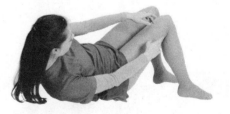

2 by pulling up and reaching your arms out toward the outside of the right knee.

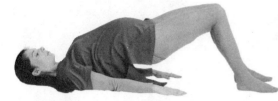

4 Next, contract your abdomen and bottom and raise your hips up off the floor in a straight line.

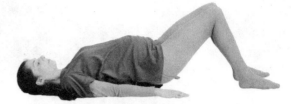

5 Hold and gently lower to the floor. Take another deep breath and then exhale slowly and repeat.

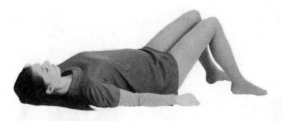

3 Slowly fold back onto the floor,

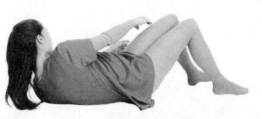

4 and repeat on the left side. Repeat three times.

An important thing to remember is to *breathe out* as your abdomen *pulls in*, and otherwise to breathe normally. **Note:** If you have separated recti muscles (as described in Postpartum Shape-Up), do *Curve-ups* with this addition: keep your hands crossed over your abdomen in order to pull the muscles toward the midline as you curl forward.

NESTING

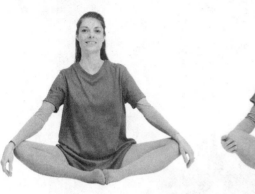

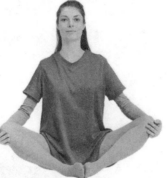

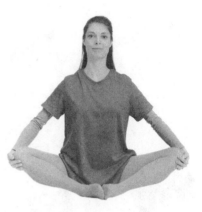

1 Sit up, placing the soles of your feet together, and bring the feet in as close as possible to maintain a comfortable balance.

2 Cup your hands underneath your knees,

3 and push up on the legs, giving resistance simultaneously as the knees push toward the floor. Hold for a few seconds.

SHOULDER CIRCLES

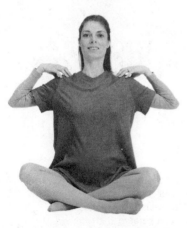

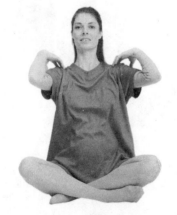

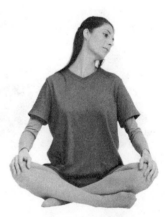

1 Sit cross-legged on the floor. Touch both hands to your shoulders,

2 and rotate your elbows backward in circles. This helps to relieve aching in your upper back due to the strain of heavy breasts.

3 Slowly circle your head to the right, then to the left.

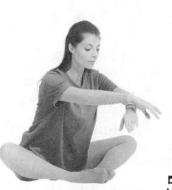

4 As you release the tension, lean slightly forward and swing your arms to cross in front of your chest,

5 and lift them straight up to the sky.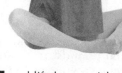

Look up and stretch your arms one at a time,

6

reaching higher with first one and then the other as if trying to pull things out of the air.

7 Then let both arms fall outward and down in arcs.

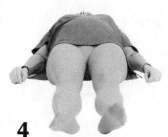

4 Breathe deeply several times, then slowly lie down and relax with your eyes closed for several minutes.

8 Tuck your hands under your knees again, and repeat the stretch.

PREGNANCY AND NUTRITION

You've got the news. No doubt about it, you're going to have a baby. The seed of life is already growing within. It's a bit early to think about it, but suitable and not-so-suitable names already pop into your head. You'll need to get a crib (or get the old one down from the attic). And sooner or later—maybe not until you sit down to dinner—something else, something *really* fundamental finally dawns on you. From this time on (actually from *before* this time), everything you take into your body will have some effect on the developing child in your womb.

You're not just waiting around for the baby to happen. Twenty-four hours a day your body is providing for your baby. And if you're to do a good "job" of it, you must care for yourself. The best way to start is by ditching the scales. (Well, at least put them in the back of a closet underneath a couple of boxes.) What? No weekly weigh-ins? Right. We want to take the emphasis off *how much* you eat and draw your attention to the importance of *what* you eat. *What* meaning healthy, wholesome, nutrient-rich foods. And from there, let nature and your appetite be your guide.

The truth is, *there is no set limit on the amount of weight any woman should gain during pregnancy*. While the medical community currently recommends gaining between 20 and 30 pounds for women of average height, that doesn't mean you should start dieting if you've gained 30 pounds. Or for that matter, that you should be stuffing yourself with so many high-calorie (and often "empty"-calorie) foods that you end up gaining to obesity. Extremes in weight gain—either very high or very low—are sometimes linked to complications and even death, according to Richard Naeye, M.D., in the *American Journal of Obstetrics and Gynecology* (September, 1979).

James Webb, M.D., an obstetrician in Jackson, Tennessee, agrees. "Gaining 50 pounds on a junk food diet may increase your chances of developing toxemia and other complications of pregnancy," he says. "A good, balanced diet with plenty of protein is your best insurance, no matter what your weight gain. . . . Unfortunately we went off the deep end years ago with those restricted diets. If you're gaining more weight eating the right kinds of food, you're definitely on the plus side."

Probably the most knowledgeable spokesperson in this regard is Tom Brewer, M.D., founder of the Society for the Protection of the Unborn through Nutrition (SPUN).

Dr. Brewer strongly believes that the prevention of birth defects starts in the kitchen, not in the delivery room. "Even if you gain 40 or 50 pounds during pregnancy while eating a nutritious, balanced diet, it won't hurt you," he told us.

We're moving away from that 20-year period where pregnant women were put on low-calorie, low-salt diets and given diuretics. "The pendulum is swinging back," says Dr. Brewer. "We're now advocating a tradition popular with our grandparents. That is, when you're pregnant, you're 'eating for two.' And if you're carrying twins, you're eating for three."

That means you've got to eat more of the foods that count. Scrap the cookies and potato chips and turn instead to natural, wholesome foods. That isn't a "diet" per se. As a matter of fact, there are some sound reasons why overweight women *shouldn't* diet during pregnancy, Dr. Brewer points out. Research shows that dieting not only restricts nutrients essential to the child, but also causes a metabolic derangement and creates an abnormal environment for the fetus, possibly impairing development of the brain and nerves—especially in the three months before birth.

Restricting your calories can also result in infants of lower birth weight. And studies do show that, in general, bigger babies are healthier babies. Moreover, there is a strong positive association between the mother's weight gain and the baby's birth weight. Maternal nutrition is, according to Dr. Brewer, "the single most important factor affecting the baby's birth weight." The trick is to gain your weight not by forcefully stuffing yourself but by eating maybe five or six small meals a day and, most important, choosing your calories wisely.

What about those "complications of pregnancy"? you may ask. How important *is* diet, anyway? The answer is: *very* important. But to know how nutrition fits in, it helps to understand the whole picture of what is happening inside your body. Only then can you conquer your own fear of "complications," and, hopefully, prevent certain hazardous conditions from occurring.

During pregnancy an organ called the placenta forms and implants itself on the back wall of the uterus to allow a transfer of essential nutrients, oxygen and waste products between the mother and the fetus. Servicing the placenta is a body of blood (much like a lake or other body of water), and nutrients pass through this blood into the baby's capillaries. From the baby, waste products are transferred by the placenta into the mother's bloodstream, and then the liver takes over, cleansing these wastes from her blood. From that point, the kidneys are responsible for excreting the wastes. Obviously, it is essential to keep providing nutrients to the placenta, which is why we stress a wholesome, balanced diet, for otherwise the growth and development of the baby will be affected.

It is also important to keep up the volume of blood needed to serve the growing placenta, and this means keeping water in the bloodstream. The more water in the blood, the greater the overall blood volume. One substance essential to holding water in the circulation is albumin, a type of protein produced by the liver. When an expectant mother isn't eating right, her liver cannot produce enough albumin. And since blood volume should increase 40 to 70 percent in the course of a normal pregnancy, maintaining a healthy liver is a top priority.

What about Salt Restriction?

If albumin levels are low, the water leaks out of the bloodstream and into surrounding tissues, causing the excessive swelling and the sudden weight gain associated with toxemia. "That's why toxemic women who begin eating more of the right kinds of food lose weight initially," Dr. Brewer explains. "They're not losing protein weight, only water weight."

Yet the majority of obstetricians still think they can reduce the sudden and rapid weight gain of toxemia by further restricting the diet and prescribing diet pills such as amphetamines to curb the appetite. To add insult to injury, they advocate low-salt diets and diuretics to bring down the swelling.

"Some degree of swelling is normal

during pregnancy," says Dr. Brewer. "Restricting the salt intake often causes the kidney apparatus to go awry and sets off high blood pressure, another symptom of toxemia. . . . No veterinarian would think of depriving a pregnant cow of salt. Pregnancy increases an animal's demand for salt."

Phyllis S. Williams, R.N., member of the board of directors for SPUN and editor for the International Childbirth Education Association, agrees. "Salt is a necessary nutrient in pregnancy," she assured us. "An adequate salt supply helps to maintain the expanded blood volume of pregnancy."

So don't be afraid to add salt. The easiest way is to salt to taste (unless there is some medical reason why you can't), or get your sodium through other foods. An adequate sodium intake is about 2,000 milligrams daily, so for your reference: a quart of skim milk has about 500 milligrams; a quart of buttermilk about 1,300; and seven ounces of tuna about 1,680.

There are other kinds of stresses on your liver throughout pregnancy, including the demanding job of clearing hormones and toxins from the bloodstream. If the liver fails to do its job properly, toxins back up in the tissues and bloodstream and could endanger the health of both you and your baby. This is especially critical during the second half of pregnancy, so you must be sure to get plenty of protein, calories, vitamins and other nutrients. From start to finish, you must consider the baby's nutritional needs, and don't be tempted to slow down toward the end of pregnancy just because you feel heavy. In the last two months of pregnancy the baby's brain is growing at its most rapid rate, so keep up the nutritious meals.

Protein, Protein, Protein

Now for the specifics: the best nutrients for you and junior. Surely protein ranks as one of the highest requirements, as it is a master builder of tissues, forming the baby's brain and the hard and soft tissues of the baby's body. It helps build the placenta and repairs your own body tissues as well. And women with a low-protein diet are twice as likely to have a miscarriage in early pregnancy as women with a high-protein diet. The Recommended Dietary Allowance (RDA) of protein for a pregnant woman is an additional 30 grams per day, the amount in one cup of uncreamed cottage cheese. A 128-pound woman over the age of 19, for example, ordinarily needs a minimum of 46 grams of protein daily. During pregnancy, her requirement jumps to 76 grams. The following foods contain about 15 grams of protein: one cup of yogurt, one cup of cooked dried beans or peas, half a cup of sunflower seeds, a quarter cup of peanut butter and about three ounces of fish or poultry.

Protein has also been found to have a function in preventing or curing metabolic toxemia of late pregnancy, a severe condition marked by high blood pressure, excess protein in the urine, extreme swelling, and fluid retention. In the severest type of toxemia, eclampsia, expectant mothers suffer convulsions (fits), coma, heart failure, fat in their livers, and bleeding into their livers. Death for both mother and baby can result.

Back in 1942, a Harvard nutritionist, Bertha S. Burke, made a study of the role of nutrition in pregnancy. She found that of women who ate a good diet consisting of 75 grams or more of protein per day, none developed toxemia. However, of women whose diet was restricted to less than 55 grams of protein, 44 percent had evidence of toxemia. The difference between a poor and a good diet for pregnancy—as far as protein goes— can be easily made up by adding a hard-boiled egg, a slice of Cheddar cheese, five dried apricots, and two handfuls of almonds to your already good daily diet.

Watch the Fat!

A much more recent study, this one at Tuskegee Institute in Alabama, links dietary fat intake to toxemia in pregnancy. A research team, headed by Ronald Chung, Ph.D., studied the diets of 65 pregnant women in their final three months of pregnancy. They found that those women who ate "significantly greater amounts of cholesterol and fat-containing foods" developed some degree of toxemia, while other women, who ingested less fat, did not.

So, go for low-fat fish and poultry, nonanimal sources of protein, and occasional cuts of lean red meat. Liver, because of its tremendous store of vitamins, minerals and protein, is also good. Relying on nonmeat sources of protein can allow you to meet the high protein requirements of pregnancy without overspending on calories or loading up on saturated fats. Many chemical residues are deposited in animal fat, and reducing meat intake means that less of these chemicals will build up in your body. These chemicals can be transferred through the placenta and in breast milk to the child. The same thing is true of any hormones, antibiotics, tranquilizers or preservatives present in meats.

To balance your nonmeat sources of protein, some careful planning is necessary. You can't just eat a cup of boiled peas—8.6 grams of protein—and expect that you're getting what you need. Vege-table proteins *must* be eaten in complementary combinations to make a completely utilized protein, one that has all eight essential amino acids present in good balance. While meat and cheese contain all of the necessary amino acids in a proportion best utilized by the body, vegetable foodstuffs such as grains and beans contain those same amino acids but in varying proportions.

Here is where the complementing comes in. Where one source, such as grain, is weak in a certain amino acid, another, such as beans, is strong. By combining the two foods at one meal, you can obtain all of the essential amino acids in the proper proportion that you need to make a complete protein.

Rather than worry about each amino acid, keep a few simple rules in mind: combine whole grains with beans, tofu, peas or lentils; combine whole grains with milk products, such as cheese; and combine beans, peas or lentils with seeds. Lots more information on complementing proteins is available in Frances Moore Lappé's well-known book, *Diet for a Small Planet* (Ballantine, 1975). Vegans—vegetarians who eat no animal products (not even cheese or milk)—have to be extra careful to balance their protein sources. If you are a vegan and are pregnant, you must also be sure to add vitamin B_{12} to your diet, probably through specially grown nutritional yeasts or supplements. The RDA for pregnant women is four micrograms, and even if you do eat meat you should make an extra effort to meet that requirement. Good sources include liver, eggs, fish and milk. (For a list of foods high in B_{12}, see Vitamins and Minerals for Women.)

Making sure you get your B vitamins should be a major consideration, so stock up on those leafy greens, wheat germ, whole grains and so forth. But be really on the lookout for vitamin B_6, or pyridoxine, because that's going to help do everything from curbing morning sickness to lifting your spirits.

Why Vitamin B_6 Is Crucial in Pregnancy

Research shows that B_6 deficiency is associated with nausea and vomiting in pregnancy, and that supplementation with B_6 can reduce—or cure—that uncomfortable condition (see Morning Sickness). B_6 is also a factor in swelling and cramping. John M. Ellis, M.D., one of the authors of *Vitamin B_6: The Doctor's Report* (Harper & Row, 1973), told us, "During my clinical experience with vitamin B_6, I have attended 225 pregnant women who received B_6 therapy. Numerous signs and symptoms appear during pregnancy that are responsive to B_6. These include painful neuropathies in the fingers and hands, swelling in the hands and feet, leg cramps, hands and arms that 'go to sleep,' and, most of all, B_6 is a factor in the prevention and treatment of toxemia of pregnancy and the convulsions of eclampsia [severe toxemia].

"All pregnant women have an increased need for vitamin B_6," says Dr. Ellis. He believes that pregnant women should have a daily supplement of at least 50 milligrams of B_6 throughout their pregnancies even though the RDA for pregnant women is only 2.5 milligrams per day.

Look to wheat germ, bananas, brewer's yeast and organ meats (chicken and beef livers) for good sources of B_6.

Dark buckwheat flour is also good, so try making buckwheat pancakes or look for bread recipes that use buckwheat. Sunflower seeds, peanuts and filberts are rich in B_6, as are whole grains in general. Poultry, especially white meat of chicken, is another source.

Beware of canned, refined and processed foods, for they all deplete vitamin B_6. And not just a little—drastically. Some 80 percent of B_6 is removed from all-purpose flour, just for one example. And precooked rice barely retains 7 percent of its original B_6 content!

Preventing Anemia during Pregnancy

During pregnancy, your blood volume increases and you store more iron, so you'll need extra dietary iron to build hemoglobin. Without sufficient iron, you will be less able to tolerate exercise, for one thing, and there is evidence that your immunity, intellectual function and intestinal nutrient absorption can all be affected.

There are some steps you can take to increase your intake of iron. One is supplementation, a course commonly followed by pregnant women in America. A leading text in nutrition, *Human Nutrition* (McGraw-Hill, 1976), gives 30 to 60 milligrams as a recommended supplement for pregnant women in their second and third trimesters. You can also eat more iron-rich foods: three ounces of liver contain 7 to 12 milligrams of iron, and one cup of prune juice contains about 1.8 milligrams. Other iron-rich foods are green, leafy vegetables, whole grain products, dried beans, wheat germ, blackstrap molasses and apricots (see also Anemia).

Another way to give your iron intake a lift is by serving spinach and other nonmeat sources of iron with some form of vitamin C, such as citrus fruit, orange juice, currants, broccoli, green peppers, tomatoes and so forth. Studies show that iron absorption can be enhanced two to five times when vitamin C is in the meal. A small amount of meat, fish or poultry also enhances iron absorption from all sources in the diet. On the other hand, you should know that milk, tea and eggs all *inhibit* the absorption of iron.

While you—and your physician— are doing your best to prevent iron deficiency anemia, another kind of anemia could very well be creeping up: megaloblastic anemia. This condition is caused by a deficiency of another B vitamin, folate, or folic acid. Your red blood cells change shape and your body may lose its ability to fight infections—quite a serious predicament! Treatment is, of course, folate supplementation, which completely cures the problem.

Since your brain and nervous system also depend on folate, if you are deficient in this B complex vitamin you may suffer from irritability and lack of appetite. And, being pregnant, a number of complications could stem from this deficiency, including toxemia, premature birth and postpartum hemorrhaging.

Aside from causing complications in the mother-to-be, folate deficiency seems to affect the baby's development. In a South African study published in *Nutrition Reports International* (November, 1974), 57 percent of children born to mothers who were severely deficient in folate during pregnancy showed abnormal or delayed development. And in a study of 35 mothers whose children had birth defects, 23 of the mothers had abnormal folate metabolism (*Lancet*, February 25, 1977).

The old standards, wheat germ and brewer's yeast, are excellent sources of folate. Make a habit of adding either to soups, stews, chopped meat preparations and baked goods. Liver is also rich in folate, and other sources include dark green, leafy vegetables (especially raw or very lightly cooked collards, spinach and beet greens), legumes, nuts, onions, asparagus and whole grain products.

Calcium for Baby's Bones and Teeth

You'll need to take in a lot more calcium if you're pregnant, for now is the time when your body really *demands* an increase. We recommend getting twice the normal (nonpregnant) 800-milligram allowance—about 1,600 milligrams— which you can do by taking in milk and other calcium-rich foods such as almonds, broccoli, cheese, canned salmon with the bones, soybeans, tofu, collards, kale and mustard greens. A quart of milk contains just under 1,200 milligrams; three ounces of salmon with bones has about 275; and a cup of skim-milk yogurt has 300. When you're pregnant, your body retains more calcium and puts out hormones that increase calcium absorption. All this to make sure your baby's bones and teeth develop in a strong and healthy fashion, and also to make sure your skeleton stores enough for breastfeeding once the baby is born. Calcium affects your muscles, too, promoting an easier delivery (see Childbirth).

Rise to the occasion and fulfill those requirements, but don't forget that vitamin D is essential for utilizing calcium (and phosphorus). Try to get at least 400 international units (I.U.) daily, about the amount added to one quart of vitamin D-fortified milk. Sunlight is, of course, a free supplement of vitamin D, so while you're outside on your walks you're likely to receive some that way. However, if you have a problem drinking milk and wonder how much vitamin D you're getting outdoors, you can turn to fish-liver oils, herring, mackerel, salmon, sardines and tuna. You *can* get too much vitamin D since it may accumulate to toxic levels in the liver, so stick to 400 I.U. or thereabouts.

Other Nutrients Are Essential, Too

All vitamins and minerals essential to good health are essential to your developing baby. But we have tried to focus here on the ones that seem most important because of a higher requirement during pregnancy or because deficiency in that nutrient is common and may very well be responsible for retarding fetal growth. We might add that vitamin A and C requirements are also higher in pregnancy, as they are for many of the B vitamins.

Vitamin K has sometimes been mentioned in connection with successful pregnancy, but if you're taking in fresh, dark green leafies or yellow vegetables, you're probably getting enough K. To make absolutely sure, include alfalfa sprouts on your luncheon salad, because that legume *has* to be one of the richest sources of vitamin K around.

Now iodine is definitely something you should think about. As your metabolism steps up during pregnancy, your thyroid has to work harder to secrete more thyroid hormone. And since the thyroid needs iodine to function properly, that mineral enters the picture in a big way. Iodized salt is one way you can get iodine, and saltwater fish is also a good source. Kelp and other seaweed products contain iodine as well, but if you're not used to cooking with seaweed, you might try kelp powder, which can easily be sprinkled like salt—in moderate amounts—on eggs, salads, vegetables and in soups.

One final note about good eating during pregnancy. If you are following our recommendations so far, a goodly amount of foods with fiber—fresh fruits and vegetables—should be already on your menu. And that fiber will really be the plus you need to keep bowel movements regular. A couple of bran muffins or a bowl of stewed prunes every now and then can't hurt, either. Also, drink more fluids—over two quarts a day through water, soups, fruit juices, etc.

Things to Avoid

It's very likely that you've been cornered by everyone and his or her grandmother telling you what you should or should not be doing now that you're pregnant. Somehow you've become fair game in open hunting season, and all the ammo your acquaintances have read in the papers, seen on TV or just "heard somewhere" is headed your way. "A glass of wine a day can't hurt, but two will." "If you smoke low-tar cigarettes, the nicotine can't affect the baby." "It's okay to drink up to eight cups of coffee." "You shouldn't drink any coffee at all." And so on. Confused? You have a right to be. Everybody's an expert—and nobody's an expert. In fact, there are a lot of things the so-called experts—the ones who do all the studies and put out the reports—don't know. So the best we can do is to tell you what kinds of substances can do you and your baby harm during pregnancy. We *can* say that we've looked long and hard at the statistics, and that there are certain things you should avoid while you're pregnant. Though it may mean a major change in your eating habits and social lifestyle or whatever, we strongly suggest that you completely cut out from your diet (or at least avoid like the plague) the following (all of which are discussed in detail under separate headings):

- *Alcohol.* Even the government, which formerly said two drinks a day was okay, is singing a different tune. The National Institute on Alcohol Abuse and Alcoholism now says that abstinence is "the safest and wisest course to follow in the interest of the best possible outcome." And well it might be. Low birth weight and abnormalities in the baby are associated with mama-to-be's drinking, and researchers in London say that even "a small amount of alcohol taken by a pregnant woman can depress the central nervous system of her fetus, as indicated by fetal breathing movements" (*Lancet,* February 17, 1979) (see Alcohol: Social Drinking).

- *Caffeine.* What? No morning cup of coffee? Nope, can't say that we'd advise it. "Caffeine readily crosses the human placenta and enters the fetal circulation," wrote three researchers from the University of Illinois. They linked spontaneous abortion, stillbirth and premature births to a high intake of caffeine (600 milligrams or about five or six cups of coffee a day) and noted that a "high rate of reproductive loss" occurred where the *man's* caffeine intake was similarly high before conception (*Postgraduate Medicine,* September, 1977). Caffeine use is also connected to breech babies and babies that are born less active and with poorer-than-average muscle tone (see Coffee, Tea and Caffeine).

- *Cigarettes.* Cigarette smoking also has a big effect on pregnancy outcome. That's because smoking limits the body's ability to deliver oxygen to the tissues, which in turn limits the oxygen going to the fetus. Also, smoking increases carbon monoxide levels in the body, which is reflected in the placenta. And, as you may have guessed, nicotine crosses the placental barrier (see Smoking).

- *Drugs.* If you can possibly avoid taking a drug while you are pregnant—even aspirin—do so. A look at our drug chart (see Drugs) will give you the nasty story on individual drugs and their effects on pregnant women. Just remember that doctors prescribing diethylstilbestrol (DES) to expectant mothers gave them little cause to believe that the drug would do harm. (Daughters born to DES-taking mothers have been found to have a higher-than-normal incidence of endometrial and vaginal cancers.)

PROLAPSED UTERUS

I was 34 years old, still a slim five feet, two inches, 93 pounds, and had my children in the early 60s when episiotomies were done routinely and considered a preventive measure against prolapse problems in the middle years. Besides, I came from a long line of peasant women who were accustomed to bearing large families. . . . So, why me?

Sometimes, the root of a prolapse problem isn't easy to trace. Usually it relates directly to childbirth—the last blow of an extremely long or tough labor. But there are more factors at fault here. In fact, a fallen uterus can just as easily be the result of a clandestine collaboration involving genetics, gravity and the aging process.

A healthy young woman's uterus is propped high atop the vagina. The cervix, or mouth of the uterus, droops into the vaginal canal for about an inch or so. But it doesn't fall further. Connective ligaments pull at it from the top, a tight, narrow vagina pushes at it from below, and a very important muscle known as the pubococcygeus (pronounced pu-bo-cocks-uh-GEE-us) muscle stretches taut from the pubic bone to the tailbone to support all the pelvic organs across the line.

The weakening of any one of these structures can cause a perfectly healthy uterus to slip down and out of its lofty position, much as a telescope collapses.

It could be a set of supportive ligaments drawn progressively lower by gravity and the excess weight of a heavy woman, a vagina that's lost its snap after accommodating a couple of children, a pubococcygeus (PC) muscle weakened by recurrent constipation and childbirth so that it resembles a loosely slung hammock, or just a weak genetic strain which leaves those ligaments vulnerable to stress. Whatever the cause, a simple exercise program can prevent prolapse problems or coax a slightly slack PC muscle back into place.

Begin with some daily yoga postures like a shoulder stand—or for more experienced yoga enthusiasts, the head stand—to give your innards a brief respite from the steady downward pull of gravity. Simply lying flat on the bed with your legs elevated by a few pillows will also help.

To strengthen the pubococcygeus muscle, try some Kegels. No, you don't eat them. They are a series of exercises devised by a surgeon, Arnold Kegel of the University of California, Los Angeles, who discovered that most of the vaginal repairs he performed could be avoided if women took care of their PC muscles.

Basically the exercises call for contracting the PC muscle—simple enough. Initially, however, the most difficult part of the exercises is locating the muscle. Since the PC muscle surrounds the urethra, vagina and rectum, contracting it will produce a tightening sensation across this entire area. Women describe it as "pulling up," or "drawing in." If you're not sure you've got the right muscle in mind, the next time you go to the bathroom, alternately stop and start your urine stream until you've emptied your bladder. Stopping urination requires contracting that muscle.

Now that you know where this muscle is located and how it feels when it's contracted, just pull it in as forcefully as you can, hold it for three to five seconds and then relax for an equal count. Do 8 to 10 repetitions approximately 5 to 10 times each day.

Once you've mastered that, try this one: imagine that your pelvic floor is a slow, flat, freight elevator with a heavy load, and it has just closed its doors on the first floor. You slowly start to tighten the muscles and the elevator moves up to the second floor. You tighten a little more and move to the third floor—hold tight for five full seconds and then move up to the fourth floor. Now you discover you can't unload yet so you *slowly* start down to the third floor as you relax just slightly. Gradually go to the second and then the first floor. Repeat the exercise 5 times and do it slowly at least 10 times a day for a total of 50 times.

It may sound like a lot of work but Kegels are actually simple and convenient exercises. They don't require equipment, a change of clothes or even a special position. You can do them sitting, standing, walking, lying down or standing on your head. So, there's no excuse for *not* working them into your daily routine.

You won't be sorry you stuck to this program, either. Regular exercise of the pubococcygeus muscle not only promotes firmer, healthier muscle tissue, but increases the blood flow to the pelvis. With better circulation your female organs will feel better and function better. You may even say goodbye to hemorrhoid problems. And talk about improving your love life!

But before we leave the impression that exercise is an easy alternative for surgery, we must point out that this program only benefits the woman with a slightly fallen uterus. More serious prolapse problems usually do not respond to mere exercise.

When Exercises Aren't Enough to Lift Your Uterus

As the uterus slips into the vaginal canal with the cervix leading the way, the cervix becomes an obstruction during intercourse. As it advances even farther, the woman may notice a heavy, dragging sensation in the pelvis and perhaps an occasional low backache. Stress incontinence (small involuntary loss of urine) can also become bothersome, particularly if the bladder is dropping down along with the uterus.

When the uterus descends so far down that it completely or nearly fills the vaginal canal, hysterectomy becomes a possible and probably the most effective solution. And in extreme cases there may not be much choice, as in this woman's case:

"I had my hysterectomy when I was 29—14 months after my last child was born. After two hard, 36-hour labors my uterus was completely prolapsed. I was in extreme pain. There was no way you could shove that uterus back in place. Anyway, we were planning to limit our family to two so there wasn't any question in my mind about whether it was the right thing to do. It was the only thing to do!"

For the woman too young or unwilling to give up her childbearing privileges or the woman too old or too ill to withstand the surgery, however, there are other alternatives.

For one thing, some women can be fitted with a pessary. This small plastic ringlike appliance (similar to the diaphragm used for contraception) acts as a support for the slipping uterus and slackened vaginal walls.

Pessaries come in various shapes and sizes to suit all degrees of prolapse. Your physician should be able to tell which type and size would best suit you.

But be forewarned, these donut-shaped devices have their shortcomings. They must be inserted by a physician, and removed regularly for cleaning, which involves repeated trips to the doctor's office —often as frequently as every six to eight weeks. Also, because they are a foreign substance and a hard piece of matter, they can cause some vaginal irritation.

But for the elderly woman who might be a poor risk for surgery these small devices are a blessing. For example, a 68-year-old woman we spoke with had been bothered by a prolapsed uterus for many years. For a long while she tried to ignore the problem, but the backaches and frequent time-outs in the john became particularly bothersome on a coast-to-coast trip—no doubt aggravated by long hours in the car. On her return, she went to her gynecologist for an exam. It wasn't difficult to diagnose her problem because the uterus was actually visible outside her vagina. Her gynecologist immediately recommended hysterectomy. But she hesitated. About 20 years previously, she had lost a kidney as a result of a serious injury, and she knew that that, plus her age, made her a pretty poor surgical risk. So she consulted a second physician— this time the head of gynecology at a prominent medical college. He didn't even mention hysterectomy. Instead he fitted her with a pessary. She returns to him twice a year to have it checked and cleaned—which to her is no trouble since she is delighted that she's been spared surgery.

In other women, a type of plastic surgery can sometimes take the place of a hysterectomy. The uterus is pulled back up to its position, the supportive ligaments repaired, and any defects in the underlying muscles of the vagina fixed. In addition, a slack or too-wide vagina can be tightened up and repairs made on a sagging bladder (cystocele) or rectum (rectocele).

In cases where the woman is older or feels that she no longer cares to have children, a hysterectomy is combined with whatever vaginal, bladder or rectal repairs have to be made. Since the repair work must be done from the bottom, most hysterectomies performed for prolapse reasons are done vaginally. Otherwise the surgeon must make two entrances—one through the abdomen to remove the uterus and another in the vagina to take care of any reconstructive work.

RESTLESS LEGS SYNDROME

"Restless legs" feels the way it sounds: restless, creeping, crawling, aching sensations deep in the muscles and bones of the legs between knee and ankle. It usually appears during extended periods of sitting—say, in the midst of a transatlantic flight or a Humphrey Bogart special—and elicits an irresistible urge to shake a leg. Pregnant women seem to be particularly susceptible— especially in the month or two before and after giving birth.

Interestingly enough, an editorial on the restless legs syndrome in the *Journal of the American Medical Association* (May 17, 1976) says that a physician "can offer little or nothing by way of treatment that the patient has not already found out for himself [or herself] by experience." By that we suppose they mean walking around to relieve the discomfort. Yet, according to several research papers we read, the root of restless legs could lie in a poor diet.

In one of those papers, M. I. Botez, M.D., of the Clinical Research Institute of Montreal and Hotel-Dieu Hospital, Montreal, Canada, describes 16 cases in which various neurological and mental disorders—including the restless legs syndrome—responded to treatment with the B vitamin folate (*European Neurology*, vol. 16, no. 1–6, 1977).

The following year, Dr. Botez published another study, this time correlating restless legs syndrome with folate deficiency in pregnancy. He enlisted the cooperation of 21 pregnant women, of whom 11 received a folate supplement and 10, a multivitamin supplement without folate. They were examined for symptoms of restless legs periodically throughout their pregnancies and again after delivery. Not surprisingly, of the 11 women who did take folate supplements only 1 suffered from restless legs, but of the 10 who did not, 8 showed symptoms of the problem.

Dr. Botez is quick to point out, however, that although the findings of this study are significant, they cannot be considered conclusive due to the small number of participants and the limited scope of the study. Nevertheless, there is good reason to suspect that a folate deficiency may be at least a part of the cause of restless legs among mothers-to-be. After all, nearly 50 percent of the ladies-in-waiting tested during another study were found to be lower in folate than nonpregnant women (*Journal of Nutritional Science and Vitaminology*, vol. 23, no. 5, 1977).

Vitamin E may also give restless legs a lift. Samuel Ayres Jr., M.D., a California dermatologist, found—quite by accident—that vitamin E helps in certain muscle disorders such as nocturnal leg cramps, abdominal cramps, and even polymyositis, a serious inflammation of the muscle. Restless legs syndrome is another muscle problem that appears to improve with vitamin E supplementation, he told us, though he admits that the exact mechanism by which the vitamin overpowers muscle problems is not known.

Whatever the reason, vitamin E does seem to help, as this letter to *Prevention* magazine illustrates:

"I was suffering from severe leg pains. I couldn't sit or lie down without lots of pain," a Texas woman wrote. "This went on for about two weeks, until I just couldn't take the pain any longer. So I went to the doctor, and he said it was 'restless legs.'

"He gave me some pills which I took for about six months, but they did not cure the condition. Then I read in *Prevention* about vitamin E for restless legs syndrome. I didn't have anything to lose so I bought some E in 1,000 international unit capsules. In two days my leg pains were gone!"

Then again, if too little folate or vitamin E isn't the problem, perhaps too much coffee is. In yet another study involving 62 persons with restless legs, caffeine and a caffeinelike drug found in chocolate surfaced as the major contributing factors (*Journal of Clinical Psychiatry*, September, 1978).

For example, a 25-year-old secretary developed restless legs syndrome shortly after she had begun to drink one cup of brewed coffee in the morning. She had never drunk coffee before. And although her coffee consumption correlated with marital stress, abstinence from caffeine alleviated the complaint despite the continued stress.

Another 46-year-old woman with restless legs, chronic anxiety and depression developed these symptoms after she was advised to use coffee liberally for another physical condition. Like the woman above, her symptoms completely vanished once coffee disappeared from her diet.

SANITARY PROTECTION

The Egyptians had a pretty neat idea—they'd roll papyrus leaves and insert them as a form of tampon. But if you were to ask your grandmother how she coped with her menstrual flow, she'd probably tell you of the messy menstrual rags held in place with knots, pins and a prayer, and the hours of soaking and scrubbing such methods entailed. For most of us, the initial encounter with commercial sanitary protection wasn't much better. Those bulky disposable napkins which required all kinds of belts-and-pins paraphernalia to keep them in place often proved more of an annoyance than they were worth.

There's no question, things have changed a lot since then. And thank goodness they have! New adhesive-stripped mini- and maxi-pads and flushable tampons have made life a lot easier. But there's still a small problem. It seems that in our zest to perfect a comfortable, convenient, leakproof and odorproof product we have occasionally outdone ourselves—and done in our health in the process.

Perhaps the most blatant example of that is the addition of deodorant to both tampons and sanitary napkins. Oh, it may smell pretty when you open the package. But these infamous chemical irritants can create a nasty rash on the vulva, or outer lips of the vagina, and do worse damage to the tender mucous lining of the vagina itself. (We discuss this in full detail under the heading Feminine Hygiene.) Also, when you consider that menstrual discharge doesn't have an odor until it comes in contact with the air and bacteria on the skin, the idea of deodorant tampons—for internal deodorizing—becomes superfluous, if not utterly ridiculous.

There may be other additives, as well—chemicals to increase absorbency, and the like—but as yet the manufacturers are not required by law to list the ingredients on the package. We contacted several manufacturers of popular brands to see whether they'd divulge that information over the phone. Some were friendly, others downright difficult—but nearly everyone refused to give us the information we were looking for. The exact makeup, they said, was "proprietary information"—you know, trade secret. About the only thing they were willing to share was the fact that most tampons and pads are primarily cotton or a rayon-cotton combination. And all are tested for safety. Let's hope so!

One company that did let us in on trade secrets (possibly because they had nothing to hide) was Johnson and Johnson—manufacturers of "o.b." tampons. According to a spokesperson for that company, the material used in their tampons is not treated in any way (other than bleaching). The absorbency then depends not on additives but rather on its basic design which was developed by a research group headed by a woman gynecologist in Europe. Be forewarned, however, "o.b." tampons come without an applicator, so if you're accustomed to those with one, these could take some getting used to.

The Superabsorbency Problem

Superabsorbent tampons pose another potential problem. A study published in *Obstetrics and Gynecology* (February, 1980) reports that excessive use of these heavy-duty tampons can produce dryness and even small sores or ulcers in the vagina.

The main hazard, however, does not appear to be in any additive or design fault, but rather in our use. Superabsorbent tampons are designed to absorb heavy menstrual flow. Consequently, they should be used only during the first two or three days of your period—and then only if the flow is exceptionally heavy. But what very often happens is that a woman who needs this kind of protection at the onset of her period will buy a box of super tampons and continue to use them throughout her menstrual period. Or another, with normal flow, may feel that superabsorbent is synonymous with less leakage or fewer changes, and chooses them because they save her time, money and worry. The trouble is, in the absence of a heavy menstrual flow, these tampons, with their built-in ability to absorb, will suck up every last trace of moisture, leaving the vaginal walls dry and subject to injury.

To avoid that kind of problem, we recommend that superabsorbent tampons be used only for exceptionally heavy menstrual flow and that women who do use them for the first few days of their period switch to regulars or pads for the last days when the flow is scant. If you worry about accidental spotting, check the diagrams on the packages of regular tampons. Those that expand in width are better able to prevent leakage.

Incidentally, regular tampons, when used improperly, may produce the same kind of effect—robbing the vaginal tissues of much-needed moisture. For that reason, don't use any tampon intermenstrually to absorb natural cervical secretions. It's also a good idea to alternate between napkins and tampons during your menstrual period. In other words, don't use tampons continuously—wear them during the day but switch to napkins at night. And finally, avoid all tampons on the last spotty days of your period.

These extra precautions may be more important to your health than you realize. Though the average woman needn't be overly alarmed, Kathryn Shands, M.D., from the Centers for Disease Control (CDC) in Atlanta, Georgia, told us there is one theory that suggests small vaginal sores or ulcers in tampon users may be the route through which bacteria enter the bloodstream, causing a rare but sometimes fatal disease called toxic-shock syndrome (TSS).

As you've no doubt heard, TSS is a new disease that begins with viruslike symptoms—headache, vomiting, fever and diarrhea—but within 48 hours may lead to a fall in blood pressure severe enough to cause kidney failure. It is caused by bacteria—*Staphylococcus*

aureus—but to date no one is sure just how it enters the bloodstream.

The interesting thing about all this is that its primary victims appear to be women. Especially young women who use tampons, and have undiagnosed symptoms of vaginitis. In three separate studies, researchers questioned 92 victims of the disease, and of them, all but 1 used tampons regularly.

It's impossible to say what role tampons play in the disease, but there is an association. As we just mentioned, many women with the disease notice some sort of vaginitis symptoms prior to their menstrual periods. Some researchers suggest that the tampon may further aggravate the situation by causing small ulcerations in the vaginal walls through which the bacteria may enter the bloodstream. But others contend that by blocking blood flow, tampons may make it easier for bacteria to grow. And still others say that the tampon itself may somehow enhance the growth of troublesome organisms.

Of course, there's always the slim possibility that the correlation between tampons and toxic-shock syndrome is just a coincidence. And anyway, we wouldn't want to suggest that every woman dispense with tampon use. After all, 70 percent of American women use tampons and yet TSS appears to be rare. At the time of this writing CDC estimates that 6 to 15 of every 100,000 women develop toxic-shock syndrome.

But to cut down your chances of becoming a statistic, don't let bothersome symptoms of vaginitis go by without a doctor's consultation. They may be symptoms of *Staphylococcus aureus*. Also, we might add, you can't go wrong by following our earlier advice concerning careful tampon use. And if by chance you have already fallen victim to TSS, don't use tampons at all. Women who've had the attack once are more likely to be stricken again—so why press your luck?

Now a word about tampon applicators: there doesn't appear to be anything physically harmful about applicators (except they can give you a nasty scratch). But environmentalists rightly criticize the use of plastic nonbiodegradable tampon applicators. Using a dozen or so tampons every month can add up to a load on the environment, they say. And let's face it, no one needs the seaside entertainment of seeing those tiny pink blimps floating up to shore. If possible, then, choose a tampon with a biodegradable cardboard applicator, or better yet, get into those that do not have any at all. With a little bit of practice, insertion will be a breeze.

For the ultimate in ecological conservation, some women's health groups are advocating the reusable menstrual sponge—sans applicator, of course. What it is, is a small piece of natural sponge that is used like a tampon except that instead of throwing it away, you rinse it out and reinsert it.

Sounds like an interesting natural alternative. But to find out just how practical they were, we decided to give them a try. Actually we were quite fired up about the concept at the onset but ended up a bit lukewarm after we had experimented with them for a cycle. There are, it seems, some basic drawbacks.

It goes without saying that insertion and removal take some getting used to. For one thing, guiding a blood-laden sponge past the constricting muscles of the vaginal opening without having it spill its contents all over the bathroom floor is a challenge that's not easy to meet. (As an aside, we've found that frequent changes and the use of a piece of dental floss threaded through the sponge aid in its removal somewhat.)

Also, the idea of reinserting the same sponge after a quick underwater rinse made us wonder just how *sanitary* this "protection" is. Besides all that, menstrual sponges are not exactly the ideal solution for the working woman or the woman who spends more than a couple of hours away from home; sooner or later she will have to face the prospect of rinsing out her sponge in a public restroom—and in full view of all those present. You can rationalize this act as a consciousness-raising experience. But many of the women we spoke with honestly admitted that the only thing they felt the act would raise is a few eyebrows.

That's not to say that it can't be done. Apparently many women do use these menstrual sponges, and quite successfully. If you would like to give them a try, check with your local health food store or drugstore.

Otherwise, the choice for sanitary protection is clearly a personal one. We feel that the most important consideration should be your health and recommend narrowing down your selection to those products without deodorants and with a minimum of other additives. Beyond that, however, it's entirely up to you whether you'll go with the external napkins, the tampons, or even the menstrual sponge. Remember, your choice should fulfill your needs and you should feel comfortable using it.

Still, there will be special instances when one type will be preferable over the other. For example, during a young woman's first menstruating year she may choose napkins over tampons since they are much easier to cope with. Napkins are also recommended for a time after childbirth while the vagina is recuperating from the trauma of delivery, and for women with vaginal infections.

Practically every spa, health club and local YWCA comes equipped with a luxury sitz spot where you can sweat or soak in temperatures exceeding 100°F. Actually, the idea of sweat bathing is nothing new. The Finnish sauna, Turkish bath, and Russian *bania* are all variations on a theme steeped in centuries-old history and custom. Today's sauna, steam bath and hot tub have evolved from that tradition—though regrettably they have become boiled-down versions of the original.

Today, few public saunas supply the bucket of water traditionally used to ladle over the hot coals. Some don't even have the coals. What we've got in most cases is a redwood-paneled walk-in closet with an electric heating element tucked into the corner. Similarly, our steam baths have shrunk from the ballroom grandeur of the Roman baths to tiny ceramic-tiled cubicles clouded with occasional gusts of steam. But it's not as bad as it seems. Although the romance is lost, at least the purpose isn't. As always, they can still get you to work up a pretty good sweat. And that is where the controversy comes in.

Seasoned sauna bathers boast feelings of exhilaration, relaxation, refreshment and total well-being. Others—usually those who've never tried it—can't imagine subjecting themselves to such torturous sweatbox conditions as would be condemned by the Geneva convention. David I. Abramson, M.D., of Oak Park, Illinois, for one, suggests that the sense of well-being people often feel after coming out is probably proportional to the discomfort they endured while in. "[It] could be compared with the great feeling of relief experienced by the patient who has been suffering from severe pain and suddenly finds that he has become free of symptoms," he says (*Journal of the American Medical Association*, January 25, 1980). Every sauna bather we've spoken with would take issue with that comment. But since elusive feelings of well-being do not lend themselves to scientific evaluation, you'll have to decide that one for yourself.

Health Benefits or Just Hot Air?

Even more important, however, is the health issue. For centuries people believed, without scientific evidence, that sweating was an extremely healthful way to cleanse the body of toxins, to stimulate circulation, to impart a fresh and youthful appearance to the skin and to prevent serious illness. Even today, many cold and flu sufferers take to the covers to "sweat it out" as a method of quickening recovery. But the question remains: can the sauna and steam room contribute to good health or are all these health claims just a lot of hot air?

Well, according to some recent evidence, the sweat bath may be more beneficial than skeptics of late have led us to believe. For example, several studies have demonstrated that the sauna and hot tub can help purify the blood. So much so that some researchers now suggest its use as an adjunct therapy to hemodialysis for kidney patients.

Apparently the sweat glands aid the kidneys' job of filtering urea from the blood. The trouble is, under today's sedentary and air-cooled conditions, we just don't sweat enough to give this perspiration-linked purification system a chance to show us what it can really do. But when we expose ourselves to a very hot environment such as the sauna, the amount of urea lost through sweat can become significant.

In one 52-year-old patient suffering from kidney failure, the sauna stimulated sweating at a rate of 21 milliliters (about 0.75 ounce) per minute. The calculated loss of urea in sweat was 2.6 grams (about 0.10 ounce) per hour and of potassium, 0.5 grams (about 0.02 ounce) per hour—which amounts to 37 percent of the urea and 60 percent of the potassium removed through an artificial kidney machine in one hour (*British Medical Journal*, July 15, 1978). Of course, that's a long time in a sweat bath, but he was under medical supervision.

Actually, the potassium lost to sweat or dialysis should be replenished, since the body needs a certain amount of this mineral for proper function. But there are other minerals—namely the harmful ones such as lead—that the body could do well without. And heavy sweating flushes those out of the system as well. In fact, a study at the University of Connecticut School of Medicine in 1973 concluded that "sauna bathing might provide a therapeutic method to increase elimination of toxic trace minerals" (*Clinical Chemistry*, vol. 19, no. 11, 1973).

In addition, the researchers conducting that study made an interesting discovery regarding mineral loss in women. They found that just because a man tends to sweat harder than a woman, it doesn't necessarily mean that he's losing more minerals. In fact, ". . . concentrations of nickel, copper, zinc and lead in sweat from the women were about two to three times those for the men."

The Weight Loss Controversy

Whether or not losing harmful minerals excites you, however, losing weight probably will. Chances are you've already heard the two sides to this argument. On the one hand, we hear that sweat bathing helps to shed pounds. And on the other, we're told that what we lose is just water weight—something we'll quickly regain at the water fountain. Which is right? Well, both are—sort of.

It's true that most of the weight you lose is water—weight that will be regained as the water is replaced. However, working up a sweat (even if you're sitting still) speeds up the body's metabolism so that you're burning calories faster than if you were lounging in air-conditioned comfort.

According to Ward Dean, M.D., an army flight surgeon who's done research on the physiological effects of sauna bathing, the body uses up about three calories for each teaspoon of water lost. Considering that the body can lose a little more than two quarts of water in one hour of heavy sweating—but that the average person probably wouldn't start sweating profusely till at least 5 minutes into a sweat bath—10 to 15 minutes in the sauna could conceivably leave you 100 to 200 calories lighter. It's not much. But, surprisingly, it's equal in calorie loss to a mile or two hoof—without all the huff and puff.

Anyway, it goes to show you that sweat bathing can offer a bit of the benefits of exercise without any of the effort. Calorie loss is just one example. Improved cardiovascular conditioning appears to be another. When you jog or swim or play racquetball, you're putting a certain amount of stress on your body by challenging your muscles to peak performance. To meet the challenge, your breathing becomes heavier, your heart beats faster, your pulse feels stronger, and your blood vessels expand so that more oxygen-rich blood can get to the muscles where it's needed. With repeated exertion, your heart and circulatory system, like your muscles, improve in strength and efficiency. To a lesser but significant degree, repeated sweat bathing does the same thing.

When you sit in a sauna, steam bath or hot tub, you're putting your body under stress, too—albeit a different kind from muscle exertion. Heat is the adversary here. And the challenge for your body is to work to keep its cool. To this end, your breathing becomes somewhat heavier, your heart beats faster, your pulse feels stronger, and the blood vessels in your skin expand in a concerted effort to get the heat out. Sweat bathing strengthens your heart and circulatory system through repeated stress just as exercise does—which is why persons with any chronic health problem such as diabetes or heart disease should get a physician's approval before *either* activity.

Of course, for overall fitness, you still can't beat good old-fashioned exercise. But, says Dr. Dean, for the disabled person in a wheelchair, the sauna could provide a good alternative way to give the heart a workout without lifting a muscle. And for the rest of us able-bodied people, the sauna could provide a nice complement to a fitness program—and possibly contribute to its most important benefit. After all, Dr. Dean told us, "Even though the sauna won't build leg muscles, no one ever died of atrophied legs. . . . But a weak cardiovascular system? Now, that's a different story!"

What's more, in addition to improving heart health, the deep heat of the sauna can help recondition tired and aching muscles so you'll be able to put more time and less teeth-clenching effort into your workouts to get the best of every exercise benefit out of them.

Another beneficiary of the sweat bath is your skin. Sweating cleanses the pores from the inside out—better than any face scrub could. What's more, a relaxing sauna followed by a brisk rub with a loofah mitt (available in many drugstores) helps to slough off dried, scaly skin and debris which may have clogged pores. Not only will you feel better, you'll also look younger. The heightened circulation to the skin imparts a rosy radiance to your cheeks. And according to Dr. Dean, it would seem logical (though it's not been proven) that this stepped-up blood flow might retard wrinkling. As for the popular belief that the sauna is more drying to the skin and hair than steam—we could find no evidence that hot air was any worse than hot water.

As an aside to one common female complaint: several of the researchers we contacted agreed that the sauna may be a useful and effective tool in the taming of menstrual cramps and other premenstrual miseries. First of all, it helps eliminate retained water, which is at the root of many premenstrual symptoms. Second, it stimulates circulation and promotes blood flow. And finally, it provides relaxation and warmth, two effective treatments for cramps.

Of course, saunas and other sweat baths are not without shortcomings. And we don't have to look far into the medical literature to find out what they are. In fact, medical doctors seem all too eager to publish observations of occasional and often obscure hazards.

As an example, the *British Medical Journal* carried one report of a 62-year-old man who suffered sauna bath burn when a door jammed and he couldn't get out (April 8, 1978). In the *Canadian Medical Journal*, an article entitled "The Sauna: A Health Hazard?" points to the danger of "sauna-takers' disease"—a severe body reaction to breathing airborne fungus originating in stagnant water of a sauna bucket (May 6, 1978). Curiously, with sauna buckets being so uncommon in American saunas—and stagnant water an unheard-of disgrace in Finnish saunas—we wonder just how many sauna takers are actually subject to sauna-takers' disease.

Sauna Bathing during Pregnancy

One article did concern us, though. Under the blaring headline, "Heat Is on Saunas as Possible Teratogens," *Medical World News* reports that women who sauna bathe during the first three months of pregnancy may subject their unborn child to severe brain damage (March 20, 1978). According to the original research paper published in the *Lancet* (March 11, 1978), however, a high fever due to illness was the primary risk factor. Five of 63 women who gave birth to severely brain-damaged children were sick with temperatures of 102°F and higher early in their pregnancy—presumably at a critical time during brain formation. In two other cases, researchers suggest that the elevated body temperature might have resulted from sauna bathing.

To find out just what kind of risk sauna bathing might pose to the mother-to-be, we contacted one of the researchers involved in this study—David Smith, M.D., professor of pediatrics at the University of Washington School of Medicine in Seattle.

"High fever was definitely the primary factor," he told us. "As for the association with sauna bathing—both cases involved prolonged exposure of 45 minutes or so. We have no indication from our studies that moderate sauna bathing has any adverse effects."

Dr. Smith went on to explain that it requires prolonged heat exposure to drive body temperature up to the 102°F thought to be the minimal level that may cause birth defects. "In the control women we studied it took at least 20 minutes before the intense heat of a sauna pushed their body temperatures to dangerous levels," he said. "Besides, few women were able to stay in till they reached that 102°F. Most felt uncomfortable after about 10 minutes, which ties in with the fact that heat-induced birth defects are rare in Finland despite Finnish women's continued sauna-bathing practices through pregnancy. They are usually careful not to exceed 6- to 12-minute exposures."

Writing in the *British Medical Journal*, a group of Finnish physicians reported that in a survey of 100 new mothers, they found that while pregnancy did not keep most women from the sauna, there was a clear trend to shorten the visits to the sauna and to reduce its temperature. Their conclusion: "Finnish people take, and have taken for at least 2,000 years, hot sauna baths once or more weekly. Our study shows similar behavior also during pregnancy. We think that there are no scientific reasons to change the habits of Finnish women who enjoy the mentally and physically refreshing effects of sauna also during pregnancy" (May 5, 1979).

We must caution, however, that there is another possible and very real danger of overdoing sweat bathing: heatstroke. In fact, not so very long ago, a California couple succumbed to this fate in their redwood hot tub. What happens is this: the body responds to extreme heat by beginning to sweat. The sweat is intended to evaporate in a cooling exercise. But when the body is immersed in hot water or trapped in an extremely hot and humid atmosphere *for too long*, it cannot perform its function. The sweat cannot evaporate and the heat builds up in the body. The heart must work extra hard to cool things off and forsakes all other body organs to shunt more blood to the skin. As you can imagine, the whole body suffers and might die without relief.

Frightening as that sounds, however, it's not the kind of thing that the experienced or knowledgeable sweat bather loses sleep over, since it's almost totally preventable. The key to safe and successful sweat bathing is moderation. That, and to a certain extent, your choice of sweat baths.

The results of several studies suggest that the dry heat of the sauna may be slightly less stressful and potentially more beneficial than the wet, humid environment of a steam bath or hot tub. When you're up to your neck in hot water or completely saturated with water and perspiration, the evaporation of sweat from the skin is markedly impaired. That means your body will be putting in double time instead of just time and a half to keep cool. In addition, the wetter your skin, the less you're going to sweat. Some time ago, researchers at Yale University School of Medicine reported that persons who exercised in a hot, humid environment for 15 minutes lost an average of 171 grams of water while those who exercised in a hot but dry environment for the same amount of time lost 191 grams (*Journal of Applied Physiology*, November, 1973). This ties in with other studies reported in the same journal which showed that sweating rates decrease during prolonged hot water baths (July, 1961), and that the rates for both evaporation and perspiration decrease as the moisture on the skin increases (March, 1979). In other words, moist environments—such as the steam bath and especially the hot tub—somewhat stifle the body's cooling mechanism and therefore pose more potential for overdoing it. At the same time, they suppress the sweat —which is, after all, the whole point of this exercise.

Tips for Safe and Satisfying Sauna Bathing

Of course, the sauna is not fail-safe either. You've got to know when to call it quits. Forget the old axiom that if a little is good, a lot is better. When it comes to sweat bathing, that attitude could get you into hot water. The sauna is a stressful place, no matter how relaxed it makes you feel. Don't overdo it! Think of it as a physical workout; you wouldn't begin a jogging program by running six miles on the first clip. Well, neither would you climb onto the highest bench and challenge yourself to an endurance test for your first crack at sauna bathing.

"You've got to take it easy your first few times—say 5 minutes or so on the lower bench," says Dr. Dean. "Then gradually work up from there using your comfort level as a guide. As soon as you feel the least bit uncomfortable, get out." And even if you think you can take more, we recommend you draw the line at 10 minutes.

Another thing—prepare yourself for the sauna just as you would for exercise. You wouldn't swim or jog on a full stomach; neither should you sauna on a salami sandwich. Wait at least an hour or two after eating. Ditto for drinking. Al-

448

cohol expands blood vessels, as does the sauna. And the two taken together can be downright devastating. Also, you probably wouldn't swim 10 laps at the pool after just having completed 6 laps on the track. So don't slump in the sauna all sweaty and exhausted from a 45-minute aerobic workout. Relax, shower, and cool off first.

In a study conducted by Albert Paolone, Ed.D., and associates at the Physical Fitness Laboratory of Exxon Corporation in New York City, 10 healthy middle-aged males were monitored during vigorous physical exercise and a follow-up 10-minute sauna. The time lag between workout and sauna warm-up was only 5 minutes—apparently not enough to bring the body temperature and heartbeat back down to normal (*Aviation, Space and Environmental Medicine*, March, 1980).

"When you exercise you build up a heat load," Dr. Paolone told us. "The trouble is, if you go into a sauna before it's dissipated, the heat load of the sauna is added to that, and there's a greater potential for overheating and heart distress. That's not to say that a sauna is dangerous. I think it can be very enjoyable. But I do recommend that a person—that is, a fairly fit person—wait about 10 to 15 minutes after exercise before entering a sauna."

Another way to figure out when the time is right, according to Dr. Paolone, is to take your pulse before exercise and again 10 minutes or so afterward. Your pulse rate should be within 20 beats of its pre-exercise rate before you subject yourself to the heat of a sauna.

Likewise, you shouldn't immediately follow a sauna bath with a hop into the hot tub—even if you've managed to sandwich a shower between them. The problem with that is that a quick flick in the shower isn't usually enough to cool

you down sufficiently. And two 10-minute sweat stints back to back could drive your body temperature up to 102°F before you know it. So, should you eventually decide to double up on exposures or mix and match sweat bath experiences during the same session, we recommend that the cool-down period between them be at least equal to the time spent heating up. In other words, if you spend 10 minutes in the sauna, take at least 10 minutes to shower and rest before a second go-round in the sauna or hot tub or Jacuzzi or whatever. And keep tabs on the time spent sweating. We recommend that women spend no longer than 10 minutes at a time in a sauna (5 to 7 minutes for a steam bath or hot tub) and no longer than 15 minutes total when combining baths in the same session.

In between and again at session's end, don't go hunting for a bank of snow or icy lake in which to plunge. While the Finns find this sudden switch from hot to cold extremely exhilarating, it's a bit much for the average American body to withstand. And for a person with heart or circulatory problems, it could be disastrous. Nevertheless, there is something to be said for following up a sauna with a cool, then briefly cold, shower. It helps to cool you off in a hurry. It heightens the effect of the experience on your circulation. And it closes the pores so that your skin doesn't immediately begin again soaking up all that environmental dirt you just showered off with your sweat.

As we mentioned earlier, heavy sweating flushes water and minerals from the system. Dr. Dean suggests that you prime yourself for the upcoming loss of water and potassium by drinking a glass of orange juice before you go into the sauna. Or you might want to substitute a banana, which is especially high in potassium, for your usual afternoon snack. Better yet, take mineral supplements—especially potassium and zinc. And be sure to drink plenty of water both before and after visits to the sauna.

Take a few accessories into the sauna with you while you bathe. In addition to the towel you'll lie on, take a dry hand towel so that you can continually wipe the perspiration from your skin. Some health clubs recommend draping a washcloth moistened with cool water across your forehead to prevent headaches.

If you're new to the sweat bath scene, test the waters a few times to see how your body responds to it. "For unexplained reasons, some people find the experience totally exhilarating and others find that it's so relaxing it puts them to sleep," Dr. Dean told us. So if you are one of those for whom the sauna is stimulating, try it first thing in the morning in place of your usual cup of coffee. If, on the other hand, it puts you to sleep, don't fight it; visiting the sauna just before bed sure beats a Nytol or hot toddy.

Sauna bathing can also be timed to complement your fitness program. Since the deep heat limbers up tight muscles, it makes an excellent warm-up for yoga, ballet or other stretching-type exercises. It also helps to relax muscles in preparation for massage.

So lie back, close your eyes, and enjoy the deep, relaxing heat. Just remember to check the door upon entering so that you won't be caught on the inside looking out when your 10-minute timer tells you it's time to take leave.

SKIN CARE

There is nothing to beautify the complexion of the face so much as frequent excursions into the mountains, climbing hills, which cause thorough perspiration and breathing; simple diet without alcohol or meat, but rather sweet fruits and sleeping in air huts.
—*The Wife as the Family Physician,*
by Anna Fischer-Dueckelmann, M.D.
(1908)

Not bad advice. In fact, unscientific and oversimplified as it may be, it makes just as much good sense today as it did earlier in this century.

In many ways, your skin is a reflection of your lifestyle. "It's the mirror of what goes on inside us, emotionally as well as physically," one dermatologist told us recently. If you spend stressful days cooped up in some office or at home with three preschoolers, and nights on the town trying to forget the days, your face may well be the first to show signs of wear. If, on the other hand, you're in the habit of jogging three miles every morning in the park and centering your diet around fresh, wholesome foods, your skin is likely to radiate a glow from within.

Actually, there's a lot more to skin care than immediately meets the eye. Beautiful skin depends on a good diet, exercise, fresh air, adequate rest and relaxation. (For more on this see also Skin Problems and Wrinkles.) The skin is also one body organ that requires gentle internal nurturing as well as proper external care.

To find out more about natural skin care for today's woman we ventured to the Irma Denson Salon in New York City—just across the street from Bloomingdale's. Vibrant, healthy skin is Irma

Denson's forte. Educated in France and trained in the fundamentals of natural skin care, she pampers her clients with lush facial treatments using all natural products made from strawberry, cucumber, pineapple, almonds and sunflower seeds as well as coaching them in the basics of at-home skin care. She shares a sampling of her healthful advice with us here.

Question: What's the biggest mistake women make in caring for their skin?
Irma Denson: There are several horrible mistakes frequently made. Probably the biggest is pulling and dragging on the face. It just amazes me how women push their faces around into all sorts of contortions in the process of washing and putting on makeup. This kind of heavyhandedness isn't necessary. In fact, it can be detrimental in that it eventually breaks down the connective fibers of the skin and accelerates wrinkling. The face, especially, must be handled very gently—soap, moisturizers and makeup applied with unvigorous, fluid strokes.

Another common mistake is going to bed with makeup on. Or, if not makeup, then with gobs and gobs of heavy cream. That's the worst thing you can do. At night, the pores must breathe and if you're smothered with makeup or a thick layer of night cream, the oxygen can't get to the skin. It's most important that at bedtime your face is impeccably clean. At the very most, apply a light layer of moisturizer around the eyes.

A third mistake women often make is that in the process of face care they neglect their neck. The neck is part of the face, and it's usually the first skin area to show signs of aging. So don't forget about it. If you wash your face, wash your neck, too. If you apply a mask to your face, apply it to your neck as well. Whatever you do to your face, always include your neck in the treatment.

How Foods Affect Our Skin

Question: How important is it for us to feed our faces a good diet?
Irma Denson: Very important. Diet has a very profound influence on the health and appearance of your skin. Some of the more obvious troublemakers include chocolate, soda and fried foods—the so-called junk foods. I try to emphasize the importance of a natural foods diet to all my clients. That is, lots of fresh fruits and vegetables for vitamins A and C, low-fat dairy products and fish for vitamin D, essential fatty acids and protein, and whole grain products for B vitamins and vitamin E. I steer clear of all fast or convenience foods myself.

Water is another dietary factor which I try to emphasize. Most people aren't drinking adequate amounts. Water helps to detoxify the body—and consequently the skin—of pollutants while bringing moisture to the skin. I'd like to tell women to drink eight glasses a day but that's a lot for the average person to handle. So, I try to get them to gradually increase their water intake by first telling them to drink three to five glasses a day.

Question: Aside from junk foods, what other internal factors affect our external covering?
Irma Denson: Alcohol is very detrimental to the skin. Smoking, too. I don't smoke but I do drink wine occasionally—or at least I *did*. A few months ago I decided to give up alcohol entirely. I haven't had any since—not even socially—and I must tell you it's made a fantastic difference in my skin.

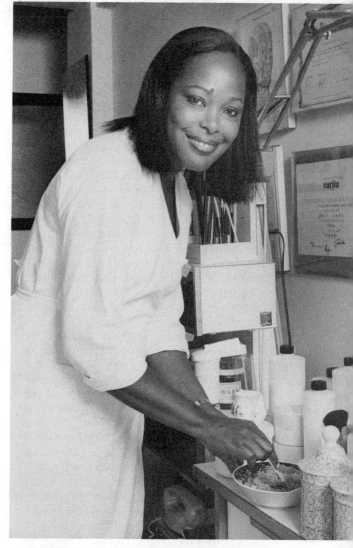

Trained in the fundamentals of healthy skin, Irma Denson pampers her clients with lush facial treatments using all natural products made from strawberry, cucumber, pineapple, almonds and sunflower seeds.

Question: Do you recommend any vitamin supplements?

Irma Denson: The B complex vitamins. Vitamin E. Cod-liver oil, which has lots of A and D, is especially good for people with dry skin that needs added moisture. And, of course, zinc.

Question: Is it really necessary to have some sort of elaborate time-consuming face care regimen?

Irma Denson: Years ago, probably not. But today, with all the air pollution—dust, dirt, smog, smoke, car exhaust—the face is really subject to all kinds of dirty, harmful elements. And it is the face, which is exposed day in and day out, that really does take the brunt of an unhealthful environment. That's why it's so important to take a little extra care with the face. It doesn't have to involve a time-consuming or expensive routine—just some special attention in your daily cleansing method, mostly, plus a little extra something once a month or so to slough off dead cells so your skin can renew itself.

The Right Way to Clean Your Face

Question: Could you explain what this special attention to our daily cleansing method would include? Is there a right and wrong way to wash the face?

Irma Denson: Oh, yes. If you scrub your face in the usual way with a bar of commercial soap, you're probably doing more harm than good. Aside from the harsh nature of the soap which I'll get into later, sudsing up in circular motions and rinsing with hot water does little more than clean off a superficial layer of dirt while leaving a residue of soap and dry skin behind.

Instead, start with a cleansing lotion or some sort of emollient cream that is available in a health food store. Pour a little bit onto a washcloth or sponge—I like a sponge with a little bit of abrasiveness—and then massage into the skin using gentle, upward motions from the center of the face to the sides. The neck should also be included using upward strokes. This loosens the dirt from the pores where it tends to accumulate. Then rinse with warm water. Actually that should be good enough for cleansing the skin. But many of my clients like the clean feeling of soap. So for them I say, let soap be the last. Use the cleansing cream first, rinse, then follow with your usual soaping up, being careful, of course, to use a mild soap.

The third step is to follow the cleansing with a nice astringent if you have oily skin, or a toner for dry skin. Just saturate a cotton ball and wipe across your face, again using fluid, upward strokes. Finally, to wash away every last trace of astringent or toner and also to close the pores, splash with cold water.

If you've never washed your face like this before, I guarantee you'll be surprised at how clean it feels!

Question: How often should you wash your face? Is it possible to wash it too much?

Irma Denson: That depends on your skin type. Obviously, if you have very dry skin you may not want to wash it as frequently as you would if you had very oily skin. Also, a lot has to do with *how* you wash your face. A woman with dry skin should avoid soap and use only a cleansing lotion, as I mentioned. If she washes her face using that method as I described, there's practically no way she can overdo it. Of course, all women are different. The important thing here is to keep your face clean, the pores closed—whatever it takes.

Question: What should we look for in a safe, mild soap?

Irma Denson: First of all, stay away from all commercial soaps. Even the ones that claim to be 99 percent pure are too harsh for our skin. One of the major drawbacks of all these supermarket varieties is that they have a highly alkaline pH which destroys the skin's delicate acid mantle. Our acid mantle helps protect us from bacteria, so it only stands to reason that we should nurture rather than destroy it. For that reason, I recommend soaps that are neutral to slightly acidic. Clay soaps are good. Oatmeal soaps are superb. Any one of the natural soaps made from pear, cucumber or strawberry are good.

Question: Are face scrubs—in which a paste made from water and a granular substance like cornmeal, almond meal, or sugar is rubbed onto the face—of any benefit?

Irma Denson: Face scrubs are excellent for sloughing off dead cells so that the skin can renew itself. You can make a face scrub using cornmeal and water but I prefer to mix the granular substance with a moisturizing lotion. Cucumber or strawberry creams are nice. The corn-meal provides the abrasion to slough off the dead cells while the lotion adds moisture to the skin. Just mix about a teaspoon or two of cornmeal with just enough moisture lotion to make a thick consistency. Or use a little honey with the cornmeal instead. Massage gently onto the skin using fluid, upward strokes. Remember to include the neck in this treatment but avoid the area around the eyes. Then rinse with warm water. This should be done at least once a week—up to three times a week if you have very oily skin.

How to Give Yourself a First-Rate Facial

Question: Can you recommend an at-home, do-it-yourself treatment similar to the kind offered professionally in salons such as yours?

Irma Denson: Certainly. It's quite easy to give yourself a facial. And you should do it at least once a month. Once a week is preferable. Start with a face scrub—a 5- to 8-minute facial massage using a cornmeal–moisture lotion mixture. Rinse with warm water. Then, to open the pores, place a hot towel over your face. Be careful that it's not too hot. Fill a basin with very warm water and sub-merge the towel in it. Wring it out thor-oughly. Then drape it over your face so it covers the under jaw and upper neck as well as the upper part of the face, but not the nose and mouth. Press the towel to your face using both hands. It should remain there for about 2 minutes. When it starts to cool off, saturate it and apply again. Do this for about 10 minutes.

Now that the pores are open, black-heads are more easily extracted. Don't squeeze them, though. You could injure the capillaries or cause them to become infected that way. Instead, push down

on the skin around them. The plugs of sebaceous matter will loosen right up and come to the surface.

The mask is next. If you have oily skin, a clay mask is good to tighten up pores and reduce oiliness. Or mix the juice of one tomato and half a lemon with a teaspoon of natural fuller's earth. Honey and wheat germ are especially good for blemishes. For dry skin, whip up an egg white until it's stiff and apply that to the face and neck. Cornstarch, honey and milk are also good for dry skin. And crushed avocado makes a ter-rific mask for dry, sensitive skin. For normal skin, I recommend plain natural yogurt. Oatmeal and brewer's yeast mixed with a little water can also be used as a mildly stimulating mask.

Again apply the mask with upward strokes, including the neck but exclud-ing the eye area. Leave it on for about 30 minutes if you have oily skin, 15 to 20 minutes for normal, and 10 minutes for dry skin. Meanwhile, relax. Lie down and cover your eyes with either cold compresses of witch hazel or slices of cucumber. Potato slices are also very good, especially for swollen eyelids.

When the mask is dry, rinse it off first with warm water, then with cold.

Now's the time to apply an astringent to close pores. To make your own astrin-gent, mix the juice of a cucumber with witch hazel in about a 1:1 ratio. (Store any unused portion in the refrigerator.) Follow this astringent with a final rinse of very cold water. And apply a mois-turizer last.

Why We All Need Moisturizers

Question: Are moisturizers for every-one? Or just women with dry skin?

Irma Denson: They're definitely for everyone. Moisturizers perform two ser-vices: they protect the skin from dirt and polluting elements, and they hydrate, or add moisture to, the skin. Notice, I said "add moisture," not add oil, and every skin type, whether dry, normal, or even oily, needs moisture.

Question: What do we look for in a good moisturizer?

Irma Denson: I like light moisturizers—lotions as opposed to heavy creams. A heavy cream can work against you in that it can suffocate the skin. The skin has to breathe—to take in oxygen. Also, creams tend to be very greasy. Another thing to keep in mind: if you have dry skin, use a moisturizer with a vegetable oil base like sesame, avocado, or olive oil—*not* mineral oil. If you have oily skin, use a water-based moisturizer; it works as effectively as an oil-based lotion but without that oily feeling.

For moisturizers, I buy commercial preparations rather than making them myself. For one thing, it's impractical to make them on a daily basis and if you don't, storage becomes a problem because they don't keep too well. It really doesn't matter, though, because there are so many good natural moisturizers on the market today made from strawberries, cucumbers, avocado and sesame oil. With vitamins added. And special ingredients like collagen (a protein), or elastin (a connective fiber), or aloe. Just browse around your health food store; I'm sure you'll be able to find something suitable.

Question: Is there a better way to apply moisturizers?

Irma Denson: Well, it's better to apply while the skin is still damp. Use only a small amount—you just want a light application. Massage in, using upward strokes on the chin, cheeks, and forehead and circular motions around the eyes, working into the bridge of the nose. It should all disappear. If it doesn't, blot off the excess and try to use less the next time around.

Question: You mentioned earlier that bedtime is not the time to slather your skin in heavy creams. When is the best time, then, to apply moisturizers?

Irma Denson: In the morning after you've washed your face. Or anytime, after you've washed your face and you plan to go outside to meet the world. The reason I say that is because our environment today tends to be laced with all sorts of pollutants. If we go outdoors, first of all, with our facial pores open, and second, with our skin unprotected, dirt and debris can become embedded in our skin. Not only does this contribute to the formation of blackheads and to an overall unattractive appearance, but it's unhealthful because the pores can become clogged so that the skin cannot breathe. So, before you go out, cleanse your face thoroughly, splash with very cold water to close the pores, and apply a moisturizer. This is especially important if you live in the city where pollution is, of course, much worse.

Question: How does skin care in the summer differ from skin care in the winter?

Irma Denson: You'll need extra moisturizing in the winter, of course, since humidity tends to be much lower in most spots. Also, an artificially heated environment tends to dry out the skin. So in the wintertime, be extra careful to protect your skin with moisturizers— even a light application at night is okay. If your home heat is especially drying, you might want to use a small cold-water vaporizer in the bedroom at night. These tend to be better than humidifiers because they're easier to clean and are less likely to breed mold.

In the summer, too, you might want to exchange your usual moisturizer for one that contains PABA (para-amino-benzoic acid), which is a natural sunscreen—especially if you spend a lot of time outdoors.

Question: Can you recommend a nice moisturizing bath?
Irma Denson: Sometimes I'll pour a quart of milk into my bath. Or I'll take 2 cups of powdered milk, ½ cup almond oil and ½ cup oatmeal and tie them up in about four layers of cheesecloth. The bag is then soaked in the bath water and also used as a scrub. This softens the skin while it moisturizes.

Question: How about an after-bath or after-shower lotion?
Irma Denson: One of the nicest I know of is fresh lemon juice. Just cut a lemon in half and rub it over your skin from head to toe. This is wonderful in the summer.

How to Smooth Out Those Rough Patches

Question: How do you deal with the rough, scaly patches on elbows and feet?
Irma Denson: That's a very good question. I personally feel that most women don't pay enough attention to their feet and elbows. But it really doesn't take so much extra effort to keep them feeling just as smooth as the rest of the skin. Many women use a pumice stone to rub away this accumulation of dead skin. I like to make a mixture of sea sand and moisture lotion and rub that in. This helps to moisturize at the same time. A loofah or dried seaweed can also be used—but only after a bath while the skin is soft and pliable.

Question: What's the best water temperature for a bath or shower?
Irma Denson: Some women find a hot bath to be very relaxing. But it's not the best thing for your skin unless, of course, you plan to follow it up with a cold shower. The trouble is, a hot bath will open up all your pores. If you don't close them again, it's like leaving the gates wide open to the elements. I recommend that bath water should be at about room temperature.

Question: How then do you feel about saunas and steam baths?
Irma Denson: The kind of sweating brought on by a sauna is a lot different from that in a hot bath. The dry heat lets the sweat flow freely from the pores, drawing debris and dead cells with it. The heat also helps to stimulate circulation. I think that they can be beneficial to the skin when done properly. By that I mean not staying in the sauna for longer than 5 to 10 minutes or the steam bath for longer than 3 to 5 minutes and following up with a cool, then cold, shower to close the pores. Moisturizers are, of course, a must afterward.

Question: Are facial saunas and steam baths equally beneficial?
Irma Denson: Sure. What you can do is bring some water to a boil on the stove, then pour it into a basin along with a handful of camomile leaves or flowers, or some mint tea leaves. Wrap your hair up in a turban towel, lean your head over the steamy and fragrant mist and place another towel over the back of your head and the bowl in a tentlike fashion. Let the steam rise up for about 10 minutes or so. This can be used in place of the hot towel during your monthly facial.

SKIN PROBLEMS

Besides those specific identifiable skin problems—like acne, liver spots, lichen planus, stretch marks and wrinkles (which we discuss under separate headings)—there's a whole host of red and rashy skin annoyances that get us every day. Skin problems dermatologists lump together under the ominous name of "dermatitis."

"Housewives' eczema" is probably the most common kind of hand dermatitis. Just dipping the hands in and out of hot, soapy water too many times a day can defat the skin, causing "dishpan hands." Frequent contact with such domestic items as bleaches, waxes, detergents, soiled diapers, or the juices of raw citrus, potatoes, tomatoes and garlic can severely irritate the skin. So can certain cosmetics, clothing, dyes, costume jewelry, paints, rubber and plastics (see Household Health Hazards).

For that reason, rubber gloves are not recommended as protection for women whose hands are *already* inflamed. Not only can excessive sweating under the gloves further harm the skin, but certain chemicals in the rubber might provoke an allergic reaction.

Once healthy skin becomes damaged and cracked, it is also more vulnerable to becoming sensitized, or allergic, to a foreign substance. And once the allergy begins, dermatitis can occur whenever and wherever an offending substance touches the sensitized person's body.

To make matters worse, some of the medications commonly used for dermatitis create yet more skin problems of their own. "Many prescribed medications, as well as many over-the-counter products, contain strong sensitizers that are easily absorbed on irritated skin," says Nia K. Terezakis, M.D., clinical assistant professor of dermatology, Louisiana State University School of Medicine. "After repeated use, they may produce secondary irritant or allergic reactions that become superimposed on the original skin disease and change its features" (*Postgraduate Medicine*, June, 1980).

Ethylenediamine, a chemical used as a stabilizer in Mycolog cream, is one of the most common sensitizers. Mycolog is often prescribed for a variety of skin problems. And although E. R. Squibb and Sons, the makers of Mycolog, told us that less than one percent of those who use the cream have an allergic reaction, one medical study showed the reaction rate to ethylenediamine as seven percent (*Minnesota Medicine*, October, 1974).

Other preparations to look out for are those that contain benzocaine or neomycin. Benzocaine is a common sensitizer found in many sunburn and poison ivy remedies. Neomycin, a common antibiotic, has been cited as a factor in six percent of all allergic skin diseases in the United States.

So what's the alternative? After all, if you're irritated by itching, oozing, weeping sores, you can't sit by and do nothing. Or can you? Dr. Terezakis thinks that may not be a bad idea. Many of these skin problems stand the best chance of recovery—with none of the complications that medications can bring—with "simple, inexpensive treatments, or better still, by *no treatment at all*," she says.

A Plan for Skin Problems

Her "simple" advice for coping with even the most complicated dermatitis includes the following:

- Use only 100 percent cotton clothing, as well as cotton sheets and pillowcases. Used sheets and towels are preferable to new ones. Wash-and-wear fabrics can be very irritating to sensitive skin.
- Do not use any laundry additives, especially fabric softeners. Low-suds detergents without additives are recommended.
- Avoid use of soaps as much as possible.
- Avoid scratching and rubbing as much as possible. Cool compresses or ice packs relieve itching faster and more safely than most medications.
- Do not use adhesive bandages or tight dressings.
- Avoid taking hot baths. They make itching worse. Cool or tepid colloidal baths (made with colloidal oatmeal, skim milk, powdered milk, cornstarch, baking soda, or a combination of some of these substances) are preferred. Soaking in tepid water, even without colloidal additives, is quite effective.
- Gently remove loose skin debris and crusts during and after baths (scabs and oozing skin are full of bacteria, and occlusive dressings—which seal the wound—provide a warm, moist environment that promotes development of infection).
- "Shake lotions" such as calamine lotion or milk of bismuth are probably the most important treatments you can find.

Otherwise, she adds, don't do anything that might add insult to injury. Avoid the use of most over-the-counter products said to relieve "symptoms" like itching and pain. Dermatitis is not just dry skin. It's damaged skin. And perhaps more than doctoring, it needs some tender nursing back to health.

SLEEP

"No small art is it to sleep," Nietzsche declared. "It is necessary to keep awake all day for that purpose." While that assessment certainly has merit, sometimes staying awake all day just isn't enough. And when that long day's journey into night continues straight through into the wee hours of the morning, it's very tempting to seek relief in tablet form.

Sleeping medications are among the most commonly used drugs—both over the counter and by prescription. Plus, when you take into account the number of tranquilizers taken to ease the daytime worries that people lose sleep over, insomnia adds up to some eye-opening profits for the drug companies. In fact, more than 25 million prescriptions for sleeping potions are written annually in the United States—with women being the number one consumers!

Trouble is, although many people depend on sleeping pills to cure them of insomnia, the drugs offer no cure.

"Some of the most important aggravators of insomnia are drugs used to treat the problem," says Thomas D. Borkovec, Ph.D., professor of psychology at Pennsylvania State University. "Most of the sleep-inducing drugs lose their effect and disrupt the stages of sleep eventually."

Studies conducted at Penn State indicate that sleeping pills can bring on chronic insomnia if used for more than two weeks. As pills lose their effectiveness, the user tends to increase the dosage, which causes a spiraling effect. Anthony Kales, M.D., of the Hershey Medical Center in Hershey, Pennsylvania, found that when 10 participants in a sleep experiment were taken off sleeping medications, they experienced intense and vivid dreams and frequent nightmares.

The Rebound Effect of Sleeping Pills

"Sleeping medications suppress the amount of the REM [rapid eye movement] stage of sleep in which dreams occur," explains Dr. Borkovec. "When a person is taken off the drugs, a REM rebound results. The person has very vivid and often horrifying dreams and the experience is much like that of an alcoholic having delirium tremens. A person often will continue taking the sleeping medications just to avoid the rebounds, which are most severe the first or second night. They diminish over the next four- or five-day period."

People who believe a little nightcap is just the ticket for dreamland should consider a different travel agency. Alcohol may send them off to dreamland, but it also shortens their stay.

"Alcohol affects sleep very adversely and should be avoided at bedtime," says Charles Pollak, M.D., co-director of the Sleep-Wake Disorders Center of Montefiore Hospital Medical Center in the Bronx. "When alcohol is first taken, it acts as a sedative. But then it metabolizes during sleep, causing a withdrawal effect. The person is aroused by it and will not sleep restfully as a result."

While some people don't drink coffee because they think the caffeine will keep them awake, others believe they won't be able to get to sleep without it. The fact is, coffee disrupts sleep, says Dr. Pollak. "People may think they tolerate it well, but the caffeine causes arousal and disturbs sleep patterns. The caffeine in teas and colas may have the same adverse effect," he adds.

Some research has been done regarding the effects on sleep of beverages such as warm milk, herbal teas and milk-cereal drinks, which are popular in Europe.

According to findings published in the *British Medical Journal* (May 20, 1972), scientific investigators in England and Scotland determined that people drinking Horlicks (a milk-cereal drink which is served warm) slept longer and were less restless through the night. The sleep-enhancing action of the beverage also became increasingly effective after several nights' use.

"People develop certain rituals for going to sleep which may serve as psychological cues to prepare them for sleep," says Richard Bootzin, Ph.D., of the psychology department at Northwestern University in Evanston, Illinois. "If you've always gone to sleep after having a cup of warm milk, the ritual may produce a strong psychological cue that works for you."

In another study investigating the relationship between late-evening eating habits and the effects of bedtime drinks on sleep, 16 people were tested using either placebo (dummy) pills; a flavored drink made from soya, egg and sucrose; warm milk; or Horlicks. Subjects who usually had little or nothing before bedtime slept better after taking the placebo pills. But those who normally had a bedtime snack slept better after drinking warm milk or Horlicks. There also was less wakefulness interrupting the first six hours of sleep after drinking Horlicks compared to either warm milk alone or the soya drink (*Proceedings of the Nutrition Society,* May, 1977).

Is there a scientific basis for such observations? Why would warm milk and milk-cereal beverages induce sleep? Those are questions that have not yet been fully answered. Some researchers believe the sleep-inducing properties of beverages such as warm milk are due to the sedative properties of a protein component or amino acid called L–tryptophan. According to Harold L. Williams, Ph.D., of the University of Oklahoma Health Sciences Center, L–tryptophan is a precursor of serotonin, a sleep-inducing substance found in the brain. "Our studies showed that people given an oral dose of tryptophan went to sleep faster and experienced an increase in slow-wave or deep sleep," says Dr. Williams. "The small intestine has enzymes which aid in transporting food products through the intestinal wall into the bloodstream. These enzymes put L–tryptophan into the bloodstream very quickly."

Since tryptophan is found in protein foods, some researchers have suggested that eating high-protein foods like milk, cheese, eggs or meat would help a person to sleep. Recent studies, however, are challenging this idea.

"The amount of L–tryptophan in foods is minimal," says Dr. Pollak. "A person would have to eat enormous quantities of meat to have an effect on sleep." And according to some researchers, even enormous quantities of high-protein foods will have no effect on sleep.

"It is true that anything that promotes serotonin is felt to be beneficial for sleep," says Carol E. Leprohon, Ph.D., of the Massachusetts Institute of Technology. "But the average person who just has trouble sleeping occasionally does not need L–tryptophan and does not need to take pills. A person might better eat something high in carbohydrates. We know that carbohydrates stimulate insulin release in the body, and insulin has a positive effect on L–tryptophan uptake into the brain."

Why aren't high-protein foods the answer? Foods that are high in protein contain other amino acids in addition to L–tryptophan, explains Dr. Leprohon, and these amino acids compete with the tryptophan for the same carrier to the brain. When you eat protein foods, you increase your intake not only of L–tryptophan but of the other amino acids as well. A person must increase the amount of L–tryptophan in the body *without* increasing the amount of the other amino acids. This may be accomplished by eating breads, cereals or other high-carbohydrate foods. "The carbohydrates stimulate insulin release into the system," she says, "and when insulin is added, the amount of other amino acids decreases in the blood, while the amount of L–tryptophan remains the same. L–tryptophan then has the advantage of getting to the brain."

Although researchers are not certain how long the process takes, Dr. Leprohon says eating a high-carbohydrate snack approximately half an hour before bedtime should be effective in inducing a restful night's sleep.

Research indicates that camomile tea also may have sleep-inducing qualities. Twelve hospital patients were given camomile tea while undergoing cardiac catheterization, a rather uncomfortable medical procedure. Of the 12 people, 10 fell into a deep sleep after drinking the tea. Although they could be aroused, they fell back asleep and remained sleeping throughout the 90-minute procedure (*Journal of Clinical Pharmacology*, November/December, 1973).

Most of us know that a good bout of exercise during the day makes it easier to fall asleep at night. But did you know that when you exercise, the *quality* of the sleep you get changes for the better? It's true. What happens is that the rhythm of your sleep changes so you spend relatively more time in a phase that sleep researchers call slow-wave sleep, or SWS. Slow-wave sleep is a very deep form of sleep which is also the most restorative, especially to the physical body. Samuel Dunkell, M.D., a New York psychoanalyst and author of the book, *Sleep Positions* (William Morrow, 1977), told us that "strenuous exercise for half an hour three times a week increases SWS. But this should not be done too close to sleep, because after strenuous exercise, the body is very stimulated. Several hours before bedtime is fine."

Arthur J. Spielman, Ph.D., a clinical psychologist specializing in sleep disorders, added that exercise done in the morning has no effect on slow-wave sleep that night. So it looks like the best time to exercise—at least as far as sleeping goes—would be, for most people, between about 4 P.M. and 8 P.M.

But here is the really interesting thing. The exercise-for-better-sleep routine works much better in people who are physically fit. Research by an Australian scientist reported in 1978 revealed that when fit and unfit people were given exercise, the amount of slow-wave sleep increased in the fit people, but not in those who weren't. Curiously, the fit people had relatively more slow-wave sleep even on days when they weren't exercising. That indicates, perhaps, that their bodies had become conditioned to restoring themselves more effectively.

Don't think that exercise won't do you any good, just because you aren't fit. All it takes is a good solid half hour of rapid walking after dinner every day for a few weeks, and you'll be getting the benefits of SWS along with all the others that come with regular exercise.

Habits are something that are pretty much out of style these days. Nobody wants to be in a rut. But when it comes to sleeping, Monte Stahl, associate director of the Sleep Disorder Center at Presbyterian Hospital in Oklahoma City, Oklahoma, told us that "an irregular bedtime is disruptive to good sleep." So try to find a time at which you are naturally and pretty consistently tired. Then hit the hay with just as much promptness as you wake up.

An especially good idea came from Wilse B. Webb, Ph.D., psychologist at the University of Florida in Gainesville. Dr. Webb told us the need for sleep varies greatly among individuals, with each person having specific requirements for sleep just as for nutrition. With nutrition, a person who functions best at a body weight of 150, let's say, can *survive* by adapting to a weight of 130. But that person won't feel up to par; a certain vitality will be absent. The same goes for sleep requirements. The individual who needs nine hours of sleep may try to crowd all his or her sleep into seven hours, but will have a continuous struggle to wake up and will frequently feel fatigued—if not downright rotten.

Moral: a woman who shortchanges herself on sleep may be cheating herself of her zest for living. Why cheat yourself of anything, let alone the enjoyment of life?

Women are *not* immune to the horrendous consequences of cigarettes. Yet many must think they are because— even in spite of today's emphatic warnings by the Surgeon General and urgent pleas from the American Lung, Heart, and Cancer Associations—more young women are taking up smoking than ever before. Granted, the total number of female smokers still lags somewhat behind the more experienced male smokers. But the mile margin is now narrowing to a hair. Between 1965 and 1979, the number of male smokers declined by 14.2 percent while the number of female smokers decreased by only 5.1 percent. What's more, studies have revealed that women are starting to smoke at an earlier age than men these days. Plus, there are more inhalers and heavy smokers among women than ever before.

Why?

Some say liberation is at least partly to blame. The move from bread baker to breadwinner has won women the social freedom to take up other previously male-oriented activities—including smoking. Women's growing independence and disposable income also make them prime targets of a vulturous advertising campaign which puts cigarette smoking on a par with the "new woman." You must have noticed that the women in cigarette ads are slim, sophisticated and liberated—and that they appear happy and vibrantly healthy. Interestingly enough, however, a cigarette model exuding all those characteristics appeared on a TV talk show recently and admitted that she *didn't* smoke. Few models do. Their looks are their livelihood and they know that

premature crow's-feet and yellowed fingernails—two ugly aftereffects of long-term cigarette smoking—could add a new and unwanted wrinkle to an aspiring career.

Cigarettes' health-robbing consequences can't be brushed off too lightly, either. But women mistakenly have felt somewhat safe from them. Let's face it, not many women worry their heads over heart attacks. And while a good number of women get a lump in their throat at the mere mention of breast cancer, few feel so much as a fleeting pang of anxiety over the prospect of lung cancer. It just doesn't happen to women, they say. But they're wrong about that—*dead wrong!*

How Smoking Endangers Women

In recent years, investigators have found that men and women with similar smoking habits stand a similar chance of dying of lung cancer or heart disease. And since more and more women are smoking, more are dying as a direct result.

The 1980 Surgeon General's Report estimates 32,000 new cases of lung cancer (among men and women) will be diagnosed and that 25,500 women will die within the year. That's four times as many women as died of lung cancer back in 1950, which makes it the third leading cause of cancer deaths in women—a more common killer than endometrial cancer! If that's not enough to shock you, consider this: at the current rate, lung cancer will surpass breast cancer as *the* leading cause of cancer deaths in women by 1985.

Clearly, cigarette smoking is no

small threat to women's health. In fact, according to the 1980 Surgeon General's Report, if you smoke more than a pack a day or have been smoking for more than 30 years, you are 10 times more likely to die of lung cancer than a nonsmoker.

Cigarette smoking may yet prove to be at the root of some cases of breast cancer as well. We already know, for example, that mother's milk can become contaminated by pollutants in food, air, and even cigarette smoke which pass from the bloodstream to the breasts. Now there is evidence that, not only during lactation, but for a good part of a woman's adult life, her breast glands continue to secrete a fluid. What's so alarming, however, is that this fluid appears to be reabsorbed by the breast tissues. And when the breast fluid contains cancer-causing chemicals, the accumulation of these chemicals in the breast could present a serious hazard. For female smokers, this threat is at least partially realized. Researchers at the University of California at San Francisco have detected significant concentrations of nicotine in the breast fluid of nonlactating women smokers. They also suggest that the cancer-causing substances in tobacco smoke probably reach the breast through similar channels (*Science*, January 20, 1978).

Don't hide your habit behind a cloak of invincibility when it comes to heart attacks, either. Women have heart attacks, too. And in a study by Dennis Slone, M.D., of the Drug Epidemiology Unit, Boston University School of Medicine, the biggest risk factor for women was not menopause or oral contraceptives or even coffee drinking, as one might suspect. It was smoking. According to Dr. Slone, the heart attack rate among women who smoked 1 to 14 cigarettes per day was nearly 4½ times greater than the rate among women who

had never smoked and who were not considered at risk. And the more cigarettes smoked, the higher the risk. In other words, for women who smoke at least 35 cigarettes a day (that's just short of two packs), the risk of heart attack increases by 21 times.

Smoking, the Pill, and Menopause

What's more, recent studies confirm that the risk of heart attack, stroke and other circulatory disorders from oral contraceptive use is further complicated by smoking. A few years ago, for example, the Boston Collaborative Drug Surveillance Program found that, for women between the ages of 37 and 46 who take birth control pills, the risk of heart attack is 14 times higher than for women in the same age group who do not take them. But what they didn't discover until later was that of the Pill users who eventually did suffer heart attacks, 92 percent were smokers. As a result of evidence such as this, the Food and Drug Administration (FDA) now requires that labeling of birth control pills warn women smokers of the double trouble.

Women's apparent increased risk of heart attack after menopause might also be linked to their smoking habits. This interesting finding came out of a mammoth study by three Boston researchers involving 3,500 middle-aged women in seven countries. What they invariably found were more smokers past menopause than nonsmokers for every age group. For example, at age 51, 79 percent of those who smoked more than a pack a day had already undergone menopause—compared to only 56 percent of those who never took a puff. Furthermore, the study suggests that the more cigarettes a woman smokes per day, the earlier her menopause is likely to occur (*Lancet*, June 25, 1977). And, says Hershel Jick, M.D., of the Boston Collaborative Drug Surveillance Program, since smoking is known to increase the risk of heart disease, and now that it also appears to throw more women prematurely into the menopause category, perhaps smoking—and not menopause per se—is responsible for the increased risk.

It would seem at first that this premature menopause syndrome might also be at the root of another correlation between cigarettes and osteoporosis. Osteoporosis, a bone-softening disorder, claims women past menopause as its primary victims. But, at least in this study, the severity of the disorder could not be explained in terms of early menopause. Rather, some other factor in the infamous cigarette was the straw that—literally—broke the woman's back.

Harry W. Daniell, M.D., examined 72 women admitted to a California hospital. All were past menopause, between the ages of 40 and 70, and all had suffered broken bones. Thirty-eight women had unexpectedly fractured a backbone while undertaking some simple, nonstrenuous activity such as lifting a turkey from the oven. The other 34 had broken their bones in car accidents or serious falls. Interestingly enough, there were significantly more smokers and heavy smokers in the first brittle bone group than in the second group with legitimate fractures. And there were more smokers in that first group of 38 than in another group of 572 women who hadn't broken a bone at all (*Archives of Internal Medicine*, March, 1976).

Dr. Daniell cites several complications of cigarette smoking as possible explanations. For one thing, he says cigarette smoking devastates lung tissues and for some reason lung disorders are commonly associated with osteoporo-

sis. Smoking also substitutes a certain amount of carbon monoxide, a deadly poison, for oxygen, an essential element for all body functions. To add insult to injury, smoking is also known to reduce the body's concentration of vitamin C, probably the body's most effective natural defense against the lethal effects of carbon monoxide.

Tobacco and Your New Baby

For younger women contemplating a family, the advice of Richard L. Naeye, M.D., of Pennsylvania State University, among others, is quit now—before conception.

Studies have repeatedly shown that smoking increases the risk of miscarriages, stillbirths and premature births. And for those babies who do come kicking into the world, having a mother who couldn't kick the habit puts them at great disadvantage. For starters, the more an expectant mother smokes, the smaller her baby is likely to be at birth. Not only will the infant weigh less, it will be shorter, with a smaller chest and head than the baby born of a nonsmoking mother. Of course, the significance of low birth weight is not fully understood. But it is believed to hinder a child in physical and intellectual development, even later in life. For example, in one study, 11-year-old children whose mothers smoked half a pack or more a day during pregnancy were still shorter than other kids their age and were three to five months behind in reading, math and general learning ability.

What's even more frightening is that we may not know half of the childhood handicaps attributable to maternal smoking. Researchers and physicians have already linked mom's habit to the mysterious killer called crib death, and to slower intellectual and physical development and hyperactivity in children. Other evidence—though still tentative to date—suggests that cigarette smoking during pregnancy might contribute to various neurological disorders, congenital heart and lung problems, and possibly even childhood cancer.

The trouble is, cigarette smoke contains over 2,000 chemical compounds and we haven't even begun to understand the effects of all of them. We do know that nicotine can pass freely from mother to the child developing in her womb, creating several threatening conditions. It constricts the blood vessels in the placenta and restricts the nourishment available to the baby. For the same reason, it may be responsible for a deadly disorder in which the placenta prematurely pulls away from the womb.

Nicotine may also contribute to lung and respiratory problems later in life. Although the fetus does not actually breathe in the womb, it does exercise its lung muscles in preparation for later breathing on its own. Fetal monitoring has demonstrated that this lung activity temporarily stops after just one cigarette—again, probably as a result of constricted blood vessels.

And finally, nicotine appears to affect baby just like mom—as a stimulant increasing heartbeat and causing fluctuations in blood pressure. Unfortunately, for junior, this could create high blood pressure and/or permanent heart damage.

Carbon monoxide is another invisible villain in cigarette smoke. It enters mother's bloodstream, taking up space that should be occupied by oxygen. Since, as was just mentioned, unborn babies do not yet have the capacity to breathe, they depend fully on mother's blood for oxygen. If a woman smokes two packs a day, the oxygen supply to her child can be reduced by 40 to 50 percent. The end result of this often shows up in lowered birth weight and perhaps slower intellectual development.

Likewise, cyanide, another dangerous chemical in tobacco, has been measured in the umbilical cord of developing fetuses exposed to mother's habit. Some researchers suggest that this may reduce both mother's and child's B_{12} supply, since this vitamin helps detoxify cyanide. And because B_{12} is necessary for the metabolism of certain sulfur-containing compounds that are vital for baby's growth and development, cyanide could be a major contributing factor in low birth weight.

The cancer-causing chemicals in cigarettes may also pose a serious threat to an unborn child. Allan Conney, Ph.D., director of biochemistry and drug metabolism at Hoffmann–LaRoche, Inc., has conducted several studies along this line in both animals and man (or woman, to be more exact). What he's found is that certain cancer-causing cigarette compounds create specific enzyme changes in the body. We don't yet know what effect these changes may have on the unborn child. But they have been noted in the developing rat fetus and in the human placenta of exposed mothers, he says.

Obviously, then, pregnancy is one of the most important times to pack up your cigarette habit. And contrary to popular opinion, it could be one of the easiest times to quit. Think about it: how many women do you know who gave up drugs, alcohol or coffee during pregnancy with nary a complaint? Probably quite a few. It happens that many women who develop morning sickness lose their taste for former cravings—

cigarettes included—and do not resume these unhealthy hangups during their entire pregnancy. Many women who quit smoking during pregnancy do not report any problems with withdrawal symptoms.

But besides that, pregnancy provides an excellent opportunity to adopt a new healthful lifestyle—both for yourself and for your yet unborn child. And since recent evidence suggests that the negative aspects of smoking may continue for some time after quitting, perhaps the best time to quit is *before* conception.

If it doesn't work out that way, there are still plenty of good reasons to quit or at least cut back during pregnancy. As mentioned, the extent of cigarette damage to unborn children is often "dose related." In other words, the more you smoke the more harm you're likely to incur on the little one. And conversely the less you smoke, the less harm.

A final plea to pregnant smokers: at the very least, don't smoke for 48 hours prior to the expected time of delivery. Anesthesiologist Judith M. Davies and associates at the University Hospital of Wales found that mothers who took a short predelivery respite from smoking had eight percent more blood oxygen available during delivery than mothers who had continued to smoke. This extra bit of oxygen, she says, could be critical during the stressful birth experience.

Nursing provides another good reason to quit. Breast milk of smoking mothers has been found to contain nicotine and significantly less vitamin C than the milk of nonsmoking mothers. Also, you might as well let your little one light up as puff smoke rings in his or her direction. Several researchers have found a relationship between parental smoking and infant respiratory infections indicating that secondhand smoke is almost as hazardous as inhaled smoke. Besides, it's a well-known fact that children of smoking households are more likely to take up the habit themselves.

Quitting Is More Difficult for Women

As you can see, women have even more to lose from cigarette smoking than men. And yet, according to recent tallies, they are less successful at quitting. No one can say for sure why that is. Bad timing maybe. According to Ellen R. Gritz, Ph.D., of the Veterans Administration Medical Center, Brentwood, and the University of California, Los Angeles, there is a tendency to put off quitting until middle age. Especially for women, the forties and fifties already present challenges aplenty—with menopause, midlife problems, and perhaps the empty nest blues. Top that off with the stress of nicotine withdrawal and it's easy to see why so many women don't make it past week one.

Women may also have more difficulty finding acceptable substitutes for smoking. Men tend to smoke for pleasure but women often smoke to cope, says Dr. Gritz. Eventually cigarettes can come to provide their major outlet from stress, depression and boredom. When they quit, they not only lose that means of coping but they're up against the emotional and physical effects of withdrawal, which can include anxiety, depression and, of course, lots and lots of stress. If they've got no alternative coping plan, they're doomed.

One very common reason for foiled female attempts to quit, however, may be weight gain. Women are much more concerned about trading pounds for puffs than men. In fact, they are often more fearful of getting fat than of getting cancer. That's not to say we condone excessive weight gain. Too many extra pounds can also be a burden to your health. But, according to one journal article, you'd have to be 125 pounds overweight to meet the health hazard of smoking just one pack of cigarettes a day! (*CA–A Cancer Journal for Clinicians*, March/April, 1979). How's that for putting things in perspective?

Nevertheless, weight gain unfortunately can follow cigarette withdrawal. Of course, not every woman who quits will gain. According to one study, perhaps half will. And again, why that is remains anyone's guess. Possible explanations range from decreased metabolic rate to increased appetite to a tendency to use eats as a substitute for puffs. There's no question that food tastes better when it's not competing with smoke.

So for many women the real question is not just "How do I quit smoking?" It's "How do I quit smoking without gaining weight?" Unfortunately, none of the how-to plans we examined adequately addressed the specific problems of the female smoker. So after talking to several physicians, psychologists, researchers and smoking experts, we combined the best advice of all of them to come up with some specific hints to help you kick the cigarette habit without tipping the bathroom scale in the process. But remember, any program is only as good as your commitment.

Getting Ready to Give It Up

The first, most important step in any smoking cessation program is *wanting* to quit. That may sound trivial but, in fact, it is probably the most important deciding factor in success or failure. Every expert we interviewed agreed—

you've really got to make up your mind to quit. If you're just lukewarm on the idea or if somebody else is the impetus in your quitting, don't bother. You're almost certain to fail before you begin. And this will only create a more cumbersome psychological hurdle when it comes time to try again.

So, carefully consider your reasons for quitting. Maybe you're planning to start a family in the near future, and your reasons have to do with an unknown family member and a new start for yourself. Or perhaps your health has been failing—you're shortwinded and nervous much of the time. Perhaps you have a family history of cancer and you don't want to add your name to the fallen limb of the family tree. Or maybe you're just fed up with a disgusting habit and would rather take a preventive stand now in favor of your health. Whatever your reasons, jot them down, then read them carefully to yourself. Are they good enough reasons to quit? Are you absolutely convinced? If so, do it.

Remember, poor timing can be an important underlying factor in failure. So consider your frame of mind. If you're unduly depressed over a divorce, death in the family, or change of address, put off quitting for another day. Also, don't take on the challenge when your mind is crowded with other pressing considerations—say, a daughter's wedding, or even the Christmas holidays. Get those occasions out of the way first. Quitting during pregnancy or menopause can be accomplished so long as you realize the extra effort it entails and prime yourself psychologically.

Surround yourself with friends who are willing to give you the psychological support you'll need. According to Dr. Gritz, although men don't always seem to benefit from outside support, women do better in programs that provide a maximum amount of social support and tend to do worse in situations where program support is low or where outside factors work against quitting. This is one reason why group sessions may be a woman's stronghold—and why we've included a list of group smoking-cessation programs.

But don't feel that you must seek the support of strangers. If your husband smokes, make a pact with him and swear off cigarettes together. Or align yourself with a close friend or friends who have also been considering quitting and make it a group challenge. If you find yourself alone in wanting to quit, don't keep it a secret. Make your wishes known to all around you and ask for their support. It's also a good idea to avoid chain-smoking companions or acquaintances—at least until you can comfortably turn down their offer of a cigarette with a "No thank you, I don't smoke." This is also a good time to spend with friends who don't smoke or cultivate new nonsmoking friends. Join a no-smoking table in the company cafeteria. Or, better yet, join a health club or YWCA and spend your lunch hour working out with a health-conscious bunch.

The Right to Become an Ex-Smoker

Then, if your commitment, timing and environment are right, quit. That is, quit in two weeks. You need time to work up to it. So set a date—say two weeks from Wednesday—circle it on your calendar, and set your sights there. If possible, arrange to take off from work or your usual schedule from Thursday through Sunday. Plan something enjoyable for those days. A long weekend at the seashore. A visit with old (nonsmoking) friends. Or

perhaps just spend the time at home working on a fun project—like furniture refinishing. Anything that will free you from your normal routine.

Till then, use the two-weeks-plus to better understand your habit and prepare yourself physically and emotionally for giving it up.

We're not going to soft-pedal quitting—smoking is a hazardous two-part hangup. First of all, some researchers now believe that nicotine is an insidiously addictive drug. While some people can sample alcohol or sleeping pills on occasion without becoming dependent, very few who have tried more than a couple of cigarettes can leave it at that. Most get hooked. Then, when you consider that the average pack-a-day smoker gets off on more than 73,000 nicotine "hits" a year and that it takes only eight seconds for the drug to seep through the lungs and into the bloodstream to the brain where it pays off its "satisfying" rewards, it's no wonder that smoking is a tough habit to crack. So be prepared.

Of course, some people claim no more than a little daytime drowsiness after quitting. But for others, withdrawal symptoms are very real. Headaches, irritability, depression, muscle aches and cramps, anxiety, visual and sleep disturbances, and a distorted sense of time perception—not to mention an intense hankering for cigarettes—have been reported by persons quitting. These symptoms usually peak around the third or fourth day and generally subside by week's end. Just hang in there.

According to Dr. Gritz, cutting back gradually as opposed to quitting "cold turkey" won't spare you these unpleasant rebound effects. In fact, since withdrawal symptoms can occur with reduced nicotine intake, cutting back could conceivably draw out the agony of withdrawal for as long as it takes you to wipe your slate clean. Why torture yourself?

Accept the fact that the first week won't be easy. Think of it as a cold. You may feel ill for a few days, but it's not terminal. You'll get over it. Like a cold, too, nicotine withdrawal can be eased along by drinking lots of liquids, especially water. Gerald Schmeling, Ph.D., a smoking researcher at Schick Shadel Hospital in Seattle, Washington, explains that drinking water flushes the nicotine out of the system. And, as an added bonus, he says, it makes you feel fuller so you're less inclined to nibble between meals.

Psyching Out the Cigarette Habit

A good attitude is a real asset at this time. If you see these physical withdrawal symptoms as a body falling to pieces, you won't hold up through the week. But if you look at the aches and painful cravings—much like the twinge of a knitting wound—as a body healing itself, you'll feel much more encouraged about your decision to quit.

Actually, though, the physiological withdrawal effects are only half the problem. The other half is psychological. And believe it or not, it's even harder to convince your mind that it can do without—particularly for women, who, as we mentioned, come to depend on a smoke to cope.

Take time during this prequitting period to analyze just why *you* smoke. Look at your smoking habits carefully. When do you smoke? What are the circumstances? That is, do you smoke when you drink alcohol or coffee, at parties, after eating, in the office or when the baby cries? What are your feelings before and after smoking?

To keep track of these feelings and circumstances, wrap a note paper around your cigarette pack, secure it with a rubber band, and replace one cigarette in the pack with a small pencil. Or keep a small note pad and pen near at hand. Then, whenever you have a smoke, record the time, place and feeling which led up to the event. It won't take more than a few days to uncover some pattern to your madness. Then think of ways to avoid these situations. For example, if your morning coffee sparks the urge for a Virginia Slims, think about a fresh-squeezed glass of orange juice instead. Likewise, if a large afternoon meal is your undoing, try a light lunch followed by a refresher break instead. Splash your face with cool water, brush your teeth with something minty and fresh, and, if you can manage it, take a quick 20- to 30-minute snooze.

Better yet, look for a completely unrelated but fully satisfying pastime. Sign up for a drawing class, or try your hand at crocheting. Or best of all, get into something that will keep you up and moving. Dancing. Yoga. Exercise at a local spa. Jogging. Bicycling. Or just walking.

Let Exercise Help You Kick the Habit

There are several reasons why starting a regular exercise program could be the biggest step you'll take toward kicking the habit. First of all, one of the greatest natural "highs" you can experience is the sensation of your body in motion. Ask anyone who jogs regularly and seriously. He or she will tell you that it's absolutely habit-forming. And what could be better than substituting a very positive healthful habit for one that is just the opposite?

Second, regular exercise discourages tobacco cravings. No one knows exactly why that is, but many individuals admit that they couldn't break the cigarette smoking habit until they first started a jogging or aerobic exercise program. Samuel Fox, M.D., former head of the American Heart Association's Exercise Committee, says, "Rare is the vigorous exerciser who will continue to smoke." Ronald M. Lawrence, M.D., president and founder of the American Medical Jogger's Association, echoes that view. "When people start jogging," he says, "they find that smoking impedes their performance—cuts down on their wind—and also that cigarettes no longer taste good." So they stop the habit. Smoking is definitely on the decline among people who jog.

Exercise also provides benefits of special interest to the female smoker. First and foremost, it burns calories and, over a period of time, it can increase your basal metabolic rate so that starting an exercise program two weeks or so before smoking your last cigarette helps offset any weight gain which might have a tendency to creep up afterward. Incidentally, there's no real evidence that exercise stimulates appetite. In fact, Dr. Schmeling assured us that if you exercise before mealtime, it acts as an appetite depressant.

Also, since it has been shown that women have a tendency to use cigarette smoking as a coping device, exercise could provide a one-way ticket to happiness and peace of mind. Several studies have revealed that exercise is a terrific pick-me-up and a fantastic antidepressant (see also Depression).

If you're not up to jogging or strenuous calisthenics, there's nothing wrong with walking. In fact, some physicians, such as John Douglass, M.D., of the Kaiser–Permanente Medical Center in

HOW EXERCISE CAN HELP YOU QUIT

For many people giving up cigarettes is like trading one bad habit for another. They quit smoking but start snacking—sometimes to the point of losing their figure. What's more, in the process of taking this step to improve their health, thay may actually feel worse than ever before—nervous, tense, tired, vaguely ill. That's where exercise comes in. According to a study of about 400 sedentary men, taking up a regular exercise program not only helped some to kick the habit but countered many negative feelings that are often associated with quitting.

Exercise Program Effects	% People
Decreased smoking	20
Decreased appetite	48
Weight loss	67
Lower stress and tension	43
Increased stamina	90
More adequate sleep and rest	37
Feelings of better health	85

SOURCE: Adapted from "Response to Physical Activity Programs and Their Effects on Health Behavior," by F. Heinzelmann and R. W. Bagley, (Public Health Rep. 85, 1970).

Los Angeles, favor walking over other aerobic exercises. It's easier on the feet and joints. And yet, when done at a brisk pace, it can contribute to improved heart and lung health, weight loss, and so forth, he says. Now you've got a good excuse to get out there and pound the pavement for 30 minutes, morning and night.

TILL YOU QUIT, TAKE THIS . . .

Vitamin A. According to a massive study in Norway, there is a strong link between the amount of vitamin A in your diet and the incidence of lung cancer. E. Bjelke of the Cancer Registry of Norway followed 8,278 men over several years and found a lower lung cancer rate among those whose diets were high in vitamin A. The researcher concludes that this vitamin may somehow modify the cancer-causing effects of certain substances in the lung (*International Journal of Cancer*, vol. 15, 1975).

Vitamin C. Vitamin C is a smoker's best shield against carbon monoxide and perhaps other cigarette poisons as well. Writing in *The Journal of Orthomolecular Psychiatry* (vol. 5, no. 1, 1976), biochemist Dr. Irwin Stone cites studies in which vitamin C detoxified carbon monoxide, arsenic compounds and cyanide—all constituents of cigarette smoke.

Vitamin E. You've read that smoking increases the risk of heart attack and stroke and may have wondered why. Actually, there are several reasons. First of all, smoking either causes or complicates atherosclerosis—a narrowing of the arteries. And second, nicotine speeds up a bodily mechanism—platelet aggregation—which may trigger the formation of a nasty blood clot called a thrombosis. This is where vitamin E comes in. Two researchers, Manfred Steiner, M.D., Ph.D., and his assistant, John Anastasi, recently found that vitamin E decreases platelet aggregation.

Vitamin B_6. The 1979 Surgeon General's Report tells us that smoking can bring on a vitamin B_6 deficiency—possibly due to an interaction between this vitamin and carbon monoxide. And since B_6 has proven invaluable to all kinds of female functions, it's important that you're not caught short.

Vitamin B_{12}. Since this vitamin is needed for the body's detoxification of cyanide, smoking results in lowered B_{12} levels in both blood and body tissues. Vitamin B_{12} is an essential nerve vitamin as well as being of utmost importance to the physical and intellectual development of a growing fetus.

Calcium or Bone Meal. Smoking accelerates osteoporosis—the loss of calcium from the bones. To counteract this effect, extra doses of calcium or bone meal are essential.

How to Control Your Weight after Quitting

Of course, we couldn't orchestrate a program on how to quit smoking without gaining weight and not mention diet. But fear not, it won't be in the calorie-counting context of other smoking-cessation programs. In fact, in our opinion, a newly nonsmoking person (who may be counting sheep to get to sleep) shouldn't be called on to count calories, too. Besides, how much you eat isn't as critical as what you eat.

For example, during the two-week prep and also after quitting day, it's a good idea to limit your intake of coffee and alcohol since these prompt cigarette smoking in many persons.

Also, you should be increasing your intake of whole plant foods like vegetables, fruits, nuts, seeds (especially sunflower seeds, which, according to Dr. Douglass, have a special suppressing effect on tobacco cravings), and whole grains. And the more of these you eat raw, the better.

For one thing, whole fruits and vegetables tend to be high in fiber with a lower concentration of calories so they will help counter any weight-gaining tendency. Second, says Dr. Douglass, by eating a natural and largely raw food diet we reacclimate our body systems. Dr. Douglass observed that people who are able to stick with a raw food diet not only lose their desire to smoke, but soon find cigarettes less tasteful. Eventually, they aren't able to tolerate the smoking habit at all. "One of my patients who had been on a 90 to 100 percent raw food diet for more than a month had a heart palpitation when he smoked a cigarette," Dr. Douglass told us. "Besides, there's something about lettuce, seeds and nuts that's out of harmony with cigarettes." Maybe it's just the idea of healthful living.

After all, once you get your body tuned up with a good diet and exercise program you'll not only be ready, you'll be willing, anxious and able to give up smoking!

SOLARIUMS

Just when we thought (and hoped) interest was fading, the sunlamp got a second wind. Suddenly, quick-tanning salons are springing up in shopping centers all over town with the same kind of appeal as the fast-food franchises before them. Not that people emerge looking like Kentucky Fried Chicken, but the salability of the product hinges on the fact that it's fast and relatively inexpensive (that is, if you compare it to a week's vacation in the Bahamas). What's worse, both fast foods and fast tans masquerade as a boon to the American experience when, in fact, they are no chum to our health and well-being.

According to the Consumer Product Safety Commission, more than 7,700 persons were treated for sunlamp-related injuries in hospital emergency rooms in 1978 (and that's *before* all this quick-tanning craze really got cranked up).

Admittedly, the majority of the skin burns and eye irritations were no doubt caused by carelessness. People have a tendency to take the precautions associated with the sunlamp all too lightly. They think that ultraviolet radiation from a sunlamp is equal in intensity to that from the sun. The truth is, the artificial light in a tanning booth may emit more than 10 times the radiation of the summer sun at high noon. Similarly, they think that they can get away with not using the goggles. But if you glance into the light for even a brief moment, you're leaving your eyes wide open for trouble. Eyes are very vulnerable to ultraviolet radiation—especially the intense light given off by a sunlamp. Looking directly at a sunlamp for only a few minutes can cause a painful though temporary condition called photokeratitis, in which the eyes burn with a sandy, gritty sensation. Overexposure can burn the cornea and result in permanent eye damage.

Another problem that can plague the sunlamp worshiper involves photosensitivity. Persons with a history of *herpes simplex* are susceptible. And in certain sensitive people, the combination of various chemical agents and the sun do not mix. The result is a nasty burn and/or skin irritation (see also Sunbathing). The chemicals we're talking about range from the antibiotic you're swallowing to the cosmetics you're slathering on your face. Of course, if you're predisposed to photosensitivity, natural sunlight is just as sure to cause this reaction as the ultraviolet rays of a sunlamp. But because of the greater intensity of the sunlamp, you're liable to come down with the symptoms much more quickly. And if you're tanning up on your coffee break or on your way to the market, there's a greater possibility that you'll be wearing makeup, or deodorant, or perfume, or one of the other offending chemicals we're talking about.

But aside from the suntanning troubles that can be avoided, there are many more that cannot. The effect of ultraviolet radiation on your skin is cumulative—that is, the more exposure you get, the greater your chances of developing premature wrinkles, discolored patches of skin and even skin cancer. In fact, in a letter to the *New England Journal of Medicine* (June 26, 1980), Richard J. Wurtman, M.D., from the Massachusetts Institute of Technology, and Frederick Urbach, M.D., from the Skin and Cancer Hospital of Temple University School of Medicine, point out something that the tanning parlors don't: that is, that these same sunlamps are widely used in scientific research to quickly generate skin cancer in animals.

In that the natural sunlight we get during leisure time outdoor activities is more than enough to supply us with all the true benefits of the sun—that is, vitamin D synthesis, a feeling of well-being, and even hormonal stimulation if that is, in fact, an effect—there really is no additional need for the sunlamp and suntanning parlors.

Besides, very few people actually tan under a sunlamp. Most turn a faint pink with a white Rocky Raccoon type of mask where the goggles have been.

But if it's the blush of color in the pale of winter that you're after, try a vigorous exercise program, like jogging or dancercise, or even a 10-minute stint in the sauna twice a week to stimulate the circulation in your skin and give your cheeks a healthy, rosy glow year-round—naturally.

SPAS

When you think "spa," what comes to mind? Fashionable turn-of-the-century Britons sipping sulfurous spring water at the pump house in Bath? Arthritic patients bathing in the warm mineral waters of Baden-Baden in West Germany?

Well, today, spas are springing up all over the United States. But the strange thing about them is that they have nothing at all to do with water—or at least with the mineral springs that made the other ones famous. Oh, they might have a few swimming pools or bubbly water baths produced artificially by the whirling jets of a Jacuzzi. But water's not what they're touting. Fitness and slimness is.

Actually, the American spa is a bit like a glorified health club. It's got the weigh-ins, the exercise routines, the equipment, the saunas, the whirlpool, the masseuses, and all the moral support you could possibly need. But because you check in for a week or two at a time (instead of the halfhearted half hour you may be putting in at your local club once or twice a week), your workouts are much more intensive. Also, because you take your meals as they are given to you—in carefully determined portions and *only* at mealtime—it's practically impossible to cheat on your diet. As you can imagine then, the results tend to be a lot more rewarding.

Of course, we can't speak for every spa. With so many scattered about over the U.S.—some good and some, no doubt, bad—it's important that you go through similar channels for choosing a spa as you would a health club (see Health Clubs). Check out the area of specialization, too. Some spas concentrate totally on weight control. Others, more health-minded, deal with fitness, natural food and holistic principles. We obviously prefer the latter. In fact, based on two very impressive experiences we had, we'd go so far as to say that if you can spare the time and the money (prices range from $500 to $2,000 a week including room and board), a visit to one of these health and fitness spots can leave you feeling like a million dollars. And, even more important, a week-long vacation there can pay off in year-long, at-home benefits.

By "benefits," we're not referring just to gains in the area of weight loss. While it's true that the majority of women we spoke with during our spa visits were there with the intent of taking off a few pounds (and by midweek, several were indeed successful at shedding 5 or 6), you don't have to be overweight or an overeater to take part in some programs. One woman we talked to actually came to the spa to *gain*

weight. Another was there to tone her tiny frame to insure a smooth line in size 4 designer jeans. Those who did come to lose had at most 20 pounds to go to reach their ideal weight—more than that and they'd probably have trouble keeping up with the vigorous program at this particular spot. Said one fellow who followed his plump but determined wife to a four-week stay at a coed spa in Mexico: "The guys at work were ribbing me about spending my vacation at a fat farm. But wait until they get a look at my pictures from the pool!"

Clearly, the label of "fat farm" doesn't stick anymore—at least at the more upbeat holistic health retreats. We met women of all ages, sizes and statures. A Massachusetts mother and daughters trio (one from New York City and the other from San Francisco) who rendezvoused to share a week of fun. A spry and white-haired woman in her late sixties who returned to the spa for her 19th visit. A couple of Canadian gals in their early thirties who took a break from husband and kids.

A New Path, Not a Reprieve

What many women don't realize, however—at least till they get there—is that fit and trim go hand in hand with a healthful lifestyle. This one-week experience isn't an end-all but a starting point for continued lifestyle improvements. After all, a 10-pound reprieve won't do you a bit of good if you go back home to your old eating habits and semi-sedentary ways. But that's where a very good spa can help. If you're the kind of person who can't quite get it together—that is, can't stick to a weight-reducing regimen long enough to lose 1 pound (let alone 20), or can't find the motivation to walk (not to mention jog) for 30 minutes each day—this health-intensive break could be just what you need to jolt you out of your old routine and give you reason and motivation to make those positive changes permanent.

Or think of it as the ultimate vacation. Removed from the demands of family or job, you have the chance to concentrate totally on yourself, to rediscover the potential you probably never knew you had, to challenge your physical capabilities to new heights, to let go of all tension and frustrations and to find out what ultimate relaxation is all about.

Even if you never much thought of yourself as the athletic type, after a full week's worth of work at a place that specializes in it, you'll be dancing to the tune of a whole different drummer.

Interestingly enough, once you get into the sunup to sundown movement routine, you won't be able to sit still. Your body will actually crave physical activity. And if you have to push yourself to get off your tush to trip the light, imagine having to hold yourself back.

Thought you never had time to exercise? It's funny, but when the will is there, the free time suddenly opens up. A morning series of eye-opening stretches becomes as routine—and necessary—as brushing your teeth. And who would rush out of the house in the morning without grooming their pearly whites?!

A week at one of these spas is a great opportunity to find just the inspiration you need for adopting a whole new set of healthful habits. After all, feeling good is the best motivation you can have. And chances are, you'll never know how good you *can* feel until you've pushed yourself to nearly peak condition—something that can't be had for less than a week's intense work, un-less, of course, you're already a serious jogger or weekday athlete.

Of course, all spas vary. And you don't have to spend a small fortune to reap million-dollar benefits. We had a tremendous experience at the Rancho La Puerta, a cold spa in Tecate, Mexico, for about $500 a week including a comfortable room with fireplace and plenty of tasty but low-cal vegetarian food. Facilities there include nine gyms, four tennis courts, three swimming pools, two saunas, one whirlpool plus running track, volleyball court, putting greens, hiking trails and 2½-mile "Parcours" trail with 20 exercise stations.

Inside the Fabulous Golden Door

But, you may be wondering, what's a day at a spa really like?

To give you an idea what a spa experience is all about, we'll take you to one of the best—right now. Located just outside of San Diego in Escondido, California, the Golden Door is an exclusive (only 32 guests at a time) and expensive (about $2,000 a week) holistic health resort which many call "the ultimate spa." You'll begin to understand why the minute you step through the golden doors—which, incidentally, aren't the entranceway to a stuffy gymnasium but the gateway to a lovely complex of Japanese gardens and teahouselike buildings nestled in a sunny valley in southern California. The setting is idyllic. The southern California climate, pleasantly warm and brilliantly clear almost all year 'round. The atmosphere, tranquil. The mood, incredibly enthusiastic and dedicated. And with three employees (including exercise instructors, masseuses, chef and beauticians) to every guest, the attention to you and to the detail such a program entails is tops.

But if you think this place is all luxury and no sweat, guess again.

6:00 A.M. Wake-up. A day at "The Door" begins at dawn with an invigorating walk-hike. Nudged from slumber by a 6:00 A.M. wake-up call, you crawl (eyes still closed) into your Golden Door warm-up suit and sneakers. Then stumble through the darkness to the mountain's base. It's cold outside. And the chill-sleep factor makes that bed you left seem more toasty and comforting than you ever imagined one could be. You trudge on despite your mind's moanings to turn back. Fortunately, several women soon join you—all headed in the same direction. At least you're not the only one up at this ungodly hour!

6:30 A.M. Morning hike. A small group has gathered. The sky brightens just enough to reveal a steep serpentine trail that slithers back and forth across

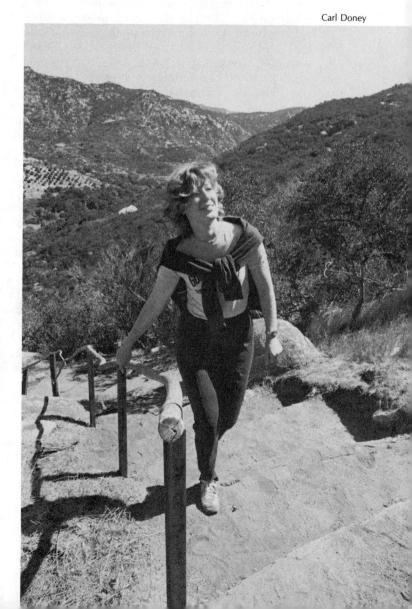

Carl Doney

On top of the world at sunrise—that's where you'll be and how you'll feel on the Golden Door's morning mountain hike.

the mountain face between massive monoliths of rock. Even through the early morning haze, the challenge is clear. Will you make it to the top?

Not today. New arrivals to the Golden Door are encouraged to begin on one of two less strenuous trails—a 1½-mile walk on level ground or a 2-mile hike over a gently sloping mountain ridge. The steeper 3-mile serpentine is reserved for more experienced fitness buffs. But by week's end, almost every guest will make it to the top—an achievement symbolic of the peak physical condition they attained in an uninterrupted week of hard work.

For most newcomers, however, the two-mile moderate trail is tough enough. Ten minutes into the hike, you've forgotten all about the cold or the warm bed you left behind. Your heart's beating faster; your breaths are getting heavier, deeper. You're actually working up a sweat and it feels good.

What's more, the sheer experience of being in this place in time is as exhilarating as the exercise you're getting while there. The air is so incredibly crisp and clean it seems to glide in and out of your lungs with no resistance. The view of earth and sky mingle in the diffused morning light to create one panoramic vista of soft tawny shades. And the mountain is perfectly still save for the music of the birds that live here and the gentle pounding of feet from the small Golden Door brigade in blue suits. It's no wonder that by the time you head down for breakfast, you not only feel awake, you feel alive.

8:00 A.M. Breakfast. At the Golden Door, most women are put on a calorie-restricted diet—700 calories a day seemed to be the most popular diet menu. But here, less food doesn't mean deprivation. What's missing in quantity is more than made up for in flavor, goodness and beauty of presentation. No empty calories served here. Today's breakfast is a perfect example. One-half of a papaya topped with a large scoop of cottage cheese and sprinkled with wheat germ and sunflower seeds and garnished with red grapes. Yes, it tastes as wonderful as it looks. And that's only the beginning. One part of the breakfast fare at the Golden Door is a special high-fiber cereal consisting of two tablespoons bran for fiber, two tablespoons wheat germ with some sunflower seeds for protein, raisins for iron and cinnamon for flavor. Mixed with a little skim milk or apple cider, this granola is considered a morning must. Finished off with a conventional cup of coffee (or tea if you wish—but no sugar or honey) this has got to rate as one of the most delectable breakfasts you've ever had.

8:30 A.M. Warm-ups. Today because the weather is so beautiful and because everyone's talking about the organic gardening done here, you opt for warm-ups in the garden. It's hard to tell just how far it is to the garden; the scenes along the way monopolize your attention. First you pass by an elaborate herb garden where the Golden Door chef plucks his seasonings fresh each day. Next you stroll through the bulb garden, a wooded area planted with a year-round display of flowering bulbs. This week, blankets of daffodils cover the forest floor with sunny splashes of yellow and white. But one of the most beautiful sites of all is the vegetable garden—seven acres of greens and grains sprawled across a sunny hillside. Lettuce of all kinds and in every stage of maturity. Spinach. Broccoli. Cauliflower. Artichokes. Five-year-old brussels sprouts plants that are a full three feet tall. All bug-free and all grown organically without the use of chemical fertilizers and pesticides.

Straw basket in garden-gloved hand, you eagerly pitch in to help harvest sugar peas for this evening's meal. For 10 minutes or so you engage in deep knee bends, toe-touches, arm stretches, and neck rotations as you search out those tender little morsels camouflaged among the leaves of green. Go ahead— pop a pod in your mouth. Still dripping with morning dew, it has the just-picked sweetness and crispness that's impossible to duplicate unless you've got your own vegetable patch at home.

9:00 A.M. Da Vinci exercises. At the Golden Door, aerobics go by the name Da Vinci, a reference to that famous man who identified large muscle groups. Da Vinci exercises use these large muscle groups in a real huff-and-puff workout. What it amounts to is kicking up your heels and keeping them airbound to the tune of some eye-opening, high-stepping music. The morning's hike had nothing over the exertion going on here. Whew!

Some Well-Deserved Beauty Pampering

10:00 A.M. Beauty break. After a shower and quick change from leotard and tights to a terry robe, you saunter over to the row of beauty rooms where a softly pillowed lounge chair awaits you. Your hands and feet are gently massaged with a lightly scented cream, then tucked away in heating-pad-like mitts and boots. Your hair is saturated with avocado oil and scooped up off your neck in loosely woven braids. Sink down into the chair, close your eyes and enjoy this little bit of pampering.

With hands lathered in massage cream, the beautician begins by massaging the tension away from your upper chest and neck. She reaches down behind your shoulder blades and gently strokes your shoulders and neck up to the base of your head. When the muscles of your neck and shoulders are somewhat freed from tension, she works her way up to your face. Working with her fingertips she massages every inch of your face ever so gently. Tapping at the frown crease between your eyebrows, smoothing away dry patches from your chin. It's too soon to tell what a difference this bit of pampering will make in the way you look, but it feels beautiful! In the 30 minutes or so that she touches you, you never felt so good. She removes the cozy covers from your hands and feet—the warmed moisture cream has left them feeling smooth and soft.

11:00 A.M. Water exercises. Now's your chance to make a splash. And don't worry about the water conditions. Even if you're the type of person who tends to test the waters with toe-first trepidation, you'll not find an objectional drop here. The exercise pool at the Golden Door is heated to between 80° and 100°F so that easing in is as easy as slipping into an evening bath. But just because the water is so warm and relaxing doesn't mean you're going to relax. To loosen up, let's jog twice around the pool's perimeter. You'll find that running in shoulder-high water is like a slow-motion dream. But it's this water resistance that boosts the usual benefits of jogging on land.

To cash in on even bigger benefits of water exercise, you have only to make use of the inflatable orange anklets, called ankies, that are tossed about the pool. Snap one around your right ankle. Like a little life-preserver, this anklet air-bag keeps your right foot bobbing atop the pool's shimmering surface.

And, incredibly, it takes quite a bit of oomph to coax that floating foot back in line with the other on the pool floor—which is precisely the idea of these exercises.

11:50 A.M. Potassium break. Cups of warmed tomato juice are distributed to the Golden Door guests while they indulge themselves in a 10-minute sunbath. What a delightful break!

12:00 noon. Spot exercises. With just enough time to towel off and swap swimsuit for sweat suit, you hurry over to the gym scheduled for spot exercises. This time, you will be working your body inch by inch, head to toe, toning every muscle, smoothing over contours.

1:00 P.M. Lunch. With the sun shining and a pleasant breeze in the air, you decide to have your lunch poolside. It arrives shortly—a lovely tray heaped high with a puffy omelet enveloping lightly steamed asparagus and fresh alfalfa sprouts. Garnished with orange and grapefruit wedges and glistening in its reflection in a tall glass of lemonade (at the Golden Door, lemonade is Perrier and fresh lemon juice sans sugar), it's got to rank as one of the most refreshing and deliciously satisfying lunches you've ever had!

Carl Doney

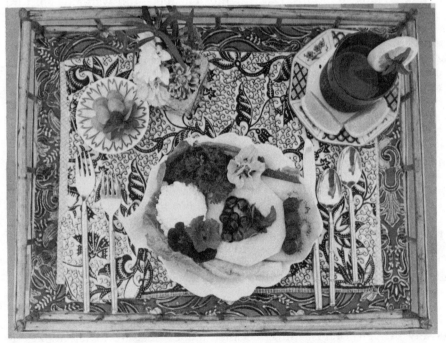

There's no mystery to the Golden Door's low-calorie—but totally satisfying—meals. The secret's in fiber-rich fruits and vegetables, fresh, crisp flavors and, of course, a lovely presentation complete with herb and flower garnishes. You can't get fat feasting your eyes!

Sauna, Massage . . . Ahhh

2:00 P.M. Massage. A leisurely lunch behind you, you saunter over to the Japanese-style bathhouse—a lovely restful environment with mosaic floor resembling river pebbles and blue stylized fish swimming silently across the walls. Slipping out of your clothes, and into a fluffy white towel, you're greeted by your masseuse—a slightly plump woman with an unrelenting smile. "Would you like to take a sauna before we start?" she asks while leading you to a dimly lit redwood room. There's nothing unusual about this sauna except that with you being the only one there, it looks rather roomy and luxurious. You lie down on the bottom bench while the friendly gal in white places a cool washcloth over your forehead. "My name is Anne; if you need anything give me a call. . . . Be back in 10 minutes," she whispers, closing the door behind her. You close your eyes and feel your every muscle sink into the bench as peace and quiet overcome you.

Time's up, Anne calls for you. She leads you over to the showers and directs you into a long hall-like shower stall. The cool water rinses off every last trace of perspiration. "Would you like to try a Scotch mist? Everyone tries it at least once," she says, flashing a frivolous grin.

"What is it? A cocktail?"

"Walk back to the far end of the shower stall, and turn around to face me. Cover your breasts with your hands." You reluctantly comply. As you turn to face her, Anne is standing like the opponent in a duel, aiming two garden hoses at you. "Ready?" she asks, and then before you have a chance to reply, zap—the sprays of water hit with the kind of tingling force it takes to flush out debris from pavement cracks. Down both legs.

"Turn to the side," Anne commands. She directs the jets of water from shoulder to ankle.

"What's this supposed to do?" you sputter.

"Stimulate circulation—doesn't it feel it?"

You've got to admit, the sting of such a concentrated and forceful stream of water sure beats the water massage shower head you had installed at home. And, if you weren't so embarrassed by the whole procedure, it would probably hurt.

"Now the back."

You dutifully make the about-face. The shooting stream strikes your back (ouch), waist, buttocks and legs. Anxious to get on with the massage, you quickly turn to the side for the finale.

Anne helps you dry off and then climb onto the massage table. You lie on your back, discreetly draped in a white sheet, as Anne begins by massaging your upper chest and reaching down across your back and neck in long, fluid strokes. Her fingers come up against a good-size muscle knot in your shoulder. "Looks like you've been bottling up a lot of stress back here," she says. "Let's see if we can work it out." She kneads, rubs and massages it. Then she concentrates her efforts on your arms—one at a time. Gently massaging each muscle and joint beginning with your fingers—each finger—she works her way up toward the shoulders. Your arm falls limp with utter relaxation. Next she tackles your toes and with the same kind of gentle persuasion brings relaxation to a part of the body that you couldn't ever imagine had once been laced with tension. She unveils your stomach and kneads your waist in a similar fashion.

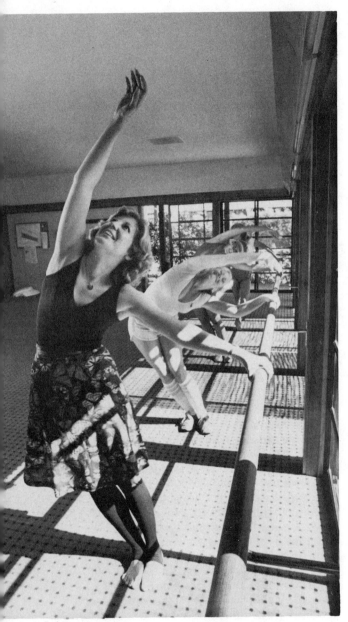

Carl Doney

Slow, easy stretches at the ballet barre keep your spine flexible, your whole body in alignment.

"Turn over."

Your whole back is in for a workout now. Anne works methodically, soothing every muscle. To finish off, she raps you from top to toe with the edge of her hands. You roll off the table—a limp and gel-like version of what got on almost an hour ago.

3:00 P.M. More aerobics. This time with Yuichi (pronounced You-ee-chee), a renowned choreographer from San Francisco. The dance floor is crowded. Everyone loves Yuichi, this silent fellow who talks totally with his graceful body movements. The music—loud and upbeat interspaced with soft and soothing—sets the pace. Yuichi leads the way with an incredible range of movements. After a short time, you feel like part of a chorus line—following his every step, dancing to the stepped-up rhythm of the music.

4:00 P.M. Stretch and relax. Time to start slowing down for day's end. At the ballet barre, the instructor leads you through a series of stretches to relax the spine, to gently stretch the neck. Slow, even stretches. Twenty-five minutes of those followed by a half hour or so of gentle relaxation—meditation. You lie on the floor and systematically tense and relax each body muscle from head to toe. Then she leads you through a visualization exercise—by the end of the class several students let out with a snore. It's that relaxing!

5:00 P.M. Herbal wrap. Back to the bathhouse where you are ushered to a dimly lit room quietly permeated with soft Japanese music. You remove your clothes and wrap up in a towel. A lady shuffles in carrying a basket of steamy sheets, lightly fragrant with lemongrass and eucalyptus. With the help of tongs, she opens one up and drapes it over a cot, then motions for you to lie down on top of it. She gathers the corners up over the top of you and proceeds to swaddle you in yet more hot sheets. Topped off with a rubber blanket to hold in the heat and finally a soft woolen blanket, you feel practically mummified—definitely not the sort of thing a closet claustrophobic would want to experience. But for most of us, the initial panic soon gives way to a soothing deep heat treatment. After about 15 minutes, you're roused from rest and unwrapped—back to your room or to the lounge to rest and prepare for dinner.

How to Eat Less and Enjoy It More

7:00 P.M. Dinner. The Golden Door's dinners are something to be experienced and savored for as long as you can—which is precisely the strategy behind the pomp and ceremony. The food is carefully prepared and beautifully presented so that half of the fun is in feasting your eyes. The portions are small and yet look larger than life because they are served on sandwich rather than dinner plates. The desserts aren't omitted, just scaled down to a token-size tablespoon or so served in a lovely blossom-shaped bowl. You can't gobble it down, either—dessert spoons at the Golden Door are demitasse size, just right for a normal number of delicate mouthfuls. Another bit of Golden Door dinner strategy: dessert is not served until a full 45 minutes has passed from the time you receive your main course.

Tonight's menu: an appetizer of lightly steamed green beans (fresh-picked from the garden) with shallots, parsley and pimiento tossed with a mild vinaigrette and served on a bed of garden lettuce; a main course consisting of half a chicken breast circled with stir-

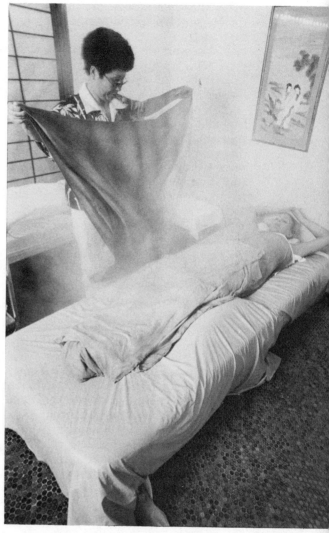

Carl Doney

Rest amidst the fragrant bouquet of steeped herbs while steaming away muscle tension. Hot herbal wraps taken at "The Door's" Japanese bathhouse provide the perfect restful ending to a high-energy day.

fried snowpeas, bean sprouts, mushrooms, and water chestnuts seasoned with sesame seeds and tamari sauce; and a dessert of lemon soufflé sweetened with fructose and garnished with kiwi fruit. Are we making your mouth water?

8:00 P.M. Evening program. Each night the Golden Door features a special presentation for its guests. A mini-class on cooking with herbs. A nutrition lecture. Tonight Deborah Szekely Mazzanti, founder of "The Door", is in town to talk about taking the lessons of "The Door" home with you.

The Golden Door's founding mother demands much of herself and expects nothing less of her guests. You'd be wise to follow her suggestions:

• *Join the sunup to sundown exercise movement,* she advises. Twenty minutes of stretching in the morning. An afternoon tennis lesson or walk in the park. An evening swim.

• *Do something active after a day's work.* Don't just slouch from the laundry room or board room to the kitchen when that five o'clock bell rings in your head. Meet your spouse for a quick game of racketball or take a solitary jog. Then shower and slip into something comfortable before preparing dinner.

• *Make meal preparation an enjoyable ritual.* Overdoing the cooking routine can lead to drudgery. Dinner shouldn't take longer than 30 minutes to prepare. And some of the more healthful methods of cooking—like stir-frying or broiling—are also the fastest (see Cooking for Health).

• *Eat for your health, not for your figure.* Simple, natural, wholesome foods tend to go easy on your waistline anyway. But the benefits they bestow on the way you look and feel far surpass anything a fad diet has to offer. And always, she says, choose fresh over canned or frozen—even if it means shopping every day.

• *Make dinner the best meal of the day* (assuming that you didn't overdo it at lunch). It's also a good time to get together with your family to chat and enjoy each other's company while savoring the food. Don't rush it.

• *Make time for relaxation.* Some people are too busy being busy, Deborah Mazzanti observes. But empty spaces in time are just as important to our health and well-being as time spent in active pursuits. Don't think of it as time wasted, she warns. Quiet, reflective moments are well spent. In fact, it is in these hours that we have our most important thoughts.

SPERMICIDES

The use of spermicides for birth control is often viewed as little more than a better-than-nothing option. Messy, risky, inconvenient, are some of the reasons women give for not using them. And yet there's something to be said for a contraceptive that's used only when you need it, that's readily available at any drugstore without a doctor's prescription, and that carries with it a minimum of health risks. So long as you can be fairly certain of its effectiveness. But how do you know?

Admittedly, the vast variety of brands and types now available can be overwhelming. You'll find the usual array of foams, creams and jellies, as well as some new, more convenient suppositories and foaming tablets. All work essentially the same. But there are fundamental differences among them—differences that can be critical to their performance and effectiveness.

Basically, spermicides protect in two ways. When inserted deep into the vagina, they form a mechanical barrier between the cervical opening and the invading sperm. At the same time, the chemical component (most commonly nonoxynol-9) coats and breaks down the surface of the sperm on contact.

On first thought, the idea of inserting any *chemical* agent into the vagina may put you off. It did us. But, try as we might, we could not find any evidence that spermicides pose a significant health hazard. (See Editor's Note at end of section.)

In the past some spermicides contained mercury compounds such as phenyl*mercuric* acetate or phenyl*mercuric* borate (which can cause serious health complications) as the active sperm-killing ingredient. But thanks to federal drug regulation, that is no longer done. However, the Food and Drug Administration does admit that they haven't actually scanned all the drugstore shelves to be sure that those brands containing mercury have been removed. So it's best to check the ingredients listed on the label for yourself to be sure mercury is not one of them.

Otherwise, the worst you can expect from the nonmercury compounds is some irritation—which is perhaps more of a problem with the foam than with the cream or jelly because of the higher concentration of nonoxynol-9. Sometimes irritations may also be due to the specific perfume used in the product. Switching brands may be all that's needed to solve the problem. And as far as your health goes, there may even be some benefits.

Fringe Benefits of Spermicides

Nonoxynol-9, the chemical used in most foams marketed in the United States, does more than kill sperm. It knocks out other vaginal invaders, like *Trichomonas* and *Candida* and even *herpesvirus*, which has been associated with cervical cancer. With their low pH, spermicides may also inhibit the growth of these bugs by keeping the vagina naturally acidic.

The first hint of that protective effect showed up in a study done by J. Barlow Martin, M.D., of the Washington University School of Medicine in St. Louis, Missouri. While testing 50 foam users for 23 weeks, Dr. Martin noticed that 8 women who had minor vaginal infections at the start of the study were free of them at the end (*Clinical Medicine*, September, 1962).

More recently, researchers at the University of Pittsburgh's Graduate School of Public Health have added to the proof that spermicides have anti-infective properties against both minor and major invaders, by showing that several spermicides decreased the infectiousness of *herpesvirus* (*American Journal of Obstetrics and Gynecology*, October 15, 1976).

A spermicide is primarily to prevent pregnancy, sure. But the fact remains that women using this method get an extra fringe benefit—better vaginal health than those using other methods like the Pill and the intrauterine device (IUD).

So why hasn't the medical establishment promoted the use of spermicides for contraception? Mostly because effectiveness studies have failed to show consistent positive results. Pregnancy rates range from 1.5 percent (as good as the Pill, IUD and the diaphragm can be) to a disappointing 29 percent. And if you don't want a baby those odds are just too risky.

But a study done at the University of Southern California School of Medicine in Los Angeles showed that spermicidal foams could be highly effective if the woman has been carefully taught the technique that best insures success. In this particular group of 2,932 women, the foam was used for about nine months. The pregnancy rate was only 3.98 percent, certainly competitive with other methods whose health risks are notorious (*Contraception,* January, 1971).

Jellies and Creams: Why Even Bother?

What's more, a comparison of all types of spermicides puts foam way on top in the effectiveness category. For one thing, foam forms the best mechanical barrier. Its consistency, which resembles shaving cream, disperses quickly to cover the necessary area. It doesn't become runny at body temperature for most women, and little seeps out during intercourse. But even more important, its potential in preventing pregnancy may well be enhanced by the fact that it has a concentration of nonoxynol-9 much higher than that found in creams and jellies.

A study of the effectiveness of creams, jellies and foams showed that jelly fared the poorest, with an average pregnancy rate of 23.1 percent. Cream's rating was 6.19 percent and the foam's was the best at 3.98 percent (*Population Reports,* January, 1975).

If you plan to use a vaginal spermicide as your only means of birth control then the aerosol foam is clearly your best bet.

Jellies and creams should be used only with a diaphragm. Some are sold especially for solo use but they are less effective than foam, so why bother? Another thing—some spermicides not specifically intended for coupling with the diaphragm may actually harm the rubber dome, although that information is not necessarily available on the package. If unsure, simply use the brand of cream or jelly recommended by the manufacturer of your particular diaphragm.

Contraceptive suppositories and tablets are not intended for use with the diaphragm, either. And as the sole method of protection, they are even less effective than jelly and cream and much less effective than foam. Problem is, suppositories and foaming tablets sometimes don't do what they're supposed to do and you're left virtually unprotected. The foaming tablet, for instance, needs vaginal secretions in order to effervesce. No moisture, no fizz. The suppositories won't melt for the same reason.

That's not to say that the foam works equally well for all women. It may be that foam disperses better in some women than in others. Or secretions from individual vaginas may help or hinder it. But it's safe to assume that a woman who's been using foam for three years or longer with no pregnancies can probably view it as a 99 percent sure method for her.

There are ways, however, to help keep the odds in your favor:

- Remember to shake the can vigorously about 20 times in order to mix the chemical with the bubbles.
- Insert the foam deep into the vagina while you're lying flat on your back. Too low and it will not cover your cervix properly. Once you insert the

foam don't get up and walk around or it may run out. If you don't have sex within half an hour of inserting the foam, you'll need another dose. The bubbles begin to go flat after that time, even if your partner doesn't.

• Don't get up immediately after sex.

The longer you lie still, the more time the spermicide has to kill the sperm. Of course, each additional sex act requires another squirt of foam. And douching is out until at least six hours after the last intercourse.

Editor's Note: As this book goes to press, a preliminary study has just been published which raises some question about the safety of spermicides—at least for an unborn child in the event pregnancy should occur. The study, conducted by Hershel Jick, M.D., director of the Boston Collaborative Drug Surveillance Program, and his colleagues, found a higher incidence of certain birth defects (2.2 percent) among 763 infants whose mothers had used spermicides near the time of conception. That compared to a 1.0 percent incidence among 3,902 infants whose mothers did not use that method of birth control for several months prior to conception (*Journal of the American Medical Association,* April 3, 1981).

The large number of children in this study makes this association noteworthy. But because there was no distinct pattern to the abnormalities, it's very possible that other factors were involved. Therefore, Dr. Jick cautions that these results should be considered tentative until more data is published. Meanwhile, to be on the safe side, he says, women who suspect they are pregnant should have a pregnancy test to be certain, then stop using spermicides. He also suggests that women discontinue using spermicides for two months prior to a planned pregnancy. Otherwise, the key is to do what you can to insure your contraceptive's highest effectiveness.

STERILIZATION

For the final word in birth control, surgical sterilization is it. But the key word here is "final," because for all intents and purposes it must be considered a 100 percent permanent method. That's why you should be 101 percent certain that it's right for you. Sterilization isn't for everyone. In fact, it's for a very select group of people—most popularly for married couples over age 30—although

more and more unmarried and childless men and women are now turning to this option.

Effectiveness ratings of 99.8 percent or better are part of the appeal, to be sure. So is the fact that never again will you be bothered by the inconvenience or long-term risks associated with some of the other methods of birth control.

Still, sterilization is not without

risks. And because of the permanent nature of these procedures, it is imperative that the decision be well thought out with all the options and risks explained in full. Sterilization is strictly voluntary, and absolutely no pressure should be exerted in the decision-making process.

While it's true that a reversal of the operation is occasionally successful, those instances are rare and it's no guarantee that fertility is restored. So don't even think about that. Instead ponder the permanency very, very carefully. If there's even the slightest possibility that the loss of a child, a divorce, a remarriage or even a first marriage may change your feelings about bearing children, then you are not ready for sterilization. On the other hand, if you are well along in your childbearing years and have no doubts, misgivings, or reservations about relinquishing your reproductive abilities forever, you're probably a good candidate. But only you can decide that.

Should you elect to do so, the next step should be deciding which partner will have the operation. For women, the sterilization procedure usually involves severing and/or sealing shut the fallopian tubes (tubal ligation) which are necessary to transport the egg from the ovaries to the uterus. The male counterpart, vasectomy, severs and seals shut the two vas deferens (the tubes that deliver sperm from the testicles to the penis). Both are permanent.

While vasectomies used to outnumber tubal ligations, that is no longer the case. In fact, by 1977, "tubals" were being performed about 50 percent more frequently than the "vas." Still, if each of you is equally comfortable with sterilization, vasectomy may be worth serious consideration. That's because the surgical procedure is less complex and therefore less risky than a tubal. The whole "operation" takes about 10 to 20 minutes and can be done in a doctor's office with a local anesthetic. The surgery is minor, as is the discomfort afterward: just a little swelling and pain in the scrotal area for a day or two.

By comparison, sterilization procedures for women are much more complicated—though, gratefully, a lot simpler than in the past. Nevertheless, even the new tubal laparoscopy, or "Band-Aid procedure" as it is fondly called, requires hospitalization and sometimes general anesthesia. In addition, because the fallopian tubes lie buried in the abdominal cavity, there's always the possibility that nearby organs might be damaged in the course of the operation. For example, in the process of sealing the tubes with a cauterizing instrument, other organs like the intestines or connective tissue might get burned, resulting in serious complications including hemorrhage or peritonitis (inflammation of the abdominal lining). That happens in about 0.2 percent of cauterizing tubals but it is hoped that the use of the newer bipolar cauterizing instrument (rather than the older unipolar model) will further decrease the chance of burns.

"Complications" of Surgery

But that's not the only complication that you may have to contend with. An internal organ can be perforated (0.3 percent of the time), the injection of carbon dioxide gas which is used to inflate the abdomen for easier viewing of the internal organs may cause cardiac irregularity (about 0.7 percent of the cases), or bleeding complications may occur (about 0.6 percent of the patients undergoing the operation).

Of course, all this can occur only if

the procedure was able to be done in the first place. Believe it or not, almost 7 out of every 1,000 tubal attempts end in failure to complete the sterilization operation. Sometimes that has to do with the skill of the surgeon but more often the surgery is cut short because of the presence of other conditions.

For example, adhesions from previous abdominal surgery or scarring of your tubes or uterus from infection may make it impossible for safe visualization and isolation of the tubes. So might extreme overweight or endometriosis.

Cauterization is a risky business even with a clear view, but with any of the complications listed above the procedure should be abandoned. Of course, it all depends on the relative severity of the disease and the expertise of your surgeon who, by the way, should discuss the possibility of failure with you before the operation.

But what about long-term complications following successful tubals or vasectomies?

For vasectomy, there's no definite evidence that any exist. But that doesn't mean there aren't any; just that it's too early to tell. One thing that does have researchers puzzled is that about one-half to two-thirds of men develop antibodies to their own sperm after a vasectomy (as if the sperm were foreign matter to be destroyed). That defensive reaction is triggered because sperm continues to be produced after vasectomy but does not have the usual outlet and so is reabsorbed by the body (at the rate of 200 million per ejaculation). The implications of this are not clear. But in a study on monkeys, several researchers found that production of antibodies injured the blood vessels. They speculate that this may speed up development of atherosclerosis.

On the other hand, tubal laparoscopy has been known to alter menstrual periods (for the worse) in some women. Whether this is a short-term or long-term complication is not known at this time. It has been suggested that these changes may be due to an altered blood supply to the ovary during the surgery, causing impaired ovarian functions.

In either case, your physician should explain in detail the different procedures available as well as the risks and benefits of each. Not to do so would be a disservice to any couple who is trying to make a decision based on the most current information available.

If you do decide on a tubal, don't be afraid to ask your surgeon about his experience with this procedure. As with all surgery, complication rates are directly related to the skill of the surgeon. One study showed that laparoscopic tubal ligation complication rates were four times higher (14.7 per 1,000 vs. 3.8 per 1,000) among women whose surgeons had done less than 100 operations.

On the other hand, improvements in techniques as well as the increased experience of surgeons have cut the risks even further in recent years.

New Methods of Sterilization

In the past, sterilization meant major abdominal surgery, general anesthesia, a five-inch incision, several days in the hospital and nearly a month of recuperation at home. Laparotomy, as this method is called, is still done today, but usually it's performed along with other necessary surgery, such as a cesarean section. While the abdomen is open it is fairly easy to locate and cut and/or tie the tubes and there's not much chance of snipping the wrong thing.

Also today, with the newer methods of sterilization—namely tubal laparoscopy—a local anesthetic can be used in many cases, eliminating the possible complications associated with general anesthesia as well as reducing recovery time.

The most popular of the newer procedures employs the use of a special instrument called a laparoscope. This nifty gadget is actually a tube with a light source which can "see" around corners. To make it even easier to see what's what, two quarts of carbon dioxide gas are used to inflate the abdominal cavity and shift the intestines out of the way.

The laparoscope is inserted through a small incision just below the navel. Through a second tiny incision just above the pubic bone another instrument is inserted which actually does the closing of the tubes.

Usually the tubes are sealed with a cauterizing instrument. By burning one to two inches of each tube it makes it virtually impossible for pregnancy ever to occur. Problem is, as we mentioned, there's also a chance of burning an organ unrelated to sterilization.

As an alternative, you may want to ask your doctor about sealing your tubes with the Hulka clip or Falope ring. Thampu Kumarasamy, M.D., of Austin, Texas, who has had extensive experience with both devices, but likes the clip better, says they are the preferred methods of sterilization today. "Not only do they pose few risks," says Dr. Kumarasamy, "but they also cause little damage to the tubes. With the Falope ring, about 2½ centimeters are involved [1 inch] while the clip (whether Hulka or another brand) only grabs about 1 centimeter or less."

Agreeing with Dr. Kumarasamy is Dr. Alan G. Gordon of the Royal Infirmary, Hull, England. He found that there was no injury in any of the 103 women who received clips. But the Falope rings caused some excessive bleeding of the tubes in about 10 percent of the women receiving them. All bleeding was controlled, however, with additional rings or clips.

No matter which method is used to seal the tubes, recovery from a laparoscopic type of tubal ligation can be expected to be brief. Most women can go home about four to six hours after surgery with only a couple of Band-Aids to mark the occasion.

Have someone else do the driving, though, whether you've had a local or a general anesthetic. For the next day or two you may experience some shoulder pain. That is due to irritation of the diaphragm from the carbon dioxide gas used to inflate your abdomen. Expect a little tenderness around the two incisions, also. After all, a cut is a cut. They may hurt for a few days but they'll heal quickly and are practically invisible after they do.

Sometimes tubal ligation can be performed through an incision in the vagina. This method is less commonly or easily performed than abdominal procedures. The chance of infection is greater, too, because of the many types of bacteria normally found in that area. Consequently, the complication rate associated with a vaginal tubal is higher than with any other method. Usually, discomfort after surgery is minimal but recovery is not as quick as with laparoscopy or mini-laparotomy. Also, intercourse must be avoided for four to six weeks after vaginal surgery—a requirement not associated with the other methods of sterilization. Actually, the lack of a visible scar (which is important to some women) is about the only major advantage.

There's another method you may

have heard about which we'll mention briefly here: mini-laparotomy. Sometimes this method can be used where laparoscopy cannot: for example, with women who've had previous abdominal surgery, or where the surgeon has not had experience using a laparoscope.

Mini-laparotomy is new to this country but is practiced throughout the rest of the world with great success. It's similar to laparotomy (the oldest method) except the incision is only 1 to 1½ inches long instead of 5 and the procedure can be done easily with a local anesthetic. No elaborate surgical equipment is necessary, just a surgeon who's had experience with the procedure so he can easily locate each tube by moving the uterus from side to side with a simple blunt instrument called an elevator. After isolating each tube he can cut or tie each one, or as we discussed earlier, use a clip or ring to seal them off.

There's a quick recovery time, too, as in the laparoscopic method. But unlike laparoscopy, no carbon dioxide gas is used and neither is the cauterizing instrument. That eliminates the risk of bowel burns and any heart irregularities which may occur (however rarely) with the use of carbon dioxide gas.

Still, this procedure is not advisable for overweight women or for those with endometriosis, pelvic infection or history of very extensive pelvic surgery.

It's hard to fathom after our lengthy discussion on safe methods of sterilization, but some doctors still advocate hysterectomy as a means to prevent future pregnancies. And yet serious complications and incidence of death are 10 to 100 times greater for women having a hysterectomy than for the simpler laparoscopic techniques (see Hysterectomy).

What If You Change Your Mind?

Now, a word about reversibility. As we mentioned earlier, you shouldn't decide on sterilization with reversal in the back of your mind, since there is still no guarantee of success. However, a significant advance has been made recently which you should know about.

It's called microsurgery, because the infinitesimal ends of the fallopian tubes (about the thickness of the lead in a pencil) are reconnected under a microscope with sutures thinner than a human hair. Surgeons doing this type of work need more than a steady hand. They need the patience of about three saints and fallopian tubes only minimally damaged during the initial sterilization process.

So far, reports of moderate success have started to trickle in. One group at Johns Hopkins Medical Center in Baltimore, Maryland, has successfully reconnected the tubes of 17 out of 26 women. According to the doctors, the rate of pregnancy is greatest during the first year after reconstruction and decreases after that, for reasons they don't understand. What they do know is that women who have been sterilized by cauterization have the least chance of being successfully reconnected. (Some say less than 10 percent.) That's because so much of the tube has been destroyed that there's not enough unburned tissue left to work with.

The doctors are more optimistic, however, about the possibilities of reversal when sterilization has been done with clips, rings, or even the older method of cutting and tying, since those procedures leave most of the tubes intact.

Surgeons in Australia have found

this to be the case, too. Reporting in the *Medical Journal of Australia* (June 14, 1980), they say that about 70 percent of those seeking reversals will have been sterilized by methods where the tubes are virtually destroyed. The remainder can be offered about a 70 percent chance of future pregnancy. But beware: tubal pregnancies occur 10 to 15 percent of the time after reconnection.

As for reversing vasectomies, the success rate ranges anywhere from 25 to 70 percent, but the new microsurgery techniques have improved those percentages just as they have for tubals. The problem is, even with the reappearance of live sperm, there's still no guarantee that they'll be able to do the job. Sperm antibodies, some feel, may account for the low pregnancy rate achieved even after "successful" reconstruction.

There's ample reason, then, why doctors should try to identify those who would be most likely to request a reversal and then counsel them to consider alternative *temporary* methods of birth control.

A recent study conducted at the Mount Sinai Hospital Medical Center of Chicago gives doctors a head start on what to look for. Of the 163 women requesting reversal, the researchers found that the average age at sterilization was only 24.4 years and many of the women were experiencing marital problems at the time it was done. With that in mind it's almost predictable that this same group of women would list remarriage as the most common reason for wanting to reverse their sterilization operation (*Ob. Gyn. News*, vol. 15, no. 15, 1980.)

Clearly, you owe it to yourself to investigate your motives for wanting sterilization in the first place. A decision made under stress is often regretted later. But a carefully thought-out decision based on sufficient information and self-awareness will lead you to choose what's most suitable for you.

STRETCH MARKS

What gives with stretch marks?

We wanted to know. And to find out we went to Albert Kligman, Ph.D., M.D., professor of dermatology at the University of Pennsylvania School of Medicine—a maverick in the research field of common everyday skin problems. If he wouldn't know, no one would.

Unfortunately, Dr. Kligman, who's spent a good deal of time investigating wrinkles, dandruff, hair loss and athlete's foot, admits that the research into stretch marks is very limited.

"You'll be astounded how very little we do know about them," he told us. "I don't know how a stretch mark forms. It's very easy to say that the fibers have ruptured, but there is no proof of that. It has something to do with increased weight which stretches the skin. It has something to do with an outpouring of hormones. That's why stretch marks often appear in adolescence and in pregnancy—two points in a woman's life when weight gain coincides with hormone fluctuations. Girls that are rounding out get stretch marks in their breasts and thighs; pregnant women find them on their breasts and stomachs. At this point, about the only advice I can offer in the way of prevention is don't gain an exorbitant amount of weight. Sorry, that's the best I can tell you."

We're sorry, too. Dr. Kligman's sage advice is all we can relay with any confidence. But since he readily admits that little is *known* of these red, then faded white incisionlike scars, it seems that the actual explanation is still up for grabs. So there's no harm in offering other theories.

For example, one theory presented at an international symposium on trace minerals held at Case Western Reserve Medical School, Cleveland, Ohio, in 1971, is that stretch marks may somehow be related to a zinc deficiency. Researchers point out that adolescence and pregnancy are two situations where weight gain is associated with stretch marks, and also two times when nutritional stores may be strained. In the late months of pregnancy, they claim, copper levels tend to be high and zinc low. Whether this imbalance also occurs in adolescence is not known. "But in the formation of elastin and collagen [the two components of skin that give it its elasticity and resiliency] there is certainly an interplay of trace metals," the researchers say.

In addition, while there is no scientific evidence to back this up either, women have long contended that keeping the skin well lubricated with some sort of emollient cream, especially during pregnancy, will help keep it soft and pliable and minimize the chances of developing stretch marks. For this purpose, cocoa butter, cod-liver oil or shark-liver oil (both excellent sources of vitamin A and D), glycerin, and lanolin have all been recommended.

SUNBATHING

Mad dogs maybe. But it's hard to believe that Englishmen go out in the noonday sun. Their unmistakable—and some would say sickly—pallor stands in sharp contrast to the seemingly healthy, bronzed bodies of every sun worshiper from Aspen to Acapulco. Still, all is not what it seems. The fact is that while sensible doses of sunlight might be beneficial, suntans are not necessarily synonymous with robust health and, according to current medical opinion, may be the one status symbol that lights the fuse for future disaster.

But before we send you running for cover, let's look at the bright side. Obviously, as anyone out on a sunny spring afternoon knows, the sun isn't all bad. It warms our bodies, brightens our moods, and colors our cheeks with a kind of natural rouge. On the scientific side, it causes a chemical in the skin to undergo a sort of metamorphosis and become a precursor of vitamin D. This precursor is then converted to vitamin D—the nutrient necessary for the proper utilization of calcium and phosphorus and thereby responsible for strengthening bones and teeth. And with women being as prone as they are to osteoporosis, a condition caused by a loss of calcium from the bone, the "sunshine vitamin" is certainly one we wouldn't want to do without.

There is also some evidence that sunlight entering through the eyes has some effect on the pituitary gland and other brain centers involved in hormone regulation. Whether this can be considered a significant health factor, no one can say for sure. But John Rock, M.D., one of the developers of the birth control pill, is fast becoming a believer.

Dr. Rock had worked in a fertility clinic for women. He saw many patients who had very irregular menstrual cycles, and in the course of treatment, discovered many and varied causes for these upsets. One of the more curious causes of menstrual irregularity, he found, was a lack of light. For some women, it seemed, proper exposure to light would regulate their cycles, with nothing else needed. Granted, that sounds a little farfetched to most of us. But Dr. Rock points out that the way many of us are living these days— tucked away in air-conditioned, windowless office buildings for much of the day—is quite different from the natural, outdoorsy state our ancestors were exposed to for millions of years. And that, he says, could make a crucial difference for some women.

Actually that comes as no surprise to John N. Ott, a light researcher and author of *Health and Light* (Devin-Adair, 1973). For one thing, he says the poultry industry has long known that light entering the eyes of chickens stimulates the birds' production of eggs through its effects on the pituitary gland. Poultrymen use lights in henhouses to maintain egg production through the short days of winter.

Further evidence that interactions between light and hormones exist in humans as well comes from a 1967 study. That research into the effect of light on the menstrual cycle suggests that through a series of mechanisms, light may induce a sudden surge of the luteinizing hormone, or LH (see Menstruation) that triggers the egg's release from an ovary each month (*American Journal of Obstetrics and Gynecology*, December, 1967).

For the moment, however, all this remains speculative. And while we wait for the conclusions of more detailed studies, be well advised that no matter how encouraging the outcome, there's still a dark side to the sun story. Mostly,

it has to do with our blind overindulgence.

For example, while prolonged exposure to sunlight won't provoke an overdose of vitamin D, there's no reason to believe that more sunning will better satisfy your recommended daily allowance. In fact, says Michael F. Holick, Ph.D., M.D., from the endocrine unit in the department of medicine, Massachusetts General Hospital, and Harvard Medical School, after one exposure to sunlight, the skin can continue to convert the vitamin D precursor to vitamin D in carefully doled-out dosages during the next three or four days without any further requirement of sunlight.

And after all, if you don't need the light, there's more than one good reason to avoid excessive exposure. In fact, researchers are building convincing cases to support limiting our time in the sun. Some believe that extended exposure to the sun may be a factor in the formation of cataracts. Others suggest that the sun can trigger migraines.

Why Look Old Before Your Time?

Of even greater concern to more people is the widely publicized finding that while sunlight has been shown to effectively help such skin conditions as acne and psoriasis, it can actually *cause* a lot more skin problems than it can curb. A painful sunburn in which reddened skin bubbles up like weathered paint is just the beginning. Weatherbeaten, dry, leathery and wrinkled skin is only a couple of sun seasons down the road. In fact, dermatologists tell us, the sun is the number one cause of prematurely aged skin.

What happens is, the sun damages the skin's collagen (a protein fiber) and elastin (a connective tissue), which together help to keep the skin taut, smooth and resilient. When we're young, this damage is quickly repaired, but as we grow older the skin loses its ability to rebuild damaged collagen and elastin fibers. The result, if you're not careful, could be a tough and somewhat corrugated complexion—not to mention a permanently sagging smile. The medical men even have a name for it—solar elastosis—that is, loss of skin elasticity due to the sun.

If you can imagine anything worse, there's this: sun-damaged skin often gives way to the development of scaly gray patches known as keratoses and ugly brown splotches commonly called liver spots. Occasionally, these pigmented patches can blossom into cancer. As a matter of fact, says Allan L. Lorincz, M.D., chief of dermatology at the University of Chicago, "the most important skin carcinogenic [cancer-causing] factor in man is sunlight exposure."

Of course, sun damage does not strike everyone equally. While no one is 100 percent immune, vulnerability hinges in part on your skin type and how readily you tan. Black or olive-skinned persons are protected to a certain extent by a darkened pigment in their skin called melanin, which can absorb harmful ultraviolet rays. Tanning is actually the result of melanin production— nature's way of building up a temporary protective sheath for those of us with lighter skins. But if you burn before you tan or burn and never tan, you're especially vulnerable to sun-induced skin cancer.

Sun intensity, of course, has some bearing on the extent of its devastation (the southwestern United States, Australia and South Africa have high incidences of sun-induced skin problems). But nevertheless, blond or red-haired persons with blue or green eyes have to be extremely careful—no matter where

they live. Ireland, for example, the land of red hair and fair complexions, has the third highest death rate from skin cancer in the world, following South Africa and Australia. The high rate exists despite the fact that Ireland is in a latitude that receives less than half the burn-causing ultraviolet radiation received by either of the other countries.

Sunlight can also react with various chemicals taken internally or applied to the skin in photosensitive persons. According to Kenneth A. Arndt, M.D., associate professor of dermatology at Harvard Medical School and chief of dermatology at Beth Israel Hospital in Boston, sun reactions commonly occur in conjunction with the use of some cosmetics, deodorant soaps, deodorants, detergents, perfumes and skin bleaches (see Liver Spots) as well as antibiotics— like tetracycline—thiazide diuretics, and tranquilizers. Though rare, oral contraceptives have also been known to react with sunlight exposure in susceptible women.

Retinoic acid, a newfound treatment for acne, appears to increase the risk of skin cancer caused by exposure to the sun (*Archives of Dermatology*, February, 1978). And that's particularly frightening in view of the fact that the persons with acne—and possibly those treated with retinoic acid—think that basking in the sun will help heal their skin.

Obviously, then, you should be extremely cautious about sunning yourself if you use any of the products just mentioned. Also, if you've ever suffered from *herpes simplex,* be forewarned that sun exposure can precipitate a recurrence or aggravate any existing sores. But beyond that, the real question remains: how do you have fun in the sun and still protect your skin from the ravages of overexposure?

One sound bit of advice is to avoid basking in the bright sunshine during the hours of 10 A.M. to 2 P.M. (or 11 to 3 daylight saving time) when the sun is at its highest intensity. Second, be especially cautious on pleasant spring days when the sun is hot but a cool breeze keeps you out longer than you should be. And third, don't underestimate the power of reflected light—from sand, concrete and even snow.

Surprising Facts about Tanning

Albert Kligman, M.D., Ph.D., an expert on sun-damaged skin, told a 1978 American Medical Association Conference on Aging Skin that sunbonnets and beach umbrellas provide less protection from the sun's rays than people think.

"A person sitting on white sand under a parasol may feel perfectly protected," Dr. Kligman said, "but light is hitting the sand, reflecting upwards and hitting normally shaded surfaces like the undersurface of the chin or arms or thighs. . . . There is more of that sort of light than we realize."

And if you think underwater adventures will keep you out of the sun's range, guess again. "The swimmer," Dr. Kligman said, "even if he makes it a practice of staying a foot under the surface, can get a sunburn since the attenuation [weakening] of ultraviolet light by water is almost zero."

A cloud cover offers uncertain protection from burning for the same reason. "A cloud is mostly water," Dr. Kligman said, "and like that water over the unwary swimmer, does allow solar radiation to go through. A thin cover of clouds might weaken sunlight by 20 percent (instead of requiring 20 minutes to get a sunburn, it can be accomplished in 30), and in three hours the unwary person is going to get fried."

Probably the biggest, and most dangerous, misconception people have about sunbathing is the idea that suntan lotions, oils and butters protect you from harmful rays of the sun. This myth may be a triumph of modern advertising, but a lot of consumers are literally getting burned as a result of it. Lotions can soothe a burn once it develops, and bronzing agents can dye you a nice brown, but unless they contain something that actually screens out ultraviolet radiation, they won't prevent a sunburn. Most of the popular suntan lotions contain no screening agent at all.

The sunscreens are out there on the pharmacy shelves, however, and the best of the lot contain one of the B complex vitamins, para-aminobenzoic acid—PABA for short.

In 1969, scientists at Harvard Medical School reported that, of 24 screening agents tested, a solution of five percent PABA in alcohol provided by far the best protection against ultraviolet radiation (*New England Journal of Medicine*, June 26, 1969). Not only was PABA discovered to be the best sunscreen, but it was found to confine its screening action to that part of the ultraviolet light spectrum that causes most of the burning. Less dangerous ultraviolet and visible light that promotes tanning got through, while the burning rays were blocked.

In the past few years, chemical derivatives (esters) of PABA have appeared on the market which outperform the original five percent PABA solution. Dr. Lorincz does not favor the esters because "there is a theoretical reason to believe that the esters can cause a higher risk of allergic sensitization.

"With a 10 percent PABA solution in alcohol, you get up to two hours of midday sun protection," he says. "You can still tan—you'll just tan more slowly."

The ability of a sunscreen to remain effective under the stress of prolonged exercise, sweating and swimming is called its "substantivity." PABA sunscreens in alcohol are considered to be quite substantive, says Dr. Lorincz. Still, when using a sunscreen, apply it both before you go out and several times during sun exposure, especially after swimming or perspiring. (And be careful when applying that it doesn't touch your swimsuit—it can stain.)

There are other possible steps you can take to reduce your susceptibility to sunburn. Researchers at the Baylor College of Medicine in Texas found that rats fed a special diet that included vitamins C and E developed a substantial resistance to the burning effects of ultraviolet light (*Clinical Research*, April, 1976). So what you eat may be as important in this regard as what you put on your skin.

Of course, you can still get a sunburn using PABA, C and E. PABA just prolongs the time you can spend in the sun; it doesn't pull you indoors when you've had enough.

SIX ALL-NATURAL SUNBURN SOOTHERS (Just in Case You Get Too Much)

- Soak in a tub of cool water. Afterward, apply cold, wet towels to the painful areas, rewetting the towels as they become warmed by the sunburn heat.
- Splash apple cider vinegar on sunburned skin and rub lightly.
- Smooth on vitamin E ointment. Or, if you haven't got the ointment on hand, squeeze out the contents of several pierced vitamin E capsules and rub into the sunburned skin. In his book, *. . .Complete Updated Vitamin E Book* (Keats, 1975), Dr. Wilfrid E. Shute writes of a young nurse who fell asleep while sunbathing and became badly burned. She suffered with fever, nausea and severe headache and was unable to work. One hour after her sunburn was covered liberally with vitamin E ointment, her fever and headache disappeared and she was back at work. Even though 20 hours had elapsed between the time she was sunburned and the vitamin E treatment, the sunburned areas did not blister or peel.
- Apply an old-fashioned barley paste, says Virginia Castleton, *Prevention* magazine's beauty editor. Grind three ounces of unpearled barley and mix with one ounce of raw honey. Blend into a smooth paste and add the unbeaten white of one egg. Gently rub into the reddened areas and leave on overnight or most of the day for best results.
- Snip off a few stems of the aloe vera plant you have growing in the kitchen for burns, press out the contents and rub the cool gelatinous liquid into the burned skin. Relief is almost instantaneous.
- Step up your intake of zinc. Zinc has a reputation for aiding wound healing. And in repeated trials zinc (in the form of oral supplements of zinc sulfate) has shown its stuff in the healing of severe burns.

UNDERWEIGHT

What's it like to be underweight? It's one problem most women wish they had. But ask a truly underweight woman what it's like and you'll get a different response. "Most people roll their eyes when I say I've been trying for years to gain weight," one woman told us. "Take it from me, though, it's not so great to be skinny. Thin, yes. But how I'd like, for once, to fill out my clothes the way other women do. Occasionally, I've been able to put on a few pounds, with great effort, only it never lasts. I'd try *anything* to gain weight if I thought it would work."

Well, fortunately, it won't be necessary to try anything drastic. Still, it's hard for most of us to realize that it's just as difficult for a lightweight to put on weight as it is for a heavyweight to lose it. Weight-loss books abound but who ever heard of a weight-gain book? It would never make the bestseller list, that's for sure.

Nevertheless, those women who are part of that silent minority deserve to know how to go about solving their problem, too.

Besides, more than your image may be at stake. Women who are too thin often fail to menstruate. While there's no evidence that this is dangerous, it can be terribly upsetting to a woman who is trying to become pregnant. Although no one can say for sure why this happens, the most plausible reason has to do with body fat. Fat has close ties with estrogen. And according to several researchers, including R. E. Frisch, Ph.D., a woman's body build must contain a particular percentage of fat (at least 17 percent) in order for estrogen production to signal the menstrual cycle to begin (*Science*, September, 1974).

But you can't gain weight if you don't have an appetite. So how's yours doing? If it's as lean as the rest of you, we may have some possible solutions.

Sometimes loss of appetite is due to loss of taste. After all, if food doesn't taste good, why bother eating? No doubt everyone, at one time or another, has experienced this when they've had a bad cold. Here, it's a temporary condition which reverses itself automatically when the cold has gone. For others, though, the problem isn't temporary nor the cure automatic. For them it may be one of nutritional deficiency.

"Copper deficiency can influence it [taste perception], vitamin A deficiency can influence it, as well as vitamin B_{12} deficiency and vitamin B_6 deficiency," says Robert Henkin, M.D., director of the Center for Molecular Nutrition and Sensory Disorders at Georgetown University Medical Center in Washington, D.C. "It's a very active system, and many vitamins and minerals impinge upon it in different ways."

Zinc, in particular, plays an important role in taste perception. Studies have shown that people who have difficulty tasting their food (hypogeusia is the technical term) often have reduced levels of zinc in their blood and saliva. That can lead to a vicious cycle, since taste loss reduces appetite and hence the likelihood of correcting the zinc deficiency through food intake alone. But when supplemental zinc is provided, full taste sensation and appetite can sometimes be restored within a month.

Selenium, too, may play a part in increasing appetite—at least in chicks. One study at Cornell University in Ithaca, New York, showed that selenium-deficient chicks increased their food intake and body weight after selenium administration (*Journal of Nutrition,* April, 1980).

Of course, just because women are sometimes referred to as "chicks" doesn't mean selenium will work for you, but it's worth a try.

Exercise, on the other hand, is obviously a plus if you want to *lose* weight. But if your problem is just the opposite it doesn't mean that you *shouldn't* indulge, only that you should slow the pace a bit. Some scientists have suggested that while intense exercising may suppress the appetite, more leisurely exercise routines may actually stimulate it. At least that's the case if we are able to translate recent animal studies into human terms.

When rats were exercised, they ate less immediately after their workouts than rats that did not exercise, but the drop in their food intake depended on how hard they worked out. When rats exercised harder for shorter periods of time, they ate less afterward than they did following more leisurely workouts, even though they burned the same number of calories (*American Journal of Clinical Nutrition,* July, 1979).

Whether your appetite needs to be stimulated or tamed a bit, your weight gain efforts should be centered around good nutritional habits. For weight gain, that means sweets are not the way to do it—not healthfully at least. Instead, try snacking on foods that are high in calories but good for you, too. At home or at work, nuts and seeds fill the bill. And nuts (cashews, filberts, Brazil nuts and

walnuts) are a good source of zinc, too. Speaking of zinc—eggs, fish, green beans, lima beans and whole grain products are all good sources. And at least some of those items could be used as snacks.

If you're at home, don't reach for potato chips—just the potato. Especially sweet potatoes. They're high in calories, loaded with nutrients and satisfy the sweet tooth fairy. So will fruit, and while you're at it, nibble some cheese, too. It's a great combination.

Remember, though, don't make your snacks so big that they interfere with your appetite for the three squares a day you normally eat, otherwise there'll be nothing gained.

And whatever you do, don't punish yourself if you slip down once in a while.

Instead reward yourself when you've accomplished a particular eating goal. This method is called self-reinforcement and has been shown to work where other methods have failed. In a study done at Southern Illinois University at Carbondale, underweight subjects in the self-reinforcement group gained significantly more pounds than either the self-punishment or control group (*Journal of Consulting and Clinical Psychology,* August, 1975). And the weight gain was maintained at a 12-week follow-up.

The nicest thing here is that only your own imagination (and pocketbook) will limit the type of reward you give yourself. Besides, it's nice to know that you can control your own body weight without overdosing on refined sugar and processed junk food.

URINARY TRACT INFECTIONS

Perhaps it stems from Eve's role in Adam's apple caper, but even today, many women would swear they're still paying dues. Vaginitis, menstrual cramps, even menopausal hot flashes—all tormenting and sometimes torturous problems—plague women only: a fact that practically smacks of divine retribution. But for some the worst punishment of all is a life sentence of cystitis, the most common type of urinary tract infection.

According to Calvin M. Kunin, M.D., of University Hospital, Columbus, Ohio, a recognized authority in this field, urinary tract infections (UTI) reportedly affect about a quarter to a third of all women between the ages of 20 and 40—three times as many women as men. And for 80 percent of the sufferers, once is not enough. The infection recurs, again and again, often to the point of utter frustration for the woman and her physician.

Any of a number of treacherous organisms including *Escherichia coli,* a bacterium commonly found in the bowel, can stage an attack on the urinary system. But since the end result is usually the same no matter which organism is involved, urinary tract infections are classified according to the *site* rather than the type of infection. *Urethritis* singles out the urethra; *cystitis* affects predominately the bladder; and *pyelonephritis* attacks the kidneys. Pyelonephritis is the most serious, but because the entire urinary system risks invasion once one part comes under attack, any type of urinary infection is potentially dangerous and should not be ignored.

Actually, it may be pretty difficult to ignore at that. The symptoms for all urinary infections are fairly similar and can become miserable enough to get even the most reluctant woman off to her physician for relief: an uncomfortable and almost continual feeling that you must urinate—even after you just have. Burning on urination and sometimes blood in the urine. Low abdominal pain and backache. Pain with intercourse. And occasionally, in more serious cases, chills, fever, lack of appetite, vomiting, and pain in the kidneys.

Why Women Are So Vulnerable

The fact that women are more susceptible to urinary infections—and that they tend to be so persistent in women—has many possible explanations. Probably the most common one involves a more vulnerable anatomy. A woman's urethra—that is, the tube that vents urine from the bladder—is obviously much shorter than a man's. That means bacteria from the outside must travel just a short distance to the bladder and from there to the kidneys.

Also, in a woman, the close proximity of the urethra, as well as the vagina, to the bacteria-ridden rectum makes contamination very convenient. In fact, it doesn't take exceptional cunning to uncover accessory situations that aid the bacterial assault on the bladder. For example, wiping your bottom from back to front can transport fecal organisms to the otherwise sterile environment of the urinary tract. Sexual intercourse may not only give bacteria a free ride to the front, but the thrusting and massaging action of the penis may actually push the bacteria up into the bladder. Hence "honeymoon cystitis"—the bladder infection that appears to be so common in new brides.

Unfortunately, though, infections do not subside after this young, tempestuous period, Dr. Kunin warns. In fact, women with a history of UTI are again prone to that problem during pregnancy. Pregnancy, it seems, provides a very ripe environment for infectious bladder bacteria to thrive. What happens is, in the last few months of pregnancy, the bladder becomes tightly sandwiched between the womb and the pubic bone so that it may not be able to empty itself completely. Stagnant urine provides a very cozy atmosphere for bacteria that may still be around from earlier bouts with bladder infections. What's worse, there appear to be some changes in the urinary tract in late pregnancy that permit those organisms easy access to the kidneys.

Thereafter, says Dr. Kunin, the prevalence of UTI in women rises with age and sexual activity. But fear not, avoiding cystitis doesn't necessarily mean mandatory celibacy.

As a matter of fact, more recent research suggests that sex plays but a secondary role in the development of recurrent urinary tract infections. And that social considerations more than anatomical ones may help explain why women are more prone to them.

Finding the Cause

In a study conducted by Leo Galland, M.D., then an assistant professor of family medicine at the State University of New York at Stony Brook, and colleagues, 84 women with a history of recurrent UTI were compared with another group of women who did not have this problem. The purpose: to determine if there were any notable differences in the sexual, hygienic, and urinating habits of women who were continually plagued by urinary tract infections and those who had never been affected.

They did find differences—but not, as you would suspect, in sexual practices. That was one area where both groups were remarkably similar. Both groups were sexually active, with the same percentage of each group engaging in intercourse as frequently as three to seven times a week. Reports of discomfort in sexual encounters were also distributed evenly between the two groups. What's more, 75 percent of both groups engaged in oral sex . . . so much for that theory!

Another theory that didn't hold much water in this study involved daily fluid intake. While physicians have long contended that drinking large quantities of water protects against UTI, it didn't seem to make any difference in this investigation. Both groups drank about the same amount of fluids each day and urinated about the same number of times.

What did appear to make the difference, however, was not how much or how many times they urinated, but *when*. Women with UTI were more likely to "hold it" for an hour or more while those who avoided the problem "went" as soon as they had the urge to do so, the researchers found. In fact, more than two-thirds of those who were in the habit of holding back said that it wasn't unusual for them to wait more than three hours before making the trip to the bathroom.

Why? Believe it or not, embarrassment in social situations was one of the more popular reasons given. Other women said they resisted using public toilet facilities, and still others ignored the urge as long as possible because it was an infringement on whatever they were doing at the time. All silly excuses when you consider the consequences!

One more thing: postponing urination *after* intercourse was also common among women with UTI. In fact, while the majority of the healthy group (68 percent) usually went to the bathroom within 10 minutes after intercourse, only a small number of cystitis sufferers (8 percent) did.

Actually, this is no breakthrough discovery. It only confirms what other studies have suggested—that retaining urine in the bladder can promote urinary tract infections. Why it does has yet to be deciphered. But the most likely reasons are that the long-term effect of this "holding pattern" may damage the bladder wall somewhat and make it more vulnerable to infection. Also, each time the bladder is full for extended periods, it exposes those weakened walls to increased concentrations of bacterial organisms (*Journal of the American Medical Association*, June 8, 1979).

Jack Lapides, M.D., of Ann Arbor, Michigan, who spent 20 years investigating the causes of urinary infections, recently explained things this way: when the bladder is distended or full, there is a decrease in blood flow through the blood vessels of the bladder. That probably delays the delivery of white blood cells and other infection fighters to that area, he says. As a result, bacteria that regularly migrate from the intestinal tract to the urinary tract and are ordinarily short-lived because of the natural defenses in the bloodstream, may have a chance to multiply and thrive.

Whatever the case, Dr. Galland does point out that when women with recurrent UTI were instructed in better bathroom habits (that is, not holding back the urge to urinate), only 15 percent of them suffered reinfection within six months.

That's quite a bit less than the 80 percent normally expected to experience a recurrence within that period of time. Very encouraging!

A preventive program, thus, begins with a more careful tuning in to nature's call. In other words, as soon as you get the urge to go, go. Make no excuse. There's no such thing as being too busy for this type of business. And if it's modesty that keeps you from leaving the room at a social gathering or board meeting, remember, stifling a blush carries far fewer health consequences than stifling the urge. Also, despite what the ads tell us, Danskins *are* just for dancing unless they come equipped with snaps at the crotch so they can be easily removed when you've got to go. The trouble is, many women today have taken to wearing leotards under their street clothes and when it comes time to go, well, it's just too much trouble. The same is true for neck-to-thigh foundation garments (you know, the bra-and-girdle-all-in-one gimmick). They're not practical.

Also, it's wise to get into the habit of emptying your bladder before and immediately after intercourse. To further protect the urethra from irritation during an aggressive bout in bed, allow plenty of time for foreplay so that you have a chance to become well lubricated first. Or, if necessary, use a lubricant like K-Y jelly.

Finally, to reduce the chances that a bacteria colony in the colon will decide to move on and take up residence in your bladder, follow some of the preventive measures described in the section Vaginitis—cystitis's sinister sister. Both of them have their beginnings in similar circumstances. For that reason, prevention of both includes the following precautions. Always wipe yourself from front to back. Keep your clothes cool and loose, which means avoid wearing nylon panties and pantyhose whenever possible, opting for cotton instead. Keep your bottom clean and dry (always wash before and after intercourse). And avoid chemical irritants such as perfumed sprays, bubble baths and scented powders.

If, in spite of these precautions, you develop what seems to be a mild case of UTI, your first line of attack is to drink plenty of water to flush your urinary tract of the invading bacteria. Eight glasses a day is the usual prescription—enough to make your urine colorless.

Why Cranberry Juice Helps

An alternative to water, says Dr. Galland, is cranberry juice. "Cranberry juice is unique and good because it contains hippuric acid, a substance that inhibits the growth of bacteria." No other juice contains it.

Another point here is that bacteria do not thrive in an acid environment. Perhaps the best way to achieve this desired effect is with a combination regimen of cranberry juice and vitamin C. A study by Kathryn E. Nickey, R.N., carried out at the University of Washington School of Nursing in Seattle showed that cranberry juice and ascorbic acid (vitamin C) had essentially the same urinary pH-lowering effect, but when taken in combination, they had the greatest acidifying effect.

If regular cranberry juice doesn't appear to help you, perhaps fresh cranberries mixed with plain yogurt is the ticket. "It is just a year since I last took any medication for bladder infection and a year since I've been free from it. This after more than 40 years of this scourge!" one woman told us. "Nothing ever really helped for long. Canned cranberry juice did nothing. But this is what helped: I ground up fresh cranberries in the food chopper, mixed in just enough honey to make it palatable, and at the first indication of trouble I started eating it with plain yogurt. The last full siege I had, the kind that hits within an hour, symptoms were greatly relieved in 6 hours and completely gone in 12. No medications!"

By the way, yogurt is an excellent food for fighting urinary as well as vaginal infections since it contains beneficial bacteria which help to keep the more harmful strains under control.

But no matter what self-help remedies you try, if symptoms persist for 24 hours, see a doctor. Remember, an infection in the bladder can quickly spread to the kidneys where it has the potential to do some real damage. Don't let it get that far before you get help.

VAGINITIS

It's incomprehensible that anything as natural as menstruation could be called a curse. But vaginitis . . . now that's a curse! The maddening itch. The malodorous discharge. The malicious recurrence just a couple of months after you'd thought you had it cleared up for good. This vexing vaginal mishap drives more women to their gynecologists than any other complaint.

Vaginitis is actually a blanket term that covers *anything* causing inflammation of the vagina. This includes the invasion of a one-celled parasite (*Trichomonas vaginalis*), bacteria (*Hemophilus vaginalis*), and a yeastlike fungus (*Can-*

dida). None are life-threatening, but all can be downright annoying.

Where might these menacing microorganisms come from?

Many physicians still maintain that a major mode of transmission is sexual intercourse with an infected bedfellow. (And you can bet that's led to more than one lewd innuendo during a gynecological exam!) Admittedly, sex has something to do with it. But it's not the whole story. In a recent study of 1,054 women with yeast infections only 414 infections were found to be sexually acquired (*British Medical Journal*, July 9, 1977). Obviously, the remaining women picked up their problem elsewhere. But where?

Some organisms, capable of ravaging tender vaginal tissues, inhabit the lower intestine with no ill effects. Unfortunately, with these troublemakers living just around the corner in the rectum, it doesn't take much to instigate a sneak attack on the vagina. And this may be one reason for the high rate of reinfection. Researchers from the department of microbiology and public health at Michigan State University took cultures from the vagina and feces of 98 women with recurrent vaginitis. In 51, both sites were infected with *Candida* (a fungus that causes the common yeast infection), while in 46 neither site showed signs of the yeast infection (*Journal of the American Medical Association*, October 24, 1977).

Presumably then, wiping yourself the wrong way (from back to front instead of the preferred front to back) after a bowel movement can transfer problem-causing bacteria from the bowel to the vagina. A shifting sanitary napkin can also spread infection, as can a misguided penis that slips by the anus on its way to the vagina.

Likewise, trouble may be lurking in the next public rest room you happen to use. No, the toilet seat isn't the primary suspect. It's the toilet bowl, says a New York physician in a letter to the editor of the *Canadian Medical Association Journal* (July 3, 1976). Suppose an infected person uses the john before you get there. In a hurry, the person neglects to flush. Now it's your turn. You sit down, do your own thing into the bowl, and droplets of the contaminated water splash upward, moistening the lips of your vagina. Voilà, you've got an itch and you can't imagine where it came from.

Sometimes it's pretty hard to avoid this pesky problem. In fact, it's possible to develop vaginitis without any outside help. Under normal conditions the vagina is host to a whole variety of microorganisms which manage to keep themselves in check and balance. But given the right—or, more precisely, the wrong—set of circumstances, one type may suddenly and uncontrollably begin to multiply.

But don't despair. There are steps you can take to heighten your defense against troublesome organisms.

Natural Defenses—How We Mess Them Up

You see, even though many factors can ignite the spark that sets off a symptomatic blaze of vaginitis, it's the climate or ecological balance within the vagina which determines whether this spark will flourish or fizzle. The vagina has a built-in defense mechanism in the form of beneficial bacteria, or microflora. In addition to keeping each other in check, some of these bacteria take the glucose, or sugar, from the vaginal wall cells and transform it into lactic acid, creating a sourly acidic environment. Unfriendly bacteria and parasites require a sweet, alkaline climate for reproduction.

Unfortunately, if you're looking for factors that disrupt vaginal ecology, you'll find plenty. Irritations caused by anything from the pink bubbly in your bath to the friction of an aggressive round in bed will set it off. Plain old lowered resistance due to lack of sleep, poor diet, emotional disturbances and anxiety can also do it. So can certain drugs such as antibiotics, gold therapy for rheumatoid arthritis, and the birth control pill; certain diseases such as diabetes; and certain conditions including pregnancy and menopause.

In addition, the pools of blood that flood the vagina during menstruation provide a sweet, alkaline medium in which certain organisms are likely to proliferate. This is one reason why many women find that their symptoms seem to multiply during or immediately after their period. Semen, says another physician in the *British Medical Journal* (January 13, 1979), also provides a playground for potentially bothersome bacteria. According to Dr. C. R. Porteous, semen is about 40 times as good a culture medium for *Candida* as blood serum, and stimulates spores to develop and irritate the vagina. Women who are plagued by repeated episodes of yeast infections may be wise to seek the double-duty protection of a condom rather than the Pill or intrauterine device (IUD).

Restoring Body Ecology

Still, your best bet is to think in terms of body ecology and use common sense to help your vagina take care of itself. If you notice that your vaginal discharge is slightly heavier, thicker, or more yellow in color than usual or that you've been feeling a little itchy lately, try a simple saltwater bath. Gideon G. Panter, M.D.,

a prominent New York City gynecologist and a faculty member at New York Hospital–Cornell Medical Center, recommends ½ cup of table salt dissolved in a bathtub of water. This solution is a good approximation of saline (normal body fluid) and is similar to your tears, which are constantly bathing and cleaning your eyes.

Soaking in this salty bath and inserting your finger into the vagina to enable the salty water to enter make an excellent first line of attack against most vaginal infections. "The saline bath will reduce the population of any invading or excessive organisms and enable your own body defense mechanism to do a better job in fighting the infection," says Dr. Panter. "Nine out of 10 times a few of these baths at bedtime will clear up the infection and save a trip to the doctor's office."

A vinegar sitz bath will help restore the acid balance and discourage further bacteria growth. Run a few inches of warm (not hot) water into a bathtub and add ½ cup of white vinegar. Then sit with your feet propped up on the sides of the tub so that the water rushes in.

Many women have also reported success in treating mild infections—and particularly yeast infections—with another ecological approach involving yogurt. "I became prone to vaginal infections of various sorts in my late twenties," one woman told us. "Nothing helped. As I grew older and near menopausal time, the condition worsened. Then I read about inserting freshly made acidophilus yogurt directly into the vagina. I tried it and, almost immediately, much of the vaginal irritation I had experienced for so long disappeared. I began this treatment three months ago and I've been delighted to find that I can travel, work, and engage in activities without the constant desire to urinate caused by vaginal infection."

Gerard T. Cicalese, M.D., associate professor of obstetrics and gynecology at New Jersey College of Medicine and Dentistry, reports that some of his patients have also improved with yogurt. "I've had a number of patients who've tried it and have had excellent results," he explains. The *Lactobacillus acidophilus* (one of the active bacteria in yogurt) helps to replenish beneficial bacteria in the vagina.

However, since many commercial yogurts do not contain this strain of bacteria, it is advisable to buy acidophilus in your health food store or drugstore. Add about two tablespoons of acidophilus powder from the capsules or crushed tablets to ½ cup of plain yogurt. Mix well. Then with a vaginal medication applicator, insert about two teaspoons of this mixture into the vagina. If you'd like, you can wash out the excess yogurt the following day.

For more stubborn cases, however, you may want to rely on medication from your physician. One word of warning, however. To clear up a persistent case of *Trichomonas* or "trich," as it's called in medical circles, most physicians favor a seven-day course of metronidazole—a drug sold in pill form under the trade name Flagyl. Flagyl wipes out trich in a week. There's only one catch. At least six animal studies have shown that Flagyl can cause cancer and chromosome damage. One study—though inconclusive—suggests that Flagyl may *not* cause cancer in humans. But in a study examining the use of Flagyl on Crohn's disease (an inflammation of the small intestine), patients receiving long-term treatment of relatively high doses of the drug showed definite changes in the genetic material of their body cells (*Lancet*, October 9, 1976).

Our advice: reserve Flagyl as a last resort. And even then, avoid it if you're pregnant, have a peptic ulcer, another infection including a yeast infection, a history of blood diseases, or a disease of the nervous system. Mixing Flagyl with alcohol can result in such side effects as headaches and nausea. During pregnancy, the combination could contribute to serious birth defects.

The natural ecological approach is still your best bet. Or, for more stubborn cases, try a combination of natural and conventional therapy.

Frequently, yeast infections are treated with an antifungal cream (nystatin or candicidin) or gentian violet, a messy purple preparation which does effectively stop the fungus. But according to Jonathan V. Wright, M.D., a practicing physician in Kent, Washington, killing off the yeast is only the first step in the cure. After all, you can't expect to grow a garden if you just yank out the weeds but don't water the plants. So the second half of the treatment is the replacement of the helpful bacteria to prevent the yeast infection from returning. To do this, he suggests using the prescribed medication for the recommended period of time, and then immediately upon completing the regimen, begin inserting yogurt as described above for five consecutive nights. Since menstruation can heighten a flareup of fungus, better wait with this regimen until you've got time to proceed with both the medication and the bacteria replacement.

How to Discourage Vaginitis

To prevent or discourage the return of vaginitis, you'll do well to follow these recommendations:

1. *Cut down on carbohydrates in your diet.* Simple carbohydrates, that is.

The sugar. The pastries. The hot fudge sundaes. Even the wine and cocktails. All that sugar boils down to a pretty unhealthy vaginal environment. Although some physicians argue that there isn't enough hardcore scientific evidence to back the low-sugar diet in the prevention of vaginitis, it does stand to reason that there is a link. To begin with, the cells of the vaginal walls contain a considerable amount of sugar (glucose, actually), all of which is derived from the carbohydrates in your diet. As these cells are shed and sloughed off, sugar is released. Now if it weren't for an ingenious built-in system in which bacteria convert this sugar into lactic acid, we'd wind up with a pretty sweet situation on our hands. Most disease-causing organisms thrive on sugar but are doomed in an acidic environment. Unfortunately, as is the case with diabetics, an overload of sugar in the system can disrupt this system of check and balance. The beneficial bacteria are outnumbered by the sugary cells being released into the environment and the sugar prevails. Vaginitis becomes a real risk.

2. *Develop a taste for yogurt.* Or pick up some *Lactobacillus acidophilus* in tablet, powder or capsule form in your health food store and include it in your daily regimen of supplements. Acidophilus does for your intestines what similarly beneficial bacteria do for your vaginal environment; it keeps the bad guy bacteria under control. And according to Michigan State microbiology researchers, "A cure for vaginitis (at least *Candida*) is not possible without prior eradication of the organisms from the gut" (*Journal of the American Medical Association*, October 24, 1977). That's where yogurt can come in handy.

3. *Avoid antibiotics.* Of course, that's easier said than done—par-

ticularly if you're plagued by a serious infection or a persistent case of acne. Antibiotics do a remarkable job of wiping out infections. But unfortunately, in the process of killing the harmful bacteria, they do a pretty good job of defeating the beneficial bacteria, including those in the vagina. So if you're prone to developing vaginitis, try to steer clear of the antibiotic route. Or, if you must submit to a course of tetracycline, replace the lost microflora by inserting yogurt directly into your vagina.

4. *Keep your clothes cool and loose.* Skintight dungarees or nylon nonventilated pantyhose can create a warm and moist vaginal environment—perfect for a colony of menacing microorganisms. So nix the nylon undies. Instead, wear cool cotton briefs or at least those with cotton sewn into the crotch. And stick with socks or knee-high nylons under slacks. Pantyhose are definitely out unless they have a set-in cotton crotch. As for those comfortable evenings at home, wear airy, loose clothing such as caftans and hostess robes. For bed, skip the pajamas and underwear. Slip into a cotton nightgown for ultimate comfort.

5. *Keep your vaginal area clean and dry.* Wash daily with a mild nonperfumed soap and water. Then pat dry and powder with cornstarch to absorb excess moisture. Also, if you can at all avoid it, don't sit around in a wet bathing suit. Make a quick change into a robe or skirt.

6. *Avoid chemical irritants.* Deodorant soaps, perfumed sprays, even that pretty pastel toilet paper and pink bubbly in your bath may prove to be potent irritants to the tender mucous membranes of the vagina.

7. *Don't douche.* There are a number of reasons why douching should *not* be a part of your personal hygiene program but the fact that it removes the protective flora of the vagina is reason

enough. In addition, anything other than a vinegar douche (and that includes a plain water or herb douche) is liable to alter the natural pH of the vagina. And those prepackaged preparations that smell like spring days (whatever that fragrance is!) or herbal bouquets can leave you with a potpourri of problems.

8. *Use a lubricant (if necessary) during intercourse.* A sterile water-soluble lubricating jelly (not petroleum jelly) works fine. And, by the way, contraceptive jellies and creams are acidic and may actually retard the growth of vaginitis organisms (see Spermicides).

VAGINITIS: Atrophic

Years ago, a woman was lucky if she lived to age 50. But, some would say, she was lucky in another respect: she'd never know the itching, irritating torment of atrophic vaginitis. Atrophic vaginitis—so called because the walls of the vagina grow thinner, or atrophy—is one bit of bad news tucked away under the happy headline that women are enjoying an increased longevity. Nevertheless, it's probably less troublesome than some inflammatory remarks would lead us to believe. And living with it is a lot easier once you know the facts.

Atrophic vaginitis is caused by a lack of estrogen, so it affects only postmenopausal women. Mind you, we said *postmenopausal* women. Unlike hot flashes, which occur during menopause at a time when estrogen levels are just beginning to fall, atrophic vaginitis (or senile vaginitis, as it is also called) usually doesn't come into the picture until estrogen levels hit rock bottom and have been there for some time. That's not until 5 to 15 years after menopause. Of course, much depends on how well the ovaries continue to function and whether your menopause is natural or surgically induced. Obviously, if the ovaries have been removed, estrogen levels drop radically and vaginitis becomes a more immediate problem. But, in either case, it takes some time till the problem becomes really troublesome.

With the loss of estrogen, the uterus gradually shrinks in size. The vagina slowly becomes shorter, narrower; it loses much of its elasticity and its lubricating capacity; the walls become as much as 26 percent thinner. Because of these changes, itching and irritation are common and sexual intercourse can be difficult, sometimes painful. Also, with the thinning of the vaginal walls, repeated penile thrusts can rub against the urethra and bladder, causing a burning sensation later on urination.

The usual treatment—estrogen—is pretty unpleasant. At first, it actually appears to be just the opposite. After all, what better way to treat a condition caused by loss of estrogen than by supplying more estrogen? At least, one would think so. But alas, all is not that simple. In fact, what we're finding now is that while the diminishing estrogen levels which accompany menopause are perfectly natural, the artificial maintenance of high levels of this hormone is pretty risky business (see Estrogen Replacement Therapy).

Even the medical men knew that. But the interesting thing is that until very recently, they believed that by applying an estrogen cream directly to the vaginal tissues you could put the benefit where you need it and avoid the risk that oral estrogen brings. Wrong. In fact, it's just the contrary.

"Estrogens placed in the vagina are absorbed more dramatically and quickly into the bloodstream than those taken by mouth," says Isaac Schiff, M.D., assistant professor of obstetrics and gynecology at Harvard Medical School. "There is a totally different biologic effect. When oral estrogens are contraindicated, it is not safe to apply them topically."

Stanley G. Korenman, M.D., professor of medicine at the University of California, Los Angeles, voices additional concerns. Namely, he wonders whether the risk of estrogen-induced endometrial cancer might be intensified by the placement of the estrogen so close to the susceptible organ. Another concern of his is that estrogen in the vaginal canal may interfere with male reproductive function. The penis takes up estrogen readily, so the hormone can make its way into the man's bloodstream as if it were taken orally.

New preparations, however, with lower concentrations of estrogen, are being tested and will be coming out soon, we were told. And since many of the problems just mentioned are dose-related, a 10-fold reduction in estrogen concentration (which is what they're testing) will markedly reduce the risk.

That's good news to many. But the question remains, is estrogen as good as they say? There is some evidence that the use of estrogen for atrophic vaginitis isn't as beneficial as commonly thought. In a study conducted in France, for example, doctors reported that estrogen can lead to a buildup of fibrous connective tissue in the vaginal walls. As a re-

sult elasticity may actually be impaired (*Ob. Gyn. News,* September 15, 1979). And that's just what you *don't* want!

But all is not as grim as it seems. For example, the French study cited above, as well as other investigations—including those by the famed Masters and Johnson team—have shown that women who have a fairly active sex life throughout the menopausal and postmenopausal years are more likely to stave off atrophic vaginitis, or at least experience a much slower shrinking of the vaginal tissues. The old axiom, use it or lose it, apparently holds true for tender vaginal tissues.

Women responding to Shere Hite's nationwide study of female sexuality, *The Hite Report* (Macmillan, 1976), also indicated that that may be the case. "I thought that menopause was the leading factor in my dry and irritable vaginal tract," one woman wrote. "My doctor thought that it was lack of hormones . . . but with my new lover, I am reborn. Plenty of lubrication, no irritation!"

If you are sexually active, and lubrication is insufficient, use a water-soluble lubricating jelly like K-Y jelly to prevent irritation.

Another ray of hope in the atrophic vaginitis dilemma comes to us from the Shute Institute in London, Ontario, Canada, where extensive vitamin E research is carried out. There, a spokesman told us, doctors have noted improvement in vaginal symptoms of postmenopausal women with the use of vitamin E vaginal suppositories while taking the same vitamin orally.

VALIUM

In one of the funniest scenes of the movie *Starting Over*, Burt Reynolds has an anxiety attack in a department store and collapses, hyperventilating, onto a conveniently waiting mattress display. His female companion, played by Jill Clayburgh, telephones Burt's brother, a physician, who rushes to the scene. By the time he arrives, however, Burt is in such a state that simple reasoning can't bring him around. In desperation, the physician-brother turns to the crowd of shoppers that has gathered at the bedside.

"Does anyone have a Valium?" he inquires.

Pocketbooks open. Pockets are probed. And before you can say "agoraphobia," every shopper within earshot has produced a plastic vial of pills.

The audience roars with laughter. But perhaps the reason this scene strikes a funny bone in most people is that it strikes a familiar note.

Valium is the king of prescription drugs and has been for at least six consecutive years. It is prescribed to more people than any other type of medication. And it is prescribed to women more than twice as frequently as to men.

What's as frightening as the numbers is the nonchalance with which doctors prescribe and patients demand it. Diazepam (the chemical name of Valium) is a muscle relaxant and an anxiety-dissolving agent which, by the manufacturer's own admission, should be reserved for unusually severe and debilitating emotional upsets. But ever since its initial success in Switzerland at calming the fears of postmenopausal women, Valium has been used as a crutch for every kind of stress—no matter how trivial. Indeed, many people believe they need tranquilizers to cope with everyday life. They consider it a preventive measure—preventing an emotional crisis before the confrontation occurs.

"Classically today, if a woman walks into her doctor's office and says, 'I'm nervous, my husband drinks too much,' the doctor will automatically give her a tranquilizer," says Joseph A. Pursch, M.D., corporate medical director for the Comprehensive Care Corporation in Orange, California. It's as if this little pill holds the magic to make everything all right, to press the creases out of every crisis, to somehow change her life for the better.

What Valium Does to Your Brain

Unfortunately, it doesn't work that way. Sure, tranquilizers offer momentary numbness, if that's what you're after. But first, consider the consequences. For one thing, Valium dulls the brain, clouds thinking and slows reflexes. It anesthetizes the emotions—all emotions, not just the bad ones. It sedates the senses—and, in doing so, can create depression where once there was only anxiety. It also interferes with serotonin, a natural brain chemical that aids in sleep. And when all that wears off, it zaps you with aftershocks that can last for weeks, even months. In fact, it's only been within recent years that we've learned just how serious these aftershocks can be. Before that, Valium was thought of as unusually safe and nonaddictive. Not any more.

Valium is more than medicine: it's a drug. And while it may sound a far cry more civilized and sophisticated than shooting up with heroin, takers of tranquilizers are actually only a hop, step and jump ahead of the street junkie. As a matter of fact, in one of the largest studies ever conducted on drug abuse, alcohol-drug interactions and Valium were mentioned in more drug-related episodes than either heroin or marijuana.

To further demonstrate the parallel between prescription tranquilizers and illegal drugs, doctors at a Senate health subcommittee testified that Valium addicts act just like any street drug user. They make appointments with different doctors to get prescriptions and rely on friends for yet more. When they run out, they suffer from withdrawal, says Conway Hunter, M.D., director of the addictive disease unit of the Peachford Hospital in Atlanta, Georgia. And withdrawal from Valium can be worse than the symptoms that drive many to the drug in the first place. Anxiety. Apprehension. Insomnia. Dizziness. Headache. Loss of appetite. And that's mild! The more severe symptoms of Valium withdrawal include nausea and vomiting, weakness and tremors, muscle twitches, seizures, psychosis, and even death. If you don't believe us, read Barbara Gordon's frightening, firsthand account in *I'm Dancing as Fast as I Can*, (Harper & Row, 1979).

Even more shocking is the fact that these symptoms are not reserved for isolated cases of drug abuse in which the person took excessive doses of the drug for extended periods of time. It can happen with moderate doses even after short-term use.

"I have seen several patients experiencing barbiturate-type withdrawal symptoms after four to six months of diazepam therapy in doses as low as 15 milligrams per day," writes David Haskell, M.D., a Cambridge, Massachusetts, physician in a letter to the *Journal of the American Medical Association* (July 14, 1975).

Drug addiction aside for the moment, let's look at some specific—and according to recent studies, significant—health hazards of tranquilizers.

For starters, researchers at Mayo Medical School and the University of Iowa College of Medicine have found that Valium may severely impair the ability to learn and remember. In a two-day trial involving 48 men and women, M. M. Ghoneim, M.D., and Ronald C. Petersen, M.D., gave customary doses of the tranquilizer to some subjects and a placebo to others, then tested their memory with five standard learning tasks. (One test, for example, required subjects to recall a list of words 15 minutes after learning them, then again a day later.)

"It was invariable—a significant impairment of memory in the subjects who received Valium," reported Dr. Ghoneim. Those dosed with the popular drug simply could not remember what they had learned as well as those whose minds remained unfogged.

"I'm astonished," Dr. Ghoneim added, "that no sufficient warning is given to patients that if they take Valium, their memory will be impaired. There are millions of people involved." His results suggest that people who engage in mental activities requiring a sharp memory—persons who hold mentally challenging jobs, for example— should be particularly careful of taking Valium, he said. What does Valium do to the mind if its use is continued for a longer period of time? Dr. Ghoneim plans future research to investigate just that question.

The Special Risk to Women

Within recent years, a veil of suspicion has also drifted over the use of Valium during pregnancy. In a letter to the prestigious British medical journal, *Lancet* (July 30, 1977), a Swedish pediatrician describes an alarming set of symptoms in a newborn called "floppy infant syndrome" and says the cause is related to the mother's use of diazepam. The child's symptoms included weakness and floppiness caused by a weakness in the skeletal muscles; sucking difficulties; a low body temperature; and occasional attacks in which the skin turned a bluish color, an obvious sign that hemoglobin was lacking in the blood. When the mother was questioned as to her general habits and condition during pregnancy, everything seemed normal. Everything, that is, except for one item: she had been taking 2 milligrams of diazepam three times a day on and off for the last three months of pregnancy. The drug had been prescribed by her obstetrician to prevent premature labor. In addition, during delivery she was given another 10 milligrams, presumably to aid relaxation. Blood samples confirmed the presence of diazepam in the baby's system—even 12 days after birth.

Actually, Valium's implication in the "floppy infant syndrome" isn't new. What is new is that a long-term, but *low* dose of the drug was sufficient to cause infant distress. Previously, these complications had only been associated with large 30-milligram doses of Valium given 15 hours or so before delivery. Apparently, repeated doses (no matter how small) can add up to trouble. Diazepam has a long half-life and can be detected in the urine up to two weeks after taking it. It's not difficult then to imagine that repeated doses can result in an accumulation of the drug in the body—and in baby's body when the drug crosses the placenta.

More concern over the use of Valium during pregnancy comes from Richard C. Strohman, Ph.D., a professor of zoology at the University of California at Berkeley. Working with chick embryos, Dr. Strohman has shown that diazepam tended to arrest the normal growth and development of muscle cells. It may seem a big step from chicks to children, but there are actually growth and developmental similarities between the two embryos, Dr. Strohman says. "Our work should at least be a warning to people using the drug."

Indeed, additional warnings come to us directly from Hoffman–LaRoche, Inc., manufacturers of Valium. In their product information handbook they carry a special warning concerning Valium use during pregnancy. It reads as follows:

> An increased risk of congenital malformations associated with the use of minor tranquilizers (chlordiazepoxide, diazepam and meprobamate) during the first trimester of pregnancy has been suggested in several studies. Because use of these drugs is rarely a matter of urgency, their use during this period should almost always be avoided. The possibility that a woman of childbearing potential may be pregnant at the time of institution of therapy should be considered.

They said it. And may we add that with everything considered, it's not a good idea to pop these pills if you're breastfeeding, either.

One more thing before we move on: Valium and cancer. Several years ago, a researcher by the name of B. A. Stoll reported that tranquilizer use was more prevalent among patients with advanced breast cancer (before diagnosis) than among those with localized tumors. Stoll also reported that tranquilizer use in women increased by two to three times after the diagnosis of breast cancer (*Risk Factors in Breast Cancer,* William Heinemann Medical Books, 1976).

Only recently, however, have we begun to understand the serious implications of his observations. Researchers at the Clinical Research Institute of Montreal in Canada noticed some time ago that diazepam had certain similarities with other cancer-promoting drugs. To test their suspicions they measured the effect of the tranquilizer on implanted breast tumors in rats. After four weeks, they report, the tumors in the diazepam-treated animals were almost three times heavier than those in the untreated rats (*Lancet,* May 5, 1979).

Of course, this is only a preliminary study and should not be considered conclusive by any means. But it does bring up a very important question—that is, whether tranquilizers given to very large numbers of women with breast cancer might somehow accelerate the growth of their tumors.

Till we get the verdict on that, we will continue to take a very strong stand against the use of Valium and other tranquilizers for minor emotional upsets and everyday stress. And so should you. For more natural ways to cope through exercise and relaxation techniques, see our section, Anxiety.

VARICOSE VEINS

At first glance, the statistics are again against us: more women develop varicose veins than men. It's true, heredity plays a major role in deciding whether our legs hold a weakened link. And a pregnancy or two can further sabotage a sloppy circulation route by increasing the blood flow to the pelvic area and then obstructing its return to the heart. But now, some scientists are saying that it's not our sex per se that's doing us in—in many cases, it's what we've been doing to our sex.

Taking birth control pills or estrogen replacement therapy during menopause increases our chances for varicose veins. So does wearing tight, restrictive clothing such as belts, girdles, control-top pantyhose, or those eye-catching (and breathtaking) "cigarette" jeans which require good gut suction and a strong set of pliers to get them zipped.

Eating a diet high in processed foods and low in fiber may likewise make us prime candidates for those swollen veins that sometimes snake down our inner thighs and lower legs. Such a diet, say several researchers, causes constipation and overloads the colon. The pressure of a loaded colon or of straining at the stool to relieve the constipation then increases the pressure of blood to the extremities and varicose veins result.

A well-known British physician agrees. He told us he became intrigued when he noted so few cases of varicose veins during 20 years of work in Africa where diets are especially high in fiber. Denis P. Burkitt, M.D., who has recently been lecturing at meetings of American physicians, says the incidence of varicose veins in India and Africa is as low as two percent. Furthermore, "rubbish" is the word he uses to describe the reasons most researchers give for the development of varicose veins— namely, multiple pregnancies, heavy lifting and man's upright posture which, along with gravity, works against the upward flow of blood. Dr. Burkitt points out that in communities where women stand erect, bear many children, and carry large burdens on their heads, varicose veins are *least* common.

He told us, "Let me tell you a thing that your textbooks in America say on varicose veins. They say it is due to the fact that man isn't adapted to standing upright. This is absolutely rubbish. People in native communities probably stand far more than the average person does in the West. Secondly, your textbooks say varicose veins are due to pregnancy. There is an *inverse* relationship geographically between pregnancies and varicose veins. When we had 1,000 pregnant women at term before delivery examined in India, 11—or 1.1 percent—had varicose veins. A study of pregnant women of the same age group in North America showed 30 percent had varicose veins. In five surveys done on varicose veins in India, not more than 3 percent of the subjects had varicose veins. And in every one of them varicose veins were commoner in men than women. So you see the idea that varicose veins are caused by pregnancy is wrong. If you have defective valves, then the pregnancy will make those noticeable. But they'll disappear again after the pregnancy."

The Link with the Low-Fiber Diet

Dr. Burkitt believes instead that varicose veins are caused primarily by constipation, which results from the Western low-fiber diet.

An American surgeon agrees with Dr. Burkitt that constipation may be at least one cause of varicose veins. Robert A. Buyers, M.D., director of surgery at Sacred Heart Hospital in Norristown, Pennsylvania, told a group of nutritionists in a 1977 speech:

All of us know about varicose veins. Every time one strains while defecating, the intra-abdominal pressure is increased. The pressure is transmitted retrograde in the legs through the veins, and this pressure exerted over years and decades in the constipated person produces dilation of the veins. The valves break down and with the help of gravity, incompetent varicose veins occur. In India and Africa, with patients on a high-fiber and vegetable diet, the incidence of varicose veins in pregnant women, for example, is less than 2 percent. In the U.S., on the other hand, the incidence reaches 40 percent during pregnancy. In Polynesia, people living in the traditional way of life have only a 2 percent incidence of varicose veins, yet the same people in the nearby Cook Islands, where they have been Americanized with Cokes, white bread and red meat, have an incidence 8 to 10 times greater.

Later, when we spoke personally to Dr. Buyers, he said most of the patients who visit him with varicose veins are beyond prevention or nonsurgical treatment and require surgery. He suggests they try a high-fiber diet after surgery to help prevent recurrence, which ordinarily occurs about 10 percent of the time, according to surgical texts.

"Without statistics and scientifically collected data—which I don't have," Dr. Buyers admitted, "it's impossible to say with certainty how the high-fiber diet works in treatment of varicose veins. The impression I get from patients, though, is that it has helped."

If, however, you do have varicose veins which don't bother you with symptoms or look bad now, the following treatments might keep them from getting worse.

Yves St. Laurent might not approve, but you'll probably feel much better if you don support elastic stockings sold in surgical supply houses. Don't prescribe elastic stockings or bandages for yourself without consulting the doctor, though. If you purchase ill-fitting stockings or wrap the bandages too tightly, you could impair circulation and make your veins worse.

Why Support Stockings Help

Elastic stockings are often prescribed for varicose veins. Usually they are only worn from just below the knee to the metatarsals (the long foot bones that end just in back of the toes). Occasionally they go clear up to the groin if the patient has varicose veins of the thighs. Measurements of various parts of your legs can be taken so that the stockings—made of elastic yarn or mercerized silk—can be made specifically for you. The stockings must exert equal pressure on the leg without cutting off the circulation at the top. Usually you will be advised to put them on before you get out of bed in the morning.

Elastic stockings may be ugly and at times uncomfortable, but they help accomplish several important goals: prevent swelling, support the veins just as the muscles do for the deep vein system, encourage pumping action, prevent blood from flowing downhill instead of uphill, collapse the stagnant pools of blood and protect thin and fragile skin and tissue from injuries. Heaviness, ach-ing, fatigue and swelling are often reduced.

Elastic bandages four to six inches wide may also be used to accomplish the same goals and relieve the same symptoms, but they are more difficult to apply since they aren't fitted for you and you have to gauge the tension yourself.

Support hose give some relief and disguise the varicosities without having the thick appearance of the elastic stockings, but two physicians we talked to said the sheer ones that look almost like regular nylons really aren't as effective as elastic stockings.

A San Francisco gynecologist who sees varicose veins in pregnant women, and often writes about women's medical problems, Lucienne Lanson, M.D., gave this advice in a telephone interview:

"Supportive stockings will make the woman more comfortable—the very sheer support hose won't give much support and the heavy surgical stockings aren't that comfortable either. A good compromise is a not-too-sheer pair of support hose."

An internal medicine specialist suggested a trade-off be made between the importance of relieving symptoms and having attractive legs. According to Victor Pellicano, M.D., founder of Centre for Medicine in Lewiston, New York, sheer support hose are not as good as the thicker ones. Either can be used. It depends on how bad the veins are and how important the cosmetic factor is to the patient. With men, it usually doesn't matter."

Concerned women might consider wearing bandages or elastic stockings at home and on days they wear slacks, and support hose on days they wear dresses.

Almost as important as what to wear is what not to wear. As we mentioned, Tight shoes or belts, girdles, clothes

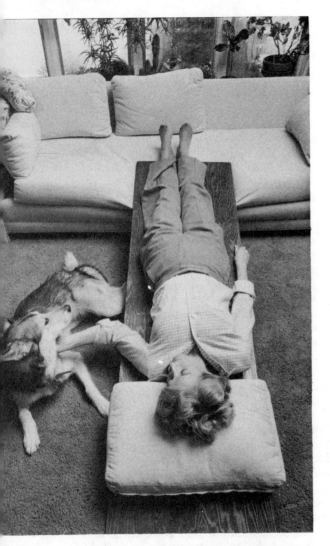

Resting on a slantboard (which needn't be anything more than a board propped up against a low piece of furniture) or elevating your feet with a few pillows is an excellent aid to varicose veins.

with elastic waistbands—anything constricting—could conceivably impair the flow of blood, especially from the waist down.

Elevation of the legs is often used with elastic stockings. The legs should be raised higher than the heart so that the blood can drain. For that reason, bedrest is far more effective than elevating the legs while sitting in a chair. A slantboard would be ideal, but a pillow at the foot or head of the bed can also be used. It may help to gently tense the calf muscle while you're resting, or to put a pillow at the foot of the bed and "walk" against it. It's probably a good idea to ask the doctor about this—people who have certain diseases of the heart, chest and esophagus shouldn't do it.

Leg elevation combined with elastic stockings is especially good for pregnant women, people with severe symptoms who don't want surgery or are poor risks for it and the elderly. It may be so effective that badly hurting legs may feel fine in the morning. Elevation can be done at periodic intervals during the day—particularly when alternated with exercise—as well as overnight.

If you overeat, stop. Fat makes varicose veins difficult to detect, and can complicate surgery and wound healing should the need arise for that. More important, fat helps cause and aggravates varicose veins because as it infiltrates connective tissues, it robs veins of their support.

If your weight is normal, you should consider getting more fiber in your diet, especially if you are constipated.

Even if lack of fiber is not a primary cause of varicose veins, a high-fiber diet is likely to be less fattening and certain to be less constipating than a low-fiber one. To get more fiber in your diet, eliminate white sugar and white flour, and pies, cakes, cookies, pastries and pastas made from them. Use whole grain flours instead. Leave the jackets on your potatoes and the skins on your vegetables. Eliminate pretzels and potato chips and other high-calorie, low-fiber snacks in favor of fresh fruits and vegetables, raw or lightly steamed.

The Advice of Nutrition-Oriented Physicians

Nutritional supplementation is not suggested for treatment of varicose veins in standard medical texts. Vitamin C and vitamin E have both been mentioned as important supplements for the disease by nutrition-oriented physicians, however. Using evidence that comes from observation of patients in his practice, Wilfrid E. Shute, M.D., of the Shute Institute in Ontario, Canada, concluded that vitamin E helps in treatment of varicose veins. He wrote in 1969:

> Our training was traditional. And so, of course, this explanation [of the possible causes of varicose veins listed earlier in the chapter] was accepted. Therefore, we at first paid little or no attention to the effects of alpha tocopherol [the active ingredient of vitamin E] on varicose veins. However, when we compared notes and found that our patients [treated with vitamin E for other ailments] were insisting that their varicose veins were getting smaller, we became interested.
> —*Vitamin E for Ailing and Healthy Hearts* (Pyramid House, 1969).

Dr. Shute goes on to describe numerous cases where vitamin E was used successfully in varicose vein cases. Dr. Pellicano, the internal medicine specialist mentioned earlier, reports similar results. "I also recommend vitamin C because it strengthens the collagen, or connective tissue," he says. "If there is no complication, such as high blood pressure, I recommend 800 to 2,400 [international] units of E daily and 1,000 to 5,000 units [milligrams] of C."

Leg exercises that use the calf muscles, such as walking, jogging, bicycling and swimming, help to pump blood back toward the heart. The rhythmic muscle contractions counteract the effects of gravity and faulty valves that cause stagnation and pooling of blood in lower legs. As calf muscles are strengthened by daily exercise, they are better able to pump blood back up toward the heart. For best results, elastic support hose or bandages should be worn during exercise.

If that suggests too athletic a program to work into your daily office or household routine, investigate the gym and pool at your local YWCA. Regular sessions there can significantly reduce the effects of long hours spent sitting at a desk or standing at a cash register.

"Pedaling" while lying on your back in bed or on the living room floor also helps to reverse blood flow by combining muscular pumping with elevation and elastic support. For someone who is not able to get outdoors for long walks or bike rides, cycling in bed for a few minutes twice a day or so may be helpful.

Inactivity and poor muscle tone make the problem worse during pregnancy, so it's a good idea to walk and do your daily dozen of the exercises you learn in childbirth preparation classes.

Vitamins and

VITAMIN A

APPROXIMATE DAILY REQUIREMENT. MOST ADULTS UNDER NORMAL CONDITIONS

5,000 I.U. Some nutritionists recommend up to 20,000 I.U. as a normal supplement. The need for A increases with greater body weight.

CONDITIONS THAT INCREASE NEED

Low bile and malabsorption problems, liver disease and damage, high intake of prepared and processed foods, low-fat diet, working in bright light, pregnancy, nursing; estrogen is considered a destroyer of A.

DEFICIENCY SYMPTOMS

Night blindness, abnormal dryness of the eyeballs, softness of the cornea, dry, rough, itchy skin, mucous membrane abnormalities.

THERAPEUTIC DOSE RANGE

Toxic level 50,000 I.U. 10,000–20,000 I.U. daily should be the maximum taken without medical supervision. Skip supplements when large amounts of liver, carrots, carrot juice or spinach are eaten. Consider that you may not require A supplements at all if you are a regular consumer of extremely A-rich foods.

May be useful when coming off the Pill if skin symptoms occur. Reduce dosage after stopping the Pill, especially if planning to have a baby.

5,000–10,000 I.U. daily may help ease arthritis pain, if blood levels of A are abnormally low.

Vitamin A sometimes helps the dry skin conditions of menopause, but some women benefit more from E, which helps them use their A better.

HORMONE INTERACTIONS

Too much estrogen keeps A from performing normally in the body.

Minerals for Women*

SYMPTOMS OF EXCESS

Loss of hair, cracked lips, dry skin, severe headaches, general weakness, blurred vision, bruising, nosebleeds, painful joints, emotional disturbances, fatigue, insomnia.

BEST FOOD SOURCES

Calf and beef liver provide enormous amounts of A, as much as 6 times the daily allowance in an average portion. Chicken liver supplies twice the daily allowance, as does a serving of chard, spinach, or turnip greens.

Other foods that contain the daily allowance, or somewhat more in an average serving, are string beans, broccoli, carrots, yellow squash, apricots, sweet potatoes and yams. A tip for calorie counters and fiber watchers: One raw carrot or ½ cup (4 oz.) of kale provides the approximate daily A requirement. The carrot has only about 20 calories, and the kale about 35. Overcooking destroys A.

INTERACTIONS WITH OTHER VITAMINS AND MINERALS

Presence of E is necessary to prevent the destruction of A in the body; A cannot be stored if choline is undersupplied. Works with B_{12}, B_2, C and E. Dietary protein is required to mobilize liver reserves of A.

OTHER COMMENTS

Vitamin A is stored largely in the liver. The half-life of A is weeks or months, meaning that it can be stored (and then mobilized from the liver by protein), so it need not be taken daily. A decreases basal metabolism.

*The information in this chart should be considered informative and not prescriptive.

SOURCES: Vitamin chart adapted from *Women and the Crisis in Sex Hormones* by Barbara Seaman and Gideon Seaman (New York: Rawson, Wade, 1977). (Used by permission.) Mineral chart compiled by Carol Munson and Susan Rosenkrantz, research associates.

NOTE: I.U. = international unit
    g. = gram (1,000 milligrams)
  mg. = milligram (1,000 micrograms)
 mcg. = microgram
 ppm = parts per million

VITAMIN B₁ (Thiamine)

APPROXIMATE DAILY REQUIREMENT. MOST ADULTS UNDER NORMAL CONDITIONS

1.5–10 mg. daily is advocated by many nutritionists for older people, the very active, and those under stress.

CONDITIONS THAT INCREASE NEED

Pregnancy, nursing, eating sugar, smoking, drinking alcohol, surgery, crash diets, taking the Pill, eating processed meats.

BEST FOOD SOURCES

Wheat germ, rice, bran, soybean flour and yeast are good sources. Other sources include vegetables, whole grains, beans, nuts and meats. Many B-rich foods are also excellent sources of fiber.

4 oz. of sunflower seed (in the hull) provide 2.3 g. of fiber, 343 calories and 1.8 mg. of B₁.

For dieters, 1 tbsp. of brewer's yeast provides most of the B₁ requirement, and only 25 calories.

THERAPEUTIC DOSE RANGE

4–15 mg. daily. Should be kept in balance with other B's unless special needs are suspected. If one B is doubled, for example, the others should be, also.

The daily allowance, or twice that, may be enough to replace B₁ lost to Pill use.

As part of the B complex, it is generally helpful for complaints stemming from Pill stoppage and menopause, and during premenstrual week and menstruation.

HORMONE INTERACTIONS

Affects the thyroid and insulin production.

DEFICIENCY SYMPTOMS

Loss of appetite, constipation, digestive disturbance, depression, irritability, inability to concentrate, numbness and prickliness in toes and feet, stiff ankles, loss of reflexes. In later stages of deficiency, nerve, muscle and heart function are affected.

Beriberi, the disease resulting from severe B_1 deficiency, occurs in two forms. In the wet form, edema (fluid retention), is paramount, and in the dry form, paralysis occurs. Death results from cardiac failure.

SYMPTOMS OF EXCESS

Edema, nervousness, sweating, rapid heartbeat, tremors, herpes, fatty liver, and allergies.

INTERACTIONS WITH OTHER VITAMINS AND MINERALS

Increases activity of B_{12}, works with pantothenic acid, niacin and riboflavin to release energy from carbohydrates. Overdose of B_1 may cause B_6 deficiency. B_1, riboflavin and B_6 work together to produce niacin.

Vitamin C decreases requirement for B_1. Tolerance to D is increased by B_1.

OTHER COMMENTS

The B vitamin most vulnerable to heat. Not stored for any great length of time and is readily excreted in the urine so it is essential to take each day. Has diuretic effect. Injections may produce allergies.

VITAMIN B₂ (Riboflavin)

APPROXIMATE DAILY REQUIREMENT. MOST ADULTS UNDER NORMAL CONDITIONS

1.7 mg., but many nutritionists consider this too low and feel the requirement should be 5 mg. for all adolescents and adults.

CONDITIONS THAT INCREASE NEED

Taking the Pill and possibly other hormones; during pregnancy, lactation and stress.

Deficiency occurs on a starchy or junk food diet, or a low-calorie, low-cholesterol, or Zen macrobiotic diet. It is difficult to attain the 1.7 mg. daily intake, much less the 5 mg. some authorities favor.

BEST FOOD SOURCES

Some sources are: almonds, asparagus, broccoli, cheese, milk, eggs, organ meats, wheat germ, whole grains, wild rice.

3 oz. of beef liver provide about 4 mg. at 195 calories. Those who fear the DES and cholesterol in liver might wish to substitute desiccated liver tablets.

4 oz. of beef heart, at about 160 calories, provide almost the daily requirement.

THERAPEUTIC DOSE RANGE

5–15 mg. daily. 10–15 mg. daily for Pill or estrogen users or those coming off hormone therapy.

Not specifically associated with hot flashes but, like other B's, may help energy and well-being at menopause.

5–10 mg. daily may help reduce arthritis pain.

Is generally helpful during premenstrual week and menstruation as part of B complex.

HORMONE INTERACTIONS

Riboflavin contributes to the normal release and activity of many hormones, including estrogen, thyroxine, insulin, pituitary and adrenal hormones.

An unusual feature of riboflavin is that it inhibits the formation of liver tumors in animals. Thus, theoretically, its depletion by the Pill could be a factor in the liver tumors associated with this contraceptive.

INTERACTIONS WITH OTHER VITAMINS AND MINERALS

Works with A and niacin in maintaining the health of the eyes; interacts closely with thiamine in monitoring thyroxine and insulin; and also works with most of the other B complex vitamins.

DEFICIENCY SYMPTOMS

Deficiencies cause damage to the mouth, lips, eyes, skin and genitalia. This sometimes appears as extended cracks on the upper or lower lip and may extend into the mucous membranes inside the mouth. Burning and itching sensations in the eyes, and scaliness of the skin—especially around the joints—may also occur; so may dandruff. Cataracts occur in severe deficiencies, and a discolored tongue or anemia are other symptoms.

SYMPTOMS OF EXCESS

Riboflavin is considered non-toxic in man. But occasionally, as with certain other vitamins, there are minor symptoms of excess which resemble deficiency symptoms. These include itching, or spontaneous sensations of burning, prickling or numbness.

OTHER COMMENTS

Normally, ⅓ of dietary amounts are excreted daily.

NIACIN

20 mg., but some nutritionists recommend 40–100 mg. a day for adolescents as well as adults.

CONDITIONS THAT INCREASE NEED

Pregnancy and nursing. The need is not increased during Pill use, perhaps because the body can manufacture its own niacin from protein, specifically tryptophan, an amino acid. It is probably not advisable for women with hot flashes to take large supplements, because flushing is also a side effect of niacin. Flushing is increased when antibiotics are taken, or when caloric intake is high. (Niacin releases energy from carbohydrates and protein as well as stimulating gastric and bile secretions.) The need for supplemental niacin is probably highest for persons whose diet is low in protein, and/or B_1, B_2 and B_6, but substantial in calories. (In the absence of B_1, B_2 and B_6, the body cannot perform its usual job of manufacturing niacin from tryptophan.)

THERAPEUTIC DOSE RANGE

For most adults 40–100 mg., but some psychiatrists use much larger amounts, experimentally, in the treatment of schizophrenia. Pill users and women with menopausal symptoms are advised not to exceed 100 mg. and to find B complex products with smaller amounts if they can. In the form of niacinamide, this vitamin is less apt to produce flushing, and should therefore be selected by women with menopausal complaints.

As part of B complex, it is generally helpful during premenstrual week and menstruation.

Sunlight sensitivity symptoms, such as skin discoloration or dryness, may be reduced by moderate supplements.

400 mg. or sometimes much more (used *only* under medical supervision) may help reduce arthritis pain.

HORMONE INTERACTIONS

Niacin is involved in the synthesis and distribution of many hormones, including estrogen, progesterone, testosterone, cortisone, thyroxine and insulin.

DEFICIENCY SYMPTOMS

Pellagra, the niacin deficiency disease, is characterized by skin eruptions, mental disturbances, digestive disorders, and deterioration of intellect.

Early symptoms of niacin deficiency are said to resemble pellagra, and may involve personality changes such as suspiciousness and hostility, skin that is sensitive to sunlight, and indigestion.

SYMPTOMS OF EXCESS

Niacin is considered to have "limited toxicity" in man. Some individuals are quite sensitive to it and may develop burning and itching skin, fatty liver, overstimulation of the central nervous system, increased pulse rate and respiration and decreased blood pressure. Unlike most of the water-soluble vitamins, it can also produce paralysis and death in laboratory animals.

BEST FOOD SOURCES

Roasted peanuts, organ meats, the white meat of poultry, fish (including tuna, halibut, and swordfish); brewer's yeast. Fruits (such as avocados, dates, figs, and prunes); whole grains, legumes and dairy products are other sources.

A serving of swordfish or chicken breast provides half your daily niacin requirement for only 150 calories. A half cup of shelled peanuts provides most of your daily fiber and niacin requirement at about 420 calories.

INTERACTIONS WITH OTHER VITAMINS AND MINERALS

Niacin works closely with almost all of the B's in food utilization, and the alleviation of deficiencies and deficiency symptoms. Many of the side effects associated with niacin deficiency cannot be corrected unless other B's are added, too. Niacin—and other B's—also cooperate with vitamins such as A, D and C in maintaining the skin, D and E in maintaining digestion and food absorption, and A and C in helping to maintain the nerves and psyche.

OTHER COMMENTS

Niacin is so essential in monitoring cholesterol metabolism that high doses of it can lower serum cholesterol. It also has a major effect on metabolic rate and temperature.

VITAMIN B₆ (Pyridoxine)

APPROXIMATE DAILY REQUIREMENT. MOST ADULTS UNDER NORMAL CONDITIONS

2.0 mg. Many nutritionists recommend 5–10 mg. routinely. Some individuals need 30–50 mg. or more routinely.

CONDITIONS THAT INCREASE NEED

Inborn deficiencies in utilizing pyridoxine are fairly common and are most apt to occur in the presence of a family history of diabetes, hypoglycemia, or malabsorption syndromes such as celiac disease. The Pill makes most users marginally depleted in pyridoxine, and many others severely depleted. Gastrointestinal disease, irradiation, and various drugs also deplete pyridoxine. The need may be increased when the diet is high in protein, for pyridoxine is instrumental in protein metabolism. The need is also increased in pregnancy and nursing.

BEST FOOD SOURCES

The typical modern diet is low in pyridoxine. Hence it is difficult for Pill users or those with inborn malabsorption problems to get enough from diet alone. Good sources include brewer's yeast, wheat bran, wheat germ, organ meats, blackstrap molasses, walnuts, peanuts, brown rice, herring (pickled, not smoked), salmon, and some fruits (bananas, avocados, grapes, pears) and vegetables (cabbage, carrots, potatoes). Cheeses and milk contain smaller amounts.

For calorie counters, generous servings of raw salmon or tuna (as prepared sashimi-style at Japanese markets and restaurants) are among the best lean sources of the daily pyridoxine requirement.

Of all the vitamins, pyridoxine seems especially hard to get from healthful dietary sources.

THERAPEUTIC DOSE RANGE

5–25 mg. is the usual therapeutic dose. Pill users often require 30–100 mg. to correct deficiency symptoms, such as depression or disturbed carbohydrate metabolism. Do not exceed 100, or at the most 300, mg. without medical supervision. Many people require twice their normal requirement of B₆ when they are under stress. A good clue to this need is dream recall. Some people need 50 mg., others as little as 5 mg., to correct malabsorption difficulties, but a few others benefit from extremely high dosages, as much as 800 or 1,000 mg.

INTERACTIONS WITH OTHER VITAMINS AND MINERALS

It is suspected that B₆ and the mineral magnesium may have a special connection, as E does with selenium. Neither vitamin can perform its job as efficiently without some boost from the pertinent mineral. Pyridoxine interacts closely with almost all of the other B vitamins, C and E. It helps K to maintain normal circulation and blood cells and helps the body adjust to stress.

HORMONE INTERACTIONS

Pyridoxine helps sustain normal maintenance of both gonadal hormones (estrogen and testosterone) and pituitary hormones (FSH and LH) in such a way that its performance is dramatically handicapped by the ingestion of estrogen preparations. The reasons remain unclear, but the evidence for this effect is overwhelming. Long-term hormone users are likely to develop seriously lowered pyridoxine levels. This vitamin also affects thyroxine, insulin, norepinephrine, and epinephrine (adrenal hormones affecting nerve condition, balance, energy, work efficiency, resistance to temperature change, stress, and the general state of the emotions) as well as growth hormone and ACTH (pituitary hormone).

DEFICIENCY SYMPTOMS

Pyridoxine is of central importance in the normal maintenance of emotional health, energy and skin; resistance to stress; and the metabolism of proteins and fats. Deficiency symptoms include severe depression and diabetic syndromes in Pill users, skin lesions, certain anemias, convulsions, extreme nervousness, weakness and lethargy. Deficiency may play a special role in the development of certain herpes infections.

Lack of dream recall is a sign of pyridoxine deficiency; and many disturbances associated with stoppage of the Pill, including skin eruptions and absence of menstruation, respond to supplementation.

SYMPTOMS OF EXCESS

Except for too-vivid dream recall and night restlessness, toxicity has not been reported at dosages below 300 mg., which is 150 times the recommended allowance. Pregnant women should be wary of doses over 50 mg. for their infants may then demonstrate withdrawal symptoms.

daily. Many vitamin products are short on B_6 because it is expensive and difficult to extract from natural foods or synthesize. Users of many B complex products may benefit from a separate pyridoxine tablet along with their general B supplement. All in all, B_6 is very tricky and individualized, especially since the need varies so much with environmental stress, as well as hormone and other drug use, inborn malabsorption problems, and dietary protein intake.

50–100 mg. is used as a specific treatment for premenstrual water retention, breast swelling and acne. In Europe 200 mg. daily for 5 days is used as a lactation suppressant, and reported to be more effective than hormones.

Women with gum and teeth problems should try supplements of at least 5–10 mg. daily. Those who think they have deficiency symptoms, which can include generally poor metabolism, water retention, and overweight as well as the other conditions mentioned, might wish to start with 25 or 50 mg. daily and cut back if sleep disturbances occur.

While it appears safe to go up to 300 mg. without medical supervision, it is inadvisable to stay on such high supplements for more than 3 months without cutting back experimentally (for a week or a month) in order to determine the effects and give any incipient toxicity a chance to wash out.

50 mg. daily may help reduce arthritis pain.

B_6 has been used to ameliorate symptoms of epilepsy and cerebral palsy, and to counteract such pregnancy side effects as nausea and headache.

OTHER COMMENTS

B_6 should never be used by patients who are under L-dopa treatment for Parkinson's disease. In obscure ways, B_6 seems to be involved in dental cavities, water and electrolyte balance and a great diversity of other symptoms. Some people feel like "new personalities" when B_6 supplements are added. They lose weight, have increased energy, recover from depressions and neurological symptoms; their skin clears and their menstruation is normalized. However, there is this danger: study results suggest that the prolonged ingestion of B_6 may lead to dependency on the vitamin.

Always take a B complex and C with it, as well as magnesium.

VITAMIN B$_{12}$ (Cyanocobalamin)

APPROXIMATE DAILY REQUIREMENT. MOST ADULTS UNDER NORMAL CONDITIONS

6 mcg.

CONDITIONS THAT INCREASE NEED

Genetic factors that block secretion in the stomach of a substance necessary for the absorption of B$_{12}$. Under these circumstances, shots instead of oral supplements may be necessary. Pregnancy and nursing, intestinal malabsorption or disease, alcoholism, cobalt deficiency, parasites, strict vegetarian diet without eggs or dairy products, aging.

Hormone users often become quite deficient in B$_{12}$, but mysteriously, anemia and other life-threatening symptoms do not seem to ensue. This is in marked contrast to the situation with pyridoxine and folate. B$_{12}$ is so closely related to protein metabolism that need may increase when protein consumption is high.

THERAPEUTIC DOSE RANGE

Highly controversial. Some doctors give weekly or twice-weekly shots of 1,000 mcg. Persons lacking the substance that aids the absorption of B$_{12}$ require enormous supplements to get the vitamin into the bloodstream, but ordinary deficiencies often respond to dosages of only a few micrograms daily. Some people say that they have much more energy and/or healthier-looking skin if they take supplements ranging from about 25–100 mcg. daily. The lower figure can be obtained in many stress or B complex vitamin formulas. To keep folate and B$_{12}$ normally balanced, it's advisable to eat a leafy vegetable every day, and liver at least once a week, desiccated liver supplements, or some other organic form without DES.

3–6 mcg. daily is sufficient for most people. Those who think they may become severely depleted with hormone use may benefit from 25–100 mcg. daily.

Pallor may improve. There are some reports of shingles being cured by B$_{12}$ therapy. The beneficial effects of B$_{12}$ on skin may be due to its helping vitamin A work better.

Never exceed more than 100 mcg. daily unless special need such as poor absorption is established.

As part of B complex B$_{12}$ is generally helpful during premenstrual week and menstruation.

DEFICIENCY SYMPTOMS

Anemia, including pale skin, heart palpitations, sore tongue, general weakness, disturbances of the spinal cord and nervous system, poor growth, altered metabolism, prickly sensations in extremities, weight loss.

SYMPTOMS OF EXCESS

Toxicity is rare. An abnormal increase in the number of red blood cells.

BEST FOOD SOURCES

Plants contain only traces, but soybeans are the best source for strict vegetarians. B_{12} occurs in all meats, especially organs such as liver, kidney, brain and heart; in egg yolk; and in sardines, salmon, crab, herring (pickled, not smoked), other fish; and cheese. B_{12} may be destroyed by cooking or food processing.

HORMONE INTERACTIONS

Abnormalities of the thyroid and parathyroid hormones are associated with B_{12} deficiencies.

Too much B_{12} might, by stimulating the parathyroid, increase the probability of osteoporosis. Its low amount in vegetarian diets could be an additional feature in the low osteoporosis rate among that group.

INTERACTIONS WITH OTHER VITAMINS AND MINERALS

Works with A, E, C, B_1, folate, pantothenic acid.

B_{12} given with folate aids in relief of fatigue. B_{12} also works with almost all of the other B vitamins.

FOLATE (Folic acid, or folacin)

APPROXIMATE DAILY REQUIREMENT. MOST ADULTS UNDER NORMAL CONDITIONS

400 mcg. Some nutritionists advocate a much higher dose of folate, as much as 2–5 mg. daily.

CONDITIONS THAT INCREASE NEED

Pregnancy, illness, alcoholism, and the use of drugs including estrogens, sulfonamides, phenobarbital, Dilantin. Taking vitamin C increases the excretion of folate. Certain intestinal bacteria destroy folate. Some people have poor natural absorption.

BEST FOOD SOURCES

The richest sources are liver or organic desiccated liver, asparagus, spinach, wheat, bran, dried beans, and brewer's yeast. Small amounts are present in all fruits, many vegetables, meat, cheese, milk and nuts. Storage and cooking (if the water is thrown out) cause substantial folate losses. Estrogen users are advised to save all their vegetable cooking water for soup. Asparagus is the best source of folate for both fiber and calorie watchers.

SYMPTOMS OF EXCESS

Scientists usually say "no toxicity reported" or "there is no known human toxicity." A few people do have allergic skin reactions. There have also been reports of increased convulsions when large doses are given to persons with seizure disorders.

THERAPEUTIC DOSE RANGE

We cannot agree with those nutritionists who say that 5 mg. daily is safe. On the other hand, there is ample evidence that Pill users, women recently off the Pill, women with menopausal symptoms or other endocrine deficiencies benefit from the pregnancy dosage of folate, which is twice the recommended allowance, or 800 mcg. Temporary dosages of 1–5 mg. daily, for only a few weeks, can reverse abnormal Pap smears and skin discolorations, as well as curing folate deficiency anemia. However, we would not advise going over 1 mg. daily, or certainly 2, except under medical supervision. We would not advise staying on a dosage of more than 1 mg. daily after symptoms improve.

As part of B complex folate is generally helpful during premenstrual week and menstruation.

Most nonprescription B complex and multiple vitamin products do not contain nearly enough folate to correct the deficiencies we

INTERACTIONS WITH OTHER VITAMINS AND MINERALS

C and folate maintain a delicate balance. On the one hand, C is needed to metabolize it properly, and works closely with it, forming red blood cells. But on the other, too much C in proportion to folate causes the latter to wash out. B₁₂ and folate are also in delicate balance, working closely together in formation of marrow and blood. For some purposes they are interchangeable. Niacin requires folate to be properly utilized. Biotin, pantothenic acid, and folate perform crucial interacting functions on the liver and other organs.

Folate, B₆, riboflavin and B₁₂ are together required for normal protein metabolism.

DEFICIENCY SYMPTOMS

Deficiency symptoms are extremely serious, including a form of anemia. Less severe deficiencies cause shortness of breath, dizziness, fatigue, intestinal disorders and diarrhea. Deficiencies during pregnancy produce hemorrhaging, miscarriage, premature birth, and a high infant mortality rate. Skin discolorations called the "mask of pregnancy" are a frequent deficiency symptom

in both expectant mothers and Pill users. Pill users, who often have folate deficiency, get anemia, bizarre changes in their cervices, and skin discolorations as a result. The higher rate of birth defects and miscarriages in women who conceive while taking or shortly after stopping the Pill is believed by some researchers to be associated with folate deficiency (and possibly vitamin A excess).

The more severe hot flashes that some menopausal and postmenopausal women experience when giving up estrogen may be a consequence of lowered folate, as well as E and C complex levels. The post-Pill syndrome including amenorrhea (absence of menstruation), may be influenced by folate deficiency, as well as deficiencies of E, other B vitamins, and zinc.

have discussed. The typical B complex product has only about 100 mcg. or sometimes none. A Pill user, for example, could not hope to correct her folate deficiency symptoms without taking 4–8 tablets containing 100 mcg. daily. Some multiple vitamins contain the recommended allowance of 400 mcg., but comparatively too much A for Pill users. Pregnancy vitamins may provide 800 mcg. of folate, but again, too much A for Pill users.

The reader who suspects she is deficient in folate can

either (1) be extremely careful about her diet; (2) ask her doctor to recommend a prescription vitamin; (3) buy separate folate tablets at a health food store or drugstore. These are usually sold in 400 mcg. dosages, and she would need to take 1 or 2 a day, along with a conventional B complex product.

May be helpful for skin problems associated with hormones or menopause, and gum and tooth problems.

HORMONE INTERACTIONS

Folate deficiency flatly eliminates the normal response of female reproductive organs to estrogen. It also has profound effects on the distribution of testosterone in men. Folate works with the growth hormone called STH.

OTHER COMMENTS

Antibody formation decreases when folate is deficient. Folate has analgesic properties, increasing the pain threshold. As sulfonamides block intestinal synthesis of folate, the vitamin, in turn, may hamper the drug.

PANTOTHENIC ACID

APPROXIMATE DAILY REQUIREMENT. MOST ADULTS UNDER NORMAL CONDITIONS

10 mg.

CONDITIONS THAT INCREASE NEED

Stress increases need.

DEFICIENCY SYMPTOMS

Nerve and muscle disturbances, tingling hands and feet, numbness, hypoglycemia, cardiovascular disorders, digestive disorders, susceptibility to infections and colds, physical weakness, depression.

INTERACTIONS WITH OTHER VITAMINS AND MINERALS

Works with biotin, folate, C, niacin, A and E. Releases energy from sugar. The body cannot utilize PABA (para-aminobenzoic acid) or choline without it.

BIOTIN

APPROXIMATE DAILY REQUIREMENT. MOST ADULTS UNDER NORMAL CONDITIONS

300 mcg.

CONDITIONS THAT INCREASE NEED

Taking antibiotics and sulfa drugs. Eating many raw eggs causes deficiencies, as the avidin in egg white ties up biotin in the intestines where it is synthesized.

DEFICIENCY SYMPTOMS

Eczema of face and body, hair loss, muscle pain, paralysis.

HORMONE INTERACTIONS

May influence cortisone, growth hormone, and testosterone.

SYMPTOMS OF EXCESS

Essentially nontoxic in man, but respiratory failure has been reported in laboratory animals.

BEST FOOD SOURCES

Meat, chicken, milk, eggs, peanuts, peas, broccoli, kale, sweet potatoes, yellow corn, whole grains and breads. Cooking losses are high.

HORMONE INTERACTIONS

Pantothenic acid is required for synthesis of several hormones, including progesterone.

THERAPEUTIC DOSE RANGE

50–100 mg. daily, especially during stress.

Due to close interactions with progesterone, it may be helpful for post-Pill infertility, menopause complaints, or even cancer prevention in recipients of hormone medication. Might also help reduce likelihood of irregularities in sugar metabolism, stroke, and heart attacks in hormone users.

As part of B complex, pantothenic acid is generally helpful during premenstrual week and menstruation.

50–100 mg. daily may help reduce arthritis pain. Some doctors prescribe much higher amounts.

OTHER COMMENTS

May have anticancer factors. Used to treat vertigo, postoperative shock, curare poisoning. Aids wound healing. Helps Addison's disease, liver cirrhosis, and diabetes.

SYMPTOMS OF EXCESS

No information available.

BEST FOOD SOURCES

Brewer's yeast and organ meats are good sources. Available in whole grains, egg yolk, fish, nuts and fruits. Losses occur through cooking.

THERAPEUTIC DOSE RANGE

About 25 mcg.

Supplements may be useful for skin problems, especially when these occur in connection with use of antibiotics or sulfa drugs.

INTERACTIONS WITH OTHER VITAMINS AND MINERALS

Ascorbic acid (vitamin C) synthesis requires biotin. Niacin cannot be metabolized if biotin is deficient. Biotin works with B_2, B_6, niacin, A and D in maintenance of skin.

OTHER COMMENTS

The severity and duration of some diseases—especially protozoan infections—is increased when biotin is deficient. Biotin is essential for normal metabolism of fat and protein.

CHOLINE AND INOSITOL

APPROXIMATE DAILY REQUIREMENT. MOST ADULTS UNDER NORMAL CONDITIONS

Recommended allowances not clarified for choline and inositol. They appear to work jointly in fat metabolism, perhaps keeping cholesterol in an emulsified state so that it cannot settle on artery walls or collect in the gallbladder.

CONDITIONS THAT INCREASE NEED

No information available.

DEFICIENCY SYMPTOMS

No information available.

HORMONE INTERACTIONS

No information available.

INTERACTIONS WITH OTHER VITAMINS AND MINERALS

No information available.

PABA (Para-aminobenzoic acid)

APPROXIMATE DAILY REQUIREMENT. MOST ADULTS UNDER NORMAL CONDITIONS

Though not accepted by all investigators as essential to human nutrition, some claim PABA is useful against the effects of aging.

CONDITIONS THAT INCREASE NEED

Exposure to sunlight in some sensitive individuals.

DEFICIENCY SYMPTOMS

No information available.

BEST FOOD SOURCES

It occurs with the other B's in natural foods such as whole grains, brewer's yeast, and organ meats, and is also applied externally as a sunscreen lotion.

HORMONE INTERACTIONS

PABA probably plays a role in the maintenance of female reproductive organs, and the normal utilization of estrogen.

INTERACTIONS WITH OTHER VITAMINS AND MINERALS

PABA is linked to folate and occurs as part of the folate molecule.

SYMPTOMS OF EXCESS

No information available.

BEST FOOD SOURCES

Fruits, meat, milk, nuts, vegetables and whole grains are good food sources of inositol. Egg yolk, beef liver and soybeans are good sources of choline. Lecithin capsules, made from soybeans, contain inositol and choline and aid in the use of vitamin E. They also contain phosphorus.

Lecithin users are advised to take calcium supplements such as dolomite with their lecithin tablets, so that phosphorus and calcium will not become unbalanced.

THERAPEUTIC DOSE RANGE

The average therapeutic dose in B complex formulas that contain these vitamins is about 100 mg. of each.

May help to control cholesterol and liver problems in users of estrogen products.

May enhance vitamin E's effects in controlling hot flashes.

May help the fat-soluble vitamins in moisturizing the skin.

Some individuals feel that choline and inositol have a soothing effect on the nerves, and there is some evidence that nerve fibers are influenced by choline. There are also reports that choline may control high blood pressure and help the liver eliminate poisons and drugs.

SYMPTOMS OF EXCESS

No information available.

THERAPEUTIC DOSE RANGE

20–30 mg. daily.

Under medical supervision, the potassium salt of PABA is sometimes used to treat arthritis and rheumatic disorders.

Since it is connected to estrogen uptake by female organs, women with signs of estrogen excess, such as premenstrual breast cysts and tenderness, or hormone-associated cancers, should probably avoid it. Perhaps DES daughters should avoid it, too.

The hormone or Pill user who is exposed to sunlight and starting to develop blotchy spots ("the mask of pregnancy") on her face may find it useful to include PABA in her supplements. By serving as a sunscreen PABA may also help delay formation of wrinkles due to collagen breakdown.

VITAMIN C

APPROXIMATE DAILY REQUIREMENT. MOST ADULTS UNDER NORMAL CONDITIONS

40–60 mg.
    200–500 mg. daily is advocated by many nutritionists.

CONDITIONS THAT INCREASE NEED

Infections, illness, allergies, exposure to pollution, stress, smoking, late pregnancy, taking the Pill, taking aspirin.

DEFICIENCY SYMPTOMS

Bruising easily, tiny hemorrhages in blood vessels under the skin, bleeding gums and dental problems, failure of wounds to heal promptly, weakness, listlessness, fatigue, aching joints, rough skin, edema (fluid retention); weakness in connective tissues that hold skin, muscles, tendons and bones together.
    Scurvy, severe C deficiency, is characterized by extreme muscular weakness, bleeding under the skin and spongy and bleeding gums.

THERAPEUTIC DOSE RANGE

Highly controversial. Linus Pauling and his followers feel that several grams daily can be beneficial, but 500–750 mg. is the usual therapeutic dose for deficiency symptoms. C should be taken in 2 or 3 separate doses. For some conditions it seems more effective when taken with the associated factors discussed under P or C Complex.
    750 mg. may be helpful for Pill or estrogen users, or those who have just come off hormone therapy.
    200–500 mg. may help those over 40 or with osteoporosis (brittle bones).
    C enhances the effectiveness of B complex in curbing premenstrual and menstrual problems.
    Women who have the special problems that benefit from C complex (e.g., excessive menstruation, hot flashes) should not take an ordinary stress formula (B complex with C). Instead, a therapeutic C complex should be taken twice daily, after breakfast and dinner, in addition to a B complex.

HORMONE INTERACTIONS

Required for the normal functioning of adrenal, pituitary and other glands.

SYMPTOMS OF EXCESS

Excess C is excreted in the urine. Occasional diarrhea, excess urination, kidney stones or abdominal pain may develop. Allergic rashes. If taking more than 750 mg. of C daily, use magnesium supplements to help prevent kidney stones. Be sure to take at least the daily requirement of folate and B_{12}, as large amounts of C can wash these out.

BEST FOOD SOURCES

Citrus fruits. Fiber and calorie watchers may wish to get some of their C from the following: broccoli (1 cup has almost 3 g. of fiber, 140 mg. of C, and only 40 calories), brussels sprouts (1 cup has 2.5 g. of fiber, 135 mg. of C, and 55 calories), and strawberries (1 cup has almost 2 g. of fiber, 88 mg. of C, and 55 calories). Cabbage, raw or cooked, is a fair source of both C and fiber, at the cost of very few calories. 1 cup of cooked cabbage, for example, provides 0.5 g. of fiber, 48 mg. of C, and 30 calories.

Cantaloupes, cauliflower, dark green, leafy vegetables, tomatoes and potatoes are also good sources.

INTERACTIONS WITH OTHER VITAMINS AND MINERALS

Needed for the metabolism of proteins and amino acids, as well as absorption and storage of iron. Helps conserve A and E, increases effectiveness of B_{12}, folate, B_6 and pantothenic acid.

OTHER COMMENTS

Stored in the adrenal cortex. Other target tissues are pituitary, ovary, connective tissue, bone, liver, teeth and gums. C maintains oxygen turnover, and is needed for normal respiration.

VITAMIN D

APPROXIMATE DAILY REQUIREMENT. MOST ADULTS UNDER NORMAL CONDITIONS

400 I.U. A few nutritionists advocate up to 4,000 or 5,000 I.U. daily for all adults, but this amount occasionally produces serious side effects.

CONDITIONS THAT INCREASE NEED

To prevent osteoporosis (brittle bones), persons over 40 require supplementation if dietary intake is low or exposure to sunlight reduced. Many adults who live in northern states, work indoors, and drink less than a quart of D-enriched millk daily are deficient in D.

D is needed to utilize calcium and phosphorus and help preserve bone mass.

DEFICIENCY SYMPTOMS

Softening of the bones (osteomalacia), rickets, loss of bone minerals, decreased blood calcium and phosphorus, osteoporosis.

THERAPEUTIC DOSE RANGE

Serious toxicity has been found at 1,800 I.U. in susceptible individuals. 800–1,200 I.U. daily should be the maximum therapeutic dosage taken without medical supervision. (Some doctors give osteoporosis patients very high doses, but they monitor the effects.) Less is needed when exposure to sunlight is increased.

400–1,600 I.U. daily for women over 40 or with symptoms of osteoporosis. Women are apt to get less D from sunlight than men because of sunscreens (to prevent wrinkles) and makeup.

400–800 I.U. daily in conjunction with dolomite or calcium pills to ease premenstrual tension and menstrual pain, especially for women with fibrocystic breast disease.

HORMONE INTERACTIONS

D deficiency (like phosphorus excess) overstimulates the parathyroid, drawing calcium from the bones and contributing to osteoporosis.

SYMPTOMS OF
EXCESS

Loss of appetite, nausea, headache, urinary problems, diarrhea, excessive thirst, weight loss, depression, irritability, psychoses, leg weakness. Death from associated calcium deposits in the kidney and lung.

BEST FOOD
SOURCES

Vitamin D-enriched milk, fish-liver oils, sardines, mackerel, herring (pickled, not smoked), salmon, tuna, shrimp and egg yolk. Low amounts in other dairy products and meats. 3 oz. of salmon (120 calories) or tuna (170 calories) or 4 oz. of shrimp (103 calories) are good sources of D for dieters.

INTERACTIONS WITH OTHER
VITAMINS AND MINERALS

Vitamins A and B_1 reduce D's potential toxicity or increase the body's tolerance for it. When taking more than double the recommended allowance of D, some A and B complex should also be added.

OTHER COMMENTS

D is formed by the action of sunlight on the skin.

VITAMIN E

30 I.U. Dosages of up to 1,600 I.U. daily are advocated by a few nutritionists. Many more advocate 50–100 I.U. daily or up to 400 or 600, but not beyond. Vitamin E consists of at least seven related chemicals named alpha, beta, gamma, delta, epsilon, zeta and eta tocopherols. The alpha form has been most studied and deemed most potent, but other forms may have as-yet-undiscovered functions. Some nutritionists feel it is necessary to take only the alpha form; others recommend taking mixed tocopherols which contain alpha plus some or all of the other variants of E.

Taking hormones, pregnancy, nursing and other stresses on reproductive system, pollution or presence of other chemical and environmental toxins, ingestion of unsaturated fats or mineral oil, menopause (hot flashes), aging, and the period after stoppage of the Pill.

Never more than 30–100 I.U. daily for persons with high blood pressure, diabetes, or rheumatic heart. Those taking digitalis should not use E without medical supervision. A normal therapeutic range that most people can handle varies from 30–600 I.U. daily. More should be medically supervised. Users of E supplements should experiment to see if they prefer the dry or oily capsules. Vitamin E is best absorbed in the presence of fat. For people who are unable to take E following a meal with fat, it may be desirable to swallow their E with 1 or 2 lecithin capsules, a soybean extract containing choline and inositol as well as large amounts of unsaturated fatty acids (or the equivalent in granules). They also contain phosphorus, which may be undesirable for persons prone to osteoporosis, such as women whose ovaries have been surgically removed or who are heavy eaters of meat. Lecithin users are advised to take calcium supplements so that phosphorus and calcium will not become unbalanced. Amenorrhea (absence of menstruation) has been effectively treated with wheat germ oil—20 drops 3 times a day for 10 days.

15–30 I.U. daily for women taking the Pill; up to 300 for women taking estrogens alone. 30–600 I.U. for women who have stopped taking the Pill or who have gone off estrogen replacement therapy.

30–600 I.U. daily for hot flashes. More (under medical supervision) for postmenopausal vaginal problems.

600 I.U. daily for fibrocystic breasts.

30–600 I.U. daily for absence of menstruation. 30–200 I.U. daily for comfort during premenstrual week and menstruation.

30–600 I.U. daily for dry or prematurely aging skin.

DEFICIENCY SYMPTOMS

Destruction of red blood cells, muscle degeneration, paralysis, hot flashes, possibly insufficient blood flow to extremities, some anemias, some reproductive disorders such as absence of menstruation; insufficient E may have adverse effects on skin health. This may be an indirect result of E's protective effect on A and other vitamins, on fat storage, or its role in protecting against toxins in the environment that damage skin.

SYMPTOMS OF EXCESS

Weight gain from increased fat storage, indigestion, possibly high blood pressure, skin rashes, sleepiness; if dose is too high, foods may seem unappetizing. At dosages of 4,000 I.U. daily taken for 3 months, diarrhea and soreness of the mouth, tongue and lips have been reported.

BEST FOOD SOURCES

Wheat germ sprinkled on cereals or salads or used in baking, whole grain bread, salads with oils such as safflower or wheat germ in the dressing.

HORMONE INTERACTIONS

Deficiency of E increases production of pituitary hormones FSH and LH; a decrease in these hormones may be the key to E's effectiveness in subduing hot flashes.

E is highly concentrated in reproductive tissues and also interacts closely with cortisone and adrenal and growth hormones.

INTERACTIONS WITH OTHER VITAMINS AND MINERALS

E interacts with, preserves, or helps utilize C, A, B_{12} and folate, K and pantothenic acid. For vegetarians, who have few dietary sources of B_{12}, E may actually substitute for it, as well as aiding in the full use of the B_{12} they do get. Capsules containing about 25 mcg. of selenium for each 200 units of E increase E's efficiency.

OTHER COMMENTS

E is stored in muscle, fat tissue and liver; 60–70% of daily dose is excreted in feces; the rest is absorbed, but has a half-life of under one week, closer to that of the water-soluble vitamins (B and C) than the other fat-soluble vitamins such as A, which has a half-life of months, or D, which has a half-life of weeks. That is why it's safer for most people to take relatively higher doses of E than A or D.

VITAMIN K

**APPROXIMATE
DAILY REQUIREMENT.
MOST ADULTS UNDER
NORMAL CONDITIONS**

30 mcg., but it is normally manufactured by intestinal bacteria.

**CONDITIONS THAT
INCREASE NEED**

Healthy people do not need to worry about K. Supplements may be required when antibiotics, sulfa drugs, or mineral oil are used, or in the presence of gallstones, liver disease, severe diarrhea, or colitis.

**DEFICIENCY
SYMPTOMS**

Normal blood clotting does not occur. Increased bleeding and hemorrhage. Vitamin K protects you from literally bleeding to death when you are injured.

HORMONE INTERACTIONS

K works with growth hormones.

**INTERACTIONS WITH OTHER
VITAMINS AND MINERALS**

K works with E.

VITAMIN P (Citrus bioflavonoids, rutin, hesperidin)

**APPROXIMATE
DAILY REQUIREMENT.
MOST ADULTS UNDER
NORMAL CONDITIONS**

The need in human nutrition has not been established.

**CONDITIONS THAT
INCREASE NEED**

Reported to be useful in conjunction with C for skin hemorrhages, gum problems, and hot flashes.

**DEFICIENCY
SYMPTOMS**

Capillary weakness that is resistant to C treatment alone.

**BEST FOOD
SOURCES**

Found in the peel and juice of citrus fruit and some vegetables.

HORMONE INTERACTIONS

May intensify some of C's normalizing effects on adrenal, pituitary and other target tissues. This may help explain its reported usefulness in hot flashes, as may its effect in strengthening capillaries.

**INTERACTIONS WITH OTHER
VITAMINS AND MINERALS**

May help prevent the destruction of C in the body.

SYMPTOMS OF EXCESS

Possible blood clots, vomiting.

BEST FOOD SOURCES

The vitamin is stable to cooking and oxidation, but is lost when foods are irradiated, as they are in some sterilization processes. K occurs in cabbage, cauliflower, soybeans, spinach, other vegetables, organ meats, strawberries and whole grains.

THERAPEUTIC DOSE RANGE

Dosages of 5 mg. or more are sometimes administered by doctors but should never be self-prescribed.

Some doctors prescribe it temporarily when they insert an IUD.

OTHER COMMENTS

Vitamin K is used to treat mothers in labor, newborn infants with neonatal hemorrhage, and persons who have been overdosed with anticoagulants, such as after a Pill-caused blood clot, or in the presence of heart disease.

K is used experimentally as a painkiller.

Vitamins K and C taken together may combat the nausea of morning sickness.

SYMPTOMS OF EXCESS

Possibly citrus allergies. Some people who can handle C alone get rashes from bioflavonoids, in natural foods or supplements.

THERAPEUTIC DOSE RANGE

Usually taken in proportion to C. For each 500 mg. of C take:
bioflavonoids—100 mg.
rutin   — 50 mg.
hesperidin   — 25 mg.

Pill users and convalescents with gum problems or easy bruising should take supplements in the amounts and proportions above.

For hot flashes the supplements should be taken in smaller amounts but in the same proportions.

For capillary problems and gum and tooth problems the smaller amounts and standard proportions should be used.

Users of the IUD and those with excessive menstruation should follow the formula above.

The P factors are clearly most helpful for people with gum disease, excessively heavy menstrual periods, and, in some cases, hot flashes. Those who use C supplements not containing the P factors should also take citrus fruit or juice to assure ingestion of some P's.

Many doctors prescribe 200–500 mg. when an IUD is inserted, and to help control spotting and heavy menstruation.

CALCIUM

APPROXIMATE DAILY REQUIREMENT. MOST ADULTS UNDER NORMAL CONDITIONS

800 mg.
Some nutritionists recommend up to 1,000 mg.

CONDITIONS THAT INCREASE NEED

Pregnancy, nursing, menopause, emotional stress, lack of exercise, and working hard in areas of high temperature increase the need for calcium. A high-protein diet may also increase the need for calcium.

DEFICIENCY SYMPTOMS

Abnormal nerve sensitivity, convulsions, loss of height, susceptibility to bone fractures (osteoporosis), and low back pain in middle-aged and elderly women, softening of the bones (osteomalacia).

THERAPEUTIC DOSE RANGE

Studies suggest postmenopausal women should consume roughly 1,500 mg. of calcium to avoid osteoporosis and osteomalacia.

An increased calcium intake may also help eliminate the pain of Paget's disease and arthritis and reduce the bone loss associated with periodontal disease (inflammation of the gums and underlying bone).

Women experiencing severe menstrual cramps report relief when they take additional calcium.

1,200 mg. a day is recommended for pregnant women and nursing mothers.

HORMONE INTERACTIONS

The body's estrogen level affects calcium absorption. In premenopausal women, who have high estrogen levels, calcium absorption is good. Postmenopausal women, on the other hand, absorb calcium poorly.

SYMPTOMS OF EXCESS

Very few people experience harmful effects from large amounts of calcium. Abnormal deposits of calcium in soft tissues usually result from concurrent low magnesium intakes rather than high calcium. A few studies suggest that extremely high intakes may interfere with the body's use of phosphorus, fat, iodine, zinc, magnesium and iron when levels of those nutrients are low.

BEST FOOD SOURCES

Milk and most other dairy products are rich sources of calcium. Because skim milk (88 calories in 1 cup) and buttermilk (88 calories in 1 cup) are low in fat and calories, they are excellent sources for dieters. Salmon (canned with bones), sardines (canned with bones), soybeans, tempeh, tofu, filberts, almonds, broccoli and dark green, leafy vegetables (collard, turnip and mustard greens and kale) are other good sources.

INTERACTIONS WITH OTHER VITAMINS AND MINERALS

Adequate levels of vitamin D and equal amounts of calcium and phosphorus are necessary for proper absorption of calcium.

Vitamin C may also aid the absorption of calcium.

High fluoride intakes deplete calcium by increasing its excretion.

Large intakes of calcium depress manganese absorption.

OTHER COMMENTS

Large amounts of protein may hinder calcium absorption. Oxalic acid in spinach, chard, rhubarb and other foods, and phytic acid in whole grains and legumes combine with calcium and impair its absorption.

CHROMIUM

APPROXIMATE DAILY REQUIREMENT. MOST ADULTS UNDER NORMAL CONDITIONS

No requirement has been established, but 50–200 mcg. has been provisionally approved by the National Research Council.

CONDITIONS THAT INCREASE NEED

Diabetes, menopause.

DEFICIENCY SYMPTOMS

Changes in sugar metabolism leading to intolerance, diabetes, and decreased storage. Also abnormal amino acid metabolism, retarded growth, and damage to the main artery from the heart associated with high cholesterol levels.

HORMONE INTERACTIONS

Chromium may augment the action of insulin.

INTERACTIONS WITH OTHER VITAMINS AND MINERALS

No information available.

COPPER

APPROXIMATE DAILY REQUIREMENT. MOST ADULTS UNDER NORMAL CONDITIONS

No requirement has been set by the National Research Council but 2–3 mg. a day is the estimated safe and adequate range.

CONDITIONS THAT INCREASE NEED

Iron deficiency anemia, high intakes of zinc or vitamin C, and a diet high in fat and sugar and low in fiber.

BEST FOOD SOURCES

Beef liver, pecans, almonds and walnuts are rich sources. Other good sources are barley, mushrooms, green leafy vegetables, dried beans, whole grains, bananas, halibut and chicken.

THERAPEUTIC DOSE RANGE

No specific information is available; however, a copper supplement may be used along with iron in the treatment of anemia.

HORMONE INTERACTIONS

The level of copper in the blood increases with pregnancy or the use of contraceptives, so that Pill or estrogen users or those recovering from hormone therapy should avoid copper supplements.

INTERACTIONS WITH OTHER VITAMINS AND MINERALS

Copper may play an important role in preventing anemia by making iron usable.

Large amounts of copper are associated with decreased vitamin A levels in the blood and a lowered absorption of zinc.

SYMPTOMS OF EXCESS

There is no current evidence of toxicity from excessive intakes of chromium. Some nutritionists are unsure about its interactions with other nutrients and discourage the use of supplements. Inhalation of chromium from industrial waste can be toxic.

BEST FOOD SOURCES

Vegetables, whole grains and fruits are good sources of chromium. Refined foods contain smaller amounts of chromium than less refined products.

THERAPEUTIC DOSE RANGE

Nutritionists suggest a minimum of 10–20 mcg. a day.

OTHER COMMENTS

Chromium plays a role in the metabolism of fats.

DEFICIENCY SYMPTOMS

Severe deficiency in adults seems to be rare although it has been observed in malnourished infants. Symptoms included poor iron absorption, a decreased number of white blood cells, loss of minerals from bone and defective red blood cell formation.

An inherited condition of faulty copper absorption, Menke's kinky hair syndrome, is characterized by slow growth, degeneration of brain tissue and stubby white hair.

Study results suggest that a high ratio of zinc to copper in the diet, or a copper deficiency, may lead to heart disease.

SYMPTOMS OF EXCESS

Intakes of copper salts at levels 10 times that found in a normal diet cause nausea and vomiting. Wilson's disease is a hereditary condition in which copper accumulates in the liver, brain, kidneys and cornea of the eyes where brown or green rings become visible.

OTHER COMMENTS

In areas where water is soft, copper may leach into household supplies from copper plumbing. Have your water tested for minerals if you think you may be getting too much copper.

FLUORINE

APPROXIMATE DAILY REQUIREMENT. MOST ADULTS UNDER NORMAL CONDITIONS

Although no requirement has been established by the National Research Council, 1.5–4.0 mg. is the estimated safe and adequate range.

CONDITIONS THAT INCREASE NEED

Pregnancy, osteoporosis (brittle bones), lack of exercise, periodontal (gum) disease, and possibly the healing of wounds.

DEFICIENCY SYMPTOMS

Lowered resistance to tooth decay.

THERAPEUTIC DOSE RANGE

Fluoridation of drinking water at a rate of 1 ppm seems to reduce tooth decay. In areas where water is not fluoridated or contains little natural fluoride, a supplement of 0.1–1 mg. is proposed for infants up to a year old, and 0.5–2.5 mg. is suggested for children up to the age of 11. Authorities disagree over whether fluoride supplements prevent tooth decay in adults.

Although 50 mg. a day may improve calcium balance, increase bone formation and prevent osteoporosis, 10 mg. or more should be taken only with instructions from a physician.

HORMONE INTERACTIONS

No information available.

IODINE

APPROXIMATE DAILY REQUIREMENT. MOST ADULTS UNDER NORMAL CONDITIONS

150 mcg.

CONDITIONS THAT INCREASE NEED

Pregnancy and nursing; living in an area where the soil is iodine-poor; eating large amounts of foods that block the absorption or use of iodine, such as rutabagas, turnips and cabbage.

DEFICIENCY SYMPTOMS

Minor deficiencies may produce lethargy, chilliness, dry skin, husky voice, fatigue, low blood pressure and weight gain.

Major deficiencies cause an enlarged thyroid gland (goiter) in adults and cretinism (mental retardation, stunted growth, thick, dry, pasty skin and a large protruding stomach) in children born to women with low iodine intake during pregnancy.

HORMONE INTERACTIONS

Iodine is an integral part of the thyroid hormone thyroxine, and plays a major part in regulating growth, development and the rate of metabolism.

SYMPTOMS OF EXCESS

Too much fluorine may cause brown stains on the teeth. If the overdose is extreme, tooth enamel may become pitted; the teeth will appear stained and corroded.

Prolonged high intake may result in large stores of fluorine in the bones and teeth. In extreme cases abnormal hardening of bone (osteosclerosis), calcification of joints, or growth retardation may occur. Death can result at levels 2,500 times higher than the recommended amounts.

Study results that suggest a link between fluoridation and cancer are inconclusive.

BEST FOOD SOURCES

Rice, buckwheat, soybeans, spinach, onions, mackerel, salmon (canned), sardines (canned), watercress and wheat germ are excellent sources.

INTERACTIONS WITH OTHER VITAMINS AND MINERALS

Fluorine protects against the effects of magnesium deficiency and with calcium helps strengthen bones and teeth. Too much fluorine, however, increases calcium and magnesium excretion.

OTHER COMMENTS

Since fluorine in the diet of a pregnant woman does little to protect the primary teeth of her unborn child against cavities, supplementary fluorine is recommended for infants in areas where the water is not fluoridated.

SYMPTOMS OF EXCESS

Too much iodine causes the thyroid gland to work overtime and the result is the same as with too little—an enlarged thyroid.

An extremely high intake may cause death.

BEST FOOD SOURCES

Saltwater fish and kelp are good sources of iodine.

THERAPEUTIC DOSE RANGE

175 mcg. a day for pregnant women and 200 mcg. a day for nursing mothers.

INTERACTIONS WITH OTHER VITAMINS AND MINERALS

Iodine plays a role in the conversion of carotene to the active form, vitamin A.

OTHER COMMENTS

The conversion of iodide to iodine, its usable form, is reduced by large amounts of PABA (para-aminobenzoic acid), part of the vitamin B complex.

IRON

APPROXIMATE DAILY REQUIREMENT. MOST ADULTS UNDER NORMAL CONDITIONS

18 mg. for women.

CONDITIONS THAT INCREASE NEED

Rapid growth, pregnancy, blood loss such as from surgery, blood donation, internal hemorrhage, or menorrhagia (heavy menstrual flow), living at high altitudes, steatorrhea (a condition in which higher than normal amounts of fat are excreted), peptic ulcers, colitis and hemorrhoids.

DEFICIENCY SYMPTOMS

Iron deficiency results in anemia, a reduction in the quantity and/or quality of red blood cells. The symptoms of anemia are pale skin, weakness and fatigue, headache, labored breathing with exertion, and heart palpitations. Other deficiency symptoms are a lowered resistance to infection, mouth soreness, decreased work capacity, behavioral changes such as apathy and irritability, and a decreased secretion of acid in the stomach.

THERAPEUTIC DOSE RANGE

IUD users often require 5 times the normal requirement of iron (about 100 mg. a day).

The use of 30–60 mg. of supplemental iron is suggested for pregnant women. Supplementation should continue for 2–3 months after the baby is born in order to replenish stores drained by pregnancy and childbirth.

Therapeutic doses for anemia may be as high as 250 mg.

HORMONE INTERACTIONS

Blood levels of iron may increase in women taking oral contraceptives.

INTERACTIONS WITH OTHER VITAMINS AND MINERALS

Vitamin C greatly enhances the absorption of iron.

Copper may stimulate the absorption of iron and may be used with iron in the treatment of anemia.

Iron decreases the absorption of manganese.

SYMPTOMS OF EXCESS

The iron content of the body is regulated by absorption on demand. When your stores of iron are low, you'll absorb more; when your supply is high, you'll absorb less.

An excessive intake of iron can cause siderosis, a condition in which excess iron accumulates in the liver and spleen (its normal storage sites), and tissue and blood levels of iron rise. People with siderosis have an increased susceptibility to infection.

Hemochromatosis is an inherited iron storage disease which affects less than $\frac{1}{10}$ of 1% of the population. These people absorb too much iron and it accumulates in tissues that don't normally store iron. Symptoms include gray skin color, breakdown of liver function, liver enlargement and scarring, diabetes and heart failure.

BEST FOOD SOURCES

Rich sources of iron are apricots, blackstrap molasses, brewer's yeast, green leafy vegetables, legumes, nuts, organ meats, sunflower seeds and wheat germ. For example, 3 oz. of liver has 7.5 mg. of iron; ½ cup of dried apricots has 3.6 mg.; 1 tbsp. of blackstrap molasses 3.2 mg.; and ½ cup of lima beans 2.2 mg.

Iron from animal sources is absorbed better than that from grains or vegetables. Combining meat with vegetable sources aids absorption.

OTHER COMMENTS

Because diets high in fiber decrease the utilization of iron, it may be wise to take iron supplements before meals.

Eating a combination of meat and vegetables enhances the absorption of iron from the vegetables by 2–3 times. The amino acid cysteine in meat is responsible for the boost.

MAGNESIUM

**APPROXIMATE
DAILY REQUIREMENT.
MOST ADULTS UNDER
NORMAL CONDITIONS**

300 mg. for women. Some nutritionists recommend 420 mg. a day.

**CONDITIONS THAT
INCREASE NEED**

Prolonged diarrhea or vomiting, magnesium-deficient liquid diets during postoperative periods, large amounts of alcohol, and the use of diuretics.

**DEFICIENCY
SYMPTOMS**

Irritability, nervousness, muscle tremors, convulsions, the calcification of soft tissues, dilation of blood vessels, foot and leg cramps, irregular pulse, muscle weakness, and skin, bone, teeth and kidney changes.

HORMONE INTERACTIONS

The hormone aldosterone (secreted by the adrenal gland) regulates magnesium excretion, while the parathyroid hormone regulates absorption.

**INTERACTIONS WITH OTHER
VITAMINS AND MINERALS**

Large amounts of fluoride or zinc deplete magnesium by increasing its excretion.

MANGANESE

**APPROXIMATE
DAILY REQUIREMENT.
MOST ADULTS UNDER
NORMAL CONDITIONS**

No requirement has been set, but 2.5–5.0 mg. has been established as a provisional safe and adequate range by the National Research Council.

**CONDITIONS THAT
INCREASE NEED**

Pill or estrogen use.

**DEFICIENCY
SYMPTOMS**

Reproductive problems, congenital defects in the fetus, growth retardation in children; also impaired sugar tolerance and abnormal formation of bone and cartilage.

HORMONE INTERACTIONS

Manganese is essential to milk production in nursing mothers. It also seems to affect the ovaries as well as the adrenals, liver and pancreas.

**INTERACTIONS WITH OTHER
VITAMINS AND MINERALS**

Manganese is involved in the conversion of vitamin B_{12} to its active form. Iron inhibits absorption, and iron deficiency increases absorption. Large amounts of calcium also decrease absorption.

SYMPTOMS OF EXCESS

Magnesium acts as a muscle relaxant; at extremely high blood levels, coma and eventually heart failure occur.

BEST FOOD SOURCES

Green leafy vegetables (kale, spinach, collard, beet and turnip greens), molasses, nuts, peas, brown rice, soybeans and whole grains are excellent sources.

THERAPEUTIC DOSE RANGE

450 mg. a day is recommended for pregnant women and nursing mothers.

OTHER COMMENTS

In areas where drinking water contains high levels of magnesium (hard water), the death rate from heart disease is lower than it is in areas with soft water.

Alcohol and diuretics increase the rate of magnesium excretion.

Phytic acid in whole grains and legumes may impair magnesium absorption.

SYMPTOMS OF EXCESS

No toxic reactions have been observed from high dietary intakes, but inhaled manganese affects the central nervous system. Toxicity is known only in workers exposed to a high concentration of manganese dust. Psychological and motor difficulties are signs of high tissue levels.

BEST FOOD SOURCES

Nuts, legumes and whole grains are rich sources; vegetables and fruits are moderately good sources.

THERAPEUTIC DOSE RANGE

Some specialists recommend that women on the Pill take 1 mg. a day.

OTHER COMMENTS

High levels of dietary protein may protect against manganese toxicity.

PHOSPHORUS

APPROXIMATE DAILY REQUIREMENT. MOST ADULTS UNDER NORMAL CONDITIONS

800 mg.
Some nutritionists suggest 1,000 mg.

CONDITIONS THAT INCREASE NEED

Pregnancy, nursing, excessive consumption of antacids and large losses of phosphorus in the urine.

DEFICIENCY SYMPTOMS

Since phosphorus is very widespread in foods, deficiencies are rare. Symptoms of low levels are fatigue, loss of appetite, and loss of minerals from bone.

INTERACTIONS WITH OTHER VITAMINS AND MINERALS

Vitamin D facilitates the absorption of phosphorus from the intestines and decreases losses in the urine.
Too much iron and magnesium interfere with absorption of phosphorus.

To be effective, many of the B vitamins must combine with phosphorus in the body.
Ideally, the intakes of calcium and phosphorus should be the same.

HORMONE INTERACTIONS

Estrogens tend to increase the phosphorus content of bones but reduce blood levels of the mineral.

POTASSIUM

APPROXIMATE DAILY REQUIREMENT. MOST ADULTS UNDER NORMAL CONDITIONS

No requirement has been established by the National Research Council, but about 2–6 g. is the estimated safe and adequate range. Some nutritionists propose 2.5 g. as a minimum requirement.

CONDITIONS THAT INCREASE NEED

Diarrhea, vomiting, use of diuretics, excessive perspiration, severe malnutrition and surgery can lead to potassium deficiency. Women who are Pill or estrogen users, those who have recently stopped taking hormones, those over 40, those with osteoporosis, or who have menstrual distress or the loss of menstruation also need more potassium.

DEFICIENCY SYMPTOMS

Muscular weakness, abnormal nerve sensitivity, heart irregularities, mental disorientation, abdominal bloating.

INTERACTIONS WITH OTHER VITAMINS AND MINERALS

Potassium acts with magnesium to relax muscles. Too little magnesium can lead to decreased retention of potassium.
Excessive intakes of sodium may have the same effect as low levels of potassium.

SYMPTOMS OF EXCESS

A high intake of phosphorus interferes with the calcium-phosphorus balance and increases the body's need for calcium.

Diets ample in meat, which is high in phosphorus, may lead to osteoporosis (brittle bones) especially if calcium intake is low.

BEST FOOD SOURCES

Foods that are rich in protein—meat, fish, poultry, eggs, milk, cheese, nuts and legumes—are also rich in phosphorus. Cereal grains, although they're high in phosphorus, are poor sources because much of the phosphorus is present as phytic acid which is not well utilized.

THERAPEUTIC DOSE RANGE

Pregnant women and nursing mothers should increase their intake to 1,200 mg.

OTHER COMMENTS

Soft drinks and other processed foods contain large amounts of phosphorus and in large quantities may disturb the calcium-phosphorus balance.

SYMPTOMS OF EXCESS

When the level of potassium in the blood is too high (often due to the failure of the kidneys to excrete it), muscular coordination is disturbed, heart irregularities develop and, in serious cases, heart attack may be the result.

HORMONE INTERACTIONS

Aldosterone, a hormone produced in the adrenal glands, regulates the excretion of potassium. Cortisone, another adrenal hormone, and prednisone, a synthetic hormone similar to cortisone, increase potassium excretion.

BEST FOOD SOURCES

Potassium is found in a wide range of foods, but because it's very soluble, large amounts may leach into cooking water.

Fruits and vegetables—apricots, bananas, oranges, cantaloupe, broccoli, potatoes—are rich sources of potassium. Beef, salmon, halibut, chicken, blackstrap molasses and brewer's yeast are other good sources.

THERAPEUTIC DOSE RANGE

About 5,150 mg. is used as the standard dose for patients on diuretic therapy.

OTHER COMMENTS

Potassium plays a major role in the regulation of body fluids, the transmission of nerve impulses and the release of insulin from the pancreas.

SELENIUM

APPROXIMATE DAILY REQUIREMENT. MOST ADULTS UNDER NORMAL CONDITIONS

No requirement has been set by the National Research Council, but 50–200 mcg. is the estimated safe and adequate range.

CONDITIONS THAT INCREASE NEED

Exposure to toxic metals—silver, mercury, cadmium (a component of cigarette smoke) and possibly lead. Aftereffects of the Pill, hot flashes or other menopause complaints.

DEFICIENCY SYMPTOMS

Recent investigations suggest that low levels of selenium may be associated with heart disease and cancer.

THERAPEUTIC DOSE RANGE

150–200 mcg. a day is the supplemental dose range suggested by one specialist. Others recommend taking only 25 mcg. Some authorities say it's advisable to take selenium with vitamin E. For example, one source suggests taking 25 mcg. for each 200 I.U. of E.

HORMONE INTERACTIONS

No information available.

SODIUM

APPROXIMATE DAILY REQUIREMENT. MOST ADULTS UNDER NORMAL CONDITIONS

No requirement has been established by the National Research Council, but 1,100–3,300 mg. is the provisional safe and adequate range. There is no evidence that large intakes of sodium are beneficial, and a low-salt diet begun early in life may protect those who risk developing high blood pressure later.

CONDITIONS THAT INCREASE NEED

Recurrent vomiting or diarrhea. Hard physical work in high temperatures may increase need because sodium is lost in perspiration. Loss should be replaced by eating foods naturally high in sodium. Studies indicate that more sodium is necessary during pregnancy and suggest that a moderate intake may actually relieve the symptoms of toxemia—high blood pressure, edema (fluid retention), blurred vision. Most people in the United States consume too much sodium, so we don't recommend increasing intake.

THERAPEUTIC DOSE RANGE

Dietary restrictions limiting sodium to 200–700 mg. a day are often recommended for hypertension and kidney disorders.

HORMONE INTERACTIONS

The hormone aldosterone regulates the sodium level in the body.

SYMPTOMS OF EXCESS

Discolored teeth, skin eruptions, brittle nails, edema (fluid retention), stomach and intestinal disorders, and partial or total loss of hair have been observed in people living in areas where environmental levels of selenium are very high.

Selenium poisoning sometimes occurs in people exposed to industrial dust containing the element.

Apparently, selenium replaces sulfur in several amino acids and inhibits the action of some proteins.

BEST FOOD SOURCES

Fish, liver and kidney are rich sources of selenium. Whole grains are also excellent, but fruits and vegetables are poor.

Selenium is volatile and may be lost during cooking.

INTERACTIONS WITH OTHER VITAMINS AND MINERALS

Selenium works with vitamin E to boost the body's immune system and to protect cells from oxidation.

OTHER COMMENTS

The requirement for selenium may rise as the dietary intake of unsaturated fats increases. Selenium resembles sulfur and frequently replaces it in sulfur-containing amino acids (the building blocks of protein). That may be why selenium is used in treating children with kwashiorkor (a protein deficiency disease).

DEFICIENCY SYMPTOMS

Dietary deficiencies are rare under ordinary circumstances.

When a combined loss of sodium and water occurs, low blood pressure, low blood volume, muscular cramps, weakness, headache, loss of appetite, a high concentration of red cells in the blood and vascular collapse can result.

SYMPTOMS OF EXCESS

Large intakes, habitually consumed, have been implicated in high blood pressure.

BEST FOOD SOURCES

Foods of animal origin—pork, liver, cheese, milk—are usually higher in sodium than those of plant origin. Processed foods often contain more sodium than natural foods. For example, potato chips have 3–10 times more sodium than baked potatoes.

INTERACTIONS WITH OTHER VITAMINS AND MINERALS

Sodium works with potassium to maintain a proper water balance in the body.

ZINC

APPROXIMATE DAILY REQUIREMENT. MOST ADULTS UNDER NORMAL CONDITIONS

15 mg.

CONDITIONS THAT INCREASE NEED

Infections, pernicious anemia (a reduced number of red blood cells caused by poor vitamin B_{12} absorption), overactive thyroid, pregnancy, nursing and the use of oral contraceptives.

DEFICIENCY SYMPTOMS

Growth retardation, delayed sexual maturation, slow wound healing, loss of sense of taste (which is usually accompanied by a loss of appetite and sense of smell), skin and hair problems, poor resistance to infection, infertility and diabetes. Zinc deficiency during pregnancy may cause fetal abnormalities.

THERAPEUTIC DOSE RANGE

20 mg. a day is recommended for pregnant women, 25 mg. a day for nursing mothers. A study of the role of oral zinc in the treatment of acne showed that a supplement of 135 mg. of zinc substantially decreased acne scars.

HORMONE INTERACTIONS

Oral contraceptives reduce zinc levels in the blood. Women with skin problems associated with menopause may require additional zinc.

INTERACTIONS WITH OTHER VITAMINS AND MINERALS

Vitamin D tends to increase the absorption of zinc. High levels of calcium and copper, on the other hand, result in decreased absorption. Zinc seems to play a role in maintaining normal blood levels of vitamin A by releasing it from storage in the liver. Zinc may also aid in the absorption of folate.

SYMPTOMS OF EXCESS

Toxicity may occur with supplementation of 2 g. or more of zinc sulfate. Symptoms include stomach irritation and vomiting. Excess ingestion of zinc may also occur from storage of food and beverages in galvanized containers. The resulting symptoms are fever, nausea, vomiting and diarrhea.

Inhalation of zinc chloride from industrial pollution has also been associated with toxicity.

Anemia from iron and copper loss may result when zinc reaches toxic levels.

BEST FOOD SOURCES

Diets high in animal protein supply large amounts of zinc, but those containing mostly carbohydrates and vegetable proteins provide much less. Good sources of zinc are meats, liver, milk, cheese, wheat germ and whole grains, eggs, nuts, green beans and lima beans. Processed foods contain little zinc.

OTHER COMMENTS

Phytic acid in whole grains and legumes interferes with zinc absorption.

However, zinc from leavened whole wheat bread is absorbed 30%–50% better than from unleavened bread.

WEIGHT CONTROL

Practically every woman we know has dieted, is dieting, or flirts with the idea of taking off a few pounds—"starting tomorrow." So why is it, with so many "losing," only a relatively small number manage to win the battle of the bulge? Quite simply, the reason is that most diets just do not work.

Let's face it, getting through six months on the average weight reduction scheme is enough to leave you slated for sainthood. It demands perfection, supernatural self-deprivation, and will-power worthy of Joan of Arc.

What's worse, most of these diet regimens wreak havoc with your health. Crash dieting, for example, is the quickest way to bring your nutritional stores crashing down to rock bottom. Many dieters become dangerously depleted in B complex factors particularly by concentrating on fruits and vegetables while going light on meat and totally avoiding "starchy" foods such as bread, spaghetti, rice, potatoes, and beans. If milk, cheese, and other dairy products have also been restricted, a B complex deficiency becomes almost a certainty.

You might be shortchanging yourself on essential minerals as well. Calcium, magnesium and iron reserves can plummet along with your weight on a sharply restricted diet.

The result of all this? Aching bones or joints (a likely result of a calcium deficiency); irritability, depression, and generally poor nerves (produced by a calcium and/or B complex deficiency); unusually severe menstrual cramps (another sign of a calcium or B vitamin deficiency); and fatigue (which can be produced by any combination of deficiencies of magnesium, iron, and B complex). Sound like anyone you know?

And as if that weren't bad enough, consider this: the type of diet which restricts your caloric intake to less than 1,000 per day or totally eliminates either fats or carbohydrates (as does the Atkins diet) can drive your metabolism to the brink of cannibalism. Your body needs a certain amount of calories each day to use for essential functions. If your diet fails to satisfy this appetite, your body may turn not only to available fat stores, but it also could devour muscle or organ protein as well. That's hardly a healthful diet plan!

But, imagine, if you can, a diet that *doesn't* demand radical changes in your taste or lifestyle or rob you of your health; one that allows flexibility and choice and provides ample calories to carry on normally; and, best of all, a diet that brings about a *permanent* weight loss.

Sound too good to be true? It's not. The trick is to concentrate on *patterns*, not pounds.

We read several good books on this "behavioral" approach to weight control. But for the following, we have drawn primarily on just one—*Lose Weight Naturally* by Mark Bricklin (Rodale Press, 1979)—because it is the most comprehensive and practical book of its type. Besides, Mark Bricklin makes losing weight interesting and fun. What other weight control book have you picked up lately that played down *what* you eat and instead stressed the importance of *why* and *when* you eat?

For many of us, says Mark, eating is

just another ugly habit like nail biting. Too often, we eat because we are bored, anxious or depressed—least of all because we are genuinely hungry. Next time you reach for a Milky Way or Egg McMuffin at midmorning ask yourself, Why? If it's for hunger, then please, be our guest. But if it's out of habit, stop right there. The calories you consume for hunger's sake are burned on request. Those that are lured into our bodies by neuroses tend to give us the outward appearance of a padded cell.

Develop Some Anti-Fattening Habits

Instead of feeding your face, calm your fears with productive, nonfattening habits. Delve into some latent interest—perhaps an old and enjoyable pastime that you had to abandon when the kids were born. Or something completely new that's a real challenge to your senses. How about jogging? As any serious runner will tell you, jogging can become an obsession—and that's good because it replaces that obsession so many of us have with food. What's more, jogging can be doubly valuable because it helps you burn calories.

Gardening is another good choice. All that stooping and bending—not to mention shuffling bundles of peat and wheelbarrows of soil—more than makes up for the deep knee bends, toe touches, and push-ups you haven't been able to find time for. Best of all, gardening gets you out of the house—and out of the kitchen—so you're not tempted by the fate that awaits you behind the refrigerator door. Besides, any activity that keeps your hands dirty keeps you from binging on a break.

Or maybe it's not boredom at all—maybe you eat because you feel guilty. Guilty because you slaved so

IDEAL WEIGHTS FOR ADULTS (Age 25 and over)

WEIGHT IN POUNDS (IN INDOOR CLOTHING)

Height (in 2-inch heels)	Small Frame	Medium Frame	Large Frame
WOMEN			
4' 10"	92–98	96–107	104–119
11"	94–101	98–110	106–122
5' 0"	96–104	101–113	109–125
1"	99–107	104–116	112–128
2"	102–110	107–119	115–131
3"	105–113	110–122	118–134
4"	108–116	113–126	121–138
5"	111–119	116–130	125–142
6"	114–123	120–135	129–146
7"	118–127	124–139	133–150
8"	122–131	128–143	137–154
9"	126–135	132–147	141–158
10"	130–140	136–151	145–163
11"	134–144	140–155	149–168
6' 0"	138–148	144–159	153–173

SOURCE: *Metropolitan Life Insurance Company. Statistical Bulletin.* October, 1977. (Based on Build and Blood Pressure Study, 1959, Society of Actuaries.)
NOTE: This chart is intended only as a general guideline; it is by no means absolute. Technically, your "ideal" weight is the one at which you feel most comfortable. Most people feel weak if their weight drops too far, sluggish if it rises too high. The key is to find the optimum weight for your own body. Don't worry if that happens to be 10 pounds more or less than the figure set forth by the Metropolitan Life Insurance Company. Another thing to consider is your proportion of fat to muscle. Muscle weighs more than fat. So it's perfectly conceivable that a woman who weighs in at a toned 130 may look slimmer and feel better than another woman of the same height who weighs maybe a few pounds less but whose body build leans more toward fat than muscle.

hard in the kitchen? Or guilty because of all those starving in India? Or just plain guilty about throwing food away? Well, here's your chance to get rid of those fattening feelings.

Step up to your refrigerator right now and select something worth trashing—preferably something with lots of calories like last night's leftover Boston cream pie. Take a good look at it and imagine what all those calories would look like on your waist or thighs or wherever you may need it least. Then say goodbye to it and toss it in the trash can. You might be surprised at how liberating an experience that little gesture can be. Do it the next time there's a slice of cake left on the plate or just one scoop of ice cream in the carton. If you're not hungry for it, don't eat it just because you feel guilty. Throw it out.

If you continually find your trash can swamped with leftovers, maybe you're cooking too much. I know, I grew up thinking food was love. So when I got married I showered my husband with food. It wasn't long before we both began putting on weight. Still I was stuck with a multitude of leftovers that invariably made their way to the hinterlands of the refrigerator never (or at least not in their edible form) to be seen again. One day, I came to the realization that I had to cut back on cooking. One-half cup of brown rice was all we ever ate, so that's all I made. One-half chicken breast each was all we really needed so if I couldn't find what I was looking for I got into the habit of ringing the bell at the meat counter and asking for a breakdown of a family pack. To fill in the appetite spaces, I made sure to toss a big salad with lots of nutritional surprises like raw broccoli, mushrooms, sprouts and watercress. We never came away from the table hungry and, as a bonus, we came away with more energy than we ever had before. But best of all, we both got back to our premarital weights—without ever having felt that we were on a diet, or ever having been deprived of food.

Out of Reach, Out of Mouth

You can also encourage weight-watching habits by putting high-calorie items and junk foods out of reach. If you must have soft drinks in the house, keep them in a secluded corner of the basement. When you want one, you'll have to walk for it. Next, organize your refrigerator so that the fattening item can be had only for a deep knee bend and a good stretch. Reserve eye-level shelves for healthy low-calorie munchies like carrots and celery and low-fat cottage cheese.

Then—and this is where you're going to have to exercise some self-discipline—allow yourself the privilege of eating *only* at the dining room table. Not in front of the TV. Not in the car. Not on the run. Whenever you're hungry (and remember, we *only* eat when we are hungry) take whatever food you've chosen to satisfy your appetite and sit down at the table with it. That goes for a carrot stick snack, too.

Think of eating as a very important activity and give it your undivided attention. Remember that the slower you eat, the *less* you're likely to eat. So chew slowly and savor each bite. If you find yourself chowing down a chicken pie like there's no tomorrow, try chopsticks to ease the pace. Or if you're right-handed, give lefty a chance; if you're left-handed, go right.

Postponing dinner for a few hours after work may give your five o'clock hunger pangs a chance to subside. Believe it or not, you'll devour that steak Diane with less famished fervor at seven or so than at five o'clock on the nose. Or better yet, make lunch your main meal. Eat light in the evening and fill up the leftover time with one of your hobbies or a brisk walk.

You're probably wondering how small changes in your lifestyle can result in big bonuses for your figure. Actually we're not promising a 10-pound drop in two weeks—nor would we want to. What we're aiming for is a modest weight reduction at first—perhaps 3 pounds a month if you're doing it by reduced food intake alone or 5 pounds a month if you're combining the dietary approach with exercise. That means a weight reduction of anywhere between 36 and 60 pounds in a year's time. Not bad—particularly when you consider that by incorporating these sensible eating patterns into your normal routine, your weight loss will be *permanent*.

Let's be more specific. No one likes to add up the calories in every apple and orange sherbet consumed. And there's no reason we have to. Instead let's begin by subtracting a few—say 300 a day.

The Easy-300 Plan for Slenderizing

Remember, the 300 calories that you will be removing must be from foods that are habitually or typically part of your daily diet. And they must fall into one of the following categories:

- Junk foods, which contribute nothing to your well-being.
- Foods that are typically consumed as snacks.
- Foods that can be divided in such a way that you can eat less of them without feeling deprived.
- Foods that are consumed as second helpings.
- Foods that don't give you a great sense of satisfaction.

CALORIC VALUES OF NATURAL VS. PROCESSED FOODS

NATURAL FOOD		CALORIES	PROCESSED FOOD		CALORIES
Carrots, sliced, cooked	½ cup	24	Carrots, canned	½ cup	35
Corn, fresh, cooked	½ cup	69	Corn, canned	½ cup	87
Peas, fresh, cooked	½ cup	57	Peas, canned	½ cup	82
Potato, baked (no butter)	1 long type	145	Potatoes, fried	1 cup	456
Whole wheat bread	1 slice	61	White bread	1 slice	74
Flank steak	4 ounces	223	Corned beef, canned	4 ounces	245
Flounder, broiled (no butter)	4 ounces	113	Fish sticks, breaded, baked	4 ounces	200
Blueberries, fresh	½ cup	45	Blueberries, canned in water	½ cup	98
Cherries, fresh	½ cup	41	Cherries, canned in syrup	½ cup	104
Grapefruit, fresh	½ medium	38	Grapefruit, canned in syrup	½ cup	89
Peach, fresh	1 medium	38	Peaches, canned in syrup	½ cup	100

SOURCE: Adapted from *Nutritive Value of American Foods in Common Units*, Agriculture Handbook No. 456, by Catherine F. Adams (Washington, D.C.: Agricultural Research Service, U.S. Department of Agriculture, 1975).

Got the idea? Of course you'll need to get yourself a good calorie-counting chart. But it shouldn't take you long to figure out where you can make up the difference. For example, by passing up that customary second slice of buttered toast at breakfast (110 calories), an extra slice of pizza for lunch (153 calories) and that last large forkful of apple pie at dinner (50 calories), you've just saved yourself 313 calories. Sometimes it's even easier: eliminate just one snack (which is eaten habitually). Did you know that one piece of marble cake contains 290 calories; one Hostess fruit pie, 460 calories; and six fig bar cookies, another 300 calories?

Another way to cut calories where you won't miss them is by turning more attention to natural foods. Natural foods (which are defined as any food to which no sugar, sweeteners, fats or oils have been added and no fiber removed) are much less fattening than processed or convenience foods. In fact, you can spare yourself 100, 200 or even more calories a day by emphasizing natural over processed (see "Caloric Values of Natural Vs. Processed Foods," page 561).

It's pretty obvious how added sugars and fats can contribute to your weight problem. But did you know that one of the major drawbacks of processed foods is that they lack fiber? Fiber is the indigestible portion of plants—the bran in the wheat and the bulky cell walls found in fresh vegetables, fruits, potatoes, beans and other natural foods. Its biggest advantage is that it fills you up on fewer calories.

A glass of apple juice isn't nearly as filling as an apple but it has just as many calories. Similarly, whole wheat bread contains about eight times more fiber than white, and you can subtract 10 calories for every whole wheat slice you substitute for white bread.

And there's an added bonus: fibrous foods actually reduce the extent to which you can absorb calories in your food. That most interesting fact was revealed in a study carried out jointly by the United States Department of Agriculture and the University of Maryland, and reported in 1978. A dozen adult men were put on a low-fiber diet for 26 days, and a high-fiber diet for another 26 days. Although their change in body weight, if any, was not reported, careful analysis revealed that on the high-fiber diet, there was a 4.8 percent decrease in calorie digestibility compared to the low-fiber diet. That's a percentage amounting to 86 fewer calories a day absorbed on a diet consisting of 1,800 calories, and 120 fewer calories a day absorbed from a diet of 2,500 calories.

As a final note on calorie variation in foods, let us remind you that all the good you do by selecting whole foods in the supermarket can be undone by how you treat those foods in the kitchen. For obvious reasons, you wouldn't take perfectly healthful and low-calorie broccoli or asparagus spears and lavish them with butter at 36 calories a pat. Or drown perfectly delectable strawberries in a dollop of whipped cream with 54 big ones. But what about those invisible calories floating in your frying pan? By tossing your potato into the deep fryer, you increase its calories by 300 percent (for more on this see section Cooking for Health).

A Little Exercise Makes Losing a Lot Easier

In describing a safe and natural method of weight control, we could stop here. After all, you can reduce simply by cutting back on your caloric intake. But if you're not stepping up your exercise program at the same time, you could be missing out on the most important reducing aid available. That's because exercise benefits our bodies in several ways. And, as figure-conscious females, we stand to gain the most.

For one thing, exercise burns calories. Let's suppose, for instance, that you are 50 years old and weigh at least 20 pounds more than you did 25 years ago. Perhaps your eating habits didn't change all that much—maybe you're even eating less—but, whether or not you realize it, your activity level has been slipping. You don't go dancing on Saturday nights anymore (250 calories). You quit your parttime waitressing job (12 hours a week at 2,280 calories). Your kids are grown and have moved out of the house, which means less household chores (say, 400 calories a week). And you've swapped your two-story "colonial"—where you climbed the stairs to bedrooms and bathroom and lugged your laundry down two flights to the basement—for the convenience of a "rancher" (climbing stairs burns more calories than almost any other activity—more than swimming, running, and so forth).

Still wondering why your weight's been creeping up on you?

Actually, exercise burns calories two ways. First, any type of physical exertion requires energy and the fuel for that energy comes from calories. Second, the kind of exercise that gets you huffin' and puffin' increases your basal metabolic rate, or the rate at which you burn calories for such basic chores as circulating

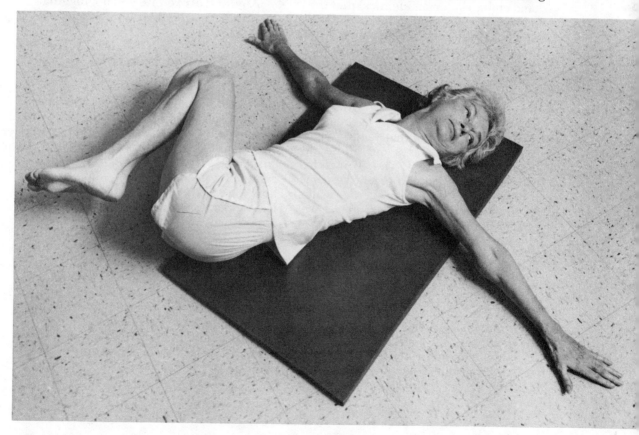

your blood, breathing, and digesting your food. And, interestingly enough, this increase in metabolic rate can continue for 30 minutes to several hours after exercise is discontinued, according to Edward Watt, Ph.D., cardiovascular physiologist at the Preventive Cardiology Clinic in Atlanta, Georgia. This explains why vigorous exercise seems to produce a calorie-loss bonus compared to very light exercise, like ironing, which does not really raise your metabolic rate.

As a woman, you should find this benefit particularly important. Maybe you've already noticed that even though your husband eats the same amount of food as you, he doesn't seem to gain weight as readily. Or maybe you were perplexed when both you and your husband embarked on an identical diet program but he beat you to his goal. Don't blame yourself. The reason may be your sluggish metabolism. Women generally have slower basal metabolic rates than men, we are told—which is one reason why vigorous exercise which helps give our metabolism a push is a girl's best friend.

Another reason is that regular vigorous exercise increases our ability to burn fat stores as fuel. The average female body is about 25 percent fat compared to 15 percent for the average male. And the older we get, the more fat we tend to store. So, exercise is important at all ages—but especially as we get on in years. It burns fat and builds lean muscle. And, even though muscle tends to weigh more than fat, the shift from fat to lean means just that; you'll be losing inches. "In my five years of running, even though I haven't lost any weight, my pants size has gone from 14 to 10," explains marathon runner Joan Ullyot, M.D. Most women, however, find that their weight and muscle tone *both* benefit from exercise.

To be honest, we can't tout exercise as a get-it-off-quick scheme. But that's actually good because the faster weight goes off, the quicker it usually comes back. And the slower it goes off, maybe, the slower it comes back. That may be even more true for weight loss through exercise than through dieting. In an important study of the effect of exercising alone, in which women lost weight at the rate of about half a pound a week, Grant Gwinup, M.D., noted that "once a certain amount of exercise had produced a certain amount of weight loss, that loss tended to be maintained with little tendency for a noticeable amount of weight to be regained" (*Archives of Internal Medicine*, May, 1975).

Any kind of exercise will do. Jogging. Tennis. Racquetball. As long as you do it often.

The Best Kind of Exercise Is the Easiest

Interestingly enough, however, the type of exercise the women in the above study took part in wasn't jogging, or strenuous calisthenics as you may have suspected. It was *walking*. And that's something all of us can do—no matter how long it's been since your last physical workout.

Walking is something that requires no special training, coordination, skill, or clothing. All you need to get started is a good, comfortable pair of shoes. Then start out gradually—maybe a 15-minute stroll around the neighborhood, gradually working up to a 30-minute walk and then an hour-long walk each day.

The number of calories you burn by walking depends on how much you weigh and where you're walking. If you are dawdling along at two miles per hour (which is the speed at which you'd be casually window shopping) you will be burning about 145 calories an hour if you weigh about 120 pounds, 185 calories if you weigh 150, and 215 calories if you're closer to 200 pounds. With moderate walking, at three miles an hour, you will burn between 235 and 350 calories depending on your weight. At four miles an hour, which is brisk walking, the kind you do when you're really serious about getting someplace, the values range between 270 and 400. If you're walking up a hill which is just steep enough to make you bend forward a little in order to balance yourself better, you would be burning up twice the number of calories that you would walking on the level.

Just because we're talking "walking," though, doesn't mean it's going to be easy. In order to lose weight by walking, you've got to walk more than 30 minutes every day. Actually, that's not asking a lot. A quick analysis of any schedule (no matter how busy) will reveal at least one half-hour period which can be better spent walking. It's something you've *got* to make time for.

With a little strategy, you can also work exercise into your routine without taking away precious time. If you drive a car to work, park a few blocks from the building and walk the extra distance. Instead of being spoiled by a laundry chute in your home, carry your dirty linen downstairs. While you're on the phone, do a few deep knee bends. Or make use of nail drying time by twisting at the waist and touching opposite toes.

Just think—simply by changing a few eating and exercise habits, you can slim down and stay there.

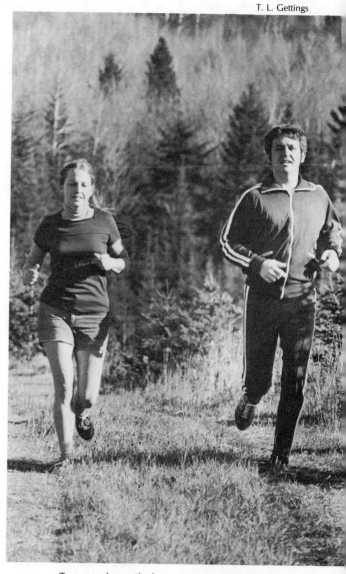

T. L. Gettings

To ease the guilt that your exercise program may be interfering with your family time, take your spouse (and children) along. Jogging, swimming, biking, even walking, are great activities to share.

CALORIE COSTS PER HOUR

ACTIVITY	WEIGHT (IN POUNDS)		
	110–125	150	180–200
CALISTHENICS	235	300	350
DANCING (in general)	240–250	270	300–450
DOMESTIC WORK Cleaning windows	180–195	210–250	295
Dinner preparation	105	135	155
Doing laundry —loading washer and dryer	125–150	160	190
—hanging clothes on line	190	245	285–300
—Ironing	160	205	235–240
Making beds	165–200	210–240	245–300
Shopping	130–150	165	195–200
Washing dishes —by hand	105	135	155
—dishwasher	60–85	110	130

SOURCES: Per-Olof Astrand and Kaare Rodahl, *Textbook of Work Physiology* (New York: McGraw-Hill, 1977). Benjamin T. Burton, *Human Nutrition*, 3d ed. (New York: McGraw-Hill, 1976). Carson C. Conrad, *How Different Sports Rate in Promoting Physical Fitness* (Washington, D.C.: President's Council on Physical Fitness and Sports, U.S. Department of Health, Education and Welfare, 1978). Helen Andrews Guthrie, *Introductory Nutrition*, 3d ed. (St. Louis: C. V. Mosby, 1975). Charles T. Kuntzleman, *Activetics* (New York: Peter H. Wyden, 1975). Charles T.

# of COMMON DAILY ACTIVITIES

EQUIVALENT ACTIVITIES AND REMARKS

1 hr. hiking with 20-lb. pack at 2 mph; ½ hr. of handball; 1 hr. swimming at easy pace. For optimum fitness, calisthenics should be combined to use muscles of the whole body in order to be as valuable as swimming, tennis, handball, etc. Begin with relaxation and limbering routine to warm up; after workout, use relaxation techniques again. Main disadvantage is that calisthenics can be boring unless done in groups or to music.

1 hr. of gardening; ¾ hr. bicycling at 10 mph. Calorie expenditure for dancing usually falls in the range of 270–460 and is governed by tempo of the music as well as individual style and enthusiasm.

1 hr. hanging clothes on line; 25 min. of rope skipping; 3 hrs. watching TV.

Basically the same as for standing only, unless you are whipping eggs, flipping a pizza shell, bending and opening drawers, etc.

2½ hr. watching TV; 50 min. waitressing. Ironing burns up considerably more calories than just standing, due to lifting and pushing the weight of the iron and hanging pressed clothes.

1 hr., 10 min. walking at 2 mph; 1 hr. of yoga; 1 hr. washing and polishing car; ¾ hr. swimming or calisthenics.

This is light shopping. Carrying heavy packages will increase calorie loss by 100.

Kuntzleman, *The Exerciser's Handbook* (New York: David McKay, 1978.) Nigel Oakley, ''Weight Control and Metabolism.'' *Cycling: The Healthy Alternative* (London: British Cycling Bureau, 1978). Roy J. Shephard, *Frontiers of Fitness* (Springfield, Ill.: Charles C. Thomas, 1971).

NOTE: Table prepared by Sharon Faelten.

ACTIVITY	WEIGHT (IN POUNDS)		
	110–125	**150**	**180–200**
DRESSING, UNDRESSING, WASHING, SHOWERING, BRUSHING HAIR	150–160	205	235
DRIVING A CAR (ranges given are automatic vs. standard)			
Light traffic	75–80	95–100	110–115
Heavy traffic	80–105	100–135	115–155
GARDENING Weeding, hoeing, digging, spading	240–305	300–390	400–450
HOUSE PAINTING	165	210	245
LAWN MOWING			
Push power mower	210	270	310
Riding mower	115	145	170
PIANO PLAYING	95	120	145
ROPE SKIPPING (75 skips/min.)	435	555	645
RUNNING			
Easy (5½ mph)	515	655	760
Moderate (8 mph)	625	800	930
Fast (11 mph)	955	1,220	1,420
Very fast (12½ mph)	1,220	1,550	1,805
SEX			
Foreplay	80	100	115
Intercourse			
—vigorous	235	300	350
—easy	105	135	155

EQUIVALENT ACTIVITIES AND REMARKS

In most cases, 1 hr. per day is taken up by these activities.

Attitude and zeal will dictate variations in calories lost here. 220 to 300 calories/hr. is a good rule of thumb, if you are hoeing beans or pampering azaleas.

1 hr. cleaning windows, light assembly-line work, or light carpentry; ¾ hr. tennis (doubles); 2¾ hr. watching TV.

Pushing your mower instead of riding on it will burn up almost twice as many calories.

A lively piece such as Liszt's "Tarantella" requires ⅓ more energy than Beethoven's "Appassionata" and 2½ times as much as Mendelssohn's songs.

1½ hr. walking at 4 mph or volleyball; 7 hr. watching TV. Do this as a "coffee break" to get your energy up and to avoid the donuts and Danish. Running shoes are advisable to avoid ankle and knee damage.

How far you run is more important than how fast you run. Unfit people should design a stretching and calisthenics program for themselves before taking up running in order to avoid knee pain, back pain, or muscle strains.

Burns slightly fewer calories than typing.
Same as hiking or swimming for the vigorous approach or piano playing for the easy approach.

ACTIVITY	WEIGHT (IN POUNDS)		
	110–125	150	180–200
SITTING	60	80	90
SLEEPING	50	65–80	80
SNOW SHOVELING (light)	475	610	710

SPORTS

	110–125	150	180–200
Bicycling (geared bike, average terrain)			
—easy (5 mph)	190	245	280
—moderate (10–12 mph)	240–325	270–415	300–475
—vigorous (13–15 mph)	515	660–720	760
Hiking (2 mph; 20-lb. pack)	235	300	350
Hill climbing	470	600	695
Skiing			
—cross-country (5 mph)	550	700	800
—downhill, excluding lifts	465	595	690
Swimming (1½ lengths)	425	540	630

EQUIVALENT ACTIVITIES AND REMARKS

1 hr. watching TV; 6 min. of handball; 20 min. of light assembly-line work or carpentry; 15 min. gardening; 13 min. walking at 4 mph.

Also equivalent to lying awake in bed. Does not vary much from basal metabolic rate.

1 hr. of handball; 2 hr. walking at 3 mph; tennis (doubles); or swimming at 20 mph at 20 yd./min.

Energy cost of sports are approximate, influenced by the vigor of the individual participant.

If you cycle 6 mi. to and from work instead of driving, taking about 30 min. each way, you could burn 15–20 lbs. of fat in a year.

4 hr. watching TV; 45 min. gardening; 1¼ hr. washing and polishing car; 1 hr. walking at 3 mph; 22 min. running at 8 mph; ½ hr. of handball; 40 min. of table tennis.

1 hr. of handball; 55 min. of moderate swimming; 3 hr. bowling; 1 hr. of downhill skiing, excluding lifts; 1¾ hr. of brisk walking.
Calorie cost is maximized by low temperatures. Excellent activity for fitness and endurance because skiing uses all major muscle groups. The amount of uphill skiing required by cross-country terrain will influence the number of calories burned.
Also uses practically all the muscle groups of the body. Should be balanced by some weight-bearing exercise such as running for all-around muscular development. If you cannot gauge your swimming speed, you can count on burning from 200 to 700 calories per hour. The butterfly stroke burns up the most calories, the crawl the least.

	WEIGHT (IN POUNDS)		
ACTIVITY	**110–125**	**150**	**180–200**
Table Tennis	355	360–450	525
Tennis (recreational) —doubles	235	300	350
—singles	335	425	495
Volleyball (recreational)	275	350	405
STANDING	105	135–140	155
TYPING	80–90	105–115	120–135
WAITRESSING	190	245	285
WALKING			
Easy (2 mph)	145	185	215
Moderate (3 mph)	235	300	350
Vigorous (4 mph)	270	345	405
YOGA	180	230	270

EQUIVALENT ACTIVITIES AND REMARKS

¾ hr. of handball; 6 hr. watching TV; 1½ hr. hiking at 2 mph with 20-lb. pack; 33 min. running at 8 mph.

Doubles: 1 hr. swimming at 20 yd./min.; 22 min. running at 8 mph.

Singles: 1 hr., 25 min. swimming at 20 yd./min.; 33 min. running at 8 mph.
Depends on how you play the game: if you run for every ball, you will burn more calories than an opponent who considers it a waste of time to run for a shot that will put him out of position.

1 hr. walking at 4 mph; 40 min. of rope skipping; 1 hr., 10 min. of calisthenics; ¾ hr. chopping wood by hand.

35 min. walking at 2 mph.

1 hr. washing and polishing car.

Calories burned by walking depend on type of surface (asphalt, grass, level, incline), type of clothing and wind resistance, as well as body weight. At approximately 3 mph, you burn 15% more calories walking on grass than on asphalt. Walking up a 15% grade burns up twice as many calories as walking on the level. Walking downstairs uses only ⅓ the calories of walking upstairs. Running upstairs demands even more calories. Climbing upstairs with a load, such as a basket of laundry, burns 11 times as many calories as walking on the level carrying the same load.

Value is due to benefits of flexibility and relaxation. Recommended as part of a warm-up routine for more vigorous activities such as running or bicycling.

WIDOWHOOD

Widowhood is one thought most of us wish we could bury beneath other future uncertainties. But the truth of the matter is, widowhood is more than just a possibility. It's a statistical *probability*. According to a report of the National Institute on Aging, by the year 2000 there will be 10 women for every 5 men over the age of 75. As it stands now, women outlive their husbands by an average of 4.3 years—that is, if they're the same age. If he has 6 years or so on her, she's liable to spend 10 years or more solo.

To explore the problems and potentials of women in widowhood (we like to think of it as the challenge of a woman's greater life expectancy), we talked with two sociologists at the Andrus Gerontology Center in Los Angeles. Leslie Morgan, Ph.D., is an assistant professor of sociology at the University of Maryland, and Carole Snow is an intern in marriage and family therapy at the University of Southern California in Los Angeles.

Question: Why should a woman want to prepare for widowhood? Wouldn't people rather not think about such things?
Dr. Morgan: That's part of the problem: there's such a denial of death that it's very hard for a married couple to sit down and discuss it objectively and plan for it. Discussing it is really a very loving thing to do, when two people recognize the fact of mortality and recognize that widowhood will probably be a reality for one of them.
Carole Snow: It's best to be prepared. There's a whole syndrome in the years following a spouse's death in which the survivor is more susceptible to illness

and injury. General malaise, including dizziness and fainting, is more common. Mortality rates are even higher among the recently widowed.

Studies show that women whose husbands committed suicide had a really bad time recovering. But those whose husbands were chronically ill before they died fared much better during their bereavement. With some warning, some psychological and emotional preparation, those women did better.

Question: But besides the fact that they have lost someone they've grown to depend on for a long time, there are other problems, aren't there?
Carole Snow: There are a lot of changes: changes in decision-making patterns, changes in responsibilities. She has to make up her own mind now.
Dr. Morgan: Grief is really only the beginning. She loses her husband, but what she really loses is a lifestyle. Quite frequently, she can't go out with the same people she used to go out with, because people go out in couples. She's the odd person out, which makes everybody uncomfortable.

Question: Yes, that's right. In fact, one study cited in a report of the National Institute on Aging found that women who have close-knit relationships with other women and who socialize in women-only groups are better able to cope with widowhood than women who socialized primarily in couples-only groups.

That ties in with what you were saying: women whose friends before widowhood were "couples" often have difficulty finding support or continued friendship in those same relationships afterwards.

Where can these women go for support?

Where Can You Turn for Support?

Dr. Morgan: That's difficult to say. A lot of the programs that are set up for widows make widowhood sound like a *disease*.

Carole Snow: And actually, what they find out in some of these programs is that people will come in for a very short time and then disappear. They don't come around anymore. What's happened is they've stopped identifying themselves as widows and started identifying themselves as women, single women. And the program no longer fulfills their needs.

Dr. Morgan: What information about widowhood that has been made available is usually very inadequate. It doesn't really explore the options people have. It doesn't paint a very realistic picture of what they can expect.

Carole Snow: They tell them to find another widow and cry together. Or they'll list page after page of sad widow stories. No one gives them alternatives!

Dr. Morgan: What we really want to get away from is the sob-story business and get into constructive things. You need to cry, but *then* what do you do?

Question: Okay, what *do* you do?

Dr. Morgan: Well, first of all, I'm not sure there's anything you can do to stave off that emotional distress, that bereavement. You have to deal with that as it comes.

Carole Snow: And even if the two people didn't get along very well, that loss still seems to be there.

Dr. Morgan: But there are other things you can do to keep your grief from becoming destructive and disabling.

Carole Snow: You can prepare for the transition in roles that occurs in widowhood. You go from married woman to widow, from part of a couple and a team to a single person.

Most widows probably have *never* lived alone. Most of them went from their father's house into their husband's. And this is their first exposure to living alone. It can be a disaster or it can be a positive experience.

Dr. Morgan: A lot of women don't know anything about their family finances. They don't know how much money their husband makes, what bills are coming in, where he keeps the key to the safe-deposit box. They don't know how or where to get the car repaired or anything else around the house. They have to learn all these things the hard way.

Carole Snow: It's like getting fired from a job you've held for 40 years—and you're not prepared for another one.

Dr. Morgan: That's right. It's a dilemma for some women whether they should move in with their children, or whether they should maintain their own house. What they need is someone to point out their options, help them take a look at their budgeting and financing and see if it's *possible* for them to keep house. But the important thing is to encourage them to make their own decisions, according to their needs, rather than merely telling them what they should and shouldn't do.

Question: Do many widows end up living with their children?

Carole Snow: Well, what happens is that the children sometimes reverse roles and try to become like *parents* to their mother.

Dr. Morgan: There's also a lot of guilt on the part of the children. They somehow expect that the widowed parent expects them to invite her to live with them. And they feel bad because they don't want to do that. In fact, she probably doesn't want to live with them any more than they want her!

Question: I think we have the problems out in the open now. Let's start solving them. What's first?

Allow Time for Grieving

Carole Snow: First, nothing. Grieving is a necessary part of the process and you have to allow yourself time for it. Don't try to be brave while you're choking back the emotions. It's important that you allow time to express yourself. Also, this is not the time to be making monumental decisions or immediate changes in your lifestyle. Wait until you can think more clearly.

Second, you have to have some acceptance of the fact that you are a widow.

You need that change in self-perception. From there, you have to define new goals *for yourself.* Before you did what he wanted to do, too. You shared goals. And you have to understand that it's possible to attain your new goals alone.

You have to reassess your emotional and financial capabilities.

Take stock of your independence. Get your *self* together. Decide what you need to do, and get moving.

The issues will be different from woman to woman. One woman might feel most the loss of a central partner or the loss of romance, so she'll deal with that. She won't even worry about getting a job. With other women, the financial issues are going to hit them right away and they're going to have to go out and get a job.

Dr. Morgan: Widowhood is looked on as a crisis and a terribly negative event. But it also presents an opportunity to do some new things, to make some changes in lifestyle through conscious decisions. That can be very exciting for some people.

Carole Snow: Widowhood *is* an awful thing. It's a loss...

Dr. Morgan: But it's not the end.

Carole Snow: But it is real. There's nothing you can do to reverse it once it happens. So why not change the stigma into an opportunity? Why not turn the loss into a different kind of gain? You've lost your husband, a big part of your life. But you haven't lost everything. You still have *you* and you can still go on.

Dr. Morgan: There's a woman I know whose husband died quite suddenly. And she has gone back to school, gotten her master's degree, and is now developing educational programs for other people. She's doing quite well.

Carole Snow: There must be hundreds of thousands of women who have never worked outside of the home in their lives—and who never thought they held a responsible job, when indeed they have: homemaker. And they've gone out and been very successful.

Question: Are there certain things people can do to *prevent* some of the overwhelming problems of widowhood, things they can do long before there's a death in the family?

Dr. Morgan: The problem has to be dealt with up front and honestly between two people, because it's good for both. He should also be considering the possibility of her death.

Question: What should they talk about when they decide to deal with it?

Dr. Morgan: They should talk about

things they would change in their lives with the other person gone. One of the hardest things to talk about is the old "Should I marry again?" question. Most people don't talk about that.

People have to realize that there is a very real possibility of living alone. And living alone and being self-sufficient is one way of living after widowhood, and also after separations and divorces, too.

Carole Snow: They should share the decision-making processes in the marriage.

Dr. Morgan: They should share information. They should write wills. Now that's a very small thing, but it can have huge implications. Another very important small thing is to set up separate bank accounts. If they have joint accounts and the husband dies, her money may be frozen and she may not be able to touch it for a long time. And that would just compound the distress. They should also share all their legal information.

My own mother and dad have done a really good thing. My father asked my mother to manage the finances. They sat down together and did their budgeting and bills and she found out where everything stood. It doesn't have to be a morbid thing. It's a sharing of responsibility; it's a positive thing. You become more competent.

Question: Sounds like a good practice for *anyone* to begin.

Dr. Morgan: Sure. It can start very simply. She can offer to help him manage the budget, help take care of the check writing every month.

Question: In other words, start making yourself into the best person you can be, *now.*

Carole Snow: And she can do that in a number of ways. If she doesn't want to get a job outside of the home, she can still take stock of her resources. She can educate herself. She can acquaint herself with as many responsibilities of the family as possible.

Take inventory of yourself. Do you like your lifestyle? Will you be able to continue it *alone*? Do you have marketable skills? Rather than spending 40 hours a week volunteering someplace, do you think you should go back to school? Some people don't even know how to look for a job! How to write a resume!

Dr. Morgan: What you do is take a look at what you want to do.

Do you want to get a job? Do you want to live differently, or live someplace else? Do you want to go out and join a political organization?

One very simple and unthreatening step is continuing education. Evening adult education is blossoming everywhere. There's everything from auto mechanics to French cooking to parapsychology. And it's a terrific opportunity for growth, to meet interesting people, and to just stimulate new things in yourself. Just go out and take a pottery course!

Carole Snow: And don't overlook possibly marketable experiences. Somebody who has been a large-scale, successful fund raiser for a charity could most likely do very well in some sort of business. Women overlook these things when writing resumes. They really *have* done things that a corporation would value.

Question: What about the husband who does not enjoy his wife setting out on these projects—the type who's very protective?

Carole Snow: Men like that are doing

their wives a tremendous disservice by protecting them. They shouldn't protect women from the harsh realities of the world. By doing this, a husband is actually throwing her out into the world unprepared. They take away from her the final protection: knowledge. Women deserve it.

Question: We're convinced. But aren't people sometimes afraid to make changes in their lives when they're reaching their fifties and sixties?

Carole Snow: Well, there's really little difference between their being 58 or 18. Except those who are 58 have more wisdom and more capabilities. But they have the same options. And people *are* starting to realize that. Time has not run out for them. It's like when you're 18, you have your whole life ahead of you. It's true at 58, too. You're not too old to do anything you might have dreamed of doing before. You always have your whole life ahead of you.

WRINKLES

"What? And erase 60 years of living!" a famous actress shot back at a suggestion that she have a face lift. Many would agree. Wrinkles give a face character. The lines define our existence. But, let's face it, sometimes it can be pretty hard to keep your chin up once you begin to notice it sag underneath.

No matter what anyone else tells you, there's nothing funny about laugh lines that remain after the joke winds down. And when the term "hang loose" refers to the skin on your face, it's enough to make you downright uptight.

That's not to say that many—or even any—of us would rush to a plastic surgeon for wrinkle repair. But we'd venture to say that, given a choice, most of us would probably opt to be without those sags and bags and creases. If only there was a simple, safe way to get rid of them—or prevent them from creeping into our expression in the first place.

With that in mind, we contacted Albert Kligman, Ph.D., M.D., professor of dermatology at the University of Pennsylvania Medical School and the country's foremost researcher in aging skin.

You may have already heard his name in connection with some other common skin problem. Dr. Kligman has made great waves in the study of everything from acne to athlete's foot. He was the one who deciphered why women tend to lose their hair just after they have a baby. And he pioneered the use of vitamin A acid in the treatment of acne.

Today, Dr. Kligman is turning his attention to another problem largely ignored by the rest of the dermatological community—wrinkles. And, as part of his efforts to find out as much as possible, he has opened a clinic for aging skin (appropriately dubbed the Clinic for Aging Skin) at the University of Pennsylvania in Philadelphia. Clearly, if anyone could tell us anything new about the age-old problem of aging skin, it would be Albert Kligman. And that he did when we recently stole a few moments of his time.

Question: Why wrinkles? Why have you devoted so much time and energy to the study of the lowly wrinkle? Surely no one ever died of wrinkles.

Dr. Kligman: No, they don't kill anybody and they're not debilitating. But I think wrinkles are a source of great human misery. And unfortunately, nobody gives a damn. The only people that care about it are the millions of people that are worrying about wrinkles. What medical people have to be concerned with is what concerns people. And there is a good deal more anxiety about wrinkles than the average practitioner, and particularly dermatologists, know about. I am looking at them because having started an aging skin clinic, I hear for the first time what people are saying. Dermatologists don't hear that. They hear if someone has a rash, or a bleeding mole, or some kind of skin disease. That's what their experience consists of—diseased skin. But a woman or a man would not go to a dermatologist and say, "My skin is beginning to wrinkle, what should I do?" They know it does not figure in medical thinking. My concern is that if it causes that much worry—and there are millions and millions of people worrying every day, affecting their moods, affecting their self-respect, causing a loss of confidence, and making them nervous—then we ought to study this!

The Incredible News about Aging and Skin

Question: But aren't wrinkles inevitable as we age?

Dr. Kligman: That's what most people think. But believe it or not, the skin doesn't show any real aging changes. You see, the skin and brain are different from the heart and kidneys and lungs and all the other organs. All those other organs reach a peak performance in adolescence. We are healthiest when we're 15 to 20, let's say—everything is at peak levels. After that time, these functions begin to decline at a pretty steady rate, something like one to two percent a year. That doesn't happen to the skin, which is why I'm so optimistic about it. The skin performs pretty much the same way from age 15 to age 50. For example, if I take a skin sample from a 15-year-old and one from a 50-year-old and measure sweating, blood supply, cell production, elasticity and so forth, I probably wouldn't be able to tell the difference—assuming of course, that the skin of the 50-year-old hasn't been insulted by living on top of Mount Everest or somewhere else with high winds and high sunlight. It's good news, you see.

Question: Well, it certainly sounds like good news. But if it's true what you say, that skin doesn't age, why are so many people concerned about aging skin? What ages the skin if not age?

Dr. Kligman: The environment is largely what produces what the average person thinks of as aging. As a matter of fact, most of what we see—the blemishes, blotches, dry spots, the benign tumors—is not due to age or the passage of time; it is due to the effect of the environment. Apart from looseness, every skin change that you can see with your eyes and feel with your hand is due to an environmental insult. It is not a natural thing.

I always show women the underside of their breast or the underside of their upper arm. That's the way the skin on their face should look. It should look that way until age 90. It ought to be smooth and soft and absolutely without a blemish, without a spot. And the only reason it isn't is that it's not protected from the environment the way the underside of the breast is.

Question: Specifically, what are the environmental factors that we should be protecting our skin from?

Dr. Kligman: Sunlight—excessive sunlight. Wind and cold. Harsh soaps. And all sorts of traumas that the skin has to endure. But mainly sunlight is the culprit here. If we paid as much attention to avoiding the sun as we do to avoiding additives in our food, we would be a race of very good-looking people. We'd look good till the day we died. Everybody would. It's just a matter of being careless. Or ignorant. Of not understanding how damaging sunlight is.

And it's not only the sunlight. Our recent research indicates that heat is also a factor. Heat penetrates, it goes right through the skin—cooking you, so to speak. When you go out on the beach, you might think you're just getting ultraviolet light but you're getting one hell of a lot of infrared radiation.

Question: But if you look at those areas of the skin—such as the underside of the breast—which aren't usually exposed to the sun, they're still absorbing the heat and yet they don't show the kind of changes you're talking about. Why is that?

Sunlight Plus Heat Add Up to Aged Skin

Dr. Kligman: Heat is not nearly as damaging as ultraviolet light—sunlight. Let's say 80 to 90 percent of the damage comes from the light. But heat intensifies the damage. In former times and again now that fuel is so expensive, we see elderly ladies who sit in front of coal or space heaters with their legs exposed. It's only heat. Yet that skin shows exactly the same damage as people who have lived under the sun. They get skin cancers. They get tumors of all kinds.

And the blotches look just as if they've been transposed from the face to the leg.

Question: In terms of aging—wrinkling—exactly how do sun and heat damage the skin?

Dr. Kligman: Sunlight and heat wreck the skin's collagen and elastin fibers. These fibers are what give skin its strength, its elasticity, its resiliency. Collagen is what keeps the skin from overextending. If I take your skin and start to pull it apart, it will stretch only to a point—that's the collagen. Now when it is stretched to the maximum and I release it, your skin will spring back—that's the elastin. Elastin is the rubber bands.

Question: Is it possible to reverse sun damage by staying out of the sun?

Dr. Kligman: That depends on the damage. Wrinkles—the result of repeated damage to collagen and elastin fibers—can't be reversed. But there is a lot of repair in blotchiness and in tumors. Premalignant tumors will very largely disappear if you get out of the sun. I see older people with lots of skin tumors go into a home—let's say the Riverview Home here in Philadelphia. They remain essentially indoors for the next 10 years and all their tumors disappear. On biopsy you can see the skin has laid down new tissues and there is a repair process going on. Their skin looks better—younger—than it did 10 years ago.

Question: Are you saying stay out of the sun at all costs?

Dr. Kligman: No, you don't have to stay out of the sun altogether. Just be careful. Use a sunscreen whenever you go outdoors. You've got to remember that the skin doesn't easily forget abuse. And the damage of the sun is cumulative, so sun protection is one habit you should adopt *throughout* your life. When a mother first takes her child out anywhere in the sunlight—in a baby carriage—she should put a sunscreen on that child. It's never too early to start preventing aging skin.

Question: Let's look at some other external factors that might also contribute to wrinkles. Does drinking alcohol accelerate the aging of skin in any way?

Dr. Kligman: Offhand, I would say yes. I can tell an alcoholic by looking at his skin. But I have no scientific evidence to back that up. The problem is that many of the alcoholics we see eat a lousy diet; they don't use sunscreens, either. And I don't know how to sort those factors out from the alcohol factor. We do know that alcohol is toxic to the brain, to the kidneys, to the liver. I think it's equally toxic to the skin.

Question: Does smoking have any effect on aging skin?

Dr. Kligman: That's another area about which we know very little. It's my personal opinion that the smoking itself doesn't do so much as the facial expressions—the constant pursing of the lips—which the act of smoking induces. You'll practically never see those vertical lines radiate from the upper lip in someone who doesn't smoke. When I see them I say, "How many did you smoke—two, three packs a day?"

How Facial Expressions Affect the Skin

Question: Is it true, then, that if you squint a lot you'll get crow's-feet or if you frown a lot you'll be stuck with a permanent crease between your brows?
Dr. Kligman: Oh, definitely.

Question: That brings to mind something our mothers threatened us with as children—that is, if we make a face, it will stay that way.
Dr. Kligman: Any facial movement—any of the emotional expressions that human beings have—are due to the contraction of muscles. Every time you make a face by contracting a muscle you throw the skin into folds. In young skin which hasn't been sun-damaged, those folds will immediately recoup. When the muscle contraction stops and you have stopped closing your eyes, for example, the skin will come back to its original position. In other words, it has tension in it and it's elastic and it's fine. In older people, especially if the connective tissue—the elastin and collagen—has been damaged, those folds do not disappear so quickly. The skin contracts, the folds appear and they just kind of slowly relax back into shape. You do that over a period of years and years throwing the skin up into these same folds—and it's a damaged skin— what you end up with are wrinkles. Wrinkles are due to repeated muscle contractions in damaged skin. That's how they appear. It takes 300 million contractions, let's say, to permanently work a fold into your skin. But you won't work it into that skin if the skin has been protected, if its elasticity is maintained by good living, by avoiding the sun.

Question: I suppose then from what you're saying, facial exercises, which are actually exaggerated facial expressions, can do more harm than good.
Dr. Kligman: You said it. First of all, they tend to throw the skin into folds as we just talked about. The other thing is that with constant contraction of the muscles, the muscles tend to get bigger. And when muscles get bigger, the skin must stretch to accommodate them.

Damaged skin that is stretched out of shape like this doesn't go back. Eventually, it sags.

Question: What about skin that has been stretched out of shape by excessive weight gain? Will it shrink back after the excess weight is lost?
Dr. Kligman: That depends on how old you are and how badly your elastin fibers have been damaged by the environment. In an older person whose skin has endured repeated sun damage, the skin is probably permanently stretched out of shape. Of course, the best thing is to watch your weight in the first place.

Question: Are there certain skin types that are more wrinkle-resistant, so to speak, than others?
Dr. Kligman: Oh, yes. The best is male skin, black skin, thick skin, oily skin.

Sex Differences, Skin Differences

Question: Why is a man's skin superior to a woman's?
Dr. Kligman: Women tend to have thinner and drier skin than men. That's just the way it is. And thin, dry skin wrinkles faster. That's why those vertical lines seen in smokers are almost exclusively seen in women smokers. Never in men. Women's thinner skin falls into permanent folds much more readily than thicker skin. In addition to that, my speculation is that women are more expressive.

Women are more generous in what they display than men to begin with. When a woman uses her face to transmit an image, it involves more muscle activity. Someday I will prove that. I think it is true. Men keep a stiff upper lip and they are supposedly more controlled. And that's why you see fewer wrinkles in men than in women.

Question: Do hormones like estrogen have anything to do with the difference?
Dr. Kligman: Probably not. We know that after menopause a woman's skin tends to get drier, her skin isn't producing as much oil as it used to. But whether the lack of estrogen is causing that, just isn't known.

Question: Does estrogen replacement therapy have any effect on oil production?
Dr. Kligman: There's no evidence that it's useful at all. In fact, I have gone so far as to apply estrogen topically to the face. It is well absorbed—so well in fact that some postmenopausal women get their periods again. But I have never been able to measure any change in the face.

Question: Why is black skin better?
Dr. Kligman: Black skin is terrific—by far the best skin that we know of all the human races. Part of the reason has to do with the pigmentation which provides a kind of built-in resistance to sun damage. But blackness is only one aspect of it. The skin biologically is different. It heals faster. Black skin will heal in half the time of white skin. It has nothing to do with pigment. It's just damn good skin.

As the white race went farther and farther north their skin got worse and worse. The Scotch-Irish skin is very bad. It dries out fast. It blisters rather than just burns. It doesn't tan. It takes forever to heal. That's why Scotch-Irish people should have special skin care programs—double thickness sunscreens, and great care about the soaps and other irritants they use.

Question: You mentioned skin thickness being a factor in skin susceptibility to wrinkles—the thicker the skin, the better. Is skin thickness determined genetically or can environmental or external factors influence it?

Dr. Kligman: It's purely genetic.

Question: Does skin thickness decrease with age?

Dr. Kligman: Yes, but not until old age. You've got to be past 60 before you'll begin to notice any change.

Question: This may seem like a silly question, but do fat people have thicker skin than thin people?

Dr. Kligman: Actually, that's a very interesting question. Nobody knows. It's a subject that I'd like to get into. There's no question that heavier people tend to have smoother skin. But we don't know whether that's because they have thicker skin or just because they have more subcutaneous tissue which pushes up the skin.

Can Exercise Help the Skin?

Question: In a Finnish study published in the *British Journal of Dermatology* (August, 1978) men in physical training were found to have thicker skin than sedentary men. Is it possible that physical exercise increases skin thickness?

Dr. Kligman: This is the only paper on the subject and it's only a preliminary study. They're working off the fact that if you are in good shape, if you exercise every day, your muscles get bigger and stronger. What these researchers are asking is, "Does the skin get thicker?" They say yes. I haven't any idea. It's conceivable that the skin is a dynamic enough organ that if you keep working out (I don't mean facial exercises but good, hard physical exercise like running) you'll increase the blood supply to the skin, which in turn will build more collagen. All that is possible.

Question: You mentioned earlier that dry skin wrinkles faster than oily skin. We know that steroid drugs are often prescribed for persons with very dry skin. Do they improve the dryness and thereby help retard wrinkles to a certain extent?

Dr. Kligman: Not at all. Steroids are harmful, especially when applied for a long time. They cause skin atrophy— that is, the tissues grow thinner, they shrink—and they harm the blood vessels so that circulation to the skin isn't what it should be.

Dr. Kligman's Prescription for Dry Skin

Question: What then do you prescribe for super-dry skin?

Dr. Kligman: Vaseline. That's it. I try to get my patients to sit in a tub for about 30 minutes twice a day and then rub themselves down with Vaseline. It's just about the only thing that works.

Question: What are the best kinds of moisturizers to prevent dry skin?

Dr. Kligman: The best creams are the very oily ones—simple emollient greases. In fact, the more greasy it is, the more effective it's going to be. If you don't like it, it's almost certain to be good for you. The things that work the best for really dry skin are awful. Vaseline. Lanolin. What they do is impregnate the outer layers of skin and keep it supple and soft so it doesn't crack.

Question: Is there any evidence that moisturizing creams containing collagen and elastin improve the skin's elasticity?

Dr. Kligman: Some women claim it works, but there's no scientific evidence whatsoever.

Question: Is there any substance to claims that creams containing placenta improve aging skin?
Dr. Kligman: Not a thing.

Question: What about nucleic acids?
Dr. Kligman: It's all nonsense.

Question: Does the vitamin A acid treatment that you use in the treatment of acne have any benefit as far as slowing down skin aging?
Dr. Kligman: Yes, it is beneficial. More from a preventive standpoint—not after all the wrinkles are formed. We know a little bit about how it works. It increases blood flow. It stimulates the skin, so to speak, and it lays down a little bit more of the gelatinlike substance that keeps the skin supple. We believe it may also help prevent tumors—precancerous skin tumors. Vitamin A is extensively used now in tumor therapy and in preventing postsurgical cancer recurrences. Like in lung cancer.... But getting back to your question, yes, it helps with aging skin. You take someone who's 40, whose skin isn't showing too much sign of age, and who is committed to sunscreens and greases—vitamin A acid will help her. It will make her skin feel better, smoother. Little wrinkles will flatten out—disappear. The skin is healthier. It'll heal better.

Question: What is vitamin A acid?
Dr. Kligman: It is a metabolite of vitamin A. Vitamin A itself as it exists in foods is not absorbed through the skin. If I put plain vitamin A on your skin nothing would happen. But vitamin A acid is absorbed and has sizable effects on skin.

Question: How often do you have to apply the vitamin A acid?
Dr. Kligman: Every day.

Question: Can you buy it in the drugstore and put it on at home?
Dr. Kligman: It's available only through prescription. Dermatologists are using it, but at this point, they're mainly prescribing it for acne. It hasn't been approved yet for aging skin.

Question: Aside from the vitamin A acid treatment, is there any way to halt or at least slow down skin aging?
Dr. Kligman: Yes. Use good sunscreens, just do all the things we've been talking about. You can slow it down.... You really can! The skin has self-recovery mechanisms even in old age.

APPENDIX:

A WOMAN'S HEALTH DIRECTORY
WHERE TO FIND HELP AND INFORMATION

SUGGESTED READING LIST

A WOMAN'S HEALTH DIRECTORY

AGING

Gray Panthers
3635 Chestnut Street
Philadelphia, PA 19104
(215) 382-3300

Aims to combat discrimination against persons on the basis of chronological age. Strives to raise the consciousness of older people (especially those over 65) as well as young people. Maintains an information and referral service. Conducts seminars and research on age-related issues. Publishes the *Network Newspaper* (bimonthly).

National Action Forum for Older Women at Stony Brook: A Center for the Health & Housing Concerns of Women over 40
School of Allied Health Professions
Health Sciences Center
State University of New York
Stony Brook, NY 11794
(516) 246-2989

Concerned with improving the quality of life for women in midlife and latelife. Aims to establish an informational resource center on the physical and mental health problems of older women. A newsletter, *Forum*, is available. Plans are underway to form a coalition of women's health groups around the United States concerned about women over 40.

National Association for Human Development (NAHD)
1750 Pennsylvania Avenue, NW
Washington, DC 20006
(202) 393-1881

NAHD is a health/social services organization which develops and implements pro-grams to assist persons in greater fulfillment of their social, economic, physical and intellectual development. Among its health promotion activities, it offers "Active People Over 60"—a health education/fitness program to encourage persons to assume greater responsibility for their own health through regular practice of self-help, self-care health habits.

National Council of Senior Citizens (NCSC)
1511 K Street, NW
Washington, DC 20005
(202) 347-8800

NCSC lobbies for health concerns of the elderly and publishes a monthly newsletter, *Senior Citizen News*. Members receive services including supplemental health insurance and drug and travel discounts. Information on nursing homes and community resources for older people is free to those who write or call.

National Institute on Aging (NIA)
Building 31, Room 5C35
National Institutes of Health
Bethesda, MD 20205
(301) 496-1752

NIA's job is to provide people with the latest medical research on aging. It offers free publications on such topics as estrogen use, special problems of older women and how to find good medical care.

National Retired Teachers
Association–American Association of
Retired Persons (NRTA–AARP)
1909 K Street, NW
Washington, DC 20049
(202) 872-4700

A mail-order pharmacy, monthly legislative bulletins, a bimonthly magazine, motel discounts and driver refresher courses are some of the services offered to members of this organization. Some health care information and referrals are available.

AGORAPHOBIA

Temple University Agoraphobia Program
3401 North Broad Street
Philadelphia, PA 19140
(215) 221-3611

Temple University has established an Agoraphobia Treatment and Research Program and has compiled a list of agoraphobia treatment facilities. To receive one send a stamped, self-addressed business envelope.

TERRAP–Menlo Park
1010 Doyle Street
Menlo Park, CA 94025
(415) 327-1312 or (415) 329-1233

Twenty-nine TERRAP (Territorial Apprehension) centers directed by Arthur Hardy, M.D., offer a method of treatment for agoraphobics. List of centers and information on the treatment program available.

ALCOHOLISM

Alcoholics Anonymous (AA)
P.O. Box 459
Grand Central Station
New York, NY 10163
(212) 686-1100

AA offers help for men and women alcoholics through group meetings. For information on a group in your area, contact AA or your state health agency on alcoholism.

National Institute on Alcohol Abuse and
Alcoholism (NIAAA)
5600 Fishers Lane
Rockville, MD 20857
(301) 443-3306

NIAAA supports prevention activities, treatment programs and rehabilitation services at the community level and in private industry. Several programs are directed at unique problems of women such as the Fetal Alcohol Syndrome, Alcoholism and Domestic Violence Programs. It operates a clearinghouse to collect and disseminate professional as well as public alcohol information. The address is National Clearinghouse for Alcohol Information, P.O. Box 2345, Rockville, MD 20852, (301) 468-2600.

Women for Sobriety, Inc. (WFS)
P.O. Box 618
Quakertown, PA 18951
(215) 536-8026

This is the only national organization to offer a complete program and line of literature exclusively for the woman alcoholic. Over 300 groups in the United States, Canada and Europe are involved in this self-help program which is based on positive thinking, metaphysics, philosophy, meditation and group dynamics. Referrals to local groups and a list of WFS literature.

ALCOHOLISM AND DRUG ABUSE

WOMEN, Inc.
570 Warren Street
Dorchester, MA 02121
(617) 442-6166

Provides treatment programs for women experiencing difficulty with drug or alcohol abuse. Offers a 24-hour residential program and a day program, with child care services. Individual and group counseling along with seminars, vocational workshops, resources and complete medical services for mother and child are also available. Mothers may go through treatment with their children.

ANOREXIA NERVOSA

American Anorexia Nervosa Association, Inc. (AANA)
133 Cedar Lane
Teaneck, NJ 07666
(201) 836-1800

Comprises a group of lay and professional people interested in the problem of anorexia nervosa. Acts as an information and referral service along with counseling and organizes self-help groups. It also maintains a speakers' bureau and collects information on research.

National Association of Anorexia Nervosa and Associated Disorders, Inc. (NAANAD)
550 Frontage Road, Suite 2020
Northfield, IL 60093
(312) 831-3438

Provides help for anorectics, their families, health professionals and others interested in the problems of anorexia nervosa. Services include counseling, referrals to doctors and treatment centers, information about eating problems, and early detection of anorexia nervosa.

BIOFEEDBACK

Biofeedback Society of America (BSA)
4301 Owens Street
Wheat Ridge, CO 80033
(303) 422-8436

Provides an open forum for the exchange of ideas, methods and results of biofeedback and related studies. The official publications of the society are *Biofeedback and Self-Regulation* and a quarterly newsletter, *Biofeedback*. A membership directory can be purchased by anyone interested in locating a biofeedback therapy center in their area.

BIRTH CONTROL

American Family Planning (AFP)
149 Lewis Road
Havertown, PA 19083
(215) 449-2006
(800) 523-5101—tollfree (outside PA)

AFP provides information and counseling on methods of birth control and abortion in hospitals and clinics nationwide.

Association for Voluntary Sterilization, Inc. (AVS)
708 Third Avenue
New York, NY 10017
(212) 986-3880

AVS offers free information on the medical and legal aspects of sterilization and provides a referral service for both men and women interested in obtaining permanent birth control.

The Couple to Couple League International, Inc. (CCL)
P.O. Box 11084
Cincinnati, OH 45211
(513) 661-7612

A nondenominational, nonprofit organization established to teach the techniques of natural family planning. The organization's manual *The Art of Natural Family Planning* is an extensive presentation of the "sympto-thermal method" by which a woman becomes aware of when she is fertile. CCL sponsors a series of four monthly meetings to teach the principles of this method. Monthly charts, basal thermometers, the manual and a teaching guide workbook are available by mail.

Planned Parenthood Federation of America, Inc. (PPFA)
810 Seventh Avenue
New York, NY 10019
(212) 541-7800

The national headquarters of this nonprofit family planning agency provides a library of information on sexuality, birth control and family planning which is open to the public. To receive free counseling and referrals for birth control, VD, abortion, sterilization, infertility and sexuality problems, check your phone book for the local Planned Parenthood branch.

BREASTFEEDING

La Leche League International, Inc. (LLLI)
9616 Minneapolis Avenue
Franklin Park, IL 60131
(312) 455-7730

A nonprofit organization founded by nursing mothers to provide support and information for women who want to breastfeed their babies. LLL groups throughout the United States, Canada and Europe hold monthly meetings where topics such as "Advantages of Breastfeeding to Mother and Baby" and "Nutrition and Weaning" are discussed. LLLI publishes a bimonthly newsletter, *La Leche League News*, and a manual, *The Womanly Art of Breastfeeding*, as well as extensive information sheets on the breastfeeding experience. LLL leaders are available for phone counseling, and a professional advisory board is available for consultation. Contact the main office for the chapter or leader in your area.

CANCER

Cancer Information Service (CIS)
National Cancer Institute
Building 31, Room 10A18
Bethesda, MD 20205
National Lines: (800) 638-6694
(800) 492-1444 (MD)
(800) 292-6201 (AK)

CIS is a network of referral offices sponsored by the National Cancer Institute and affiliated with the nation's top cancer research and treatment centers. Its "Hotline" counselors answer a variety of questions and provide the names of treatment centers. The CIS staff also informs callers about local self-help groups and service organizations.

Foundation for Alternative Cancer Therapies, Ltd.
(212) 741-2790

Encourages the testing of all viable, biological cancer treatments through sponsorship of research, annual conventions, seminars, and the publication of *Cancer Forum*. Information is provided on nontoxic cancer treatments, and a referral service to clinics, centers, and/or doctors using a biological and nutritional approach to the restoration of body chemistry is available. (Telephone inquiries preferred.)

Northwest Cancer Association
P.O. Box 3216
Bellevue, WA 98009
(206) 232-1698

Disseminates information on nontoxic cancer treatments. A book and tape library is open to the public and a yearly convention is sponsored on nontoxic cancer treatments. Information on alternative cancer treatments, including the names of doctors and clinics using such treatments, is available to anyone.

CANCER (BREAST)

Breast Care Advisory Center
P.O. Box 224
Kensington, MD 20795

Gives information and has a referral service for breast cancer patients. (Mail inquiries preferred.)

National Surgical Adjuvant Breast Project (NSABP)
University of Pittsburgh
Pittsburgh, PA 15260
Hotline: (412) 624-2671

This agency, sponsored by The National Cancer Institute, has been established to study the cure rates for all types of treatment procedures, including surgery, currently being done for breast cancer. Its hotline telephone number can put patients in touch with treatment centers close to their homes, which can provide treatment information for their specific problem.

Reach to Recovery (American Cancer Society)
777 Third Avenue
New York, NY 10017
(212) 371-2900

A rehabilitation program for women who have had breast surgery, designed to help them meet their physical, psychological and cosmetic needs. Referred by a physician, trained volunteers who have had a mastectomy visit new mastectomy patients in the hospital to offer rehabilitation information, exercise equipment, a temporary breast form and psychological support.

CHILDBIRTH

American Society for Psychoprophylaxis in Obstetrics (ASPO)
1411 K Street, NW, Suite 200
Washington, DC 20005
(202) 783-7050

ASPO is a national nonprofit association that promotes the Lamaze method of prepared childbirth and the ideals of family-centered maternity care in cooperation with the medical community, maternal and child health professionals and parents. In addition to certifying quality teachers in the Lamaze method, ASPO is concerned with the family's experience of pregnancy and birth, as well as preparing parents for the demands of childrearing through films, support groups and informative materials on parenting. Special attention is paid to involving the entire family in the birth process as evidenced in the film, "Fathers," recently introduced by ASPO. *Genesis* is the Association's bimonthly newsletter. Information on childbirth classes and other services can be obtained from the national headquarters or from chapters located in several cities across the country.

Home Oriented Maternity Experience (H.O.M.E.)
  511 New York Avenue
  Takoma Park
  Washington, DC 20012
(301) 587-4664

An educational association providing information and support to couples desiring a safe home or home-oriented birth experience. Publishes *Home Oriented Maternity Experience: A Comprehensive Guide to Homebirth* and a newsletter, *News from H.O.M.E.* Names of resources and sources of community help all over the United States and Canada are available to those interested, as is information on speakers and childbirth classes.

International Childbirth Education Association (ICEA)
  P.O. Box 20048
  Minneapolis, MN 55420
(612) 854-8660

ICEA promotes positive family involvement in childbirth and infant care. Member groups and individual members offer classes in preparation for childbirth and will make referrals to hospitals, birthing centers and doctors. ICEA also sponsors conferences and workshops, publishes a number of periodicals and books pertaining to family-centered maternity care and maintains the ICEA Bookcenter which offers an extensive list of publications on all aspects of childbirth education and family-centered maternity care.

National Association of Parents and Professionals for Safe Alternatives in Childbirth (NAPSAC)
  P.O. Box 267
  Marble Hill, MO 63764
(314) 238-2010

A consumer advocate organization, NAPSAC publishes books on childbirth including the *NAPSAC Directory of Alternative Birth Services and Consumer Guide,* listing over 3,200 birth centers, midwives and homebirth doctors. NAPSAC also sponsors conferences and professional training workshops. Quarterly newsletter available to members.

CHILDBIRTH (CESAREAN)

C/SEC, Inc. (Cesareans/Support, Education and Concern)
  66 Christopher Road
  Waltham, MA 02154
(617) 547-7188

C/SEC aims to provide information and change attitudes toward cesarean childbirth. It certifies cesarean instructors in the eastern United States. C/SEC literature includes information on vaginal birth after cesarean. Members receive a quarterly newsletter and discounts on publications.

CIRCULATION

National Heart, Lung, and Blood Institute
  Building 31, Room 4A21
  Bethesda, MD 20205
(301) 496-4236

Provides information on the effects of smoking, exercise, alcohol and stress on the heart, lungs and blood. Major prevention and education programs address such risk factors as hypertension, diabetes, elevated cholesterol levels, excess salt and congenital abnormalities.

CONSUMER INFORMATION

Consumer Information Center
18th and E Streets, NW
Washington, DC 20405
(202) 566-1794

The Center's job is to get consumer information on a wide variety of subjects from the various government agencies out to the public. For a free catalog of available literature write: Consumer Information Center, Pueblo, CO 81009.

Food and Drug Administration (FDA)
Consumer Communications
5600 Fishers Lane
Rockville, MD 20857
(301) 443-3170

Handles consumer complaints in labeling or safety of medical devices, ray-emitting devices (sunlamps, microwave ovens and televisions), drugs and cosmetics, as well as food. Literature on adverse reaction to drugs is free, and the magazine *FDA Consumer* is available from the Superintendent of Documents, U.S. Government Printing Office, Washington, DC 20402.

Federal Trade Commission (FTC)
Bureau of Consumer Protection
6th and Pennsylvania Avenue, NW
Washington, DC 20580
(202) 523-3727

Seeks to prevent false advertising in food, drugs and cosmetics. Complaints to the FTC should be submitted in writing and clearly documented.

COUNSELING

Women in Transition (WIT)
112 South 16th Street
Philadelphia, PA 19102
(215) 563-9556/57

This organization has established a telephone hotline for counseling, information and referrals in an effort to help women who are experiencing marital distress, separation, divorce or widowhood. WIT also provides supportive counseling to displaced homemakers, and training to professionals and other community-based personnel interested in providing similar services at their own site.

Family Service Association of America
44 East 23rd Street
New York, NY 10010
(212) 674-6100

Counseling services for family problems may be found by looking under "Family Services" in the telephone directory's white pages or under "Social Services" in the Yellow Pages. A publications list is available through the main office.

DES

DES Action National
Long Island Jewish–Hillside Medical Center
New Hyde Park, NY 11040
(516) 775-3450

Acts as a clearinghouse for information on DES, provides peer support for DES mothers and daughters and medical referrals where available. Groups have been formed in other areas of the country.

HEART DISEASE

American Heart Association
7320 Greenville Avenue
Dallas, TX 75231
(214) 750-5300

Provides information on heart disease, high blood pressure, diet, exercise, smoking, rehabilitation, birth defects, etc.

HERPES

American Social Health Association (ASHA)
260 Sheridan Avenue
Palo Alto, CA 94306
(415) 321-5134

ASHA provides information on venereal disease and has started a support and information service for victims of *herpes simplex* virus. For more information, send a stamped, self-addressed envelope to: HELP, Box 100, Palo Alto, CA 94302.

HYPOGLYCEMIA

Adrenal Metabolic Research Society of the Hypoglycemia Foundation, Inc.
153 Pawling Avenue
Troy, NY 12180
(518) 272-7154

An association interested in furthering scientific investigation into the knowledge of metabolic aspects of hypoglycemia and hyperinsulinism through laboratory research and publication. Attempts are made to apply such knowledge to the prevention and treatment of these problems. Information from medical literature is provided about hypoglycemia, allergies, addiction, alcoholism, etc. A quarterly newsletter entitled *Homeostasis* and information on the work of John Tintera, M.D., is also available. Referrals are made to physicians throughout the United States who support the Foundation's philosophies.

JOGGING

National Jogging Association
2420 K Street, NW
Washington, DC 20037
(202) 965-3430

Encourages and fosters individual, family and club jogging and running among people of all ages and levels of fitness in the belief that such a program can lead to improved health and a greater sense of well-being. Publishes *The Jogger,* informational booklets on running, and provides information on all aspects of jogging, aerobic fitness and sportsmedicine to interested persons. Referrals are made to medical specialists interested in sportsmedicine and running.

MASSAGE

American Massage & Therapy Association
P.O. Box 1270
Kingsport, TN 37660
(615) 245-8071

A national association with state chapters interested in organizing all professional and ethical massage therapists; in upgrading the image of massage through legislation, educational standardization, and professionalism; and in informing the general public about certified massage therapists. Holds regional and national conferences, provides literature describing massage and the association, and provides a referral to its members.

MEDICAL INFORMATION

American College of Obstetricians and Gynecologists (ACOG)
1 East Wacker Drive, Suite 2700
Chicago, IL 60601
(312) 222-1600

ACOG will supply information on women's health including pregnancy, hysterectomy and hormones. Write directly to the Resource Center at the above address to request ACOG booklets. Please enclose a self-addressed, stamped envelope.

Center for Medical Consumers and Health Care Information, Inc.
237 Thompson Street
New York, NY 10012
(212) 674-7105

The Center encourages consumers to make a critical evaluation of the information they receive from health professionals. To this end, it provides a free medical health library, publishes *Health Facts*, a bimonthly newsletter, and operates a phone-in tape service on over 140 subjects.

MENTAL HEALTH

Know, Inc.
P.O. Box 86031
Pittsburgh, PA 15221
(412) 241-4844

This women's educational group publishes articles concerning a variety of women's issues, including information on choosing a counseling method. Send 25¢ for a list of their publications.

National Institute of Mental Health (NIMH)
5600 Fishers Lane
Rockville, MD 20857
(301) 443-4515

For referrals to community mental health services, NIMH programs and publications, contact the National Clearinghouse for Mental Health Information, 5600 Fishers Lane, Room 11A-21, Rockville, MD 20857.

The National Mental Health Association
1800 North Kent Street
Arlington, VA 22209
(703) 528-6405

A nationwide, voluntary, nongovernmental organization dedicated to the promotion of mental health, the prevention of mental illness and the improved care and treatment of the mentally ill. Its 850 chapters and divisions and more than one million citizen volunteers work toward these goals through a wide range of activities in social action, education, advocacy and information. Local Mental Health Associations assist members of their communities by making appropriate referrals to mental health services and provide the public with information concerning mental health and mental illness.

MIDDLE AGE

Midlife Counseling Associates
1321 South Eliseo Drive
Kentfield, CA 94904
(415) 461-0900

A Bay-area group which addresses the special needs of middle-aged women, such as career exploration and change, shifts in personal relationships, menopause and widowhood. It conducts small support-discussion groups, offers individual counseling and coordinates Bay-area conferences of women's groups.

MIDWIFERY

The American College of Nurse-Midwives
  1012 14th Street, NW, Suite 801
  Washington, DC 20005
(202) 347-5445

A professional organization for nurse-midwives in the United States dedicated to improving the independent management of women and normal newborns within the health care system. Certifies nurse-midwives and provides an informational forum through its many publications including the bimonthly *Journal of Nurse Midwifery* and a newsletter called *Quickening*. Referrals are made to practicing nurse-midwives in specified geographical areas.

MIGRAINE

National Migraine Foundation
  5214 North Western Avenue
  Chicago, IL 60625
(312) 878-7715

The Foundation is a voluntary health agency initially supported by the American Association for the Study of Headache which publishes the journal *Headache*. It supports headache research, acts as a clearinghouse for headache information and has a referral service for headache sufferers. Members receive the quarterly publication, *National Migraine Foundation Newsletter*.

MOTHERHOOD

Mothers Are People Too (MAPT)
  1411 K Street, NW, Suite 200
  Washington, DC 20005
(202) 783-7050

A national service offered by the American Society for Psychoprophylaxis in Obstetrics (ASPO) whose main purpose is to create discussion groups that focus on emotional reactions and adjustments to recent motherhood. Advises as to the location of local groups.

NUTRITION

Center for Science in the Public Interest (CSPI)
  1755 S Street, NW
  Washington, DC 20009
(202) 332-9110

A nonprofit organization that investigates and researches issues in the area of nutrition and the American diet. A monthly newsletter publishes information on the role the government and industry play in shaping food safety and quality. Other books and pamphlets covering such topics as food additives, school lunch programs, and politics and nutrition are also available.

Price–Pottenger Nutrition Foundation
  P.O. Box 2614
  La Mesa, CA 92041
(714) 582-4168

The Foundation publishes Dr. Weston Price's book, *Nutrition and Physical Degeneration*, rents and sells films, videotapes, and other printed information and research on nutrition and human health. Quarterly publications are available to members giving updates on recent findings, many of which relate directly to feminine well-being and optimal nutrition during pregnancy and childhood.

United States Department of Agriculture (USDA)
Office of Governmental and Public Affairs
Washington, DC 20250
(202) 447-2791

The USDA publishes a great deal of information on the nutrient content of foods, including the authoritative work *Composition of Foods: Raw, Processed, Prepared*, Agriculture Handbook No. 8. One popular publication is the booklet *Nutritive Value of American Foods in Common Units*, Agriculture Handbook No. 456, which is a handy listing of the nutrient content of foods by serving size. For a list of publications write to the Publications Distribution Center at the above address.

PREGNANCY

American Foundation for Maternal and Child Health
30 Beekman Place
New York, NY 10022
(212) 759-5510

The Foundation is a watchdog agency sponsoring educational conferences on obstetric practices and drugs used by women during pregnancy and in childbirth and their effects on the health of the mother and the subsequent development of the offspring. It offers leaflets such as "Getting What You Want for Your Childbirth Experience" and "The Pregnant Patient's Bill of Rights." Send a stamped, self-addressed envelope when corresponding.

Society for the Protection of the Unborn through Nutrition (SPUN)
17 North Wabash Avenue, Suite 603
Chicago, IL 60602
(312) 332-2334

SPUN encourages a holistic approach to pregnancy with an emphasis on nutritional standards that would discourage low-salt, weight-control diets and the use of drugs during pregnancy. It provides free literature, conducts weekend seminars, publishes a bimonthly newsletter, and makes referrals to nutrition-oriented obstetricians and midwives in the United States.

RAPE

National Center for the Prevention and Control of Rape
National Institute of Mental Health
5600 Fishers Lane
Rockville, MD 20857
(301) 443-1910

Funds research into the causes and methods of preventing rape and sexual assault. The Center provides funding for direct services through rape crisis centers and other programs, and publishes the *National Directory: Rape Prevention and Treatment Resources* as well as other literature including *Rape and Older Women: A Guide to Prevention and Protection*. The *Acquaintance Rape Prevention* film series is also available. For information, write to the above address, Room 15–99.

SMOKING

Office on Smoking and Health
Technical Information Center
Park Building, Room 116
5600 Fishers Lane
Rockville, MD 20857
(301) 443-1690

Call or write for free information on the health hazards of smoking and how to quit.

VEGETARIANISM

Vegetarian Information Service, Inc.
  P.O. Box 5888
  Washington, DC 20014
(301) 530-1737

An organization formed to collect, organize and disseminate information on all aspects of vegetarianism. Advises public officials and mass media representatives on the benefits of a vegetarian way of life through testimonies, conferences, and letters. A medical bibliography of scientific information on vegetarianism is available.

VITAMIN E

The Shute Institute for Clinical and Laboratory Medicine
  10 Grand Avenue
  London, Ontario, Canada N6C 1K9
(519) 432-1884

This foundation is the "world headquarters" for the therapeutic use of vitamin E based on the pioneering work of Drs. Evan and Wilfrid Shute. Primary focus is on the treatment of coronary artery disease and problems of poor circulation, burns, diabetes and women's health problems. Nutrition, exercise and orthomolecular medicine play a prominent role in the clinic's treatment methods. Inquiries are answered from both professionals and laypersons interested in obtaining information on any aspect of vitamin E research.

WOMEN'S HEALTH GROUPS

Boston Women's Health Book Collective
  Box 192
  West Somerville, MA 02144
(617) 924-0271

This group coauthors *Our Bodies, Ourselves* and *Ourselves and Our Children,* both excellent reference books on women's health and being parents. Royalty monies from the books are used to support women's health projects and collect information on health, which is available on request. It also coauthors the book, *International Women and Health Resource Guide,* which lists books, articles, films and organizations concerned with women's health. Pamphlets on menstruation and sexually transmitted diseases are available.

Feminist Women's Health Center/Woman's Choice Clinic
  15251 West Eight-Mile Road
  Detroit, MI 48235
(313) 341-5666

A medical self-help organization designed to help women be in control of their reproduction and health care, and to provide immediate health care services to women at reasonable costs. A self-help clinic and pregnancy screening are among its many activities.

Health Policy Advisory Center (Health/PAC)
  17 Murray Street
  New York, NY 10007
(212) 267-8890

Another watchdog agency, Health/PAC distributes informative literature on women's health issues. It also publishes the *Health/ PAC Bulletin,* which has a women's health column covering current topics.

National Women's Health Network (NWHN)
224 7th Street, SE
Washington, DC 20003
(202) 543-9222

NWHN is the nation's only consumer organization on women and health. It has a resource center on women's health issues and provides a DES litigation information service. It serves the consumer by pressuring federal regulatory agencies and testifying at congressional hearings. A bimonthly publication on the latest health information for women is sent to members.

Reproductive Rights National Network
41 Union Square, West, Room 206
New York, NY 10003
(212) 675-2651

This activist network of over 35 women's health and organizing groups works on a broad range of reproductive rights issues including abortion, sterilization abuse and reproductive health in the workplace. The organization gives referrals to other progressive women's support groups throughout the country, and members are welcome.

BIRTH CONTROL

The Art of Natural Family Planning, by John and Sheila Kippley. Cincinnati: Couple to Couple League International, 1979.

The Birth Control Book, by Howard I. Shapiro. New York: St. Martin's Press, 1977.

A definitive guide to all forms of contraception with the pros and cons of each. Written by a gynecologist associated with Planned Parenthood and the National Organization for Women.

Contraceptive Technology 1980–1981, by Robert A. Hatcher et al., 10th rev. ed. New York: Irvington, 1980.

Written by the authors of *My Body, My Health* and other experts in the field of gynecology, this provides up-to-date information on all forms of contraception.

A Cooperative Method of Natural Birth Control, by Margaret Nofziger. Summertown, Tenn.: The Book Publishing Company, 1976.

A beautifully illustrated guide to natural birth control which incorporates temperature and mucus observations and the rhythm method. Gives many examples of charts and additional information on the menstrual cycle. Also the publishers provide a kit including a basal body thermometer and charts with the book on request.

The Ovulation Method of Birth Regulation: The Latest Advances for Achieving or Postponing Pregnancy—Naturally, by Mercedes Arzú Wilson. New York: Van Nostrand Reinhold, 1980.

BREAST PROBLEMS

Breast Cancer: A Nutritional Approach, by Carlton Fredericks. New York: Grosset & Dunlap, 1977.

Breast Self-Examination, by Albert R. Milan. New York: Workman, 1980.

First, You Cry, by Betty Rollin. New York: J. B. Lippincott, 1976.

A firsthand account of a woman's brush with breast cancer. Focuses on the emotional consequences.

Post-Mastectomy: A Personal Guide to Physical and Emotional Recovery, by Win Ann Winkler. New York: Hawthorn Books, 1976.

Why Me? What Every Woman Should Know about Breast Cancer to Save Her Life, by Rose Kushner. New York: New American Library, 1977.

Written by a breast cancer victim, this book emphasizes the importance of knowing what options are available and where to go for the most appropriate cancer treatment.

COOKING FOR HEALTH

Bread Winners, by Mel London. Emmaus, Pa.: Rodale Press, 1979.

The Deaf Smith Country Cookbook, by J. F. Ford et al. New York: Macmillan, 1973.

The Fish-Lovers' Cookbook, by Sheryl and Mel London. Emmaus, Pa.: Rodale Press, 1980.

The Green Thumb Cookbook, by the editors of *Organic Gardening and Farming* magazine and edited by Anne Moyer. Emmaus, Pa.: Rodale Press, 1977.

Laurel's Kitchen: A Handbook for Vegetarian Cookery and Nutrition, by Laurel Robertson et al. Petaluma, Calif.: Nilgiri Press, 1976.

The Natural Healing Cookbook, by Mark Bricklin and Sharon Claessens. Emmaus, Pa.: Rodale Press, 1981.

The New York Times Natural Foods Cookbook, by Jean Hewitt. New York: Quadrangle, 1971.

Recipes for a Small Planet, by Ellen B. Ewald. New York: Ballantine, 1975.

The Seasonal Kitchen: A Return to Fresh Foods, by Perla Meyers. New York: Holt, Rinehart and Winston, 1973.

The Supermarket Handbook: Access to Whole Foods, by Nikki Goldbeck and David Goldbeck. New York: Harper & Row, 1973.

A handbook designed to guide you to healthful foods in the supermarket.

The Vegetarian Epicure, by Anna Thomas. New York: Alfred A. Knopf, 1972.

The Vegetarian Epicure: Book Two, by Anna Thomas. New York: Alfred A. Knopf, 1978.

DRUGS

Drug-Induced Nutritional Deficiencies, by Daphne A. Roe. Westport, Conn.: Avi Publishing, 1976.

In-depth coverage of nutritional disorders caused by such drugs as antibiotics, sedatives, contraceptives and cholesterol-lowering agents.

Hazards of Medication, by Eric W. Martin et al. 2d ed. Philadelphia: J. B. Lippincott, 1978.

A major textbook covers adverse reactions, contraindications and interactions of most drugs.

Here's to Your Health: The Sobering Facts about Social Drinking, by Joyce Hoffman and the editors of *Prevention* magazine. Emmaus, Pa.: Rodale Press, 1980.

I'm Dancing as Fast as I Can, by Barbara Gordon. New York: Harper & Row, 1979.

Startling firsthand account of a woman's experience with Valium addiction.

Keep Off the Grass: A Scientific Enquiry into the Biological Effects of Marijuana, by Gabriel G. Nahas. Elmsford, N.Y.: Pergamon, 1979.

The People's Pharmacy, by Joe Graedon. New York: St. Martin's Press, 1976.

Important consumer information on drugs. Plus practical tips on drug usage, how to minimize side effects and insure effectiveness.

Turnabout: Help for a New Life, by Jean Kirkpatrick. Garden City, N.Y.: Doubleday, 1978.

A woman's account of her bout with alcoholism and the struggles that led her to develop a treatment program that addressed the special needs of the woman alcoholic.

We Mind If You Smoke, by Don C. Matchan. New York: Pyramid, 1977.

A consumer's guide to the many methods available to help the smoker quit.

FITNESS

Aerobic Dancing, by Jacki Sorensen with Bill Bruns. New York: Rawson, Wade, 1979.

The Complete Woman Runner, by the editors of *Runner's World* magazine. Mountain View, Calif.: World, 1978.

Getting Strong: A Woman's Guide to Realizing Her Physical Potential, by Kathryn Lance. New York: Bobbs-Merrill, 1978.

A fitness program that focuses on building strength through weight training utilizing household objects.

New Age Training for Fitness and Health, by Dyveke Spino. New York: Grove Press, 1980.

A fresh look at fitness and athletic training that emphasizes the positive frame of mind essential for a healthy lifestyle. Incorporates relaxation and visualization techniques. Special chapters on women and training.

Rating the Exercises, by Charles T. Kuntzleman and the editors of *Consumer Guide.* New York: William Morrow, 1978.

Running for Health and Beauty: A Complete Guide for Women, by Kathryn Lance. New York: Bobbs-Merrill, 1977.

Savitri's Way to Perfect Fitness through Hatha Yoga, by Savitri Ahuja. New York: Simon & Schuster, 1979.

The Secrets of the Golden Door, by Deborah Szekely Mazzanti. Rev. ed. New York: Bantam, 1979.

Founding director of California's famed Golden Door spa shares her secrets of fitness, health and beauty. Included is a four-week high-energy, low-cal menu program.

Starbodies: The Women's Weight Training Book, by Franco Columbu and Anita Columbu. New York: E. P. Dutton, 1978.

Total Glow: Dr. Rona's Unbeatable Health Program Incorporating Nutrition, Exercise, Relaxation, by Luanne Rona. Wilmington, Del.: Enterprise, 1978.

A holistic health program involving exercise, relaxation and good nutrition written by a woman physician.

Total Woman's Fitness Guide, by Gail Shierman and Christine Haycock. Mountain View, Calif.: World, 1979.

The U.S. Air Force Academy Fitness Program for Women, by Jack Galub. Englewood Cliffs, N.J.: Prentice-Hall, 1979.

Women's Running, by Joan Ullyot. Mountain View, Calif.: World, 1976.

GENERAL HEALTH

Dr. Wright's Book of Nutritional Therapy: Real-Life Lessons in Medicine without Drugs, by Jonathan V. Wright. Emmaus, Pa.: Rodale Press, 1979.

Nutrition-oriented doctor and *Prevention* magazine columnist, Dr. Wright outlines many actual cases and therapies involving problems such as allergies, depression, diabetes, arthritis, gynecological problems and many others.

Headaches: The Drugless Way to Lasting Relief, by Harry C. Ehrmantraut. Brookline, Mass.: Autumn Press, 1980.

High Level Wellness: An Alternative to Doctors, Drugs and Disease, by Donald B. Ardell. Emmaus, Pa.: Rodale Press, 1977.

Approaches lifestyle in a holistic way with an emphasis on integrating nutritional awareness, physical fitness, stress management, environmental sensitivity and self-responsibility to achieve a feeling of optimal well-being.

How to Get the Best Health Care for Your Money: The Family Guide to New Choices in Health Care, edited by Lori Breslow. Emmaus, Pa.: Rodale Press, 1979.

Oh, My Aching Back: A Doctor's Guide to Your Back Pain and How to Control It, by Leon Root and Thomas Kiernan. New York: David McKay, 1973.

A prominent orthopedic surgeon describes in detail what the back is all about. Explains both diagnostic and treatment procedures for back problems and provides helpful daily advice on overcoming and preventing chronic back pain.

The Practical Encyclopedia of Natural Healing, by Mark Bricklin. Emmaus, Pa.: Rodale Press, 1976.

A comprehensive, easy-to-understand guide to natural health care, providing detailed, documented information on preventing and treating over 140 health problems from acne and arthritis to warts and yeast infections. By the Executive Editor of *Prevention* magazine.

The *Prevention* Guide to Surgery and Its Alternatives, by the editors of *Prevention* magazine. Emmaus, Pa.: Rodale Press, 1980.

A consumer's guide to surgery and possible alternatives. Includes suggestions on how to avoid developing the conditions that may lead you to the operating table.

GYNECOLOGY

Cystitis: The Complete Self-Help Guide, by Angela Kilmartin. New York: Warner Books, 1980.

Every Woman's Guide to Hysterectomy: Taking Charge of Your Body, by Dee Dee Jameson and Roberta Schwalb. Englewood Cliffs, N.J.: Prentice-Hall, 1978.

Combining personal experience with medical facts, this book offers advice, information and encouragement to women undergoing hysterectomy. Includes information on alternative treatments.

Female Complaints: Lydia Pinkham and the Business of Women's Medicine, by Sarah Stage. New York: W. W. Norton, 1979. An historical account that looks at the story of Lydia Pinkham and her famed Vegetable Compound for female complaints within the context of changing attitudes toward female sexuality at the turn of the century.

From Woman to Woman, by Lucienne Lanson. New York: Alfred A. Knopf, 1975.

A gynecological reference guide written by a woman gynecologist. Question and answer format.

Men Who Control Women's Health: The Miseducation of Obstetrician-Gynecologists, by Diana Scully. Boston: Houghton Mifflin, 1980.

A treatise on the women's health care system and the role men play in it. Enlightening firsthand experience of a woman researcher who spent hundreds of hours observing ob-gyn specialists in training at two major medical centers.

Menstruation, by Hilary C. Maddux. New Canaan, Conn.: Tobey, 1975.

My Body, My Health: The Concerned Woman's Guide to Gynecology, by Felicia H. Stewart et al. New York: John Wiley & Sons, 1979.

Written by three gynecologists and a health educator in the field. An easy-to-understand textbook of gynecology.

Our Bodies, Ourselves, by the Boston Women's Health Book Collective. 2d ed. New York: Simon & Schuster, 1976.

A landmark book on health and social issues that concern women. One of the first books to emphasize self-help in the area of women's health.

Vaginal Health, by Carol V. Horos. New Canaan, Conn.: Tobey, 1975.

Women and the Crisis in Sex Hormones, by Barbara Seaman and Gideon Seaman. New York: Rawson Associates, 1977.

An in-depth look into estrogen, its use, and its adverse effects on the female body. Also, alternatives to estrogen therapy offered.

HERBS

The Herb Book, by John B. Lust. Sini Valley, Calif.: Benedict Lust, 1974.

An excellent reference catalog with over 2,000 listings. Includes botanical, medical and historical information with details on methods of preparation and the many uses of herbs.

Herb Gardening in Five Seasons, by Adelma Grenier Simmons. New York: Hawthorn Books, 1964.

Hygieia: A Woman's Herbal, by Jeannine Parvati. Berkeley, Calif.: Bookpeople, 1978.

The Rodale Herb Book: How to Use, Grow, and Buy Nature's Miracle Plants, edited by William H. Hylton. Emmaus, Pa.: Rodale Press, 1974.

MENOPAUSE AND THE OLDER WOMAN

Breaking Out of the Middle-Age Trap, by Leslie A. Westoff. New York: New American Library, 1980.

This perceptive and reassuring guide, based on over 100 case histories, outlines the problems and focuses on the many opportunities available to middle-aged women.

A High Old Time or How to Enjoy Being a Woman over Sixty, by Lavinia Russ. New York: Warner, 1973.

A lighthearted look at growing older, with tips on how to age gracefully.

The Menopause Book, by Barrie Anderson et al. New York: Hawthorn Books, 1977.

Eight doctors—specialists in gynecology, psychiatry and internal medicine, all women—provide honest, sound and thorough answers to questions women have about menopause.

Menopause: A Positive Approach, by Rosetta Reitz. Radnor, Pa.: Chilton, 1977.

One woman's extensive study of menopausal women. Special emphasis on nutritional aids to relieve uncomfortable symptoms.

Nutrition and the Later Years, by Ruth B. Weg. Los Angeles: University of Southern California Press, 1978.

Presents scientific information relevant to nutritional needs during the later years of life. Nutritional inadequacies are reviewed as they relate to daily life and the development of problems such as diverticulitis, diabetes and osteoporosis.

Surviving the Change: A Practical Guide to Menopause, by Joan Israel et al. Detroit: Cinnabar, 1980.

The View in Winter: Reflections on Old Age, by Ronald Blythe. New York: Harcourt Brace Jovanovich, 1979.

A unique inquiry into aging made up of conversations with older people from all walks of life. Written by an English historian and storyteller.

Women of a Certain Age: The Midlife Search for Self, by Lillian Rubin. New York: Harper & Row, 1979.

Based on her own experiences as well as those of other women, a sociologist examines middle age, its problems and opportunities.

MIND AND BODY

Active Loving: Discovering and Developing the Power to Love, by Ari Kiev. New York: T. Y. Crowell, 1979.

A practical guide to a deeper understanding of your ability to love, through realizing that in order to find and sustain love, you must first be loving.

The Best Little Girl in the World, by Steven Levenkron. Chicago: Contemporary Books, 1978.

A study of young women suffering from anorexia nervosa written by a psychologist.

The Broken Heart: The Medical Consequences of Loneliness, by James J. Lynch. New York: Basic Books, 1977.

The Golden Cage: The Enigma of Anorexia Nervosa, by Hilde Bruch. Cambridge, Mass.: Harvard University Press, 1978.

Husbands and Wives: A Nationwide Survey of Marriage, by Anthony Pietropinto and Jacqueline Simenauer. New York: Times Books, 1979.

The Massage Book, by George Downing. New York: Random House, 1972.

My Mother, My Self: The Daughter's Search for Identity, by Nancy Friday. New York: Delacorte Press, 1977.

Passages: Predictable Crises in Adult Life, by Gail Sheehy. New York: E. P. Dutton, 1976.

A perceptive and reassuring study of the patterns of adult life. Focuses on the crises and how you can use them to grow to your full potential.

Personal Habit Control: How to Achieve Health and Happiness through Permanent Control over Your Habits, by Peter M. Miller. New York: Simon & Schuster, 1978.

Psychology of Women, edited by Juanita Williams. New York: W. W. Norton, 1979.

A collection of essays on the many different aspects of women and their behavior.

Rape, by Carol V. Horos, New Canaan, Conn.: Tobey, 1974.

The Relaxation Response, by Herbert Benson. New York: William Morrow, 1975.

Shows how a simple, meditative technique can help you relieve inner tensions, deal more effectively with stress, lower blood pressure, and improve your general physical and emotional health. Written by a physician.

Stress and the American Woman, by Nora Scott Kinzer. Garden City, N.Y.: Doubleday, 1979.

Unfinished Business: Pressure Points in the Lives of Women, by Maggie Scarf. Garden City, N.Y.: Doubleday, 1980.

This enlightening book looks at six decades in a woman's life—from the teens through to the sixties—and the physical and psychological points that characterize each. Based on case histories.

Widow, by Lynn Caine. New York: William Morrow, 1974.

A moving, personal account of the problems the author experienced when her husband died of cancer.

Widows and Widowhood: A Creative Approach to Being Alone, by James A. Peterson and Michael P. Briley. New York: Association Press, 1977.

The Womanly Art of Self-Defense: A Commonsense Approach, by Kathleen Keefe Burg. New York: A & W Publishers, 1979.

The Women's Yellow Pages: Original Sourcebook for Women, edited by Carol Edry and Rosalyn Gerstein. Boston: The Public Works, 1978.

Provides information and advice on a variety of topics, complete with addresses of additional sources for help. At the time of writing, only the New England edition is available.

NUTRITION

The Complete Book of Minerals for Health: All-New Edition, by Sharon Faelten and the editors of *Prevention* magazine. Emmaus, Pa.: Rodale Press, 1981.

The Complete Book of Vitamins, by the staff of *Prevention* magazine. Rev. ed. Emmaus, Pa.: Rodale Press, 1977.

Diet for a Small Planet, by Francis Moore Lappé. New York: Ballantine, 1975.

An excellent and complete account of how to insure proper protein balances from non-meat foods to produce high-grade protein nutrition at least equivalent to meat proteins. An extensive recipe section provides deliciously clear examples of what foods complement each other to achieve protein richness.

Dr. Wilfrid E. Shute's Complete Updated Vitamin E Book, by Wilfrid E. Shute. New Canaan, Conn.: Keats, 1975.

Noted heart specialist and leading researcher of vitamin E offers his experiences and others' in the treatment of a variety of ailments using vitamin E.

Eater's Digest: The Consumer's Factbook of Food Additives, by Michael F. Jacobson. Garden City, N.Y.: Doubleday, 1972.

Introductory Nutrition, by Helen Andrews Guthrie. 4th ed. St. Louis: C. V. Mosby, 1979.

An introductory textbook written by a professor of nutrition. A helpful, ready reference.

Nutritive Value of American Foods in Common Units, Agriculture Handbook No. 456, by Catherine F. Adams. Washington, D.C.: Agricultural Research Service, U.S. Department of Agriculture, 1975.

This invaluable reference book outlines, in several hundred pages of charts, the nutritional value of American foods. Provides calorie, protein, vitamin and mineral content of every food from avocados to zucchini, canned, fresh or frozen.

Vitamin B$_6$: The Doctor's Report, by John M. Ellis and James Presley. New York: Harper & Row, 1973.

From the doctor who pioneered research into the problems caused by B$_6$ deficiency comes this excellent summary of his work. Details his experiences with the use of B$_6$ in alleviating problems associated with pregnancy, menstruation and menopause.

PREGNANCY AND CHILDBIRTH

Birth without Violence, by Frederick Leboyer. New York: Alfred A. Knopf, 1975.

Famed obstetrician Frederick Leboyer presents radical yet surprisingly simple techniques for easing newborns through the trauma of birth.

The Cesarean Birth Experience, by Bonnie Donovan. Boston: Beacon Press, 1977.

A practical, comprehensive and reassuring guide for parents and professionals.

Cesarean Childbirth: A Handbook for Parents, by Christine Wilson and Wendy Roe Hovey. Garden City, N.Y.: Doubleday, 1980.

The Complete Pregnancy Exercise Program, by Diana Simkin. New York: New American Library, 1980.

Coping with a Miscarriage: Why It Happens and How to Deal with Its Impact on You and Your Family, by Hank Pizer and Christine O'Brien Palinski. New York: Dial Press, 1980.

Directory of Alternative Birth Services and Consumer Guide, by Penny Simkin. Marble Hill, Mo.: The National Association of Parents and Professionals for Safe Alternatives in Childbirth, 1978.

Essential Exercises for the Childbearing Year: A Guide to Health and Comfort before and after Your Baby Is Born, by Elizabeth Noble. Boston: Houghton Mifflin, 1976.

Having a Cesarean Baby, by Richard Hausknecht and Joan Rattner Heilman. New York: E. P. Dutton, 1978.

A reassuring—and enlightening—look at new approaches to cesarean deliveries.

Healthy Pregnancy the Yoga Way, by Judi Thompson. Garden City, N.Y.: Doubleday, 1977.

Husband-Coached Childbirth, by Robert A. Bradley. Rev. ed. New York: Harper & Row, 1974.

Obstetrician and promoter of natural childbirth, Dr. Bradley focuses on the active role of the husband as "labor coach."

Immaculate Deception: A New Look at Women and Childbirth in America, by Suzanne Arms. Boston: Houghton Mifflin, 1975.

Looks at the way the experience of childbirth has been dominated by the medical profession when it is women themselves who are in charge of the birth process. Emphasizes the freedom to choose the method and place of birth.

Mother Care: Helping Yourself through the Emotional and Physical Transition of New Motherhood, by Lyn DelliQuadri and Kati Breckenridge. Los Angeles: J. P. Tarcher, 1978.

The New Pregnancy: The Active Woman's Guide to Work, Legal Rights, Health Care, Travel, Sports, Dress, Sex and Emotional Well-Being, by Susan S. Lichtendorf and Phyllis L. Gillis. New York: Random House, 1979.

Now That You've Had Your Baby, by Gideon G. Panter and Shirley Motter Linde. New York: David McKay, 1976.

An obstetrician's guide to exercise, nutrition and emotional well-being in the postpartum period.

Ourselves and Our Children, by the Boston Women's Health Book Collective. New York: Random House, 1978.

A parents' guide to parenting. Written by the authors of *Our Bodies, Ourselves.*

The Post Partum Book: How to Cope with and Enjoy the First Year of Parenting, by Hank Pizer and Christine Garfink. New York: Grove Press, 1979.

The Pregnancy-After-30-Workbook, edited by Gail Sforza Brewer. Emmaus, Pa.: Rodale Press, 1978.

A practical approach to pregnancy geared for the over-30 mother—but with sound advice for women of all ages.

What Every Pregnant Woman Should Know: The Truth about Diets and Drugs in Pregnancy, by Gail Sforza Brewer with Tom Brewer. New York: Random House, 1977.

Women Can Wait: The Pleasure of Motherhood after Thirty, by Terri Schultz. Garden City, N.Y.: Doubleday, 1979.

You Can Breastfeed Your Baby, Even in Special Situations, by Dorothy Patricia Brewster. Emmaus, Pa.: Rodale Press, 1979.

A comprehensive guide to breastfeeding which covers unusual situations and problems such as breastfeeding a premature baby or twins and how to allow for breastfeeding when traveling or working.

SEXUALITY

Afterplay: A Key to Intimacy, by James Halpern and Mark A. Sherman. New York: Stein & Day, 1979.

An interesting examination of what couples do *after* sex and how it can affect a love relationship.

The Hite Report: A Nationwide Study on Female Sexuality, by Shere Hite. New York: Macmillan, 1976.

A fascinating study that incorporates the experiences of 3,000 women who answered questionnaires on their sexuality.

SKIN AND HAIR CARE

The Complete Hair Book: The Ultimate Guide to Your Hair's Health and Beauty, by Philip Kingsley. New York: Grosset & Dunlap, 1979.

A Consumer's Dictionary of Cosmetic Ingredients, by Ruth Winter. Rev. ed. New York: Crown, 1976.

Consumer's Guide to Cosmetics, by Tom Conry with the Science Action Coalition. Garden City, N.Y.: Doubleday, 1980.

Cosmetics: What the Ads Don't Tell You, by Carol Ann Rinzler. New York: T. Y. Crowell, 1977.

A Guide to Natural Cosmetics, by Connie Krochmal. New York: Quadrangle, 1973.

The Handbook of Natural Beauty, by Virginia Castleton. Emmaus, Pa.: Rodale Press, 1975.

WEIGHT CONTROL

Activetics, by Charles T. Kuntzleman. New York: Peter H. Wyden, 1975.

A weight loss program that emphasizes activity, any activity, over dieting as a means to lose weight. Focuses on daily activities such as washing dishes, raking leaves, taking evening walks and many more.

Fat and Thin: A Natural History of Obesity, by Anne Scott Beller. New York: Farrar, Straus & Giroux, 1977.

Lose Weight Naturally, by Mark Bricklin. Emmaus, Pa.: Rodale Press, 1979.

The no-diet, no-nonsense approach to permanent weight control. Utilizes behavior modification and self-hypnosis techniques.

Permanent Weight Control: A Total Solution to the Dieter's Dilemma, by Michael J. Mahoney and Kathryn Mahoney. New York: W. W. Norton, 1976.

Rating the Diets, by Theodore Berland and the editors of *Consumer Guide.* New York: New American Library, 1979.

A comparative look at many popular diets. Rates the diets according to effectiveness, nutritive value and potential hazards.

INDEX

HEALTH RECORDS